Autoimmune Diseases of the Skin: Pathogenesis, Diagnosis and Management

Autoimmune Diseases of the Skin: Pathogenesis, Diagnosis and Management

Editor: Deb Willis

AMERICAN
MEDICAL PUBLISHERS
www.americanmedicalpublishers.com

AMERICAN
MEDICAL PUBLISHERS
www.americanmedicalpublishers.com

Cataloging-in-Publication Data

Autoimmune diseases of the skin : pathogenesis, diagnosis and management / edited by Deb Willis.
p. cm.
Includes bibliographical references and index.
ISBN 978-1-63927-903-6
1. Skin--Diseases. 2. Skin--Diseases--Pathogenesis. 3. Skin--Diseases--Diagnosis.
4. Skin--Diseases--Treatment. 5. Autoimmune diseases. I. Willis, Deb.
RL72 .A98 2023
616.5--dc23

American Medical Publishers,
41 Flatbush Avenue,
1st Floor, New York,
NY 11217, USA

ISBN 978-1-63927-903-6 (Hardback)

Contents

Preface

An autoimmune disease is a health condition in which the body's immune system attacks the healthy tissues and organs instead of the harmful ones. This condition negatively impacts several parts of the body including the skin. There are several types of autoimmune skin diseases, namely, Behcet's disease, dermatitis herpetiformis, dermatomyositis, lichen planus, scleroderma, ocular cicatricial pemphigoid, vasculitis, pemphigoid and pemphigus. Some common symptoms of autoimmune skin diseases are rashes, blisters, lesions, fatigue, and scaly patches. Generally, a biopsy is performed and blood tests can also be done for the diagnosis of autoimmune skin diseases. The treatment methods for these diseases vary according to the type of skin condition. Systemic corticosteroids and immunosuppressive treatments are commonly used to treat pemphigus and pemphigoid. Dapsone and a gluten free diet can be used to treat the condition of dermatitis herpetiformis. This book provides comprehensive insights into the pathogenesis, diagnosis and management of autoimmune skin diseases. With state-of-the-art inputs by acclaimed experts, it targets students and medical professionals.

The researches compiled throughout the book are authentic and of high quality, combining several disciplines and from very diverse regions from around the world. Drawing on the contributions of many researchers from diverse countries, the book's objective is to provide the readers with the latest achievements in the area of research. This book will surely be a source of knowledge to all interested and researching the field.

In the end, I would like to express my deep sense of gratitude to all the authors for meeting the set deadlines in completing and submitting their research chapters. I would also like to thank the publisher for the support offered to us throughout the course of the book. Finally, I extend my sincere thanks to my family for being a constant source of inspiration and encouragement.

Editor

1

Geospatial Correlation of Amyopathic Dermatomyositis with Fixed Sources of Airborne Pollution

David R. Pearson[1*] *and Victoria P. Werth*[2,3]

[1] Department of Dermatology, University of Minnesota Medical School, Minneapolis, MN, United States, [2] Corporal Michael J. Crescenz VA Medical Center, Philadelphia, PA, United States, [3] Department of Dermatology, Perelman School of Medicine, University of Pennsylvania, Philadelphia, PA, United States

***Correspondence:**
David R. Pearson
pearsond@umn.edu

Objective: Dermatomyositis (DM) may result from exogenous triggers, including airborne pollutants, in genetically susceptible individuals. The United States Environmental Protection Agency's 2011 National Air Toxics Assessment (NATA) models health risks associated with airborne emissions, available by ZIP code tabulation area (ZCTA). Important contributors include point (fixed), on-road, and secondary sources. The objective of this study was to investigate the geospatial distributions of DM and subtypes, classic DM (CDM) and clinically amyopathic DM (CADM), and their associations with airborne pollutants.

Methods: This retrospective cohort study identified 642 adult DM patients from 336 unique ZCTAs. GeoDa v.1.10 was used to calculate global and local Moran's indices and generate local indicator of spatial autocorrelation (LISA) maps. All Moran's indices and LISA maps were permuted 999 times.

Results: Univariate global Moran's indices for DM, CDM, and CADM prevalence were not significant, but LISA maps demonstrated differential local spatial clustering and outliers. CADM prevalence correlated with point sources (bivariate global Moran's index 0.071, pseudo-$p = 0.018$), in contrast to CDM (−0.0053, pseudo-$p = 0.46$). Bivariate global Moran's indices for DM, CDM, and CADM prevalence did not correlate with other airborne toxics, but bivariate LISA maps revealed local spatial clustering and outliers.

Conclusion: Prevalence of CADM, but not CDM, is geospatially correlated with fixed sources of airborne emissions. This effect is small but significant and may support the hypothesis that triggering exposures influence disease phenotype. Important limitations are NATA data and ZCTA population estimates were collected from 2011 and ZCTA of residence may not have been where patients had greatest airborne pollutant exposure.

Keywords: dermatomyositis, pollution, environmental, geospatial analysis, Moran index

INTRODUCTION

The pathogenesis of dermatomyositis (DM) is incompletely understood, but may result from diverse exogenous exposures that trigger disease in genetically susceptible individuals, including drugs, infections, and environmental factors such as ultraviolent radiation (UVR) and airborne pollutants (1 18). Important subtypes include classic DM (CDM), which demonstrates clinical and laboratory evidence of myositis, and clinically amyopathic DM (CADM), diagnosed when patients do not have symptomatic myositis and have only minimal or no objective findings of myositis (19, 20). There is evidence that disease phenotype has been associated with specific exposure patterns (5, 8, 10, 21).

The United States Environmental Protection Agency (EPA), an independent agency of the United States federal government that aims to protect human health and the environment, provides publicly available data on airborne emissions in the United States at the level of ZIP code tabulation areas (ZCTA) (22). ZCTAs are geographic representations of the United States Postal Service ZIP code service areas, and were developed by the United States Census Bureau to tabulate summary statistics over geographic areas. In 2015, the EPA released the most recent version of the National Air Toxics Assessment (NATA) based on 2011 emissions. NATA is a screening tool designed to provide information on potential risks of breathing air toxics (22). Emission levels of 181 air toxics (such as benzene, formaldehyde, and diesel particulate matter) were measured, then modeled to predict overall health risks and applied over geographic areas (22). Important contributors include *point* sources, which denote emissions from larger, stationary industrial and commercial facilities, *on-road* sources, produced by vehicles on roads, and *secondary* sources, which are formed from the chemical reactions of other emitted pollutants (22). Since DM has been associated with airborne pollutants, this dataset may be useful in analyzing exposure patterns (11–13).

Geospatial analysis is a statistical approach to analyze data over a geographic region, with applications in environmental science, public health, and other fields. Geospatial statistical techniques, including global and local Moran's indices, can be used to evaluate clustering and dispersion patterns, and have found increasing use in medicine (23–25). These techniques have not been applied to the study of DM due in part to the low incidence and prevalence of disease. The relatively large cohort at the University of Pennsylvania provides an opportunity to use geospatial analysis to assess exposure patterns in DM.

The objective of this study was to investigate the geospatial distributions of DM and its subtypes and their associations with airborne pollutants in the greater Philadelphia metropolitan area.

METHODS

Patient Selection

This retrospective cohort study spanned January 1, 2000 through December 31, 2017. Data collection was complete July 31, 2018. Adult patients ≥18 years of age seen in dermatology or rheumatology clinics at the University of Pennsylvania with a United States ZCTA of primary residence listed in their medical record and a diagnosis of DM, encoded by International Classification of Disease (ICD) 9th and 10th revision codes (710.3 and M33.0X, M33.1X, M33.9X, respectively) were included. Patients were identified using PennSeek, a custom, secure implementation of Oracle's web-based Endeca Information Discovery platform adapted by the University of Pennsylvania Data Analytics Core. PennSeek allows for targeted keyword searches using Boolean logic of unstructured or semi-structured medical documents that reside in the main Penn Medicine electronic health record and ancillary systems, described in detail elsewhere (26). After assembling the cohort, individual patient charts were reviewed to verify diagnosis, exclude erroneously coded patients, and extract variables of interest.

2011 NATA Dataset

2011 NATA risk estimates including total airborne, point, on-road, and secondary source risks were taken from the EPA's dataset, organized by ZCTA (22).

Variables

DM subtype was assigned based on the treating clinician's note. In cases of ambiguity or disagreement, evidence of myositis was determined by patient-reported symptoms plus an objective sign (elevated creatinine kinase or aldolase or consistent EMG, MRI, or muscle biopsy). Patients who fulfilled these criteria were labeled as CDM and those lacking labeled as CADM. Demographics and ZCTAs were extracted from the medical record. Prevalence was calculated using United States Census Bureau (USCB) 2007-2011 American Community Survey population estimates, organized by ZCTA (27).

Analysis

Continuous variables are presented as median (interquartile range, IQR) and categorical data are presented as count (percentage). Heatmaps were created with Tableau Public version 10.4 (Tableau Software, Inc. 2018. Seattle, Washington).

Geospatial analysis was performed by calculation of the global Moran's index, an inferential statistic which estimates spatial autocorrelation and falls between -1 and $+1$ (28). More positive or negative values correspond to greater spatial clustering or competitive dispersion, respectively (28). To test the null hypothesis of random spatial distribution, empiric significance is computed by permutation to yield a pseudo-p-value (28). A pseudo-p-value differs from an analytic p-value because it is a summary of the results of the reference distribution, and is dependent on the number of permutations used (28). In order to visualize spatial clustering, local indicators of spatial autocorrelation (LISA) maps were created using local Moran's index calculations (29). This statistic identifies significant locations as high-high or low-low spatial clusters and high-low or low-high spatial outliers relative to neighboring regions (29). In both indices, neighbor less regions are excluded from analysis.

Bivariate global and local Moran's indices were calculated in the same fashion; global indices measure spatial autocorrelation between an outcome variable in one geographic region and a second variable in neighboring regions, and local indices were mapped with bivariate LISA (BiLISA) maps (30).

GeoDa version 1.10 was used for geospatial analyses. Shapefiles were obtained from the USCB 2017 ZCTA boundary files and the weights matrix was assigned first-order queen contiguity (neighboring regions share common edges or vertices). All global and local univariate and bivariate Moran's indices and LISA and BiLISA maps were permuted 999 times. A pseudo-$p < 0.05$ was set as significant.

Ethics

This study was carried out in accordance with the recommendations of the University of Pennsylvania Institutional Review Board (protocol number 828959), which waived the requirement of written informed consent from subjects. Written consent was waived due to the retrospective nature of the study and minimal risk it posed to subjects. The protocol for this study conforms to the ethical guidelines of the Declaration of Helsinki. The protocol was approved by the University of Pennsylvania Institutional Review Board.

RESULTS

Of 205,084 adult patients seen in dermatology or rheumatology clinics at the University of Pennsylvania from January 1, 2000 through December 31, 2017, PennSeek identified 653 patients. Upon individual chart review, 9 patients were excluded for diagnoses other than DM and 2 were excluded for absence of a ZCTA in their medical record, resulting in 642 patients who met inclusion criteria.

Baseline characteristics of the patient cohort are noted in **Table 1**. The median age at symptom onset was 49 (IQR 37, 58) years. Most patients were female (532, 82.8%), white (476, 74.1%), and diagnosed with CDM (439, 68.4%), though a notable fraction had CADM (203, 31.6%). Data on year of symptom onset was available for 630 patients (98.1%) and divided into approximate quartiles. One hundred fifty-nine patients (25.2%) developed symptoms in 2005 or earlier, 176 patients (27.9%) between 2006 and 2009, 153 patients between 2010 and 2013, and 142 patients (22.5%) from 2014 to the end of the study period.

Three hundred thirty-six unique ZCTAs represented a total underlying population of 8,110,198 (**Table 1**, **Data Sheet 1**). The median prevalence of DM per ZCTA was 8.6 (IQR 4.6, 15.2) per 100,000. When ZCTAs outside of the greater Philadelphia metropolitan area were excluded, the median prevalence of DM was 9.2 (IQR 5.2, 16.3) per 100,000. The median total airborne risk per ZCTA was 43 (IQR 37, 48) per million, including 1.24 (IQR 0.64, 1.67) per million from point sources, 9.13 (IQR 6.56, 12.18) per million from on-road sources, and 18.10 (IQR 16.47, 19.17) per million from secondary sources.

Heatmaps of the prevalence of DM and subtypes CDM and CADM in the greater Philadelphia metropolitan area are illustrated in **Figure 1**, divided into sextiles. Many ZCTAs with high prevalence of DM and CDM were observed in the western and northern metropolitan area. CADM prevalence is lower overall and aligns along a northeast-southwest axis. **Figure S1** shows heatmaps of the onset year by quartile, with no clear patterns of clustering or outliers.

TABLE 1 | Baseline characteristics of adult dermatology and rheumatology patients with dermatomyositis (DM) seen at the University of Pennsylvania between January 1, 2000 and December 31, 2017, with median 2011 NATA risk calculations.

Metric	Cohort (n = 642)
Median age at symptom onset, years (IQR)	49 (37, 58)
Female sex	532 (82.8%)
PATIENT-REPORTED RACE/ETHNICITY	
White	476 (74.1%)
Black	76 (11.8%)
Asian, American Indian, or Alaskan Native	20 (3.1%)
Other	70 (10.9%)
DM SUBTYPE	
CDM	439 (68.4%)
CADM	203 (31.6%)
SYMPTOM ONSET YEAR QUARTILES (n = 630)	
2005 or earlier	159 (25.2%)
2006–2009	176 (27.9%)
2010–2013	153 (24.3%)
2014–2017	142 (22.5%)
ZCTA	
Unique ZCTAs	336
2010 Census population	8,110,198
Median DM prevalence per ZCTA (IQR), per 100,000	8.6 (4.6, 15.2)
Median DM prevalence per Phl metropolitan ZCTA (IQR), per 100,000 (n = 607)	9.2 (5.2, 16.3)
MEDIAN 2011 NATA RISK PER ZCTA, PER MILLION	
Total airborne risk (IQR)	43 (37, 48)
Point source risk (IQR)	1.24 (0.64, 1.67)
On-road source risk (IQR)	9.13 (6.56, 12.18)
Secondary source risk (IQR)	18.10 (16.47, 19.17)

CADM, clinically amyopathic dermatomyositis; CDM, classic dermatomyositis; DM, dermatomyositis; IQR, interquartile range; NATA, National Air Toxics Assessment; Phl, Philadelphia; ZCTA, zip code tabulation area.

Geospatial Analysis

Univariate global Moran's indices for the prevalence of DM, CDM, and CADM were not significant (**Table 2**), but LISA maps demonstrated differential local spatial clustering and outliers (**Figure 2**), as indicated by the presence of high-high (red) and low-low clustering (bright blue), and high-low (pink) and low-high (light blue) outliers. DM and CDM shared several clustered and outlier ZCTAs, and differed notably from CADM, which demonstrated high-high clustering along a northeast-southwest axis. High-low outliers occurred predominantly in ZCTAs of low relative population.

The prevalence of CADM vs. point sources showed a significant bivariate global Moran's index (0.071, pseudo-p = 0.02), and BiLISA mapping demonstrating western metropolitan high-high clustering and eastern metropolitan low-low clustering (**Figure 3a**). In contrast, the prevalence of CDM vs. point sources was not significant (−0.0053, pseudo-p = 0.46), and BiLISA mapping demonstrating western low-high outliers and eastern low-low clustering (**Figure 3b**). Bivariate global Moran's indices for the prevalence of DM, CDM, and CADM vs. other airborne toxics were not significant, and BiLISA mapping revealed similar local spatial clustering and outliers between subtypes (**Figure S2**).

Univariate global Moran's indices for both DM onset year (by quartile) and median age at symptom onset were not significant (data not shown).

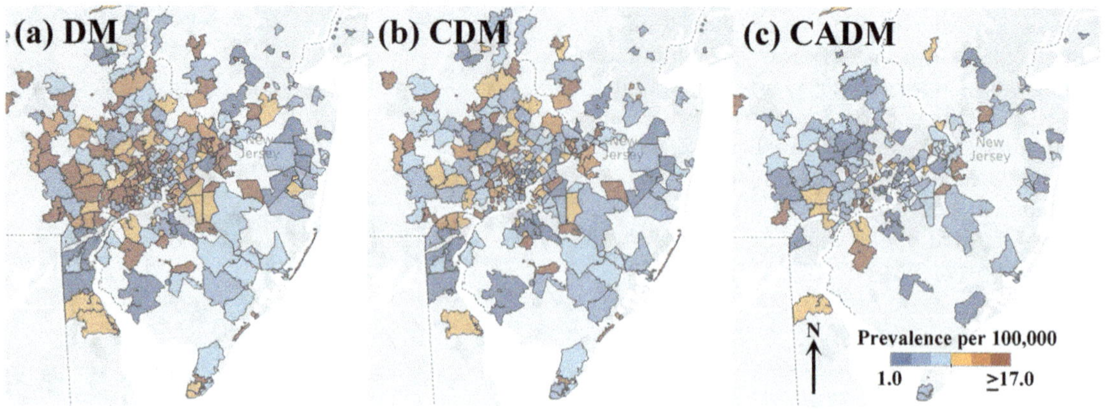

FIGURE 1 | Heatmaps of prevalence per 100,000 of the full cohort of dermatomyositis (DM) patients **(a)**, and subtypes classic DM (CDM, **b**) and clinically amyopathic DM (CADM, **c**) in the greater Philadelphia metropolitan area (legend inset: low prevalence, blue; high prevalence, orange). Many ZCTAs with high prevalence of DM and CDM are observed in the western and northern metropolitan area. CADM prevalence is lower across the region and aligns along a northeast-southwest axis.

TABLE 2 | Univariate global Moran's indices of the prevalence of dermatomyositis (DM) and subtypes, and bivariate global Moran's indices of DM prevalence vs. 2011 NATA metrics.

Outcome variable	Lagged variable	Global Moran's index	Pseudo p-value
DM prevalence	Univariate	0.0054	0.16
	Total airborne risk*	0.0080	0.34
	Point sources*	0.0019	0.36
	On-road sources*	0.0057	0.15
	Secondary sources*	0.0036	0.46
CDM prevalence	Univariate	0.0051	0.16
	Total airborne risk*	0.0080	0.33
	Point sources*	−0.0053	0.46
	On-road sources*	0.0082	0.28
	Secondary sources*	−0.00076	0.47
CADM prevalence	Univariate	0.064	0.06
	Total airborne risk*	−0.0015	0.49
	Point sources*	**0.071**	**0.02**
	On-road sources*	−0.025	0.18
	Secondary sources*	0.043	0.09

CADM, clinically amyopathic dermatomyositis; CDM, classic dermatomyositis; DM, dermatomyositis; NATA, National Air Toxics Assessment.
**Bivariate global Moran's index.*
Bold values indicate significant finding.

DISCUSSION

In this retrospective study of 642 DM patients, we found a significant geospatial correlation between exposure to point sources of airborne pollutants and CADM. Other airborne toxics including overall calculated airborne risk, on-road, and secondary sources did not correlate with DM, CDM, or CADM prevalence.

The association between point sources and CADM is modest but significant, as seen by the magnitude of the global Moran's index. Since DM has been associated with a variety of exogenous triggers besides airborne toxics, it is not surprising that this exposure does not account for all cases. It is noteworthy that CDM was not correlated with point sources, supporting the hypothesis that the type of triggering exposure may influence disease phenotype.

Past studies have demonstrated associations between specific exogenous triggers and serotype, which is known to correlate with clinical phenotype (31–33). The intensity of UVR exposure has been strongly associated with the proportion of CDM patients expressing anti-Mi-2 antibodies (odds ratio [OR] 6.0), while anti-TIF1-γ antibodies have been negatively correlated with latitude (OR 0.96) (8, 21). HLA alleles associated with anti-Mi-2 and anti-TIF1-γ antibodies were also negatively associated with latitude (21). Anti-MDA-5 antibodies were inversely associated with population of city of residence and appeared to cluster along rural areas near the Kiso River in Japan (10). Hydroxyurea may induce a DM-like eruption that spares muscles, while other drugs may induce a CDM-like presentation and viral infections may trigger juvenile DM (5, 34).

This study has important limitations. It is a retrospective cohort from a tertiary referral facility in a heavily-populated urban center. The ZCTA of residence listed in the patient's chart may not have been the location where greatest airborne pollutant exposure occurred and does not factor transportation routes or job location. The listed ZCTA may not have been where DM onset occurred, especially in longstanding cases. Reference data were taken from available years: ZCTAs were collected from medical records in 2018, ZCTA shapefiles were based on 2017 USCB boundary files, NATA metrics were calculated from data collected in 2011, and ZCTA population estimates were collected from 2007 to 2011 in the USCB American Community Survey. Both population estimates and airborne pollutant levels may have changed since 2011, though more recent, reliable data was not available.

It is important to note that NATA metrics are risk assessments based on collected airborne emissions and do not reflect exposure to all compounds, all pathways of exposure, or accurately model

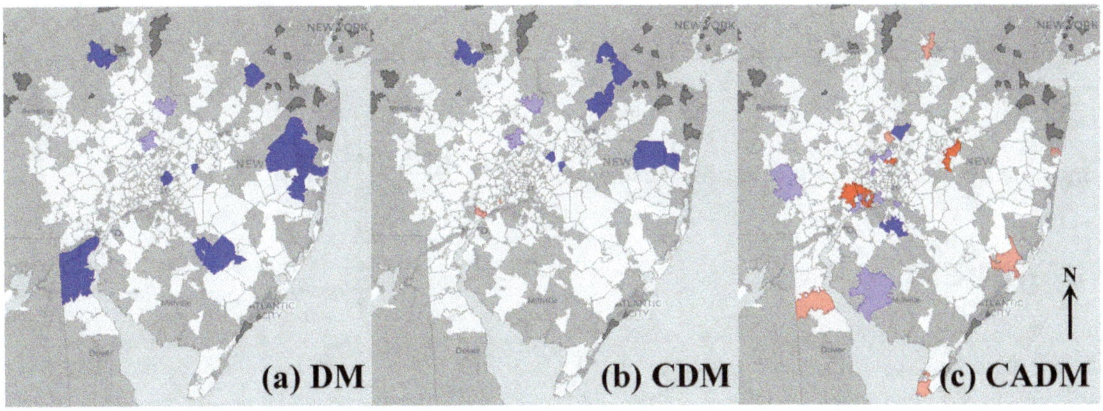

FIGURE 2 | Local indicators of spatial autocorrelation (LISA) maps for prevalence of the full cohort of dermatomyositis (DM) patients **(a)**, and subtypes classic DM (CDM, **b**) and clinically amyopathic DM (CADM, **c**). High-high (red) and low-low (bright blue) spatial clusters, and high-low (pink) and low-high (light blue) spatial outliers relative to neighboring regions are identified. Geospatially non-significant (white) and neighborless (dark gray) regions are visible. Differential spatial clustering is most notable between CDM **(b)** and CADM **(c)**.

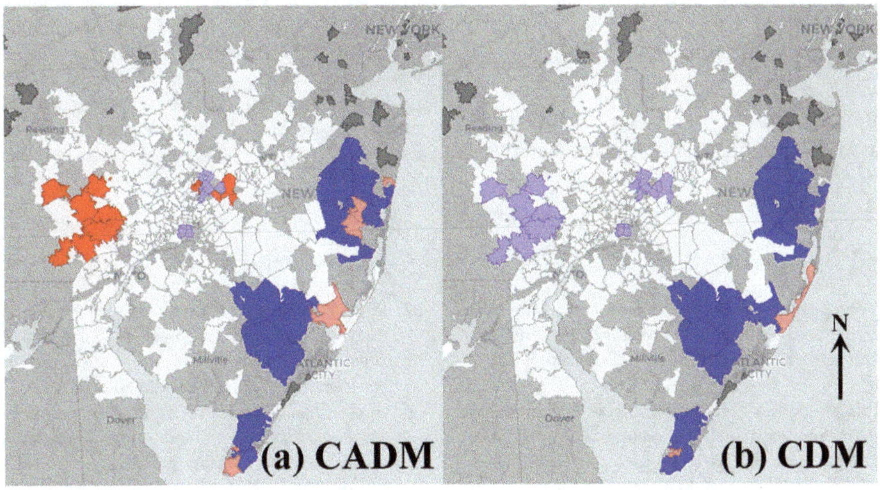

FIGURE 3 | Bivariate local indicators of spatial autocorrelation (BiLISA) maps for prevalence of clinically amyopathic dermatomyositis (CADM, **a**) and classic dermatomyositis (CDM, **b**) vs. point sources. High-high (red) and low-low (bright blue) spatial clusters, and high-low (pink) and low-high (light blue) spatial outliers relative to neighboring regions are identified. In CADM **(a)**, western metropolitan high-high clustering and eastern metropolitan low-low clustering is prominent, while in CDM **(b)**, western low-high outliers and eastern low-low clustering is notable. Geospatially non-significant (white) and neighbor less (dark gray) regions are visible.

episodic emissions (22). Risk assessments by source represent pooled data from many pollutants, and the contributed risks of individual compounds were not assessed. Furthermore, these data apply to geographic areas and groups, rather than specific locations or individuals (22).

The prevalence of DM found in this study is lower than previously reported (35). This estimate is not population-based and likely underestimates the true prevalence in the greater Philadelphia metropolitan area. During the 18-year time period of this study, there were 5 major academic medical centers and a large number of group and individual dermatology and rheumatology practices, many of whom see DM patients not included here.

While the spatial distribution of onset of DM symptoms changed over time, specific regions did not cluster by onset year. DM frequency remained approximately stable when comparing the 4-year intervals from 2006 to 2009, 2010 to 2013, and 2014 to 2017. However, DM, especially CADM, is frequently delayed in diagnosis or misdiagnosed and presentation to a tertiary referral center may result in additional delay, so patients with more recent onset may be unaccounted for (36).

Identifying exogenous triggers for DM is challenging given the heterogeneity of both exposure and the underlying disease. Geospatial analysis is a candidate method for studying geographic patterns of exposure and may have applications examining infectious triggers, pollutants, demographics, and other factors. Future population-based studies may better estimate these associations. Further exploration of the geospatial distribution of DM phenotype by serology, malignancy association, or the presence of interstitial lung disease may also be useful for determining risk factors and understanding disease pathogenesis.

In conclusion, in this retrospective cohort study we found prevalence of CADM, but not CDM, is geospatially correlated with larger, geographically fixed sources of airborne pollution. This effect is small but significant and may support the hypothesis that triggering exposures may influence disease phenotype in DM.

ETHICS STATEMENT

This study was carried out in accordance with the recommendations of the University of Pennsylvania Institutional Review Board (protocol number 828959), which waived the requirement of written informed consent from subjects. Written consent was waived due to the retrospective nature of the study and minimal risk it posed to subjects. The protocol for this study conforms to the ethical guidelines of the Declaration of Helsinki. The protocol was approved by the University of Pennsylvania Institutional Review Board.

AUTHOR CONTRIBUTIONS

DP and VW contributed conception and design of the study. DP collected the primary data, performed the statistical analysis, and wrote the first draft of the manuscript. DP and VW contributed to manuscript revision and read and approved the submitted version.

SUPPLEMENTARY MATERIAL

Data Sheet 1 | Unique ZCTAs and corresponding census populations and DM counts, calculated prevalences, and NATA risk estimates are shown. On the far right, counts of DM are listed by year of symptom onset. CADM, clinically amyopathic dermatomyositis; CDM, classic dermatomyositis; DM, dermatomyositis; NATA, National Air Toxics Assessment; ZCTA, zip code tabulation area.

Figure S1 | Heatmaps of new-onset cases of dermatomyositis in the greater Philadelphia metropolitan area in 2005 or earlier **(a)**, 2006–2009 **(b)**, 2010-2013 **(c)**, and 2014–2017 **(d)** (legend inset: lower count, light blue; higher count, dark blue). Geospatial analysis did not demonstrate clustering or dispersion.

Figure S2 | Bivariate local indicators of spatial autocorrelation (BiLISA) maps for prevalence of the full cohort of dermatomyositis (DM) and subtypes classic DM (CDM) and clinically amyopathic DM (CADM) vs. total airborne risk (**a–c**, respectively), on-road sources (**d–f**, respectively), and secondary sources (**g–I**, respectively). High-high (red) and low-low (bright blue) spatial clusters, and high-low (pink) and low-high (light blue) spatial outliers relative to neighboring regions are identified. Geospatially non-significant (white) and neighbor less (dark gray) regions are visible. Note the similarities in both spatial clustering and outliers between DM, CDM, and CADM. All global Moran's indices were non-significant.

REFERENCES

1. Hengstman GJD, Van Venrooij WJ, Vencovsky J, Moutsopoulos HM, Van Engelen BGM. The relative prevalence of dermatomyositis and polymyositis in Europe exhibits a latitudinal gradient. *Ann Rheum Dis.* (2000)59:141–2. doi: 10.1136/ard.59.2.141
2. Neil Crowson A, Magro CM, Dawood MR. A causal role for parvovirus B19 infection in adult dermatomyositis and other autoimmune syndromes. *J Cutan Pathol.* (2000)27:505–15. doi: 10.1034/j.1600-0560.2000.027010505.x
3. Okada S, Weatherhead E, Targoff IN, Wesley R, Miller FW. Global surface ultraviolet radiation intensity may modulate the clinical and immunologic expression of autoimmune muscle disease. *Arthritis Rheum.* (2003)48:2285–93. doi: 10.1002/art.11090
4. Packman LM, Lipton R, Ramsey-Goldman R, Shamiyeh E, Abbott K, Mendez EP, et al. History of infection before the onset of juvenile dermatomyositis: results from the National Institute of Arthritis and Musculoskeletal and Skin diseases research registry. *Arthritis Care Res.* (2005)53:166–72. doi: 10.1002/art.21068
5. Seidler AM, Gottlieb AB. Dermatomyositis induced by drug therapy: a review of case reports. *J Am Acad Dermatol.* (2008)59:872–80. doi: 10.1016/j.jaad.2008.05.034
6. Dastmalchi M, Grundtman C, Alexanderson H, Mavragani CP, Einarsdottir H, Helmers SB, et al. A high incidence of disease flares in an open pilot study of infliximab in patients with refractory inflammatory myopathies. *Ann Rheum Dis.* (2008)67:1670–7. doi: 10.1136/ard.2007.077974
7. Orbach H, Tanay A. Vaccines as a trigger for myopathies. *Lupus.* (2009)18:1213–6. doi: 10.1177/0961203309345734
8. Love LA, Weinberg CR, McConnaughey DR, Oddis CV, Medsger TA, Jr., Reveille JD, et al. Ultraviolet radiation intensity predicts the relative distribution of dermatomyositis and anti-Mi-2 autoantibodies in women. *Arthritis Rheum.* (2009) 60:2499–504. doi: 10.1002/art.24702
9. Rider LG, Wu L, Mamyrova G, Targoff IN, Miller FW. Environmental factors preceding illness onset differ in phenotypes of the juvenile idiopathic inflammatory myopathies. *Rheumatology.* (2010) 49:2381–90. doi: 10.1093/rheumatology/keq277
10. Muro Y, Sugiura K, Hoshino K, Akiyama M, Tamakoshi K. Epidemiologic study of clinically amyopathic dermatomyositis and anti-melanoma differentiation-associated gene 5 antibodies in central Japan. *Arthritis Res Ther.* (2011) 13:6. doi: 10.1186/ar3547
11. Orione MA, Silva CA, Sallum AM, Campos LM, Omori CH, Braga AL, et al. Risk factors for juvenile dermatomyositis: exposure to tobacco and air pollutants during pregnancy. *Arthritis Care Res.* (2014)66:1571–5. doi: 10.1002/acr.22358
12. Blanc PD, Järvholm B, Torén K. Prospective risk of rheumatologic disease associated with occupational exposure in a cohort of male construction workers. *Am J Med.* (2015)128:1094–101. doi: 10.1016/j.amjmed.2015.05.001
13. Bernatsky S, Smargiassi A, Barnabe C, Svenson LW, Brand A, Martin RV, et al. Fine particulate air pollution and systemic autoimmune rheumatic disease in two Canadian provinces. *Environ Res.* (2016)146:85–91. doi: 10.1016/j.envres.2015.12.021
14. Wright NA, Vleugels RA, Callen JP. Cutaneous dermatomyositis in the era of biologicals. *Semin Immunopathol.* (2016)38:113–21. doi: 10.1007/s00281-015-0543-z
15. Limaye V, Smith C, Koszyca B, Blumbergs P, Otto S. Infections and vaccinations as possible triggers of inflammatory myopathies. *Muscle Nerve.* (2017)56:987–9. doi: 10.1002/mus.25628
16. Mamyrova G, Rider LG, Ehrlich A, Jones O, Pachman LM, Nickeson R, et al. Environmental factors associated with disease flare in juvenile and adult dermatomyositis. *Rheumatology.* (2017)56:1342–7. doi: 10.1093/rheumatology/kex162
17. Thompson C, Piguet V, Choy E. The pathogenesis of dermatomyositis. *Br J Dermatol.* (2017) 179:1256–62. doi: 10.1111/bjd.15607
18. Zeidi M, Chansky P, Werth V. Acute onset/exacerbation of dermatomyositis and Sjogrens Syndrome following ingestion of IsaLean® herbal supplement: clinical and immunostimulatory findings. *J Invest Dermatol.* (2018)138:S75. doi: 10.1016/j.jid.2018.03.449
19. Bohan A, Peter J. Bohan A, Peter J. Polymyositis and dermatomyositis. *N Engl J Med.* (1975)292:344–7. doi: 10.1056/NEJM197502202920807

20. Sontheimer RD. Dermatomyositis: an overview of recent progress with emphasis on dermatologic aspects. *Dermatol Clin.* (2002)20:387–408. doi: 10.1016/S0733-8635(02)00021-9
21. Parkes J, Rothwell S, Oldroyd A, Chinoy H, Lamb J, (MYOGEN) MGC. Genetic background may contribute to the latitude-dependent prevalence of dermatomyositis and anti-TIF1-γ autoantibodies in adult patients with myositis. *Arthritis Res Ther.* (2018)20:117. doi: 10.1186/s13075-018-1617-9
22. United States Environmental Protection Agency. *National Air Toxics Assessment.* Available online at: https://www.epa.gov/national-air-toxics-assessment (accessed March 26, 2019).
23. Toledo CRS de, Almeida AS de, Chaves SA de M, Sabroza PC, Toledo LM, Caldas JP. Vulnerability to the transmission of human visceral leishmaniasis in a Brazilian urban area. *Rev Saude Publica.* (2017)51:49. doi: 10.1590/s1518-8787.2017051006532
24. Dantas AP, De Azevedo UN, Nunes AD, Amador AE, Marques M V., Barbosa IR. Analysis of suicide mortality in brazil: spatial distribution and socioeconomic context. *Rev Bras Psiquiatr.* (2018)40:12–8. doi: 10.1590/1516-4446-2017-2241
25. Bagheri N, Wangdi K, Cherbuin N, Anstey KJ. General practice clinical data help identify dementia hotspots: a novel geospatial analysis approach. *J Alzheimers Dis.* (2017)61:1. doi: 10.3233/JAD-170079
26. Small AM, Kiss DH, Zlatsin Y, Birtwell DL, Williams H, Guerraty MA, et al. Text mining applied to electronic cardiovascular procedure reports to identify patients with trileaflet aortic stenosis and coronary artery disease. *J Biomed Inform.* (2017)72:77–84. doi: 10.1016/j.jbi.2017.06.016
27. United States Census Bureau. *American Fact Finder: American Community Survey.* Available online at: https://factfinder.census.gov/faces/nav/jsf/pages/programs.xhtml?program=acs. Published 2018.
28. Anselin L. *Global Spatial Autocorrelation (1): Moran Scatter Plot and Spatial Correlogram.* Available online at: https://geodacenter.github.io/workbook/5a_global_auto/lab5a.html#fn3 (accessed March 26, 2019).
29. Anselin L. Local Indicators of Spatial Association—LISA. *Geogr Anal.* (1995)27:93–115. doi: 10.1111/j.1538-4632.1995.tb00338.x
30. Anselin L. *Global Spatial Autocorrelation : Bivariate, Differential and EB Rate Moran Scatter Plot.* Available online at: https://geodacenter.github.io/workbook/5b_global_adv/lab5b.html (accessed March 26, 2019).
31. Daly ML, Gordon PA, Creamer D. Cutaneous features of dermatomyositis associated with myositis-specific antibodies. *Br J Dermatol.* (2017)176:1662–5. doi: 10.1111/bjd.15020
32. Best M, Jachiet M, Molinari N, Manna F, Girard C, Pallure V, et al. Distinctive cutaneous and systemic features associated with specific antimyositis antibodies in adults with dermatomyositis: a prospective multicentric study of 117 patients. *J Eur Acad DermatolVenereol.* (2018) 32:1164–72. doi: 10.1111/jdv.14759
33. Wolstencroft PW, Fiorentino DF. Dermatomyositis clinical and pathological phenotypes associated with myositis-specific autoantibodies. *Curr Rheumatol Rep.* (2018) 20:5. doi: 10.1007/s11926-018-0733-5
34. Manlhiot C, Liang L, Tran D, Bitnun A, Tyrrell PN, Feldman BM. Assessment of an infectious disease history preceding juvenile dermatomyositis symptom onset. *Rheumatology.* (2008) 47:526–9. doi: 10.1093/rheumatology/ken038
35. Bendewald MJ, Wetter DA, Li X, Davis MDP. Incidence of dermatomyositis and clinically amyopathic dermatomyositis: a population-based study in Olmsted County, Minnesota. *Arch Dermatol.* (2010) 146:26–30. doi: 10.1001/archdermatol.2009.328
36. Da Silva D, Patel B, Werth V. Dermatomyositis: a diagnostic dilemma. *J Am Acad Dermatol.* (2018) 79:371–3. doi: 10.1016/j.jaad.2017.12.074

2

Role of the Pruritic Cytokine IL-31 in Autoimmune Skin Diseases

Bernhard F. Gibbs, Nikolaos Patsinakidis and Ulrike Raap *

Division of Experimental Allergy and Immunodermatology, University of Oldenburg, Oldenburg, Germany

Correspondence:
Ulrike Raap
raap.ulrike@klinikum-oldenburg.de

Many autoimmune skin diseases, such as bullous pemphigoid (BP), psoriasis and certain types of chronic urticaria, are associated with intensive pruritus. While histamine and neuropeptides have previously been ascribed to play a role in itch that accompanies these diseases, recent evidence suggests that the pruritogenic cytokine interleukin (IL)-31 is a major driver of pruritic responses. IL-31 was originally shown to be produced by activated helper T cells, particularly Th2 cells, mast cells, macrophages and dendritic cells. However, more recent evidence demonstrated that eosinophils are a major source of this cytokine too, particularly in bullous pemphigoid. Basophils have also been shown to express the cytokine which, through autocrine action, strongly supports the production of other Th2-type cytokines from these cells. These investigations suggest that the dynamic recruitment of eosinophils and basophils in some autoimmune skin diseases could play an important role in the severity of IL-31-mediated itch. Furthermore, these studies suggest that IL-31, in addition to its pruritic actions, also has potential immunomodulatory roles in terms of supporting Th2-type immunity, which often underpins IgE-associated autoimmune diseases (such as bullous pemphigoid and urticaria) as well as allergies. While the role of IL-31 in psoriasis remains to be clarified, current evidence shows that this cytokine plays a major role in BP, chronic spontaneous urticaria and dermatomyositis. This suggests potential use of IL-31 receptor-blocking therapeutic approaches (e.g., Nemolizumab) for the treatment of IL-31-associated disorders.

Keywords: IL-31, itch, autoimmunity, bullous pemphigoid, psoriasis, eosinophils, basophils

INTRODUCTION

IL-31 was first described by Dillon et al as a T cell-derived cytokine that was predominantly produced by The cells (1). Interestingly, mice which overexpressed IL-31 were observed to develop severe pruritus, alopecia and skin lesions (1). Furthermore, animal models of airway hypersensitivity exhibited increased IL-31 receptor expressions and these expressions, as well as those of IL-31 receptors in the skin, were also verified in respective human tissues (1). Human and mouse IL-31 share 31% amino acid homology and the genes for this cytokine are, respectively, located on chromosome 12q24.31 and chromosome 5 (1).

IL-31 is a member of the gp130/IL-6 family of cytokines and is a four helix bundle cytokine that acts as a ligand for the heterodimeric IL-31 receptor A (IL-31RA), a novel type I cytokine receptor, and the oncostatin M receptor (OSMR), the latter of which increases IL-31 binding affinity to IL-31RA. Both of these IL-31 receptors are expressed on a variety of different cell types including T cells, dorsal root ganglia (DRG), keratinocytes, dendritic cells, eosinophils, basophils, and macrophages (2–7). The functional activity of IL-31 appears to depend on the expression of both the IL-31RA and OSMR since, in basophils, we recently demonstrated that blocking of either receptor type decreases IL-31-induced IL-4 and IL-13 release (7).

Subsequent signaling following receptor complex binding involves the Janus kinase–signal transducer and activator of transcription pathway, the phosphoinositide-3-kinase–Akt pathway as well as the mitogen-activated protein kinase pathway (4, 8–10). IL-31 signaling controls a wide range of biological functions and immunomodulatory effects, such as the release of chemokines, proinflammatory cytokines, regulation of cell proliferation and stimulation of DRG sensory neurons which are responsible for induction of itch [reviewed in (11, 12)].

GENERAL PROPERTIES OF IL-31 IN SKIN DISEASES

In dermatological diseases, IL-31 is of particular interest in terms of itch and inflammation as well as impaired skin-barrier function arising from IL-31-induced tissue remodeling (13, 14). The cytokine was not only found to induce severe pruritus in mice, where levels of IL-31 correlated with scratching behavior, but a NC/Nga mouse model of atopic dermatitis demonstrated the potential therapeutic benefit of blocking anti-IL-31 antibodies (1, 15, 16). Before the discovery of IL-31, histamine was widely considered to be the most important pruritic mediator and the relative lack of therapeutic control of itch by H1-antihistamines was ascribed following the discovery of additional H4-receptor input in pruritus [reviewed in (17)]. This is partly supported by a recent successful clinical trial using an H4-receptor antagonist in atopic dermatitis (18), indicating potential future combinational H1- and H4-receptor antagonist/inverse agonist approaches. However, recent data from human clinical trials using nemolizumab (CIM331), a humanized antibody against interleukin-31 receptor A, clearly indicates that IL-31 is an important mediator of itch in humans too (19, 20).

Alongside its pruritogenic actions, IL-31 has a proinflammatory role too due to the upregulation of proinflammatory gene expressions in T cells, including CCL2 and granulocyte colony-stimulating factor (21). Interestingly, CCL2 has recently been implicated in driving basophil trafficking in systemic lupus erythematosus (SLE) and in severe allergic reactions (22, 23). IL-31 release by CD4+ T cells is mostly restricted to Th2 cells, although Th1 cells can produce this cytokine *in vitro* following exposure to IL-4 (21). Epidermal keratinocytes are also a major target for IL-31, where it induces chemokine gene expressions for GRO1α (CXCL1), I-309 (CCL1), MIP-1β (CCL4), TARC (CCL17), MIP-3β (CCL19), MDC (CCL22), and MIP-3 (CCL23), [(1), reviewed in(11)]. Furthermore, Singh et al. showed that IL-31 increased epidermal basal-cell proliferation in mice resulting in thickening of the epidermal skin layer but increased transepidermal water loss (14). This impairment of skin barrier function occurs due to IL-31 decreasing filaggrin expression in human keratinocytes (24). Interestingly, reduced filaggrin expressions are strongly associated with atopic dermatitis and have been shown to enhance *Staphylococcus aureus* colonization (24, 25).

Increased levels of IL-31 have now been shown in various inflammatory skin diseases including prurigo nodularis (12), atopic dermatitis (26–28), contact eczema (29), chronic spontaneous urticaria (CsU) (30), as well as in a subset of patients with mastocytosis (31). In an animal model of atopic dermatitis anti-IL-31 treatment significantly reduced scratching in mice (16), underlining the important role of IL-31 in mediating pruritus. This seems to apply to humans too, where IL-31 levels were shown to correlate with disease severity in atopic dermatitis (27, 28). Interestingly, CsU patients respond to omalizumab therapy which was recently shown to be associated with reduced IL-31 serum levels (32). This suggests that this IL-31 may be modulated by IgE-dependent mechanisms and this further highlights the potential of anti-IL-31 as a therapeutic approaches as well as targeting IgE-positive effector cells.

IL-31 IN AUTOIMMUNE SKIN DISEASES

IL-31 has thus far been shown to play a prominent role in common inflammatory skin diseases, such as atopic dermatitis, particularly in relation to pruritus. However, since pruritus is also a major feature in bullous pemphigoid, chronic spontaneous urticaria (CsU) and other autoimmune diseases there is a potential role for IL-31 in some of these diseases too.

Chronic Spontaneous Urticaria

It has long been recognized that autoimmune mechanisms are an important component of CsU [reviewed in (33)]. CsU is defined by the rapid appearance of pruritic wheals lasting <24 h but which may occur repeatedly over a period of at least 6 weeks. The autoimmune association in CsU is either due to IgE mediated autoallergy against thyroid peroxidase or IgG auto-antibodies against the α-subunit of the high-affinity IgE receptor(FcεRI) and, more rarely, against IgE. All of these possible autoimmune mechanisms activate mast cells and basophils, cells which have been centrally implicated with CsU (34–36).

While mast cells and basophils are the main sources of histamine, antihistamine treatment in patients with CsU does not fully eliminate itch, suggesting that IL-31 may have some input in pruritic mechanisms associated with CsU. Indeed, we observed increased IL-31 serum levels in CsU patients, although these levels were generally lower than those seen in atopic dermatitis patients (30). These observations have recently been confirmed by Lin et al. who demonstrated significantly higher levels of IL-31 in CsU patients with most severe pruritus intensity compared to milder forms but not with urticarial activity *per se* (37). This supports the notion that IL-31 contributes to itch rather than other aspects of disease activity.

In our own investigations, we subsequently discovered that the main cellular sources of IL-31 in skin lesions of CsU patients are basophils (7). Basophils produced and released IL-31 in response to IgE-dependent stimulation and were even more responsive in terms of secreting the cytokine following incubation with the bacterial peptide *N*-Formylmethionyl-leucyl-phenylalanine (7). Basophils also expressed both IL-31 and OSMR receptors, and

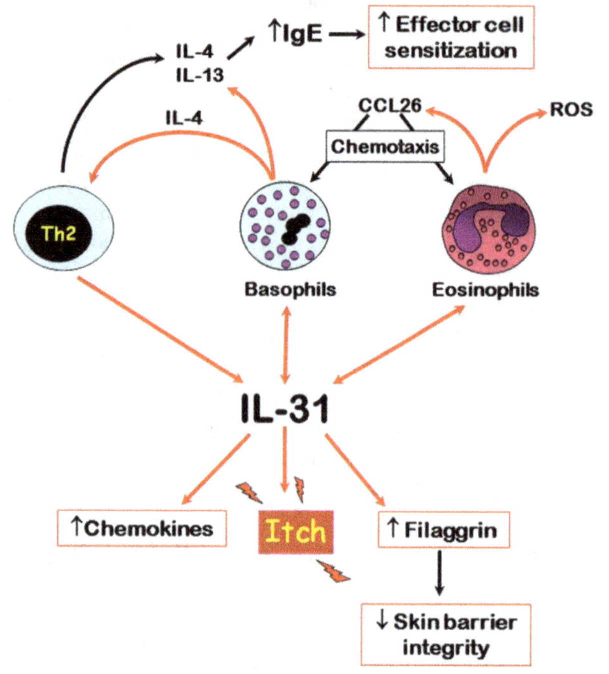

FIGURE 1 | Overview of the main cellular sources and potential roles of IL-31 in autoimmune skin diseases. Red arrows denote direct effects, black indirect effects. Double arrows denote autocrine activation.

were responsive to IL-31 stimulation which gave rise to release of the archetypal Th2-type cytokines IL-4 and IL-13 from these cells. Surprisingly, however, IL-31 failed to cause degranulation of basophils, as determined by the expression of the degranulation markers CD63 and CD203c as well as histamine release (7).

Since basophils are predominant sources of both IL-31 and histamine, inhibition of basophil function is of therapeutic interest in controlling itch-related symptoms in CsU. Furthermore, basophils not only significantly infiltrate the skin in CsU (38) but are also crucial contributors of IL-4 and IL-13 which support IgE class-switching and, in the case of IL-4, also Th2 immunity [reviewed in (39)]. IgE-dependent basophil activation can be therapeutically targeted with the monoclonal antibody omalizumab, which prevents free-circulating IgE from binding to cells such as basophils and also mast cells, leading to the down-regulation of cell-surface FcεRI expressions as well as the degree of IgE sensitization. Since the autoimmune component of CsU is thought to involve autoantibodies against either FcεRI or IgE a reduction of cell-surface IgE and/or FcεRI due to omalizumab presents an important therapeutic strategy. Indeed, omalizumab has been used successfully to treat patients with CsU (40, 41). The fact that IL-31 levels are also reduced following omalizumab treatment further supports the role of basophils in CsU (32). This is underlined by reports of a rapid reduction *in vivo* of both FcεRI and IgE expressions on basophils due to omalizumab (42). While mast cells may also be targeted by omalizumab, the reductions in FcεRI receptor density resulting from omalizumab therapy are known to occur sooner in basophils than for skin mast cells, possibly due to a greater turnover of basophils compared to their skin tissue-fixed mast cell counterparts (43).

In addition to our observations regarding IL-31 inducing Th2-type cytokine release from basophils, we found that the cytokine also facilitates basophil chemotaxis (7). This indicates that IL-31 plays a role in the orchestration and accumulation of basophils in inflammatory skin diseases such as CsU. Since basophils are majorly involved in the pathogenesis of CsU, targeting IL-31 directly (e.g., by nemolizumab) may prevent both IL-31-mediated basophil recruitment as well as the autocrine effects of this cytokine in stimulating the release of IL-4 and IL-13 from basophils. Such approaches using nemolizumab (CIM331) have recently been tested successfully (also in terms of reducing itch) in atopic dermatitis in both humans and other primates (19, 20, 44–46). Similarly, the anti-canine-IL-31 monoclonal antibody, lokivetmab, has been used to treat atopic dermatitis in dogs (47–49). However, the potential clinical benefits of anti-IL-31 monoclonal antibodies have yet to be reported for CsU (and indeed other autoimmune skin diseases).

Bullous Pemphigoid

The autoimmune blistering skin disease, bullous pemphigoid (BP), is accompanied by severe pruritus, thus suggesting possible involvement of IL-31. Indeed, Salz et al reported high IL-31 levels in BP blister fluids as well as an association of this cytokine with granulocytes (50). More recently, we also showed that IL-31 is expressed in the lesional skin of BP patients, particularly in eosinophils from skin tissue and also within blister fluids (51). Moreover, eosinophils were demonstrated to be the major cellular source of IL-31 in BP and isolated peripheral blood eosinophils secreted substantial amounts of IL-31 (51). Similarly to basophils, IL-31 also has chemotactic effects on eosinophils and additionally stimulates these cells to release reactive oxygen species and the chemokine CCL26 (5).

It is, however, as yet unclear whether BP patients display elevated serum levels of IL-31, since the currently published literature has reported conflicting observations. Our own investigation showed only minor elevations in serum IL-31 levels vs. non-BP controls (51) compared to Salz et al (50), who observed significant increases, and Kulczycka-Siennicka et al. (52), who reported reduced levels of the cytokine. Despite these different observations regarding IL-31 serum levels, it is clear that eosinophils are one of the major sources for the increased IL-31 levels in BP blister fluids, which often contain a highly enriched accumulation of eosinophils. Because BP patients experience pruritus particularly in lesional skin the increases in IL-31 levels in blister fluids offer a plausible explanation for this localized itch.

Basophils have also been reported to be associated with BP (53) but their potential contribution to IL-31 in this disease is not yet known. Eosinophil-derived IL-31 may possibly participate in the trafficking of basophils to lesional tissues affected by BP and this may further be supported by IL-31-induced CCL26 release from eosinophils (5). Furthermore, there are several case reports of successful therapy of BP using omalizumab, suggesting potential basophil involvement (54–56). However, Freire et al recently showed that the mast cells and eosinophils make up most of the IgE-expressing cells in BP skin (57) and both cell types are widely reported to participate in various autoimmune skin diseases [reviewed in (58, 59)]. It is thus conceivable that the clinical benefit of omalizumab therapy may largely due to a reduction in eosinophil and mast cell function.

Psoriasis

It was originally thought that IL-31 does not play a role in psoriasis, based on comparisons of cellular expressions of the cytokine (both at mRNA level and immunoreactivity) together with controls (12, 29, 60). However, more recent investigations have reported that serum IL-31 levels are significantly elevated in psoriasis and that chronic itch associated with psoriatic skin is accompanied by increased transcription of IL-31 (61, 62). Narbutt et al further showed that IL-31 serum levels were significantly reduced after narrowband UVB phototherapy, coinciding with a substantial reduction in pruritus in these patients (61). This study indicates that itch accompanying psoriasis might be associated with IL-31. Interestingly, skin mast cells have been shown to express elevated IL-31 in psoriatic skin compared to healthy controls (63). In contrast, however, Czarnecka-Operacz et al. failed to observe any correlation between itch severity in psoriasis and IL-31 (64). On balance, and despite the possibility that it may contribute to pruritic forms of the disease, the currently published literature does not yet provide a clear consensus regarding the role of IL-31 in psoriasis *per se*.

Autoimmune Connective Tissue Diseases Affecting the Skin

Pruritus is a prominent symptom in several autoimmune connective tissue diseases such as lupus and dermatomyositis, although these diseases can affect multiple organ systems and are often supervised by dermatologists. In lupus erythematosus there is currently only sparse evidence to suggest a role of IL-31 and, as yet, no reports specifically dealing with cutaneous forms of this autoimmune disease. Although pruritus does often accompany cutaneous lupus erythematosus it is usually mild in severity and (65), possibly indicating that IL-31 is not a major player in this disease. In systemic lupus erythematosus (SLE) IL-31 serum levels were not shown to be significantly increased compared to healthy controls (66). However, in stark contrast, a more recent study reported significant increases in IL-31 serum levels in SLE as well as identification of IL-31 polymorphisms that were associated with SLE in the Chinese population (67). While the role of IL-31 in SLE is still unclear these IL-31 polymorphisms may nonetheless serve as novel genetic markers of susceptibility to SLE (67).

Dermatomyositis is another autoimmune disease that involves the skin and is sometimes involves considerable pruritus(68), although the muscles and sometimes the lungs can also be affected. In a recent article, Kim et al showed that itch correlated with increased cutaneous severity where IL-31 and IL-31RA gene expressions in lesional skin were upregulated compared with either non-lesional skin or that from healthy controls (69). IL-31 mRNA expression also positively correlated with itch score and immunoreactivity for IL-31 and IL-31RA was greater in lesional skin. Furthermore, lesional dermatomyositis skin contained significantly more IL-31-producing cells, of which CD4+ cells were the most abundant IL-31-expressing cell type (70).

Alopecia Areata

In addition to its role in pruritic skin diseases, IL-31 was originally also associated with alopecia areata, an autoimmune disease involving inflammation of the hair follicles and a loss of immune privilege [reviewed in (70)]. However, although IL-31 and hair loss was described in mice (1) it was not subsequently observed in patients with alopecia areata (60).

CONCLUDING REMARKS

The published literature to date shows that IL-31 is differentially associated with autoimmune skin diseases, especially those where pruritus is a major symptom, such as CsU and bullous pemphigoid. Here, recent evidence shows that basophils and eosinophils are major sources of this cytokine, respectively, especially within affected skin tissues. However, the input of other IL-31-producing cells, especially CD4+ T cells, in these autoimmune diseases still needs to be elucidated in terms of IL-31-mediated immunomodulatory roles. IL-31 possibly plays a role in the trafficking of basophils to affected tissue sites because of its known actions in supporting the release CCL2 and CCL26 chemokines. Basophil-derived IL-4, the release of which is also driven by IL-31, may support the development of Th2 cells and subsequent further IL-31 production. The interplay of IL-31 and various immune cells that are known to play a role in autoimmune skin diseases is summarized in **Figure 1**. Overall, IL-31 is a crucial driver for pruritus in certain autoimmune skin diseases and the recent development of blocking antibodies offers exciting new therapeutic opportunities to combat itch-related symptoms.

AUTHOR CONTRIBUTIONS

All authors listed have made a substantial, direct and intellectual contribution to the work, and approved it for publication.

ACKNOWLEDGMENTS

The authors would like to thank the Deutsche Forschungsgemeinschaft for providing research funding (Translationale Pruritusforschung RA 1026/3-1).

REFERENCES

1. Dillon SR, Sprecher C, Hammond A, Bilsborough J, Rosenfeld-Franklin M, Presnell SR, et al. Interleukin 31, a cytokine produced by activated T cells, induces dermatitis in mice. *Nat Immunol.* (2004) 5:752–60. doi: 10.1038/ni1084
2. Bando T, Morikawa Y, Komori T, Senba E. Complete overlap of interleukin-31 receptor A and oncostatin M receptor beta in the adult dorsal root ganglia with distinct developmental expression patterns. *Neuroscience.* (2006) 142:1263–71. doi: 10.1016/j.neuroscience.2006.07.009

3. Horejs-Hoeck J, Schwarz H, Lamprecht S, Maier E, Hainzl S, Schmittner M, et al. Dendritic cells activated by IFN-gamma/STAT1 express IL-31 receptor and release proinflammatory mediators upon IL-31 treatment. *J Immunol.* (2012) 188:5319–26. doi: 10.4049/jimmunol.1101044
4. Kasraie S, Niebuhr M, Baumert K, Werfel T. Functional effects of interleukin 31 in human primary keratinocytes. *Allergy.* (2011) 66:845–52. doi: 10.1111/j.1398-9995.2011.02545.x
5. Kunsleben N, Rüdrich U, Gehring M, Novak N, Kapp A, Raap U. IL-31 induces chemotaxis, calcium mobilization, release of reactive oxygen species, and CCL26 in eosinophils, which are capable to release IL-31. *J Invest Dermatol.* (2015) 135:1908–11. doi: 10.1038/jid.2015.106
6. Kasraie S, Niebuhr M, Werfel T. Interleukin (IL)-31 induces pro-inflammatory cytokines in human monocytes and macrophages following stimulation with staphylococcal exotoxins. *Allergy.* (2010) 65:712–21. doi: 10.1111/j.1398-9995.2009.02255.x
7. Raap U, Gehring M, Kleiner S, Rüdrich U, Eiz-Vesper B, Haas H, et al. Human basophils are a source of - and are differentially activated by - IL-31. *Clin Exp Allergy.* (2017) 47:499–508. doi: 10.1111/cea.12875
8. Diveu C, Venereau E, Froger J, Ravon E, Grimaud L, Rousseau F, et al. Molecular and functional characterization of a soluble form of oncostatin M/interleukin-31 shared receptor. *J Biol Chem.* (2006) 281:36673–82. doi: 10.1074/jbc.M607005200
9. Chattopadhyay S, Tracy E, Liang P, Robledo O, Rose-John S, Baumann H. Interleukin-31 and oncostatin-M mediate distinct signaling reactions and response patterns in lung epithelial cells. *J Biol Chem.* (2007) 282:3014–26. doi: 10.1074/jbc.M609655200
10. Dambacher J, Beigel F, Seiderer J, Haller D, Göke B, Auernhammer CJ, et al. Interleukin 31 mediates MAP kinase and STAT1/3 activation in intestinal epithelial cells and its expression is upregulated in inflammatory bowel disease. *Gut.* (2007) 56:1257–65. doi: 10.1136/gut.2006.118679
11. Zhang Q, Putheti P, Zhou Q, Liu Q, Gao W. Structures and biological functions of IL-31 and IL-31 receptors. *Cytokine Growth Factor Rev.* (2008) 19:347–56. doi: 10.1016/j.cytogfr.2008.08.003
12. Sonkoly E, Muller A, Lauerma AI, Pivarcsi A, Soto H, Kemeny L, et al. IL-31: a new link between T cells and pruritus in atopic skin inflammation. *J Allergy Clin Immunol.* (2006) 117: 411–7. doi: 10.1016/j.jaci.2005.10.033
13. Ständer S, Weisshaar E, Raap U. Emerging drugs for the treatment of pruritus. *Expert Opin Emerg Drugs.* (2015) 20:515–21. doi: 10.1517/14728214.2015.1051964
14. Singh B, Jegga AG, Shanmukhappa KS, Edukulla R, Khurana Hershey GH, Medvedovic M, et al. IL-31-driven skin remodeling involves epidermal cell proliferation and thickening that lead to impaired skin-barrier function. *PLoS ONE.* (2016) 11:e0161877. doi: 10.1371/journal.pone.0161877
15. Takaoka A, Arai I, Sugimoto M, Yamaguchi A, Tanaka M, Nakaike S. Expression of IL-31 gene transcripts in NC/Nga mice with atopic dermatitis. *Eur J Pharmacol.* (2005) 516:180–1. doi: 10.1016/j.ejphar.2005.04.040
16. Grimstad O, Sawanobori Y, Vestergaard C, Bilsborough J, Olsen UB, Gronhoj-Larsen C, et al. Anti-interleukin-31-antibodies ameliorate scratching behaviour in NC/Nga mice: a model of atopic dermatitis. *Exp Dermatol.* (2009) 18:35–43. doi: 10.1111/j.1600-0625.2008.00766.x
17. Gutzmer R, Gschwandtner M, Rossbach K, Mommert S, Werfel T, Kietzmann M, et al. Pathogenetic and therapeutic implications of the histamine H4 receptor in inflammatory skin diseases and pruritus. *Front Biosci.* (2011) 3:985–94. doi: 10.2741/s203
18. Werfel T, Layton G, Yeadon M, Whitlock L, Osterloh I, Jimenez P, et al. Efficacy and safety of the histamine H4 receptor antagonist ZPL-3893787 in patients with atopic dermatitis. *J Allergy Clin Immunol.* (2018) 143:1830–7.e4. doi: 10.1016/j.jaci.2018.07.047
19. Nemoto O, Furue M, Nakagawa H, Shiramoto M, Hanada R, Matsuki S et al. The first trial of CIM331, a humanized antihuman interleukin-31 receptor A antibody, in healthy volunteers and patients with atopic dermatitis to evaluate safety, tolerability and pharmacokinetics of a single dose in a randomized, double-blind, placebo-controlled study. *Br J Dermatol.* (2016) 174:296–304. doi: 10.1111/bjd.14207
20. Ruzicka T, Hanifin JM, Furue M, Pulka G, Mlynarczyk I, Wollenberg A, et al. Anti-interleukin-31 receptor A antibody for atopic dermatitis. *N Engl J Med.* (2017) 376:826–35. doi: 10.1056/NEJMoa1606490
21. Stott B, Lavender P, Lehmann S, Pennino D, Durham S, Schmidt-Weber CB. Human IL-31 is induced by IL-4 and promotes TH2-driven inflammation. *J Allergy Clin Immunol.* (2013) 132:446–54. doi: 10.1016/j.jaci.2013.03.050
22. Pan Q, Feng Y, Peng Y, Zhou H, Deng Z, Li L, et al. Basophil recruitment to skin lesions of patients with systemic lupus erythematosus mediated by CCR1 and CCR2. *Cell Physiol Biochem.* (2017) 43:832–39. doi: 10.1159/000481609
23. Korosec P, Turner PJ, Silar M, Kopac P, Kosnik M, Gibbs BF, et al. Basophils, high-affinity IgE receptors, and CCL2 in human anaphylaxis. *J Allergy Clin Immunol.* (2017) 140:750–58. doi: 10.1016/j.jaci.2016.12.989
24. Cornelissen C, Marquardt Y, Czaja K, Wenzel J, Frank J, Lüscher-Firzlaff J, et al. IL-31 regulates differentiation and filaggrin expression in human organotypic skin models. *J Allergy Clin Immunol.* (2012) 129:426–33. doi: 10.1016/j.jaci.2011.10.042
25. van Drongelen V, Haisma EM, Out-Luiting JJ, Nibbering PH, El Ghalbzouri A. Reduced filaggrin expression is accompanied by increased *Staphylococcus aureus* colonization of epidermal skin models. *Clin Exp Allergy.* (2014) 44:1515–24. doi: 10.1111/cea.12443
26. Bilsborough J, Leung DY, Maurer M, Howell M, Boguniewicz M, Yao L, et al. IL-31 is associated with cutaneous lymphocyte antigen-positive skin homing T cells in patients with atopic dermatitis. *J Allergy Clin Immunol.* (2006) 117:418–25. doi: 10.1016/j.jaci.2005.10.046
27. Raap U, Wichmann K, Bruder M, Stander S, Wedi B, Kapp A, et al. Correlation of IL-31 serum levels with severity of atopic dermatitis. *J Allergy Clin Immunol.* (2008) 122:421–23. doi: 10.1016/j.jaci.2008.05.047
28. Raap U, Weissmantel S, Gehring M, Eisenberg AM, Kapp A, Folster-Holst R. IL-31 significantly correlates with disease activity and Th2 cytokine levels in children with atopic dermatitis. *Pediatr Allergy Immunol.* (2012) 23:285–88. doi: 10.1111/j.1399-3038.2011.01241.x
29. Neis MM, Peters B, Dreuw A, Wenzel J, Bieber T, Mauch C, et al. Enhanced expression levels of IL-31 correlate with IL-4 and IL-13 in atopic and allergic contact dermatitis. J *Allergy Clin Immunol.* (2006) 118:930–37. doi: 10.1016/j.jaci.2006.07.015
30. Raap U, Wieczorek D, Gehring M, Pauls I, Stander S, Kapp A, et al. Increased levels of serum IL-31 in chronic spontaneous urticaria. *Exp Dermatol.* (2010) 19:464–66. doi: 10.1111/j.1600-0625.2010.01067.x
31. Hartmann K, Wagner N, Rabenhorst A, Pflanz L, Leja S, Forster A, et al. Serum IL-31 levels are increased in a subset of patients with mastocytosis and correlate with disease severity in adult patients. *J Allergy Clin Immunol.* (2013) 132:232–35. doi: 10.1016/j.jaci.2012.11.008
32. Altrichter S, Hawro T, Hanel K, Czaja K, Luscher B, Maurer M, et al. Successful omalizumab treatment in chronic spontaneous urticaria is associated with lowering of serum IL-31 levels. *J Eur Acad Dermatol Venereol.* (2016) 30:454–55. doi: 10.1111/jdv.12831
33. Philpott H, Kette F, Hissaria P, Gillis D, Smith W. Chronic urticaria: the autoimmune paradigm. *Intern Med J.* (2008) 38:852–7. doi: 10.1111/j.1445-5994.2008.01673.x
34. Altrichter S, Peter HJ, Pisarevskaja D, Metz M, Martus P, Maurer M. IgE mediated autoallergy against thyroid peroxidase - a novel pathomechanism of chronic spontaneous urticaria? *PLoS ONE.* (2011) 6:e14794. doi: 10.1371/journal.pone.0014794
35. Rauber MM, Pickert J, Holiangu L, Möbs C, Pfützner W. Functional and phenotypic analysis of basophils allows determining distinct subtypes in patients with chronic urticaria. *Allergy.* (2017) 72:1904–11. doi: 10.1111/all.13215
36. Church MK, Kolkhir P, Metz M, Maurer M. The role and relevance of mast cells in urticaria. *Immunol Rev.* (2018) 282:232–47. doi: 10.1111/imr.12632
37. Lin W, Zhou Q, Liu C, Ying M, Xu S. Increased plasma IL-17, IL-31, and IL-33 levels in chronic spontaneous urticaria. *Sci Rep.* (2017) 7:17797. doi: 10.1038/s41598-017-18187-z
38. Ying S, Kikuchi Y, Meng Q, Kay AB, Kaplan AP. TH1/TH2 cytokines and inflammatory cells in skin biopsy specimens from patients with chronic idiopathic urticaria: comparison with the allergen-induced late-phase cutaneous reaction. *J Allergy Clin Immunol.* (2002) 109:694–700. doi: 10.1067/mai.2002.123236

39. Varricchi G, Raap U, Rivellese F, Marone G, Gibbs BF. Human mast cells and basophils-How are they similar how are they different? *Immunol Rev.* (2018) 282:8–34. doi: 10.1111/imr.12627
40. Magerl M, Staubach P, Altrichter S, Ardelean E, Krause K, Metz M, et al. Effective treatment of therapy-resistant chronic spontaneous urticaria with omalizumab. *J Allergy Clin Immunol.* (2010) 126:665–6. doi: 10.1016/j.jaci.2010.05.047
41. Maurer M, Altrichter S, Bieber T, Biedermann T, Bräutigam M, Seyfried S, et al. Efficacy and safety of omalizumab in patients with chronic urticaria who exhibit IgE against thyroperoxidase. *J Allergy Clin Immunol.* (2011) 128:202–9. doi: 10.1016/j.jaci.2011.04.038
42. Metz M, Staubach P, Bauer A, Brehler R, Gericke J, Kangas M, et al. Clinical efficacy of omalizumab in chronic spontaneous urticaria is associated with a reduction of FcεRI-positive cells in the skin. *Theranostics.* (2017) 7:1266–76. doi: 10.7150/thno.18304
43. Beck LA, Marcotte GV, MacGlashan D, Togias A, Saini S. Omalizumab-induced reductions in mast cell Fce psilon RI expression and function. *J Allergy Clin Immunol.* (2004) 114:527–30. doi: 10.1016/j.jaci.2004.06.032
44. Fioranelli M, Roccia MG, Lotti T. Therapy with anti-interleukin-31 receptor A antibody for atopic dermatitis. *Dermatol Ther.* (2017) 30:e12490. doi: 10.1111/dth.12490
45. Kabashima K, Furue M, Hanifin JM, Pulka G, Wollenberg A, Galus R, et al. Nemolizumab in patients with moderate-to-severe atopic dermatitis: Randomized, phase II, long-term extension study. *J Allergy Clin Immunol.* (2018) 142:1121–30. doi: 10.1016/j.jaci.2018.03.018
46. Oyama S, Kitamura H, Kuramochi T, Higuchi Y, Matsushita H, Suzuki T, et al. Cynomolgus monkey model of interleukin-31-induced scratching depicts blockade of human interleukin-31 receptor A by a humanized monoclonal antibody. *Exp Dermatol.* (2018) 27:14–21. doi: 10.1111/exd.13236
47. Tamamoto-Mochizuki C, Paps JS, Olivry T. Proactive maintenance therapy of canine atopic dermatitis with the anti-IL-31 lokivetmab. can a monoclonal antibody blocking a single cytokine prevent allergy flares? *Vet Dermatol.* (2019) 30:98–104. doi: 10.1111/vde.12715
48. Michels GM, Walsh KF, Kryda KA, Mahabir SP, Walters RR, Hoevers JD, et al. A blinded, randomized, placebo-controlled trial of the safety of lokivetmab (ZTS-00103289), a caninized anti-canine IL-31 monoclonal antibody in client-owned dogs with atopic dermatitis. *Vet Dermatol.* (2016) 27:505–e136. doi: 10.1111/vde.12364
49. Moyaert H, Van Brussel L, Borowski S, Escalada M, Mahabir SP, Walters RR, et al. A blinded, randomized clinical trial evaluating the efficacy and safety of lokivetmab compared to ciclosporin in client-owned dogs with atopic dermatitis. *Vet Dermatol.* (2017) 28:593–e145. doi: 10.1111/vde.12478
50. Salz M, Haeberle S, Hoffmann J, Enk AH, Hadaschik EN. Elevated IL-31 serum levels in bullous pemphigoid patients correlate with eosinophil numbers and are associated with BP180-IgE. *J Dermatol Sci.* (2017) 87:309–11. doi: 10.1016/j.jdermsci.2017.07.019
51. Rüdrich U, Gehring M, Papakonstantinou E, Illerhaus A, Engmann J, Kapp A, et al. Eosinophils are a major source of interleukin-31 in bullous pemphigoid. *Acta Derm Venereol.* (2018) 98:766–71. doi: 10.2340/00015555-2951
52. Kulczycka-Siennicka L, Cynkier A, Waszczykowska E, Wozniacka A, Zebrowska A. The role of Intereukin-31 in pathogenesis of itch and its intensity in a course of bullous pemphigoid and dermatitis herpetiformis. *Biomed Res Int.* (2017) 2017:5965492. doi: 10.1155/2017/5965492
53. Ito Y, Satoh T, Takayama K, Miyagishi C, Walls AF, Yokozeki H. Basophil recruitment and activation in inflammatory skin diseases. *Allergy.* (2011) 66:1107–13. doi: 10.1111/j.1398-9995.2011.02570.x
54. Dufour C, Souillet AL, Chaneliere C, Jouen F, Bodemer C, Jullien D, et al. Successful management of severe infant bullous pemphigoid with omalizumab. *Br J Dermatol.* (2012) 166:1140–2. doi: 10.1111/j.1365-2133.2011.10748.x
55. London VA, Kim GH, Fairley JA, Woodley DT. Successful treatment of bullous pemphigoid with omalizumab. *Arch Dermatol.* (2012) 148:1241–3. doi: 10.1001/archdermatol.2012.1604
56. Menzinger S, Kaya G, Schmidt E, Fontao L, Laffitte E. Biological and clinical response to omalizumab in a patient with bullous pemphigoid. *Acta Derm Venereol.* (2018) 98:284–6. doi: 10.2340/00015555-2845
57. Freire PC, Muñoz CH1, Stingl G. IgE autoreactivity in bullous pemphigoid: eosinophils and mast cells as major targets of pathogenic immune reactants. *Br J Dermatol.* (2017) 177:1644–53. doi: 10.1111/bjd.15924
58. Diny NL, Rose NR, Čiháková D. Eosinophils in autoimmune diseases. *Front Immunol.* (2017) 8:484. doi: 10.3389/fimmu.2017.00484
59. Fang H, Zhang Y, Li N, Wang G, Liu Z. The autoimmune skin disease bullous pemphigoid: the role of mast cells in autoantibody-induced tissue injury. *Front Immunol.* (2018) 9:407. doi: 10.3389/fimmu.2018.00407
60. Nobbe S, Dziunycz P, Mühleisen B, Bilsborough J, Dillon SR, French LE, et al. IL-31 expression by inflammatory cells is preferentially elevated in atopic dermatitis. *Acta Derm Venereol.* (2012) 92:24–8. doi: 10.2340/00015555-1191
61. Narbutt J, Olejniczak I, Sobolewska-Sztychny D, Sysa-Jedrzejowska A, Słowik-Kwiatkowska I, Hawro T, et al. Narrow band ultraviolet B irradiations cause alteration in interleukin-31 serum level in psoriatic patients. *Arch Dermatol Res.* (2013) 305:191–5. doi: 10.1007/s00403-012-1293-6
62. Nattkemper LA, Tey HL, Valdes-Rodriguez R, Lee H, Mollanazar NK, Albornoz C, et al. The genetics of chronic itch: gene expression in the skin of patients with atopic dermatitis and psoriasis with severe itch. *J Invest Dermatol.* (2018) 138:1311–7. doi: 10.1016/j.jid.2017.12.029
63. Niyonsaba F, Ushio H, Hara M, Yokoi H, Tominaga M, Takamori K, et al. Antimicrobial peptides human beta-defensins and cathelicidin LL-37 induce the secretion of a pruritogenic cytokine IL-31 by human mast cells. *J Immunol.* (2010) 184:3526–34. doi: 10.4049/jimmunol.0900712
64. Czarnecka-Operacz M, Polanska A, Klimanska M, Teresiak-Mikołajczak E, Molinska-Glura M, Adamski Z, et al. Itching sensation in psoriatic patients and its relation to body mass index and IL-17 and IL-31 concentrations. *Postepy Dermatol Alergol.* (2015) 32:426–30. doi: 10.5114/pdia.2015.56097
65. Samotij D, Szczech J, Kushner CJ, Mowla MR, Danczak-Pazdrowska A, Antiga E, et al. Prevalence of pruritus in cutaneous lupus erythematosus: brief report of a multicenter, multinational cross-sectional study. *Biomed Res Int.* (2018) 2018:3491798. doi: 10.1155/2018/3491798
66. Zhang M, Xu WD, Zhu Y, Wen PF, Leng RX, Pan HF, et al. Serum levels of cytokines in systemic lupus erythematosus: association study in a chinese population. *Z Rheumatol.* (2014) 73:277–80. doi: 10.1007/s00393-013-1274-y
67. Huang HT, Chen JM, Guo J, Lan Y, Wei YS. The association of interleukin-31 polymorphisms with interleukin-31 serum levels and risk of systemic lupus erythematosus. *Rheumatol Int.* (2016) 36:799–805. doi: 10.1007/s00296-016-3422-6
68. Shirani Z, Kucenic MJ, Carroll CL, Fleischer AB Jr, Feldman SR, Yosipovitch G, et al. Pruritus in adult dermatomyositis. *Clin Exp Dermatol.* (2004) 29:273–6. doi: 10.1111/j.1365-2230.2004.01510.x
69. Kim HJ, Zeidi M, Bonciani D, Pena SM, Tiao J, Sahu S, et al. Itch in dermatomyositis: the role of increased skin interleukin-31. *Br J Dermatol.* (2018) 179:669–78. doi: 10.1111/bjd.16498
70. Rajabi F, Drake LA, Senna MM, Rezaei N. Alopecia areata: a review of disease pathogenesis. *Br J Dermatol.* (2018) 179:1033–48. doi: 10.1111/bjd.16808

3

Blue and Long-Wave Ultraviolet Light Induce *in vitro* Neutrophil Extracellular Trap (NET) Formation

Elsa Neubert[1,2†], Katharina Marie Bach[1†], Julia Busse[1], Ivan Bogeski[3], Michael P. Schön[1,4], Sebastian Kruss[2,5] and Luise Erpenbeck[1]*

[1] Department of Dermatology, Venereology and Allergology, University Medical Center Göttingen, Göttingen, Germany, [2] Institute of Physical Chemistry, Göttingen University, Göttingen, Germany, [3] Institute of Cardiovascular Physiology, University Medical Center Göttingen, Göttingen, Germany, [4] Lower Saxony Institute of Occupational Dermatology, University Medical Center Göttingen, Göttingen, Germany, [5] Center for Nanoscale Microscopy and Molecular Physiology of the Brain (CNMPB), Göttingen, Germany

***Correspondence:**
Luise Erpenbeck
luise.erpenbeck@med.uni-goettingen.de

† These authors have contributed equally to this work

Neutrophil Extracellular Traps (NETs) are produced by neutrophilic granulocytes and consist of decondensed chromatin decorated with antimicrobial peptides. They defend the organism against intruders and are released upon various stimuli including pathogens, mediators of inflammation, or chemical triggers. NET formation is also involved in inflammatory, cardiovascular, malignant diseases, and autoimmune disorders like rheumatoid arthritis, psoriasis, or systemic lupus erythematosus (SLE). In many autoimmune diseases like SLE or dermatomyositis, light of the ultraviolet-visible (UV-VIS) spectrum is well-known to trigger and aggravate disease severity. However, the underlying connection between NET formation, light exposure, and disease exacerbation remains elusive. We studied the effect of UVA (375 nm), blue (470 nm) and green (565 nm) light on NETosis in human neutrophils *ex vivo*. Our results show a dose- and wavelength-dependent induction of NETosis. Light-induced NETosis depended on the generation of extracellular reactive oxygen species (ROS) induced by riboflavin excitation and its subsequent reaction with tryptophan. The light-induced NETosis required both neutrophil elastase (NE) as well as myeloperoxidase (MPO) activation and induced histone citrullination. These findings suggest that NET formation as a response to light could be the hitherto missing link between elevated susceptibility to NET formation in autoimmune patients and photosensitivity for example in SLE and dermatomyositis patients. This novel connection could provide a clue for a deeper understanding of light-sensitive diseases in general and for the development of new pharmacological strategies to avoid disease exacerbation upon light exposure.

Keywords: neutrophilic granulocytes, NET formation, UV-Vis light, inflammation, ROS formation, riboflavin

INTRODUCTION

Neutrophilic granulocytes (hereafter referred to as neutrophils) are able to expel fibril networks of decondensed chromatin, decorated with a variety of antimicrobial substances, in a process termed neutrophil extracellular trap (NET) formation or NETosis (1). Initially, NETosis was described as an immune defense strategy against intruding pathogens, distinct from phagocytosis and the release of cytotoxic substances. Apart from their role in the defense within the innate immune system, the dysregulation of NETosis appears to be involved in the pathology of various diseases (2) such as rheumatoid arthritis (3), systemic lupus erythematosus (SLE) (4), psoriasis (5, 6), thrombosis (7), atherosclerosis (8), and cancer (9). The activation mechanisms and underlying cascades of NETosis depend highly on the particular stimulus (10, 11). Additionally, neutrophils and therefore also neutrophils undergoing NETosis, are very sensitive to environmental cues that affect, for example, adhesion (12–15).

In most scenarios, the cell undergoes a characteristic sequence of morphological changes during NETosis including chromatin decondensation, cytoskeleton degradation, cell rounding, and softening, which ultimately lead to NET expulsion and cell death ("suicidal" NETosis) (16, 17). Initially, active enzyme-dependent mechanisms dominate these processes. For instance, the initiation of chromatin decondensation often involves the release of neutrophil elastase (NE) and myeloperoxidase (MPO) from the neutrophilic granules and subsequent translocation to the nucleus (18, 19). Following initiation of chromatin decondensation, which represents the point of no return in NETosis, further progression until the NET release is mainly driven by the material properties of the NETotic cell such as the entropic swelling of its chromatin (17).

Interestingly, a connection between dysregulated NET formation and the production of autoantibodies against NET components has been described in several diseases including SLE, rheumatoid arthritis and small-vessel vasculitis (20, 21). Mechanistically, NET formation in this context often relies on the activity of peptidylarginine deiminase 4 (PAD4), which citrullinates histones contributing to chromatin decondensation (22–25). This hypercitrullination has been linked to the development of autoantigens against citrullinated histones, for instance in the pathogenesis of rheumatoid arthritis (26). Interestingly, autoimmune disorders such as systemic lupus erythematosus (SLE) or dermatomyositis, can also be triggered and/or aggravated by light. Although for these diseases both the increased propensity for NET formation as well as the marked light sensitivity is well-documented (27–30), the connection between these two phenomena remains elusive.

Electromagnetic radiation of wavelengths above ultraviolet C (UVC) light passes the ozone layer of the stratosphere and can thus reach the human skin (31). Within the human skin, light intensity is modified by reflection, absorption as well as scattering and its penetration depth increases with higher wavelengths (32–34). However, the actual penetration of each wavelength also strongly depends on the specific skin composition, as well as body region, age, gender, skin type, pigmentation, and therefore ethnicity.

High-energy UV light causes severe skin damage. This has been linked not only to photodermatoses but also to phototoxic and photoallergic reactions, skin cancer and photoaging (35, 36). Many of these reactions are mediated by highly reactive radicals and/or reactive oxygen species (ROS) originating from the excitation of photosensitive substances (37). Prominent examples are flavin-based molecules originating from riboflavin (also known as vitamin B2) (38). Under physiological conditions, these reactions are kept in balance by antioxidants, but they can be strongly dysregulated in the context of diseases and after persistent exposure to UV light.

Additionally, light can have several direct effects on neutrophils. Irradiation with UVB light has been reported to recruit neutrophils into upper layers of the skin and has been linked to photoaging (35, 39). Furthermore, increased apoptosis rates of neutrophils occur upon direct irradiation with high doses of UVB or UVC (40, 41) and UVC light can also induce a unique form of NADPH oxidase (NOX)-independent NETosis (named apoNETosis) (41). However, the connection between NET formation and light in a physiologically relevant setting with light which penetrates deeper into the skin such as UVA or blue light, has not been investigated. Thus, a deeper understanding of direct effects of light on immune cells could greatly add to our understanding of light-induced or -aggravated diseases and facilitate the development of therapeutic strategies.

MATERIALS AND METHODS

Isolation of Neutrophils

All experiments with human neutrophils were approved by the Ethics Committee of the University Medical Center (UMG) Göttingen (protocol number: 29/1/17). Neutrophils were isolated from fresh venous blood of healthy donors. Beforehand, all donors were fully informed about possible risks, and their informed consent was obtained in writing. The consent could be withdrawn at any time during the study. Blood was collected in S-Monovettes EDTA (7.5 ml, Sarstedt), and neutrophils were isolated according to previously published protocols based on histopaque 1119 (Sigma Aldrich) as well as Percoll (GE Healthcare) density gradients (17, 42). Neutrophils were resuspended in $HBSS^{-Ca2+/Mg2+}$ and further diluted in the desired medium as described in the appropriate methods sections and figure legends. Purity of the cell preparation was >95% as assessed by cytospin (Cytospin 2 centrifuge, Shanson) and Diff Quick staining (Medion, Diagnostics).

Irradiation of Neutrophils With LED Light

Neutrophils were suspended in either Roswell Park Memorial Institute (RPMI) comp. [RPMI without phenol red (Gibco) + 0.5% heat-inactivated (at 56°C) fetal calf serum (hiFCS, Biochrom GmbH, Merck Millipore)] ± 10 mM HEPES (Roth) or Hank's balanced salt solution (HBSS) comp. [$HBSS^{+Ca2+/Mg2+}$ without phenol red (Lonza) containing 0.5% hiFCS and glucose (AppliChem) equalized to RPMI]. If applicable, these media were supplemented with 0.2 or 2 mg/l riboflavin (Sigma-Aldrich) and 1 mM tryptophan (Sigma-Aldrich) as indicated in the figure captions. Cells were seeded at 10,000 cells per well in $CELLview^{TH}$ black glass-10-well-slides (Greiner bio-one) and left to settle for 30 min (37°C, 5% CO_2). Afterward, the appropriate medium was added, and cells were irradiated with the indicated LED-light at 37°C (ibidi heating system). Cells were irradiated in the heating chamber from below with LEDs of 375 nm (ultraviolet light, M375L3 Mounted LED, Thorlabs GmbH), 470 nm (blue light, M470L3 Mounted LED, Thorlabs GmbH), or 565 nm (green light, M565L3 Mounted LED, Thorlabs GmbH), which were attached to an uncoated convex lens (PLANO-CONVEX LA1131, f = 50.0 mm, uncoated, Thorlabs GmbH) and a T-cube LED Driver (Thorlabs GmbH). For evaluation of light dose-dependent effects, cells were irradiated with cumulative doses of 3.5, 18, 35, and 70 J/cm^2 at 375 nm or 21, 54, 107, and 214 J/cm^2 at 470 nm. The light doses were calculated with respect to the actual power of the LED as measured with the PM12-122 Compact USB Power Meter (Thorlabs GmbH), taking into account the actual distance between the light source and the cells as well as the light transmission through the CELLviewTH glass-10-well-slides according to the manufacturer's specifications. For experiments with an equal light energy-dose or photon flux, the light-doses or duration of exposure, respectively, were adjusted for 470 and 565 nm, the reference value was irradiation with 70 J/cm^2 at 375 nm. Exclusive treatment with the indicated medium without irradiation was used as a negative control and activation with 100 nM PMA (Sigma Aldrich) as a positive control. Before, during, and after activation with light or PMA, the cells were carefully shielded from other light sources. After the activation, the cells were incubated for 3 h, and NETosis was stopped by fixing the cells in 2% paraformaldehyde (PFA, Roth). Before further staining, the cells were kept at 4°C.

Inhibitor Experiments

For inhibition experiments, cells were isolated, settled in RPMIcomp. supplemented with 10 mM HEPES and activated as described above. Inhibitors or ROS scavengers were added at least 20 min (in case of MitoTEMPO 1 h) before cell irradiation with 70 J/cm^2 of 375 nm or 214 J/cm^2 of 470 nm, at 37°C. For an additional control experiment, Trolox and catalase/SOD were added separately after irradiation. The cells were then incubated for an additional 3 h without an additional washing step in the presence of the inhibitors to allow for NET formation and fixed by 2% PFA. Pure medium or 100 nM PMA without irradiation were used as negative and positive controls, respectively. The following inhibitors and ROS scavengers were used in this study: GW-311616A hydrochloride (iNE, Axon Medchem) at 5 µM, 4-aminobenzoic acid hydrazide (4-ABAH, Cayman chemicals) at 100 µM, z-VAD-FMK (Promega) at 20 µM, necrostatin-1 (Nec-1, Enzo) at 50 µM, Y-27632-dihydrochloride (Abcam) at 20 µM, Cl-amidine (Merck Millipore) at 200 µM, MitoTEMPO (Sigma-Aldrich) at 5 µM, diphenyleneiodonium chloride (DPI, Sigma-Aldrich) at 1 µM, Trolox (Sigma-Aldrich) at 50 µM, PEG-catalase at 2,000 U/ml (Sigma-Aldrich), and a mixture of catalase (filtered, Worthington) and superoxide dismutase (SOD, Sigma Aldrich/Merck) at 2,000 and 50 U/ml, respectively.

NET Quantification

To investigate levels of NETosis, cells were washed twice with PBS (Sigma-Aldrich) and, subsequently, neutrophilic DNA was stained with 1.62 µM Hoechst 33342 (Thermo Fisher Scientific) for 15 min. After staining, the cells were stored in PBS for further analysis. For blinded quantification, six microscopic fluorescence images (16×) were obtained in a standardized manner (Axiovert 200 equipped with EC Plan-Neofluar Ph1 and DAPI filter Set 49, Zeiss, software: Metamorph 6.3r2., Molecular Devices or Micro Manager 1.4) using the camera CoolSNAP ES (Photometrics). The number of decondensed vs. condensed nuclei was counted in these images using ImageJ 1.46r (National Institutes of Health), and the relative number of decondensed nuclei/expelled NETs was determined as a percentage of total cells ('NETotic cells') according to previously published studies (17, 43). Relative rates of NETotic cells were normalized to NETs after light-irradiation without any inhibitor ("Rel. number NETotic cells"). The amount of released NETs was determined by counting SYTOX Green-positive cells with decondensed nuclei.

Live Cell Imaging/Discontinuous Irradiation of Neutrophils

Neutrophils (5 × 10^6 per ml in RPMI + 0.5% FCS or HSA + 10 mM HEPES) were seeded in ibidi channel slides (µ-Slide I$^{0.6}$ Luer, ibidi) and stained with 1.62 µM Hoechst and, if indicated, 5 µM SYTOX Green (life technologies) at 37°C for 10 min. Cells were irradiated with broad-spectrum UVA light (300–400 nm) for 3 min using the DAPI filter Set 49. For life cell imaging, NET formation was observed in real time for 3.5 h with a frame rate of one picture per min (Uniblitz stutter driver, model VCM-D1, Visitron Systems) and a 15 ms exposure time. To exclude the toxic effects of the photo-activation of Hoechst, a control experiment was performed without DNA staining during live cell imaging. In this case, NET rates were determined by Hoechst staining directly after 3.5 h. For The SYTOX Green/Hoechst double staining, NETosis was observed for 3 h with a frame-rate of 15 min per image. Images were recorded at 10× or 16× magnification. Images in the center of the light beam and in non-irradiated areas were obtained in a standardized pattern and in a blinded manner, and NETosis rates were determined as described above. The representative combined panorama image in **Figure 1** was obtained with the Plugin MosaicJ for ImageJ (44).

Immunofluorescence Staining

To confirm colocalization of MPO with decondensed chromatin and histone citrullination as a marker for NETosis, activated cells were analyzed by immunofluorescence according to previously published protocols (17). Here, a permeabilization buffer containing 0.1% tritonX and a BSA-based blocking solution (from TSA-kit, Perkin Elmer) was used. Cells were stained with the primary monoclonal anti-human antibody against myeloperoxidase (IgG1, mouse, clone:2C7, ab25989, 1:500, Abcam) and the polyclonal antibody against citrullinated histone 3 (H3Cit, rabbit, ab5103, 1:500, Abcam) and visualized with the polyclonal anti-mouse Alexa488 secondary antibody (IgG, goat, 1:300, #4408, Cell Signaling Technology) or the anti-rabbit Alexa555 secondary antibody (IgG, goat, 1:500, A211428, Life technologies), respectively. Directly before mounting with fluorescence mounting medium (Dako), DNA was stained with Hoechst. Colocalization of MPO, H3Cit and DNA was imaged at 100× magnification by confocal fluorescence microscopy (IX83, Olympus; software: Olympus Fluoview Ver.4.2, Olympus). All pictures were recorded at equal exposure times for MPO and H3Cit within the same experiment, to ensure comparability.

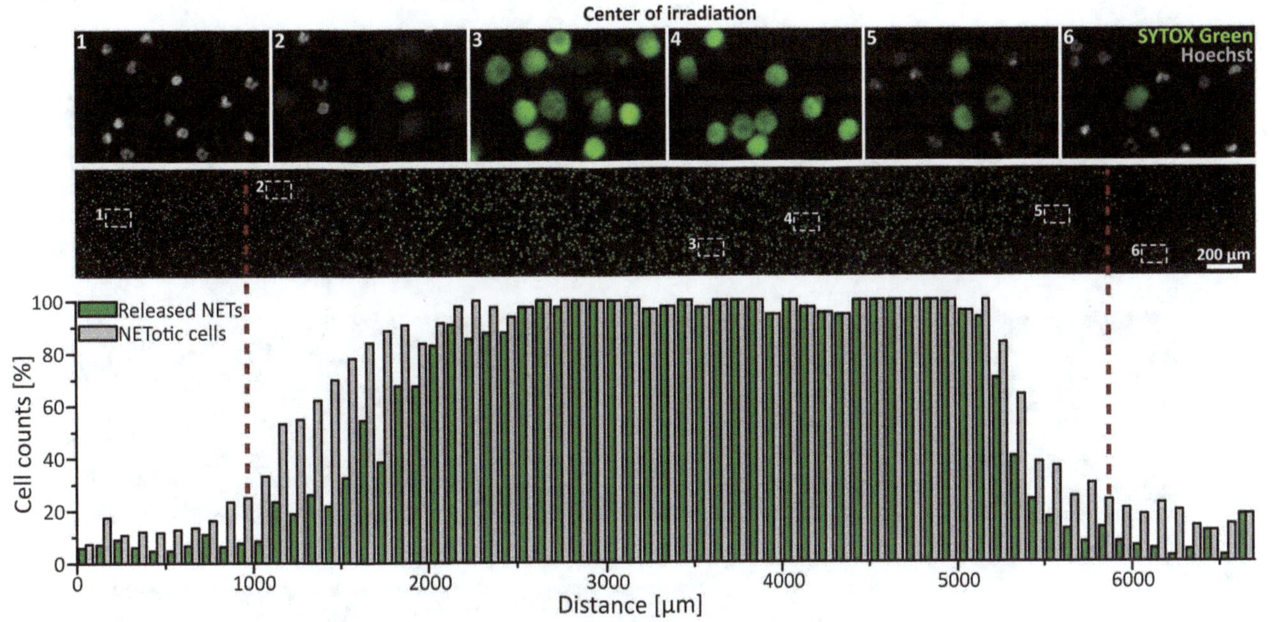

FIGURE 1 | UVA light-induced, locally restricted decondensation of chromatin. UVA light (300–400 nm, ~60 J/cm^2) leads to chromatin decondensation and expulsion of the chromatin into the extracellular space as indicated by SYTOX green positive staining of decondensed chromatin. This effect is locally restricted to the area of irradiation. Irradiation: 3 min to induce NET formation + intermittent irradiation during live-cell imaging (3 h; frame rate: 15 min/image). Cells were kept in RPMIcomp. + 10 mM HEPES.

ROS (H_2O_2) Detection/AmplexRed Assay

Cells were seeded at 10,000 cells per well in RPMIcomp. + 10 mM HEPES, HBSScomp. or HBSScomp. + 2 mg/l riboflavin + 1 mM tryptophan and activated at 70 J/cm^2 of 375 nm light. After activation, 5 μl samples of the supernatant were taken at defined time points (0, 10, 20, or 30 min) close to the slide bottom for reactive oxygen species (ROS) detection. As controls, cells in all three media were either left without irradiation, only media was irradiated, or cells were treated with 100 nM PMA without irradiation. The obtained samples were diluted in a black 96-well-plate (BRANDplates, BRAND GMBH) with PBS containing 50 μM of AmplexRed reagent (Thermo Fisher Scientific), a highly sensitive probe for H_2O_2, and 0.5 U/ml horseradish peroxidase (HRP, Sigma-Aldrich/Merck). Additionally, 10 U/ml SOD (Sigma Aldrich/Merck) were added, to ensure complete detection of ROS by transformation of superoxide radicals to H_2O_2. During the sample collection, cells were gently rocked to ensure equal distribution of ROS. For all samples, the fluorescence intensities of the formed resorufin were measured with the microplate reader Clario Star (software 5.40.R3, BMG labtech), and the results were processed with the software MARS (version 3.32, BMG labtech). Absolute H_2O_2 concentrations were determined *via* calibration with H_2O_2 (Roth) in HBSScomp. After ROS detection, cells were further incubated for a total of 3 h before terminating the activity with 2% PFA, and the number of NETotic cells was determined.

Light Absorption by Riboflavin

The absorbance spectrum of riboflavin (Sigma-Aldrich) was obtained in PBS against PBS alone with the UV-VIS-NIR spectrometer (JASCO V-670, Spectra Manager Software) using a 10 mm-path cuvette.

Statistics

Statistical analysis was performed using GraphPad Prism (version 6.0 for Mac or Windows, GraphPad Software Inc.). If applicable, GAUSS distribution was confirmed by the Shapiro-Wilk normality test. Significance was confirmed on unnormalized data by a two-tailed paired t-test or a one-way ANOVA/Bonferroni's multiple comparisons test with $^{*}p < 0.05$, $^{**}p < 0.01$, $^{***}p < 0.001$, $^{****}p < 0.0001$. Error = mean ± standard error of the mean (SEM) or standard deviation (SD), as indicated.

RESULTS

UVA and Blue Light Induce NETosis Dose-Dependently

To investigate whether UVA light is sufficient to activate NETosis, freshly isolated human neutrophils were irradiated for 3 min with physiologically relevant broad-spectrum UVA light in a standard microscopy setup (wavelengths 300–400 nm, ~60 J/cm^2). Morphological changes of the nuclei were recorded using Hoechst staining over 3.5 h in real-time (**Supplementary Movie**). Neutrophilic chromatin readily decondensed over time, rounded up and finally formed cloud-like structures of decondensed chromatin 1–2 h after exposure to light. This characteristic rearrangement of chromatin is consistent with previously published live-cell studies of NETosis (17, 45–47). The fully decondensed chromatin stained positive for SYTOX Green within 3 h, indicating cell membrane rupture and NET release.

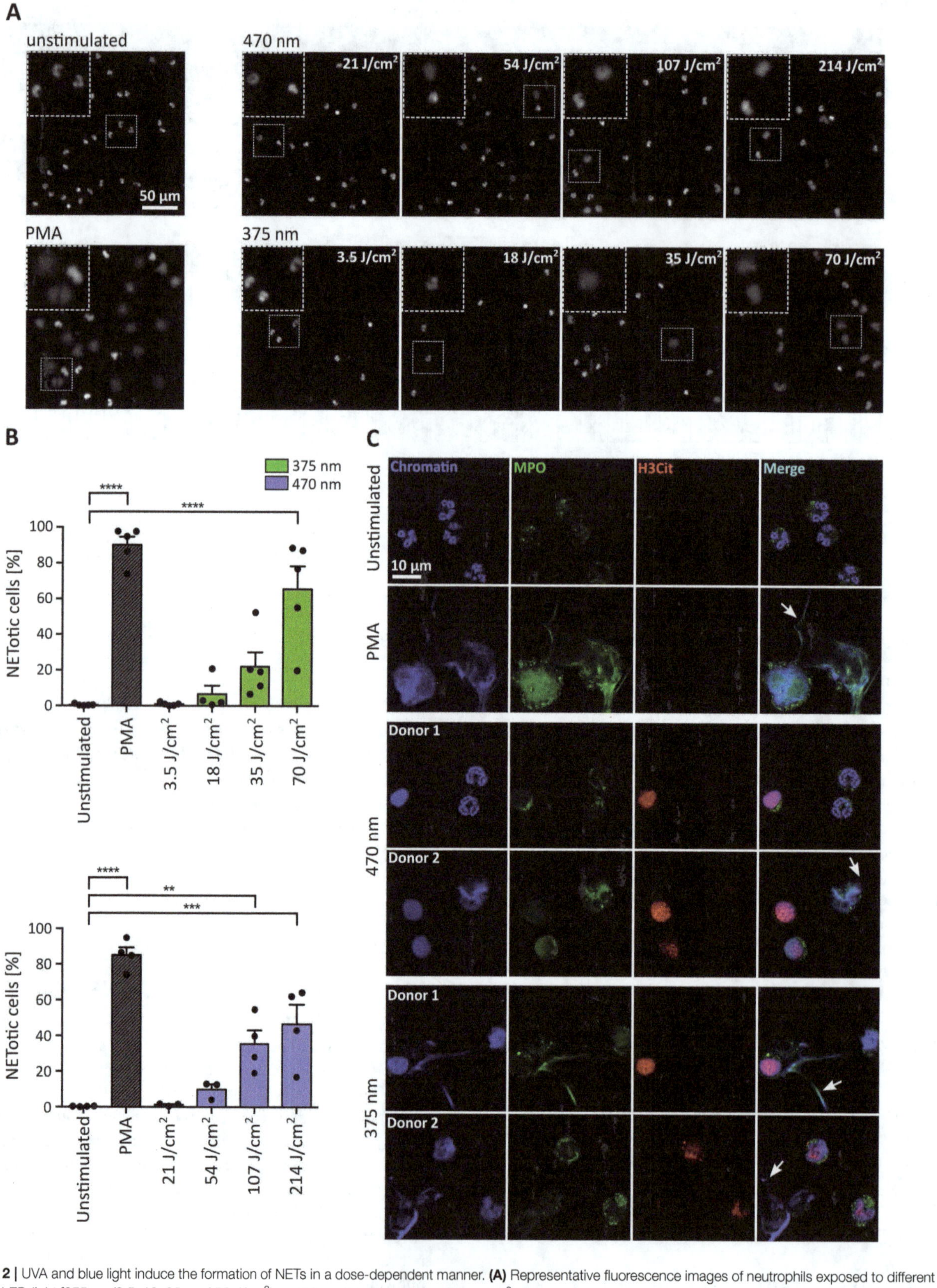

FIGURE 2 | UVA and blue light induce the formation of NETs in a dose-dependent manner. **(A)** Representative fluorescence images of neutrophils exposed to different doses of LED-light [375 nm (3.5, 18, 35, and 70 J/cm²) or 470 nm (21, 54, 107, and 214 J/cm²)]. Decondensation of chromatin, stained by Hoechst, clearly increases

(Continued)

FIGURE 2 | with duration of light exposure. **(B)** NET rates significantly increase for both tested LEDs with light doses. Statistics: one-way-ANOVA with Bonferroni's multiple comparisons test (tested against unstimulated cells). $^{**}p < 0.01$, $^{***}p < 0.001$, $^{****}p < 0.0001$. $N = 3$–5 independent experiments. Error bars = SEM. **(C)** Histone 3 becomes citrullinated (red/Alexa555) in early stages of chromatin decondensation (blue/Hoechst) after irradiation with both wavelengths. The decondensed chromatin colocalizes with MPO (green/alexa488) most prominently within the released NET fibers (arrows), similar to PMA-induced NETs. Confocal microscopy imaging of fixed samples. Cells were kept in RPMIcomp. + 10 mM HEPES.

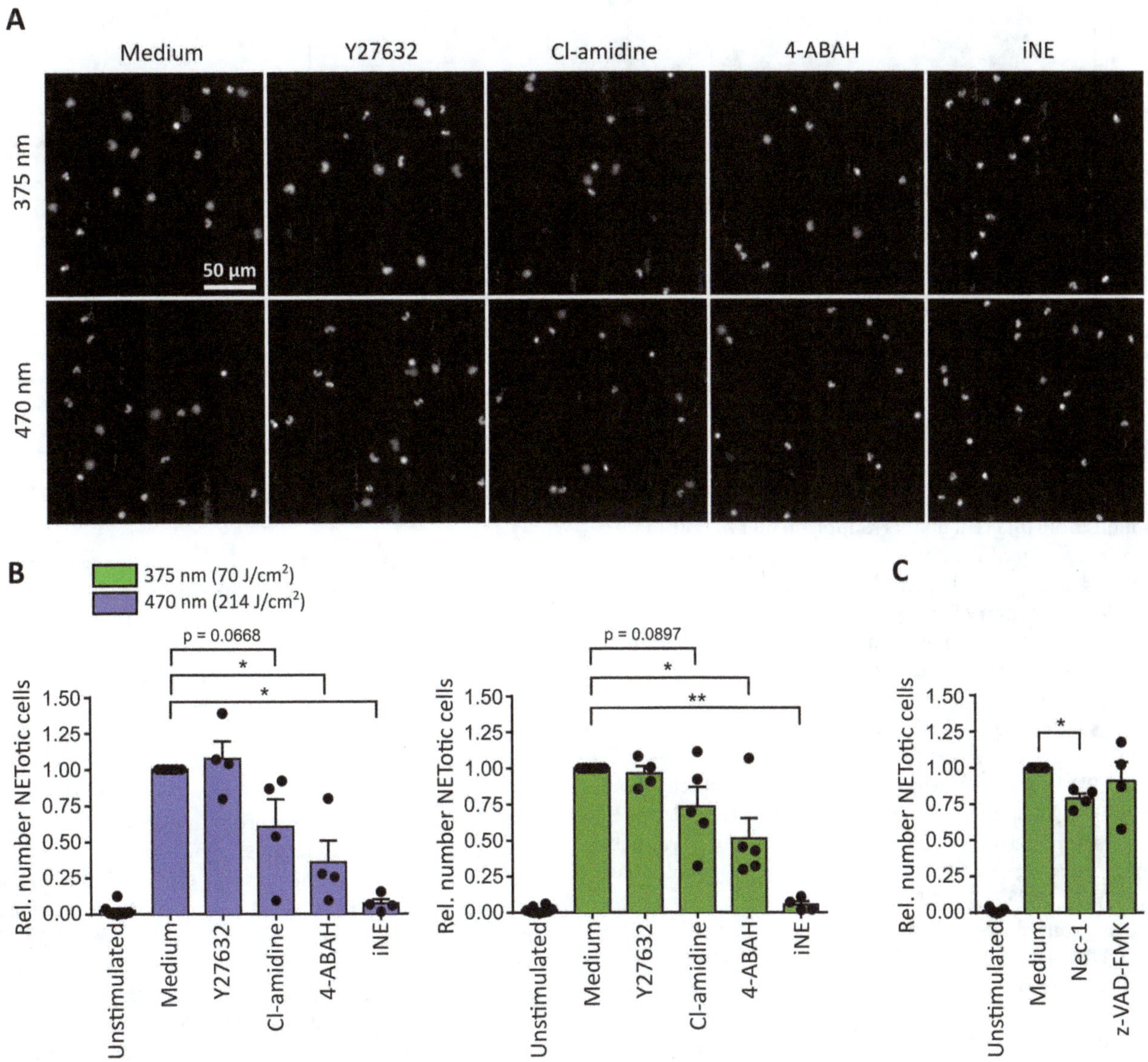

FIGURE 3 | Neutrophil elastase (NE) and myeloperoxidase (MPO) are indispensable for light-induced NETosis. **(A)** Representative images of neutrophil nuclei stained by Hoechst after exposure to UVA (70 J/cm^2 of 375 nm) or blue light (214 J/cm^2 of 470 nm) in the presence of specific inhibitors. NETosis is clearly reduced upon inhibition of MPO (4-ABAH, 100 µM), NE (GW-311616A, iNE, 5 µM) and, to a lower extent, of PAD enzymes (Cl-amidine, 200 µM). However, neutrophils are still able to undergo NETosis in the presence of ROCK 1/2 inhibition by Y-27632 (20 µM). **(B)** Quantification of NETotic cells after irradiation with LED-light of 375 or 470 nm, respectively, in the presence of Y-27632, Cl-amidine, 4-ABAH, or iNE. The inhibition of MPO and NE significantly reduces light-induced NET formation. Inhibition of PAD-enzymes decreases the number of NETotic cells induced by LED-light. However, NETosis appears independent of ROCK 1/2 activity. Statistics: two-tailed paired *t*-test. $^{*}p < 0.05$, $^{**}p < 0.01$. N = 4–5 independent experiments. Error bars = SEM. Cells kept in RPMIcomp. + 10 mM HEPES. **(C)** Light-induced NETosis (70 J/cm^2 of 375 nm) occurs independently of z-VAD-FMK (20 µM, pan-caspase inhibitor) and is reduced by Nec-1 (50 µM, RIP1 kinase inhibition). Statistics: two-tailed paired *t*-test. $^{*}p < 0.05$. $N = 4$ independent experiments. Error bars = SEM. Cells were kept in RPMIcomp. + 10 mM HEPES.

The counting of decondensed nuclei led to slightly higher cell counts than SYTOX Green-positive cells since not all NETotic cells had already released the final NET into the medium. This was particularly prominent in the transition zone between irradiated and non-irradiated regions. Strikingly, this dramatic effect was restricted to the light-exposed area and did not

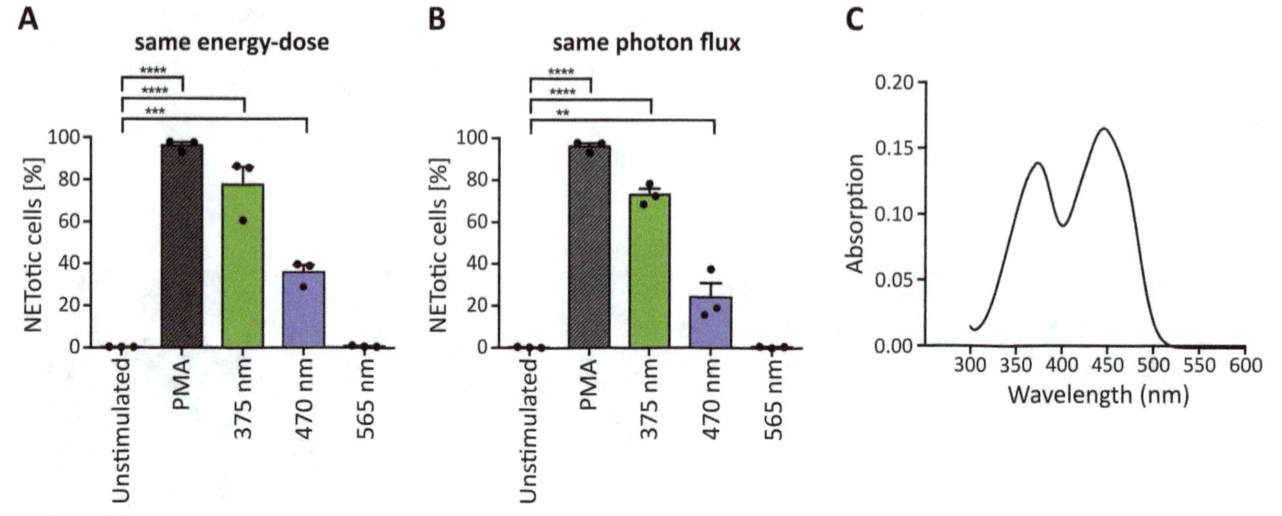

FIGURE 4 | Wavelength-dependency of NET formation correlates with light absorption of riboflavin. UVA and blue light significantly induce NET formation at **(A)** the same energy-dose and **(B)** the same photon flux, whereas green light (565 nm) does not induce NETosis under either condition. Statistics: repeated measure one-way-ANOVA with Bonferroni's multiple comparisons test (tested against unstimulated cells). $^{**}p < 0.01$, $^{***}p < 0.001$, $^{****}p < 0.0001$. $N = 3$ independent experiments. Error bars = SEM. Cells kept in RPMIcomp. + 10 mM HEPES. **(C)** Riboflavin absorbs light in the UVA-blue light region with maxima at 373 and 445 nm. At 375 nm, the absorption is slightly higher (0.138), than at 470 nm (0.130).

occur in unexposed areas (**Figure 1**) and was reproducible with neutrophils from different donors (**Supplementary Figure 1**). To exclude light-induced cytotoxic effects of the Hoechst staining, neutrophils were stained after the full incubation period as control (**Supplementary Figure 1**).

For the initial experiments in **Figure 1**, broad-spectrum UVA (300–400 nm) light was used, and cells were observed over 3–3.5 h with a combination of continuous and intermittent light exposure during live-cell imaging. To verify the obtained results in a more controlled fashion, we established a precisely defined LED-light-based setup and irradiated the cells from below with light of distinct wavelengths and doses (**Figure 2**). Cells were exposed to 3.5, 18, 35, or 70 J/cm^2 of UVA light (375 nm) and 21, 54, 107, or 214 J/cm^2 of visible blue light (470 nm). The LED-light clearly induced chromatin decondensation dose-dependently starting with significant rates of NETosis at 70 J/cm^2 for 375 nm and at 107 J/cm^2 for 470 nm, respectively (**Figures 2A,B**). Interestingly, the morphology of NETs induced by LED-light slightly differed from PMA-induced NETs. Light-induced NETs, as well as the remaining cell body, appeared smaller compared to NETs stimulated with PMA. These differences possibly originate from the strong PMA-induced cell adhesion, which typically occurs in early stages of NETosis. For both tested wavelengths, the decondensed chromatin colocalized with MPO, a typical feature of NET formation (**Figure 2C**). Additionally, a clear citrullination of histone 3 (H3Cit) could be observed. This citrullination typically appeared during early stages of chromatin decondensation whereas MPO seemed to colocalize more with strongly decondensed chromatin and was especially prominent in the released NET fibers (**Figure 2C**).

Light-Induced NETosis Depends on MPO and NE

One of the hallmarks of NET formation is the strong dependency on enzyme activity, especially in the first phase of NETosis, enabling histone modification and, consequently, chromatin decondensation (17). The involved enzymes can vary among different stimuli. In most cases, the activation of granular enzymes such as NE and MPO or members of the PAD family, particularly PAD4, are indispensable (11). Therefore, we inhibited the activity of various enzymes known to be involved in chromatin decondensation or that are required for associated signaling cascades of well-described activators of NETosis.

For both tested wavelengths a significant reduction of NETosis was observed in the presence of the MPO-inhibitor 4-aminobenzoic acid hydrazide (4-ABAH, 100 μM) (48) or the NE-inhibitor GW-311616A (iNE, 5 μM) (49) (**Figures 3A,B**). Both inhibitors efficiently blocked the decondensation of chromatin (**Figure 3A**), thus indicating that decondensation in light-induced NETosis depended on MPO and NE activity as reported for PMA-induced NETosis (18, 19). Additionally, inhibition of PAD activity by Cl-amidine (200 μM) (50) reduced NET formation after irradiation with light of both wavelengths by around 25-50% (**Figure 3B**). Therefore, it is likely that the activity of PAD enzymes can enhance light-induced NETosis by modifying proteins, particularly histones, by citrullination (23, 51, 52). Dependency on Rho-associated coil kinase 1 and 2 (ROCK 1/2) activity, which is implicated in cytoskeleton regulation, has only recently been linked to PMA-induced NETosis (17). Nonetheless, irradiation of neutrophils in the presence of Y-27632 (20 μM) blocking the ATP binding site of ROCK 1/2 (53), showed no effect on NETosis rates in response to light (**Figure 3B**). It is important to note that inhibitors were still functional after irradiation with UVA light as demonstrated in PMA-induced NET formation (**Supplementary Figure 2**).

In order to exclude that the observed effects were associated with neutrophil apoptosis, the involvement of caspases after UVA irradiation was investigated. To this end, cells were irradiated in the presence of the pan-caspase inhibitor z-VAD-FMK (20 μM) (54). Indeed, the involvement of apoptotic pathways was not detected. In contrast, a contribution of the receptor-interacting protein kinase (RIPK) 1/3-mixed lineage kinase domain-like protein (MLKL)-necroptosis-pathway, which has been reported for instance in PMA-induced NETosis (55), could not be excluded. Inhibition by the RIP1 kinase inhibitor necrostatin-1 (Nec-1, 50 μM) (56) decreased the rate of NETotic cells by ~25% (**Figure 3C**).

Altogether, these findings suggest that UVA and blue light induce NETosis in an MPO- and NE-dependent manner. This process can be supported by PAD enzymes and appears to be independent of caspase activity.

Light-Induced NETosis Is Mediated by Riboflavin Excitation and Subsequent ROS Generation

The penetration of light through the human skin depends strongly on the wavelength. Approximately 10–15% of UVA light and 40–50% of blue light can pass the epidermis and reach deeper layers (33, 34). In principle, light of higher wavelengths penetrates deeper into the skin (33). To evaluate whether light of higher wavelengths is also sufficient to induce NET formation, we irradiated neutrophils with light up to 700 nm (565 nm LED; green light), of which more than 60% reach the dermis and in part, even the subcutaneous tissue (34, 57). To make comparisons possible, cells were irradiated with the same light energy-dose (**Figure 4A**) and the same photon flux for each wavelength (**Figure 4B**). The calculations were based on 70 J/cm^2 375 nm-LED light. Interestingly, at the same energy-dose and same photon flux, neutrophils did not undergo NETosis after exposure to green light, whereas irradiation with UVA or blue light revealed robust NETosis (**Figures 4A,B**). However, irradiation with 375 nm induced higher rates of NETotic cells compared to 470 nm. Possible explanations for this phenomenon include the slightly higher absorption of riboflavin at 375 nm (0.138 vs. 0.130) as well as the higher energy of the photons at 375 nm, leading to higher energy within the riboflavin molecule and subsequent excitation.

Several substances, which are present at high concentrations in human skin, can absorb light in the UV-VIS region and were reported to enhance light-mediated tissue damage. One of the most prominent and well-documented photosensitizer is riboflavin (38, 58). Riboflavin is present in tissues with permanent light exposure such as the skin and eyes [3 and 1.7 mg/kg dry matter, respectively (38)] and has multiple essential biological functions. Most prominently, it acts as a precursor for FAD and FMN in flavoprotein-dependent processes (58, 59). Photosensitizing mechanisms of riboflavin are based on the absorption of UVA and blue light with maxima at 373 and 445 nm as confirmed within this study in line with previously published data (60) (**Figure 4C**). Riboflavin is excited to a stable triplet-state *via* a short-lived singlet-state. The excited triplet-state can directly react with oxygen (type II photoreaction) or with reactive substrates (type I photoreaction) to radicals or radical anions. These radicals can then further react with molecular oxygen to hydrogen peroxide (H_2O_2) or hydroxyl radicals *via* superoxide anion radicals (38, 61, 62) (for a potential type I photoreaction with tryptophan see **Supplementary Figure 3**). Importantly, riboflavin is present in the culture medium RPMI at 0.2 mg/l and was previously linked to an increased phototoxicity in culture media in *in vitro* studies. Such reactions were observed for instance in combination with the culture buffer 4-(2-hydroxyethyl)-1-piperazineethanesulfonic acid (HEPES) (63) or amino acids like tryptophan and tyrosine supplemented to RPMI (64).

Given the wavelength-dependency of NETosis, the absorption spectra of riboflavin (**Figure 4**) and the fact that H_2O_2 as a ROS can induce NETosis (16, 65–67), it appeared likely that the observed light-induced NETosis was mediated by the excitation of riboflavin and subsequent ROS production. To test this hypothesis, we first scavenged ROS by the cell-permeable vitamin E derivate Trolox at a concentration of 50 μM (68). Indeed, scavenging ROS with Trolox significantly reduced NET formation in response to UVA irradiation (**Figure 5A**). To further analyze this mechanism, extra- and intracellular ROS generation were addressed separately. Extracellular ROS was scavenged by a mixture of catalase and superoxide dismutase (SOD) (2,000 U/ml and 50 U/ml, respectively) (69, 70), NADPH oxidase-derived ROS was blocked by diphenyleneiodonium chloride (DPI, 1 μM) (71) and mitochondrial-derived ROS was inhibited by MitoTEMPO (5 μM) (72). While the inhibition of NADPH oxidase- and mitochondrial ROS generation showed no effect on the obtained NETosis rates, scavenging extracellular ROS by catalase and SOD abrogated NETosis completely (**Figure 5A**). This result strongly supported the hypothesis that extracellular substrate-mediated production of ROS facilitated light-induced NETosis. Furthermore, the addition of the catalase-SOD-mixture after the irradiation was still fully sufficient to inhibit NETosis (**Supplementary Figure 4A**) excluding the fact that side products of catalase or SOD themselves induced by UVA irradiation were responsible for the observed effect. These results also highlight the differences between the here-studied light-induced NET formation and the "classical" PMA-induced NETosis. In contrast to light-induced NETosis, the formation of NETs in response to PMA depended on the activity of the NADPH-oxidase, which is in agreement with several previous reports (16) and was independent of mitochondrial ROS generation. Additionally, we observed a decreased NETosis rate following PMA stimulation after scavenging extracellular ROS and/or intracellular H_2O_2 (**Supplementary Figure 4B**). However, H_2O_2 scavenging was not sufficient to completely block NETosis. Therefore, especially the activity of NADPH oxidase and the subsequent ROS-mediated signaling appears to be a requisite for PMA-induced NETosis.

In a second step, we studied the mechanism of extracellular ROS generation in greater depth. As described above, aromatic amino acids such as tryptophan can react with excited

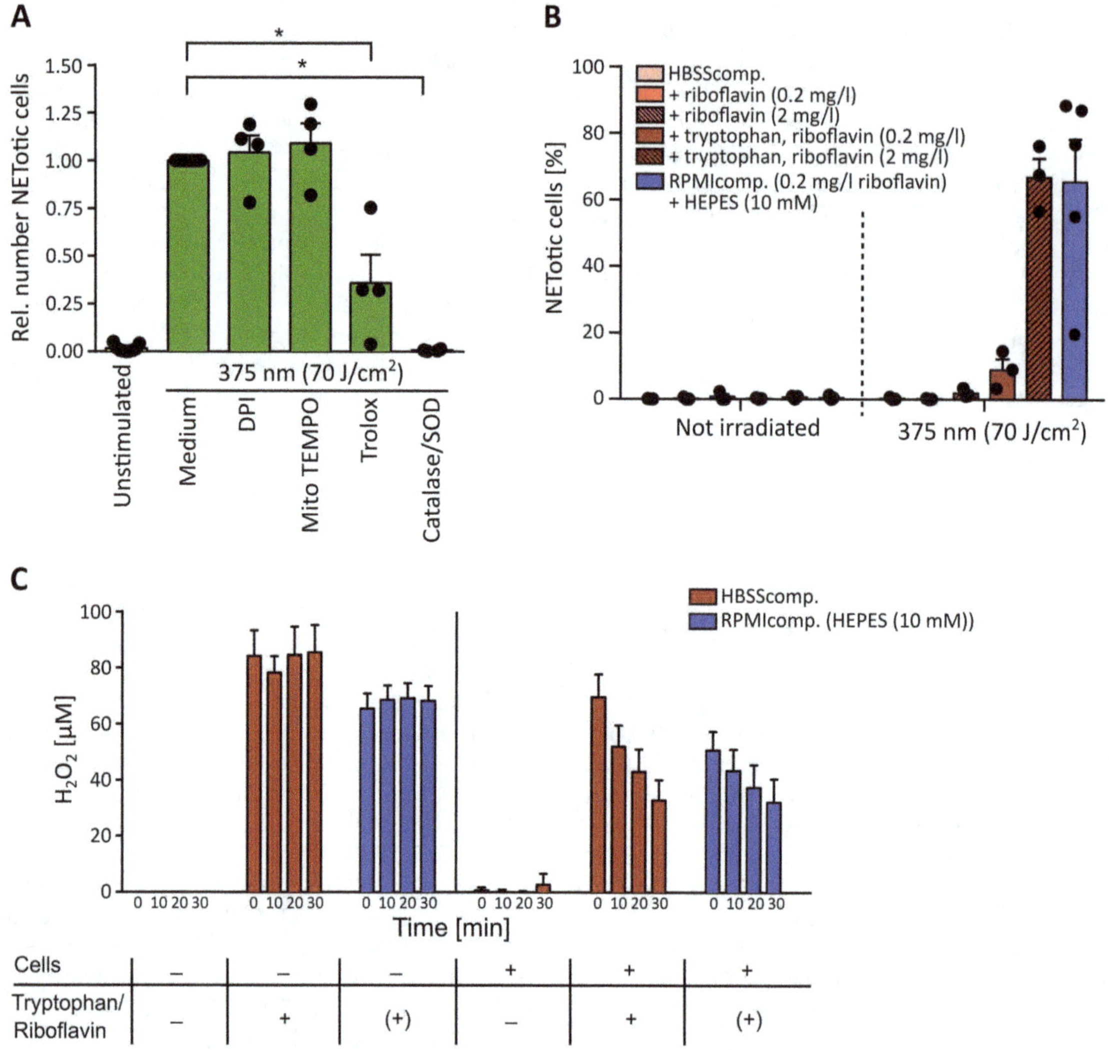

FIGURE 5 | Light-induced NETosis depends on extracellular reactive oxygen species (ROS) generation. **(A)** Light-induced NETosis is significantly inhibited by the ROS scavenger Trolox (50 μM) and by exclusively scavenging external ROS by a combination of catalase/SOD (2,000 and 50 U/ml). NETosis appears to be independent of intracellular ROS production by NADPH oxidase, as shown by inhibition with DPI (1 μM) or mitochondrial ROS, inhibited by MitoTEMPO (5 μM). Statistics: two-tailed paired *t*-test. $^{*}p < 0.05$. $N = 4$ independent experiments. Error bars = SEM. Cells were kept in RPMIcomp. + 10 mM HEPES. **(B)** 70 J/cm^2 of 375 nm light clearly induces NET formation in HBSScomp. + riboflavin (2 mg/l) + tryptophan (1 mM). The obtained NET rates are comparable with NETosis induced in RPMIcomp. (containing 0.2 mg/l riboflavin) + 10 mM HEPES. In contrast, irradiation in HBSScomp. alone or supplemented only with riboflavin (0.2 or 2 mg/l) does not lead to NET formation. $N = 3$–5 independent experiments. Error bars = SEM. **(C)** Induction of extracellular H_2O_2 levels by light measured by AmplexRed. Irradiation of HBSScomp. (red) + 2 mg/l riboflavin + 1 mM tryptophan or RPMIcomp. (0.2 mg/l riboflavin, 0.024 mM tryptophan) + 10 mM HEPES (blue) induces stable extracellular H_2O_2 levels between 60 and 100 μM. Similar H_2O_2 levels are measurable after irradiation of neutrophils in these two media. In the presence of neutrophils, the H_2O_2 levels are continuously reduced over 30 min to around 30–40 μM. In HBSScomp. without riboflavin and tryptophan, neither direct irradiation nor irradiation in the presence of neutrophils causes any increase in H_2O_2 levels. "+" = addition of 2 mg/l riboflavin and 1 mM tryptophan. "(+)" = 0.2 mg/l riboflavin and 0.024 mM tryptophan within RPMI. $N = 3$–4 independent experiments. Error bars = SEM.

riboflavin/flavoproteins. As essential components of proteins, these amino acids are frequently expressed in human skin and can, therefore, contribute to ROS formation triggered by riboflavin excitation. To precisely evaluate the contribution of tryptophan to NET formation, neutrophils were irradiated in the culture buffer HBSS containing 0.5% FCS (HBSScomp.) and supplemented with 0.2 or 2 mg/l riboflavin, a reasonable physiological range of riboflavin within human skin (38), in the presence or absence of 1 mM tryptophan. Indeed, in comparison to non-irradiated cells, UVA light exposure resulted in marked NETosis in the presence of both riboflavin and tryptophan. This effect was increased with the higher riboflavin concentration. In contrast, no NET formation was observed in pure HBSScomp. or in buffer supplemented exclusively with riboflavin (**Figure 5B**). These results strongly support the hypothesis that riboflavin mediated NET formation increases in the presence of additional substrates like tryptophan. Interestingly, a similar effect was observed for HEPES-buffer in RPMIcomp. NET rates markedly

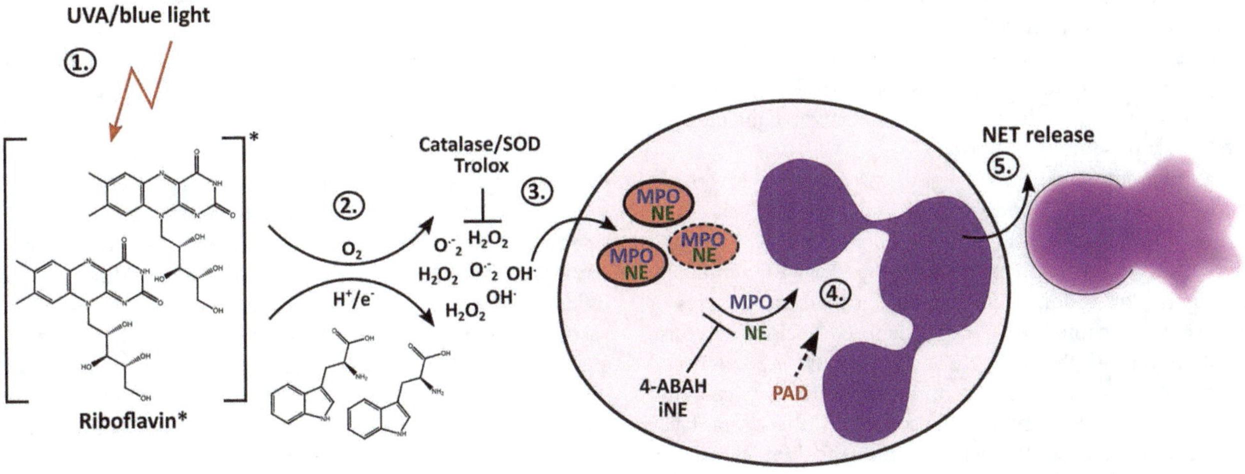

FIGURE 6 | Proposed mechanism of light-induced NETosis. (1) Riboflavin absorbs UVA and blue light and is excited to the triplet state. (2) Tryptophan or other substrates (e.g., HEPES-buffer, tyrosine) transfer electrons or protons to triplet-riboflavin, which leads to ROS production. (3) Extracellular ROS generation (e.g., $H_2O_2/OH^{\cdot}$ or $O^{\cdot-}_2$) by excited riboflavin in the presence of reactive substrates is required for further progression of NET formation. Extracellular ROS is scavenged by Trolox or catalase/SOD. (4) Extracellular ROS most likely activates the translocation of granular enzymes like NE and MPO to the nucleus, which leads to the decondensation of chromatin. The activation of NE and MPO is mandatory for chromatin decondensation and can be inhibited by 4-ABAH and iNE. Citrullination by PAD enzymes can presumably enhance decondensation. (5) After full decondensation, cells release the NET.

increased in the presence of HEPES, the standard medium condition used for this study, compared to RPMIcomp. without HEPES (**Supplementary Figure 5A**).

To confirm this hypothesis, extracellular ROS levels were measured after irradiation in the above-described solutions in an AmplexRed assay. In line with the observed NET rates (**Figure 5B**), irradiation with UVA light led to dramatically increased extracellular H_2O_2 levels in both RPMIcomp. + HEPES as well as HBSScomp. + riboflavin (2 mg/l) + tryptophan (**Figure 5C**). Sole irradiation of these two media compositions consistently resulted in stable H_2O_2 levels of 60–100 μM. In contrast, irradiation of supplement-free HBSScomp. as well as culturing of cells in media without irradiation did not lead to H_2O_2 production (**Figure 5C; Supplementary Figure 5B**). As a control, extracellular H_2O_2 levels were determined after activation with 100 nM PMA. As depicted, lower levels of extracellular H_2O_2 were observable after PMA treatment, which increased over time (**Supplementary Figure 5B**) (70). Importantly, in this experimental setup, we obtained NET rates comparable to the rates displayed in **Figure 5B** after UVA irradiation of cells in RPMIcomp. + HEPES or HBSScomp. + riboflavin (2 mg/l) + tryptophan (**Supplementary Figure 5C**). Overall, these results support the hypothesis that ROS-mediated UVA/blue light-induced NET formation is a consequence of riboflavin excitation. Our findings indicate that excited riboflavin reacts with biological substrates such as tryptophan and thus causes ROS production.

DISCUSSION

UVA and blue light penetrate human skin, and the energy-rich UV light in particular, can cause severe tissue injury *via* immunological and inflammatory effects (73). Both UVA and blue light from the sun reach the earth's surface and penetrate the human epidermis.

It has been shown that *in vitro* irradiation of neutrophils with UVB (40) or UVC light (74) can cause cell death and that exposure to UVA light can enhance ROS production (75). Activation of NETosis has also been considered in response to UVC light (41) However, the exact mechanisms behind it and the influence of blue and long-wave UV light on NET formation remains enigmatic. We have discovered that light of the UVA or blue spectrum is able to induce the release of NETs. The formation of NETs in this scenario depends on extracellular ROS, which are generated through the excitation of riboflavin in conjunction with substrates such as tryptophan. During the "classical" NETosis cascade, NE and MPO are typically released from neutrophil granules and translocate to the nucleus where they promote chromatin decondensation. According to our findings, light-induced NET formation also depends on MPO and NE. Additionally, inhibition of PAD activity by Cl-amidine during irradiation with UVA or blue light clearly showed reduction in NET formation, and histones were citrullinated after light irradiation with both wavelengths. Therefore, the citrullination of histones most likely contributes to decondensation of chromatin in this setting. Altogether, these results imply that this novel light-mediated NET formation culminates in the initiation of the "classical" pathway of suicidal NETosis by engaging the enzymes MPO, NE and PAD4 (**Figure 6**), as extensively described for different stimuli throughout the last years (11).

Interestingly, in response to near infrared (980 nm) laser light, a ROS-dependent form of NET formation has recently been reported (76), which was shown to involve autophagy signaling. In spite of the fact that NETs have been shown to impair wound healing (43), this laser light-mediated NET formation was suggested to be particularly relevant in the context of photobiostimulation with 980 nm diode lasers used to improve wound healing (76). However, the exact mode of action of the laser light remains unclear. The question whether autophagy is implicated in the here-described mechanism of light-induced NETosis warrants further studies.

In a different study, UVC light was reported to trigger apoptosis and/or NOX-independent suicidal NETosis in a dose-dependent manner (41). Highly energetic UVC light had triggered NETosis dependent on mitochondrial ROS and p38 MAPK activation. Additionally, certain biochemical features of apoptosis accompanied UVC-dependent NETosis. Therefore, the authors termed this new NETosis pathway "ApoNETosis" (41). Of note, one must bear in mind that naturally occurring UVC light is almost completely absorbed by the ozone-layer (31) and thus does not reach the human skin. Moreover, while artificial light sources are able to generate UVC light, this would not be expected to penetrate in high amounts across the stratum corneum of the skin. Thus, the physiological relevance of UVC light in the context of NETosis remains disputable. Nevertheless, there may be some relevance for *ex vivo* neutrophil studies.

The mechanism we described here is NOX-independent, similarly to "ApoNETosis." However, UVA or blue light-induced NETosis does not involve mitochondrial ROS production, but clearly depends on MPO and NE activation (**Figures 3, 5A**). The release of NE from the azurosome depends on MPO activity and NADPH-dependent ROS generation (19). In this study, we detected a high extracellular light-induced ROS production in riboflavin-containing media, which was stable for over 30 min after irradiation (**Figure 5C**). This result indicates that riboflavin excitation together with reactive substrates induces high levels of stable ROS species like H_2O_2 (77). H_2O_2 can easily diffuse into the cell and could therefore directly activate the release of serine proteases from the neutrophilic granules. Thus, in NETosis induced by extracellular ROS, additional production of ROS via NADPH-oxidase would not be required, which explains our observation that light-induced NETosis was independent of NADPH.

Importantly, the production of H_2O_2 in these media (especially RPMI + HEPES) and the subsequent release of NETs has to be considered for live cell imaging of neutrophils, especially when working with light of the blue or UVA spectrum. Choosing media without light-sensitive substances would avoid light-induced, ROS-mediated NETosis *ex vivo*.

Typically, in non-inflamed skin, neutrophils closest to the skin surface are found within the superficial arterio-venous plexus of the papillary dermis (57). The transmission of light depends on the local skin composition, but one can estimate that 10–15% of UVA light and 40–50% of blue light reach the upper papillary dermis (33, 34).

In our study, we observed NET formation after irradiation of neutrophils starting with 18 J/cm^2 of 375 nm and 54 J/cm^2 of 470 nm LED-light (**Figure 2**). These doses correspond to around 40 h (375 nm) or 9 h (470 nm LED spectrum) sun exposure at the specific wavelength, respectively. However, under real-life conditions one must consider the complex spectrum of sunlight, which is not limited to single wavelengths, as well as factors such as the thickness of the local ozone-layer, location on earth, weather, irradiation angle, level above the sea as well as time of day and season which will affect light penetration (31). Also, UVA and blue light-induced NET formation may play a more important role in pathological situations of skin if patients suffer from a generally heightened propensity for light-induced NET formation. Additionally, neutrophils may be more strongly affected by light, for example if they are present in higher layers of the skin under inflammatory conditions. Indeed, inflammatory skin diseases are often associated with enhanced vasodilation, perivascular inflammatory infiltrates and even neo-angiogenesis. In many cases, this is associated with an enhanced infiltration of neutrophils and other inflammatory cells into the epidermis, which would again facilitate light-induced NET formation. Additionally, exposure to UV-Vis light particularly of the UVB region appears to directly recruit neutrophils into upper layers of the skin (39). This phenomenon has been proposed to be mediated for instance by the production of cytokines like IL-8 or TNFα by other cell types such as keratinocytes and fibroblasts in response to UVB irradiation (78, 79).

In healthy skin, ROS levels are closely regulated by enzymatic and non-enzymatic antioxidant like glutathione-peroxidase and catalase, vitamin C, and vitamin E. As human skin contains significant amounts of riboflavin, ROS generation by excitation of riboflavin and subsequent reaction with active substrates (e.g., in a type I photoreaction) including aromatic amino acids is very likely (38, 62, 64, 80, 81). Nonetheless, the antioxidants systems mentioned above balance out these reactions under normal circumstances. In the context of diseases, this complex antioxidant system can be dysregulated or exhausted. For instance, extensive or continuous exposure of sunlight causes increased ROS levels with associated inflammation and tissue damage, even in healthy individuals (82). This ROS-associated oxidative tissue damage is mostly mediated by the deeper-penetrating UVA portion of the spectrum.

Interestingly, increased redox stress has been documented in autoimmune disorders (83). For instance, SLE appears to be frequently associated with high oxidative stress indicated by decrease in antioxidant systems, general increased ROS levels as well as elevated antibodies against oxidatively modified proteins (84). In fact, neutrophils from SLE patients reveal higher oxidative burst (85) with decreased intracellular antioxidant systems (86), what makes them less resistant toward extracellular ROS generation.

Additionally, neutrophils of patients suffering from psoriasis and SLE were reported to be generally primed for NETosis (5, 87) and NETosis is clearly involved in the pathogenesis of many chronic inflammatory and autoimmune diseases (2). For example, autoantigens against NET components were detected in SLE (88). Furthermore, impaired clearance of NETs has been described in the pathogenesis of SLE, leading to an accumulation of potential autoantigens in the form of NET components (89).

Most likely, both conditions–ROS imbalance and an increased propensity for NET formation–will add to one another and result in a ROS-mediated inflammatory loop. To what extent NETosis induced by light contributes to this cycle, has to be investigated within *in vivo* studies.

Several autoimmune diseases, most prominently the above-mentioned systemic and cutaneous lupus erythematosus as well as dermatomyositis, show severe photosensitivity. Patients suffering from lupus, whether acute, subacute, or chronic, develop new cutaneous lesions after sun exposure. Even an exacerbation of SLE like fatigue or joint pain has been well-documented after light-exposure (28). Nevertheless, the exact pathophysiological mechanism has not been unraveled yet and involves a differential interplay between different light-induced effects (28).

Most likely, the abnormal response of lupus patients to light is not a monocausal one but given the importance of NETs in this disease and other autoimmune disorders it appears likely that a connection between light exposure and NET formation is an important factor. The question of whether neutrophils of lupus and dermatomyositis patients are *per se* more prone to light-induced NETosis and whether these reactions can be prevented warrant further translational studies. In this context, the question as to what extent light-induced NETs are targets for autoantibody formation, also remains a highly interesting one.

Altogether, it is important to bear in mind that, according to our calculations, NET formation in response to moderate doses of light is most likely not a frequent event and that in healthy individuals NETs are usually rapidly cleared by DNases and subsequent phagocytosis (90, 91). Thus, it is unlikely that exposure to modest doses of sunlight in healthy individuals will lead to a profound inflammatory reaction. However, the here-presented mechanism could be highly important in pathological conditions, such as those discussed above.

On the other hand, light-mediated, ROS-dependent NETosis may also be instrumentalized in a clinical setting to help fight bacteria in bacterial keratitis, as a recent study has impressively shown. Here, the combination of UVA light with riboflavin was used in the "photochemical" therapy of bacterial keratitis due to its bactericidal effect (92). Furthermore, one may speculate whether at least a part of the effect of photodynamic therapy (PDT), can be explained by NET generation. Visible light irradiation, especially of the red but also blue light spectrum, is used in combination with photosensitizers such as aminolevulinic acid (ALA) or methyl aminolevulinate (MAL) in the therapy of basal cell carcinomas, Bowen's disease, and actinic keratosis (*carcinoma in situ*) (93). This therapy is based on the excitation of the photosensitizer porphyrin originating from ALA or MAL and subsequent ROS generation similar to what we have reported in this study for riboflavin. Therefore, the highly interesting question remains whether NETosis can also be activated by ROS generation in this therapeutic context.

In conclusion, we show that UV-Vis light causes ROS-dependent NET formation, which most likely bears great clinical relevance for important diseases such as SLE and dermatomyositis.

ETHICS STATEMENT

The studies involving human participants were reviewed and approved by Ethics Committee of the University Medical Center (UMG) Göttingen. The patients/participants provided their written informed consent to participate in this study.

AUTHOR CONTRIBUTIONS

EN and KB performed most experiments, co-wrote the paper, and designed the study together with LE. LE supervised the project. JB provided selected data sets. SK, MS, and IB provided crucial scientific input as well as technical support. All authors proofread and edited the final manuscript.

ACKNOWLEDGMENTS

We thank Zhang Xin for technical support with the ROS measurements. We thank Hedwig Stanisz-Bogeski, Maren Steinhoff, Andreas Janshoff, and Claudia Steinem for fruitful discussions and support.

REFERENCES

1. Brinkmann V, Reichard U, Goosmann C, Fauler B, Uhlemann Y, Weiss DS. Neutrophil extracellular traps kill bacteria. *Science.* (2004) 303:1532–5. doi: 10.1126/science.1092385
2. Sollberger G, Tilley DO, Zychlinsky A. Neutrophil extracellular traps: the biology of chromatin externalization. *Dev Cell.* (2018) 44:542–53. doi: 10.1016/j.devcel.2018.01.019
3. Sur Chowdhury C, Giaglis S, Walker UA, Buser A, Hahn S, Hasler P. Enhanced neutrophil extracellular trap generation in rheumatoid arthritis: analysis of underlying signal transduction pathways and potential diagnostic utility. *Arthritis Res Ther.* (2014) 16:R122. doi: 10.1186/ar4579
4. Leffler J, Gullstrand B, Jonsen A, Nilsson JA, Martin M, Blom AM, et al. Degradation of neutrophil extracellular traps co-varies with disease activity in patients with systemic lupus erythematosus. *Arthritis Res Ther.* (2013) 15:R84. doi: 10.1186/ar4264
5. Hu SC-S, Yu H-S, Yen F-L, Lin C-L, Chen G-S, Lan C-CE. Neutrophil extracellular trap formation is increased in psoriasis and induces human β-defensin-2 production in epidermal keratinocytes. *Sci. Rep.* (2016) 6:31119. doi: 10.1038/srep31119
6. Schön MP, Erpenbeck L. The interleukin-23/interleukin-17 axis links adaptive and innate immunity in psoriasis. *Front Immunol.* (2018) 9:1323. doi: 10.3389/fimmu.2018.01323

7. Jimenez-Alcazar M, Rangaswamy C, Panda R, Bitterling J, Simsek YJ, Long AT, et al. Host DNases prevent vascular occlusion by neutrophil extracellular traps. *Science.* (2017) 358:1202–6. doi: 10.1126/science.aam8897
8. Warnatsch A, Ioannou M, Wang Q, Papayannopoulos V. Inflammation. Neutrophil extracellular traps license macrophages for cytokine production in atherosclerosis. *Science.* (2015) 349:316–20. doi: 10.1126/science.aaa8064
9. Erpenbeck L, Schön MP. Neutrophil extracellular traps: protagonists of cancer progression? *Oncogene.* (2016) 36:2483–90. doi: 10.1038/onc.2016.406
10. Kenny EF, Herzig A, Kruger R, Muth A. Diverse stimuli engage different neutrophil extracellular trap pathways. (2017) 6:e24437. doi: 10.7554/eLife.24437
11. Papayannopoulos V. Neutrophil extracellular traps in immunity and disease. *Nat Rev Immunol.* (2018) 18:134–47. doi: 10.1038/nri.2017.105
12. Kruss S, Erpenbeck L, Schön MP, Spatz JP. Circular, nanostructured and biofunctionalized hydrogel microchannels for dynamic cell adhesion studies. *Lab Chip.* (2012) 12:3285–9. doi: 10.1039/c2lc40611j
13. Kruss S, Erpenbeck L, Amschler K, Mundinger TA, Boehm H, Helms H-J, et al. Adhesion maturation of neutrophils on nanoscopically presented platelet glycoprotein Ibα. *ACS Nano.* (2013) 7:9984–96. doi: 10.1021/nn403923h
14. Neubert E, Senger-Sander SN, Manzke VS, Busse J, Polo E, Scheidmann SEF, et al. Serum and serum albumin inhibit *in vitro* formation of neutrophil extracellular traps (NETs). *Front Immunol.* (2019) 10:12. doi: 10.3389/fimmu.2019.00012
15. Erpenbeck L, Gruhn AL, Kudryasheva G, Guenay G, Meyer D, Neubert E, et al. Effect of adhesion and substrate elasticity on neutrophil extracellular trap formation. *Front. Immunol.* (2019). doi: 10.1101/508366
16. Fuchs TA, Abed U, Goosmann C, Hurwitz R, Schulze I, Wahn V, et al. Novel cell death program leads to neutrophil extracellular traps. *J Cell Biol.* (2007) 176:231–41. doi: 10.1083/jcb.200606027
17. Neubert E, Meyer D, Rocca F, Günay G, Kwaczala-Tessmann A, Grandke J, et al. Chromatin swelling drives neutrophil extracellular trap release. *Nat. Commun.* (2018) 9:3767. doi: 10.1038/s41467-018-06263-5
18. Papayannopoulos V, Metzler KD, Hakkim A, Zychlinsky A. Neutrophil elastase and myeloperoxidase regulate the formation of neutrophil extracellular traps. *J Cell Biol.* (2010) 191:677–91. doi: 10.1083/jcb.201006052
19. Metzler KD, Goosmann C, Lubojemska A, Zychlinsky A, Papayannopoulos V. A myeloperoxidase-containing complex regulates neutrophil elastase release and actin dynamics during NETosis. *Cell Rep.* (2014) 8:883–96. doi: 10.1016/j.celrep.2014.06.044
20. Radic M, Marion TN. Neutrophil extracellular chromatin traps connect innate immune response to autoimmunity. *Semin Immunopathol.* (2013) 35:465–80. doi: 10.1007/s00281-013-0376-6
21. Lee KH, Kronbichler A, Park DD, Park Y, Moon H, Kim H, et al. Neutrophil extracellular traps (NETs) in autoimmune diseases: a comprehensive review. *Autoimmun Rev.* (2017) 16:1160–73. doi: 10.1016/j.autrev.2017.09.012
22. Neeli I, Khan SN, Radic M. Histone deimination as a response to inflammatory stimuli in neutrophils. *J Immunol.* (2008) 180:1895–902. doi: 10.4049/jimmunol.180.3.1895
23. Leshner M, Wang S, Lewis C, Zheng H, Chen XA, Santy L, et al. PAD4 mediated histone hypercitrullination induces heterochromatin decondensation and chromatin unfolding to form neutrophil extracellular trap-like structures. *Front Immunol.* (2012) 3:307. doi: 10.3389/fimmu.2012.00307
24. Lewis HD, Liddle J, Coote JE, Atkinson SJ, Barker MD, Bax BD, et al. Inhibition of PAD4 activity is sufficient to disrupt mouse and human NET formation. *Nat Chem Biol.* (2015) 11:189–91. doi: 10.1038/nchembio.1735
25. Tatsiy O, Mcdonald PP. Physiological stimuli induce PAD4-dependent, ROS-independent NETosis, with early and late events controlled by discrete signaling pathways. *Front Immunol.* (2018) 9:2036. doi: 10.3389/fimmu.2018.02036
26. Khandpur R, Carmona-Rivera C, Vivekanandan-Giri A, Gizinski A, Yalavarthi S, Knight JS, et al. NETs are a source of citrullinated autoantigens and stimulate inflammatory responses in rheumatoid arthritis. *Sci Transl Med.* (2013) 5:178ra140. doi: 10.1126/scitranslmed.3005580
27. Garcia-Romo GS, Caielli S, Vega B, Connolly J, Allantaz F, Xu Z, et al. Netting neutrophils are major inducers of type I IFN production in pediatric systemic lupus erythematosus. *Sci Transl Med.* (2011) 3:73ra20. doi: 10.1126/scitranslmed.3001201
28. Kim A, Chong BF. Photosensitivity in cutaneous lupus erythematosus. *Photodermatol Photoimmunol Photomed.* (2013) 29:4–11. doi: 10.1111/phpp.12018
29. Zhang S, Shu X, Tian X, Chen F, Lu X, Wang G. Enhanced formation and impaired degradation of neutrophil extracellular traps in dermatomyositis and polymyositis: a potential contributor to interstitial lung disease complications. *Clin Exp Immunol.* (2014) 177:134–41. doi: 10.1111/cei.12319
30. Lood C, Blanco LP, Purmalek MM, Carmona-Rivera C, De Ravin SS, Smith CK, et al. Neutrophil extracellular traps enriched in oxidized mitochondrial DNA are interferogenic and contribute to lupus-like disease. *Nat Med.* (2016) 22:146–53. doi: 10.1038/nm.4027
31. Gueymard CA, Myers D, Emery K. Proposed reference irradiance spectra for solar energy systems testing. *Solar Energy.* (2002) 73:443–67. doi: 10.1016/S0038-092X(03)00005-7
32. Anderson RR, Hu J, Parrish JA. Optical radiation transfer in the human skin and applications in *in vivo* remittance spectroscopy. In: Marks R, Payne PA, editors. *Bioengineering and the Skin.* Dordrecht: Springer (1981).
33. Anderson RR, Parrish JA. The optics of human skin. *J Invest Dermatol.* (1981) 77:13–9. doi: 10.1111/1523-1747.ep12479191
34. Svobodova A, Vostalova J. Solar radiation induced skin damage: review of protective and preventive options. *Int J Radiat Biol.* (2010) 86:999–1030. doi: 10.3109/09553002.2010.501842
35. Rijken F, Kiekens RC, Bruijnzeel PL. Skin-infiltrating neutrophils following exposure to solar-simulated radiation could play an important role in photoageing of human skin. *Br J Dermatol.* (2005) 152:321–8. doi: 10.1111/j.1365-2133.2004.06335.x
36. D'orazio J, Jarrett S, Amaro-Ortiz A, Scott T. UV radiation and the skin. *Int J Mol Sci.* (2013) 14, 12222–12248. doi: 10.3390/ijms140612222
37. Pattison DI, Davies MJ. Actions of ultraviolet light on cellular structures. *EXS.* (2006) 131–57. doi: 10.1007/3-7643-7378-4_6
38. Cardoso DR, Libardi SH, Skibsted LH. Riboflavin as a photosensitizer. Effects on human health and food quality. *Food Funct.* (2012) 3:487–502. doi: 10.1039/c2fo10246c
39. Lee PL, Van Weelden H, Bruijnzeel PL. Neutrophil infiltration in normal human skin after exposure to different ultraviolet radiation sources. *Photochem Photobiol.* (2008) 84:1528–34. doi: 10.1111/j.1751-1097.2008.00380.x
40. Sweeney JF, Nguyen PK, Omann GM, Hinshaw DB. Ultraviolet irradiation accelerates apoptosis in human polymorphonuclear leukocytes: protection by LPS and GM-CSF. *J Leukoc Biol.* (1997) 62:517–23. doi: 10.1002/jlb.62.4.517
41. Azzouz D, Khan MA, Sweezey N, Palaniyar N. Two-in-one: UV radiation simultaneously induces apoptosis and NETosis. *Cell Death Discov.* (2018) 4:51. doi: 10.1038/s41420-018-0048-3
42. Brinkmann V, Laube B, Abu Abed U, Goosmann C, Zychlinsky A. Neutrophil extracellular traps: how to generate and visualize them. *J Vis Exp.* (2010). doi: 10.3791/1724
43. Wong SL, Demers M, Martinod K, Gallant M, Wang Y, Goldfine AB, et al. Diabetes primes neutrophils to undergo NETosis, which impairs wound healing. *Nat Med.* (2015) 21:815–9. doi: 10.1038/nm.3887
44. Thevenaz P, Unser M. User-friendly semiautomated assembly of accurate image mosaics in microscopy. *Microsc Res Tech.* (2007) 70:135–46. doi: 10.1002/jemt.20393
45. Brinkmann V, Goosmann C, Kuhn LI, Zychlinsky A. Automatic quantification of *in vitro* NET formation. *Front Immunol.* (2012) 3:413. doi: 10.3389/fimmu.2012.00413
46. Gupta S, Chan DW, Zaal KJ, Kaplan MJ. A high-throughput real-time imaging technique to quantify NETosis and distinguish mechanisms of cell death in human neutrophils. *J Immunol.* (2017) 200:869–79. doi: 10.4049/jimmunol.1700905
47. Van Der Linden M, Westerlaken GHA, Van Der Vlist M, Van Montfrans J, Meyaard L. Differential signalling and kinetics of neutrophil extracellular trap release revealed by quantitative live imaging. *Sci Rep.* (2017) 7:6529. doi: 10.1038/s41598-017-06901-w
48. Kettle AJ, Gedye CA, Winterbourn CC. Mechanism of inactivation of myeloperoxidase by 4-aminobenzoic acid hydrazide. *Biochem J.* (1997) 321:503–8. doi: 10.1042/bj3210503
49. Macdonald SJ, Dowle MD, Harrison LA, Shah P, Johnson MR, Inglis GG, et al. The discovery of a potent, intracellular, orally bioavailable, long duration inhibitor of human neutrophil elastase–GW311616A a development candidate. *Bioorg Med Chem Lett.* (2001)

11:895–8. doi: 10.1016/S0960-894X(01)00078-6
50. Luo Y, Arita K, Bhatia M, Knuckley B, Lee YH, Stallcup MR, et al. Inhibitors and inactivators of protein arginine deiminase 4: functional and structural characterization. *Biochemistry*. (2006) 45:11727–36. doi: 10.1021/bi061180d
51. Nakashima K, Hagiwara T, Yamada M. Nuclear localization of peptidylarginine deiminase V and histone deimination in granulocytes. *J Biol Chem*. (2002) 277:49562–8. doi: 10.1074/jbc.M208795200
52. Wang Y, Wysocka J, Sayegh J, Lee YH, Perlin JR, Leonelli L, et al. Human PAD4 regulates histone arginine methylation levels via demethylimination. *Science*. (2004) 306:279–83. doi: 10.1126/science.1101400
53. Narumiya S, Ishizaki T, Uehata M. Use and properties of ROCK-specific inhibitor Y-27632. *Methods Enzymol.* (2000) 325:273–84. doi: 10.1016/S0076-6879(00)25449-9
54. Slee EA, Zhu H. Chow SC, Macfarlane M, Nicholson DW, Cohen GM. Benzyloxycarbonyl-Val-Ala-Asp (OMe) fluoromethylketone (Z-VAD.FMK) inhibits apoptosis by blocking the processing of CPP32. *Biochem J.* (1996) 315(*Pt* 1):21–4. doi: 10.1042/bj3150021
55. Desai J, Mulay SR, Nakazawa D, Anders H-J. Matters of life and death. How neutrophils die or survive along NET release and is "NETosis" = necroptosis? *Cell Mol Life Sci.* (2016) 73:2211–9. doi: 10.1007/s00018-016-2195-0
56. Degterev A, Hitomi J, Germscheid M, Ch'en IL, Korkina O, Teng X, et al. Identification of RIP1 kinase as a specific cellular target of necrostatins. *Nat Chem Biol.* (2008) 4:313–21. doi: 10.1038/nchembio.83
57. Swerlick RA. The structure and function of the cutaneous vasculature. *J Dermatol.* (1997) 24:734–8. doi: 10.1111/j.1346-8138.1997.tb02527.x
58. Pinto J, Rivlin R. *Riboflavin (Vitamin B2). Handbook of Vitamins.* 5th ed. (2013).
59. Powers HJ. Riboflavin (vitamin B-2) and health. *Am J Clin Nutr.* (2003) 77:1352–60. doi: 10.1093/ajcn/77.6.1352
60. Gore DM, Margineanu A, French P, O'brart D, Dunsby C, Allan BD. Two-photon fluorescence microscopy of corneal riboflavin absorption. *Invest Ophthalmol Vis Sci.* (2014) 55:2476–81. doi: 10.1167/iovs.14-13975
61. Heelis PF. The photophysical and photochemical properties of flavins (isoalloxazines). *Chem Soc Rev.* (1982) 11:15–39. doi: 10.1039/cs9821100015
62. Martin CB, Tsao M-L, Hadad CM, Platz MS. The reaction of triplet flavin with indole. A study of the cascade of reactive intermediates using density functional theory and time resolved infrared spectroscopy. *J Am Chem Soc.* (2002) 124:7226–34. doi: 10.1021/ja0123711
63. Keynes RG, Griffiths C, Garthwaite J. Superoxide-dependent consumption of nitric oxide in biological media may confound *in vitro* experiments. *Biochem J.* (2003) 369:399–406. doi: 10.1042/bj20020933
64. Wang RJ, Nixon BR. Identification of hydrogen peroxide as a photoproduct toxic to human cells in tissue-culture medium irradiated with "daylight" fluorescent light. *In Vitro.* (1978) 14:715–22. doi: 10.1007/BF026 16168
65. Zawrotniak M, Kozik A, Rapala-Kozik M. Selected mucolytic, anti-inflammatory and cardiovascular drugs change the ability of neutrophils to form extracellular traps (NETs). *Acta Biochim Pol.* (2015) 62:465–73. doi: 10.18388/abp.2015_1055
66. Behnen M, Moller S, Brozek A, Klinger M, Laskay T. Extracellular acidification inhibits the ROS-dependent formation of neutrophil extracellular traps. *Front Immunol.* (2017) 8:184. doi: 10.3389/fimmu.2017.00184
67. Nadesalingam A, Chen JHK, Farahvash A, Khan MA. Hypertonic saline suppresses NADPH oxidase-dependent neutrophil extracellular trap formation and promotes apoptosis. *Front Immunol.* (2018) 9:359. doi: 10.3389/fimmu.2018.00359
68. Hamad I, Arda N, Pekmez M, Karaer S, Temizkan G. Intracellular scavenging activity of Trolox (6-hydroxy-2,5,7,8-tetramethylchromane-2-carboxylic acid) in the fission yeast, Schizosaccharomyces pombe. *J Nat Sci Biol Med.* (2010) 1:16–21. doi: 10.4103/0976-9668.71667
69. Jancinova V, Drabikova K, Nosal R, Rackova L, Majekova M, Holomanova D. The combined luminol/isoluminol chemiluminescence method for differentiating between extracellular and intracellular oxidant production by neutrophils. *Redox Rep.* (2006) 11:110–6. doi: 10.1179/135100006X116592
70. Bjornsdottir H, Welin A, Michaelsson E, Osla V, Berg S, Christenson K, et al. Neutrophil NET formation is regulated from the inside by myeloperoxidase-processed reactive oxygen species. *Free Radic Biol Med.* (2015) 89:1024–35. doi: 10.1016/j.freeradbiomed.2015.10.398
71. Ellis JA, Mayer SJ, Jones OT. The effect of the NADPH oxidase inhibitor diphenyleneiodonium on aerobic and anaerobic microbicidal activities of human neutrophils. *Biochem. J.* (1988) 251:887–91. doi: 10.1042/bj2510887
72. Bordt EA, Polster BM. NADPH oxidase- and mitochondria-derived reactive oxygen species in proinflammatory microglial activation: a bipartisan affair? *Free Radic Biol Med.* (2014) 76:34–46. doi: 10.1016/j.freeradbiomed.2014.07.033
73. Clydesdale GJ, Dandie GW, Muller HK. Ultraviolet light induced injury: immunological and inflammatory effects. *Immunol Cell Biol.* (2001) 79:547–68. doi: 10.1046/j.1440-1711.2001.01047.x
74. Frasch SC, Nick JA, Fadok VA, Bratton DL, Worthen GS, Henson PM. p38 mitogen-activated protein kinase-dependent and -independent intracellular signal transduction pathways leading to apoptosis in human neutrophils. *J Biol Chem.* (1998) 273:8389–97. doi: 10.1074/jbc.273.14.8389
75. Li C, Shi X, Chen M, Xu G, Su X, Jiang P, et al. Ultraviolet light A irradiation induces immunosuppression associated with the generation of reactive oxygen species in human neutrophils. *J Innov Optl Health Sci.* (2016) 09:1650001. doi: 10.1142/S1793545816500012
76. Migliario M, Tonello S, Rocchetti V, Rizzi M, Reno F. Near infrared laser irradiation induces NETosis via oxidative stress and autophagy. *Lasers Med Sci.* (2018) 33:1919–24. doi: 10.1007/s10103-018-2556-z
77. Mahns A, Melchheier I, Suschek CV, Sies H, Klotz LO. Irradiation of cells with ultraviolet-A (320–400 nm) in the presence of cell culture medium elicits biological effects due to extracellular generation of hydrogen peroxide. *Free Radic Res.* (2003) 37:391–7. doi: 10.1080/1071576031000064702
78. Strickland I, Rhodes LE, Flanagan BF, Friedmann PS. TNF-alpha and IL-8 are upregulated in the epidermis of normal human skin after UVB exposure: correlation with neutrophil accumulation and E-selectin expression. *J Invest Dermatol.* (1997) 108:763–8. doi: 10.1111/1523-1747.ep12292156
79. Bashir MM, Sharma MR, Werth VP. TNF-alpha production in the skin. *Arch Dermatol Res.* (2009) 301:87–91. doi: 10.1007/s00403-008-0893-7
80. Silva E, Ugarte R, Andrade A, Edwards AM. Riboflavin-sensitized photoprocesses of tryptophan. *J Photochem Photobiol B.* (1994) 23:43–8. doi: 10.1016/1011-1344(93)06984-B
81. Shen L, Ji HF. A theoretical study on the quenching mechanisms of triplet state riboflavin by tryptophan and tyrosine. *J Photochem Photobiol B.* (2008) 92:10–2. doi: 10.1016/j.jphotobiol.2008.03.005
82. Wagener FADTG, Carels CE, Lundvig DMS. Targeting the redox balance in inflammatory skin conditions. *Int J Mol Sci.* (2013) 14:9126–67. doi: 10.3390/ijms14059126
83. Glennon-Alty L, Hackett AP, Chapman EA, Wright HL. Neutrophils and redox stress in the pathogenesis of autoimmune disease. *Free Radic Biol Med.* (2018) 125:25–35. doi: 10.1016/j.freeradbiomed.2018.03.049
84. Shah D, Mahajan N, Sah S, Nath SK, Paudyal B. Oxidative stress and its biomarkers in systemic lupus erythematosus. *J Biomed Sci.* (2014) 21:23. doi: 10.1186/1423-0127-21-23
85. Perazzio SF, Salomao R, Silva NP, Andrade LE. Increased neutrophil oxidative burst metabolism in systemic lupus erythematosus. *Lupus.* (2012) 21:1543–51. doi: 10.1177/0961203312461060
86. Li KJ, Wu CH, Hsieh SC, Lu MC, Tsai CY, Yu CL. Deranged bioenergetics and defective redox capacity in T lymphocytes and neutrophils are related to cellular dysfunction and increased oxidative stress in patients with active systemic lupus erythematosus. *Clin Dev Immunol.* (2012) 2012:548516. doi: 10.1155/2012/548516
87. Villanueva E, Yalavarthi S, Berthier CC, Hodgin JB, Khandpur R, Lin AM, et al. Netting neutrophils induce endothelial damage, infiltrate tissues, and expose immunostimulatory molecules in systemic lupus erythematosus. *J Immunol.* (2011) 187:538–52. doi: 10.4049/jimmunol.1100450
88. Carmona-Rivera C, Kaplan MJ. Detection of SLE antigens in neutrophil extracellular traps (NETs). *Methods Mol Biol.* (2014) 1134:151–61. doi: 10.1007/978-1-4939-0326-9_11
89. Hakkim A, Fürnrohr BG, Amann K, Laube B, Abed UA, Brinkmann V, et al. Impairment of neutrophil extracellular trap degradation is associated with lupus nephritis. *Proc Natl Acad Sci USA.* (2010) 107:9813–8. doi: 10.1073/pnas.0909927107
90. Farrera C, Fadeel B. Macrophage clearance of neutrophil extracellular traps is a silent process. *J Immunol.* (2013) 191:2647–56. doi: 10.4049/jimmunol.1300436

91. Kolaczkowska E, Jenne CN, Surewaard BG, Thanabalasuriar A, Lee WY, Sanz MJ, et al. Molecular mechanisms of NET formation and degradation revealed by intravital imaging in the liver vasculature. *Nat Commun.* (2015) 6:6673. doi: 10.1038/ncomms7673
92. Makdoumi K, Mortensen J, Sorkhabi O, Malmvall BE, Crafoord S. UVA-riboflavin photochemical therapy of bacterial keratitis: a pilot study. *Graefes Arch Clin Exp Ophthalmol.* (2012) 250:95–102. doi: 10.1007/s00417-011-1754-1
93. Wan MT, Lin JY. Current evidence and applications of photodynamic therapy in dermatology. *Clin Cosmetic Invest Dermatol.* (2014) 7:145–63. doi: 10.2147/CCID.S35334

4

Formyl Peptide Receptor 2 Activation Ameliorates Dermal Fibrosis and Inflammation in Bleomycin-Induced Scleroderma

Gyu Tae Park[1], *Yang Woo Kwon*[1], *Tae Wook Lee*[1], *Seong Gyu Kwon*[1], *Hyun-Chang Ko*[2], *Moon Bum Kim*[2] *and Jae Ho Kim*[1,3*]

[1] Department of Physiology, Pusan National University School of Medicine, Yangsan-si, South Korea, [2] Department of Dermatology, Pusan National University School of Medicine, Yangsan-si, South Korea, [3] Research Institute of Convergence Biomedical Science and Technology, Pusan National University Yangsan Hospital, Yangsan-si, South Korea

***Correspondence:**
Jae Ho Kim
jhkimst@pusan.ac.kr

Systemic sclerosis is a profibrotic autoimmune disease mediated by the dysregulation of extracellular matrix synthesis. Formyl peptide receptor 2 (Fpr2) is a G protein-coupled receptor that modulates inflammation and host defense by regulating the activation of inflammatory cells, such as macrophages. However, the role of Fpr2 in the development and therapy of scleroderma is still unclear. The present study was conducted to investigate the effects of Fpr2 activation in the treatment of scleroderma fibrosis. We found that intradermal administration of WKYMVm, an Fpr2-specific agonist, alleviated bleomycin-induced scleroderma fibrosis in mice and decreased dermal thickness in scleroderma skin. WKYMVm-treated scleroderma skin tissues displayed reduced numbers of myofibroblasts expressing α-smooth muscle actin, Vimentin, and phosphorylated SMAD3. WKYMVm treatment attenuated macrophage infiltration in scleroderma skin and reduced the number of M2 macrophages. The therapeutic effects of WKYMVm in scleroderma-associated fibrosis and inflammation were completely abrogated in Fpr2 knockout mice. Moreover, WKYMVm treatment reduced the serum levels of inflammatory cytokines, such as tumor necrosis factor-α, and interferon-γ, in the scleroderma model of wild-type mice but not in Fpr2 knockout mice. These results suggest that WKYMVm-induced activation of Fpr2 leads to alleviation of fibrosis by stimulating immune resolution in systemic sclerosis.

Keywords: systemic sclerosis, scleroderma, fibrosis, Fpr2, WKYMVm

INTRODUCTION

Systemic sclerosis or scleroderma is a multiple autoimmune and inflammatory connective tissue disease, resulting in extensive tissue fibrosis in multiple organs. Prominent skin and organ fibrosis is a hallmark feature of scleroderma and is accompanied by fibro-proliferative vasculopathy and immune dysfunction (1, 2). Activated fibroblasts or myofibroblasts, characterized by increased expression of α-smooth muscle actin (α-SMA) and Vimentin, are the key effector cells in scleroderma. Differentiation of fibroblasts into myofibroblasts increases the production of extracellular matrix components, such as collagen, with subsequent development of fibrosis (1, 3). Fibroblast recruitment and differentiation to myofibroblasts are regulated by a combination of autocrine and paracrine profibrotic mediators. Despite significant therapeutic advancements in the treatment of scleroderma, no effective therapy is currently available.

It has been reported that differentiation of tissue-resident fibroblasts to myofibroblasts is promoted by pro-inflammatory mediators which are secreted by macrophages and monocytes (4). Activated macrophages are classified into two major subtypes, M1, and M2 phenotypes (5). M1 type macrophages release pro-inflammatory cytokines, such as TNF-α, interleukin-1β, interleukin-12, and interleukin-23 during inflammation (6). Whereas, M2 macrophages, which are pro-fibrotic/anti-inflammatory, suppress inflammation, and play a key role in tissue fibrosis by secreting TGF-β (7). In fibrosis, inflammatory cytokines induce activation of M2 macrophages expressing transforming growth factor-β (TGF-β), which activate fibroblast differentiation to myofibroblasts (7–9). Accumulating evidence suggests that scleroderma is initiated by chronic inflammation, and that increased infiltration and sustained activation of immune cells are responsible for the extensive fibrosis in scleroderma (3) Moreover, it has been reported that scleroderma can be alleviated by resolution of inflammatory responses (8).

The formyl peptide receptors (FPRs), belonging to the G protein-coupled receptor family, play an important functional role in host defense and inflammation by regulating the activation of phagocytes (10). FPRs are mainly expressed in phagocytes, such as neutrophils, monocytes, and macrophages, and are also functionally expressed in different cell types, such as fibroblasts (11). Three FPRs (FPR1, FPR2/ALX, and FPR3) have been identified in humans, and Fpr1 and Fpr2 have been found in mice as counterparts to human FPR1 and FPR2, respectively, (12). An increasing body of evidence suggests that FPR2 plays a key role in immune resolution. It has been reported that FPR2 is activated by various ligands, such as pro-resolving eicosanoids (lipoxins and resolvins), and a synthetic hexapeptide, Trp-Lys-Tyr-Met-Val-D-Met-NH2 (WKYMVm). It was recently reported that three FPR receptors are overexpressed in scleroderma fibroblasts compared with that in normal fibroblasts (13, 14). Moreover, WKYMVm treatment has been shown to promote differentiation of fibroblasts to myofibroblasts and matrix deposition *in vitro*, suggesting a deteriorating effect of Fpr2 activation in scleroderma. However, the role of Fpr2 in the progression of scleroderma remains elusive.

In the present study, we explored the effect of the Fpr2 agonist WKYMVm on fibrosis and inflammation in the scleroderma animal model, and clarified the role of Fpr2 in WKYMVm-induced therapeutic effect on scleroderma using Fpr2 knockout mice.

MATERIALS AND METHODS

Materials

BLM was purchased from Tokyo Chemical Industry chemicals (Tokyo, Japan). The synthetic peptide, WKYMVm, was synthesized at Anygen (Kwangju, Republic of Korea), and its purity was estimated to be >98%. Anti-α-SMA antibody (ab5694) and anti-CD163 antibody (ab182422) were purchased from Abcam PLC (Cambridge, UK). Anti-CD68 antibody (MCA1957GA) was purchased from AbD Serotec (Raleigh, NC, USA). Anti-NOS2 antibody (SC-650) was purchased from Santa Cruz Biotechnology, Inc. (Dallas, TX, USA). Anti-phospho-SMAD3 antibody (44-246G), Anti-Arginase-I antibody (PA5-29645), Anti-TLR2 antibody (PA5-20020) was purchased from Thermo Fisher Scientific (Waltham, MA, USA). Anti-Vimentin Antibody (MAB-2105SP), Recombinant TGF-β1 (240-B-002) protein was purchased from R&D Systems (Minneapolis, MN, USA). Mouse enzyme-linked immunosorbent assay (ELISA) kits for TNF-α (430904), and INF-γ (430804) were purchased from BioLegend (San Diego, CA, USA). QuickZyme Total Collagen Assay kit was purchased from QuickZyme Biosciences (Leiden, Netherlands).

Scleroderma Animal Model

BLM powder was dissolved in PBS buffer at a concentration of 1 mg/mL and sterilized by filtration. To establish the scleroderma animal model, C57BL6/J wild-type and Fpr2 knockout mice (6-weeks-old, weighing 22–24 g, male) were subcutaneously injected with 100 μL BLM solution (1 mg/mL) at a single location on the shaved backs (1 cm^2) of mice for 6 weeks using a 27-gauge needle. The injection was carried out daily for 3 weeks to initially induce scleroderma, followed by subsequent administration of 100 μL PBS containing both BLM (1 mg/mL) and WKYMVm (1 μM) for an additional 3 weeks. As a control experiment, BLM solution without WKYMVm was injected into the scleroderma skin tissues. The therapeutic effects of WKYMVm on scleroderma were examined by histological analysis of the scleroderma skin tissues of mice.

Histological Analysis and Measurement of Total Collagen Content

For histological analysis of scleroderma tissues, animals were sacrificed, and tissue samples were excised. The skin samples were fixed in 4% paraformaldehyde overnight, and embedded in paraffin. The specimens were sectioned and stained with hematoxylin & eosin (H&E) for determination of dermal thickness, and five areas in one section were randomly selected for this purpose. For determination of the amount of collagen deposition, tissue sections were stained with Masson's Trichrome staining. The images of stained tissue sections were scanned using Axio Scan.Z1 (Carl Zeiss Microscopy, Germany) at ×100 magnification. Using Image J, dermal thickness distance between the epidermal-dermal junction and the dermal-subcutaneous fat junction was measured on H&E-stained images. Collagen density in skin specimens was quantified by using Image J analysis of Masson's Trichrome staining. Collagen deposition in scleroderma skin tissues was measured by a hydroxyproline assay kit (QuickZyme Total Collagen Assay kit) according to the manufacturer's protocol.

Abbreviations: α-SMA, α-smooth muscle actin; BLM, bleomycin; ELISA, Enzyme-linked immunosorbent assay; FPR2, Formyl peptide receptor 2; IFN-γ, interferon-γ; PBS, phosphate buffered saline; TGF-β1, transforming growth factor-β1; TNF-α, tumor necrosis factor-α; Wm, WKYMVm.

Immunohistochemistry

Formalin fixed, paraffin-embedded skin sections were stained with antibodies against α-SMA, Vimentin, and phospho-SMAD3 for staining of myofibroblasts. Anti-ILB4 antibody and anti-CD68 antibody were used for staining of endothelial cells and macrophages, respectively. Anti-NOS2 and anti-TLR2 antibodies were used for staining of M1 macrophages, and M2 macrophages were stained by anti-CD163, and anti-Arginase-I. The tissue specimens were then incubated with Alexa Fluor 488 goat anti-rabbit, Alexa Fluor 568 goat anti-rabbit, or Alexa Fluor 488 goat anti-rat antibody, followed by washing and mounting in Vectashield medium containing 4′,6-diamidino-2-phenylindole (DAPI) for staining of nuclei. The stained sections were visualized under a laser confocal microscope (Olympus FluoView FV1000). The numbers of α-SMA^+ILB4^-, $Vimentin^+$, and $Vimentin^+$p-$SMAD3^+$ myofibroblasts, and the numbers of $CD68^+$ macrophages, M1 type ($CD68^+NOS2^+$ and $CD68^+TLR2^+$), M2 type ($CD68^+$Arginase-1^+ and $CD68^+CD163^+$) macrophages were quantified in high-power field using ImageJ software. Four randomly selected microscopic fields from three serial sections in each tissue block were examined by two independent observers blinded to the experimental conditions.

ELISA Analysis

To measure the levels of inflammatory cytokines in the peripheral blood of mice, blood was collected from scleroderma and therapeutic mice by cardiac puncture using a 27G syringe and allowed to clot at 4°C overnight. Serum was collected after removal of the clot and centrifuged at 1,000 × g for 30 min in 4°C. The levels of TNF-α and INF-γ were assayed using an ELISA kit (BioLegend) according to the manufacturer's instructions. The absorbance values were measured at 450 nm by an ELISA reader and interpolated with a standard curve.

Statistical Analysis

The results of multiple observations are presented as mean ± SD. Student's two-tailed unpaired *t*-test was used to determine statistical significance of two groups. For multivariate data analysis, group differences were assessed with one-way or two-way ANOVA, followed by Scheffé's *post hoc* test.

RESULTS

WKYMVm Treatment Reduces Fibrosis in Bleomycin-Induced Scleroderma

To explore the effect of Fpr2 activation in scleroderma, we established a scleroderma murine model by subcutaneous injection of bleomycin (BLM) for 3 weeks. Subcutaneous injection of BLM alone resulted in increased dermal thickness and collagen deposition that paralleled with a reduction of subcutaneous adipose layer, which was replaced by connective tissues containing collagen. To explore the effects of Fpr2 activation on therapy of scleroderma, the BLM-induced scleroderma mice were subcutaneously co-administrated with both BLM, and WKYMVm for additional 3 weeks. Subcutaneous injection of WKYMVm significantly reduced the dermal thickness associated with BLM-induced scleroderma at 1 μM concentration (**Figures 1A,B**). Moreover, BLM-induced scleroderma skin exhibited excessive deposition of thick collagen fibers extending into the subdermal adipose tissue and subcutaneous injection of BLM and WKYMVm markedly alleviated skin fibrosis and collagen deposition, as demonstrated by Masson's Trichrome staining (**Figures 1A,C**). Consistently, the levels of hydroxyproline, which is associated with collagen as an indicator of the severity of fibrosis (15), increased in BLM-induced scleroderma skin, and administration with WKYMVm significantly reduced the BLM-increased hydroxyproline content in skin (**Figure 1D**). WKYMVm treatment significantly decreased the BLM-induced dermal thickness, collagen density, and hydroxyproline levels at 0.5 μM and maximally reduced those values at 1 μM concentration (**Figure S1**). Moreover, the BLM-induced increase of dermal- thickness and collagen deposition was time-dependently alleviated by administration of WKYMVm for additional 3 weeks (**Figures 2A–D**).

It has been reported that fibroblast activation or myofibroblast differentiation plays a key role in the progression of scleroderma (1). To explore the effects of WKYMVm on myofibroblast differentiation, we performed immunostaining of the scleroderma skin specimens with antibodies against α-SMA and Vimentin, which are markers for myofibroblasts (16, 17). α-SMA is expressed in not only myofibroblasts but also blood vessels expressing ILB4, an endothelial marker. Therefore, the number of α-SMA^+ILB4^- cells was counted for determination of myofibroblast differentiation. BLM treatment increased the number of α-SMA^+ILB4^- cells, and WKYMVm treatment abrogated the BLM-induced increase of α-SMA^+ILB4^- cells (**Figures 3A,C**). Moreover, the number of Vimentin-positive myofibroblasts also increased in BLM-treated skin, and WKYMVm treatment decreased the BLM-induced increase of Vimentin-positive cells (**Figures 3B,D**). TGF-β-dependent SMAD3 phosphorylation has been reported to play a key role in myofibroblast differentiation during the progression of fibrotic diseases (18). Therefore, we next quantified the number of Vimentin- and p-SMAD3-double positive myofibroblasts. The number of $Vimentin^+$p-$SMAD3^+$ myofibroblasts increased in the BLM-induced scleroderma model, and WKYMVm treatment markedly reduced the BLM-induced increase of $Vimentin^+$p-$SMAD3^+$ cell number (**Figures 3B,E**). Consistently, BLM treatment increased the mRNA level of tissue inhibitor of metalloproteinase-1, which plays a key role in scleroderma-associated fibrosis (19), and WKYMVm treatment reduced the BLM-induced expression of tissue inhibitor of metalloproteinase-1 (**Figure S2A**).

To explore whether Fpr2 activation directly regulates the differentiation of fibroblasts to α-SMA-positive myofibroblasts, we next examined the effects of WKYMVm on myofibroblast differentiation induced by TGF-β1, which is a well-known ligand that induces myofibroblast differentiation (20). TGF-β1-induced α-SMA expression in fibroblasts was not affected by treatment with WKYMVm (**Figure S3**), suggesting that WKYMVm does not directly inhibit TGF-β1-induced differentiation of fibroblasts to myofibroblasts. Taken together, these results suggest that WKYMVm-induced activation of Fpr2 alleviated BLM-induced

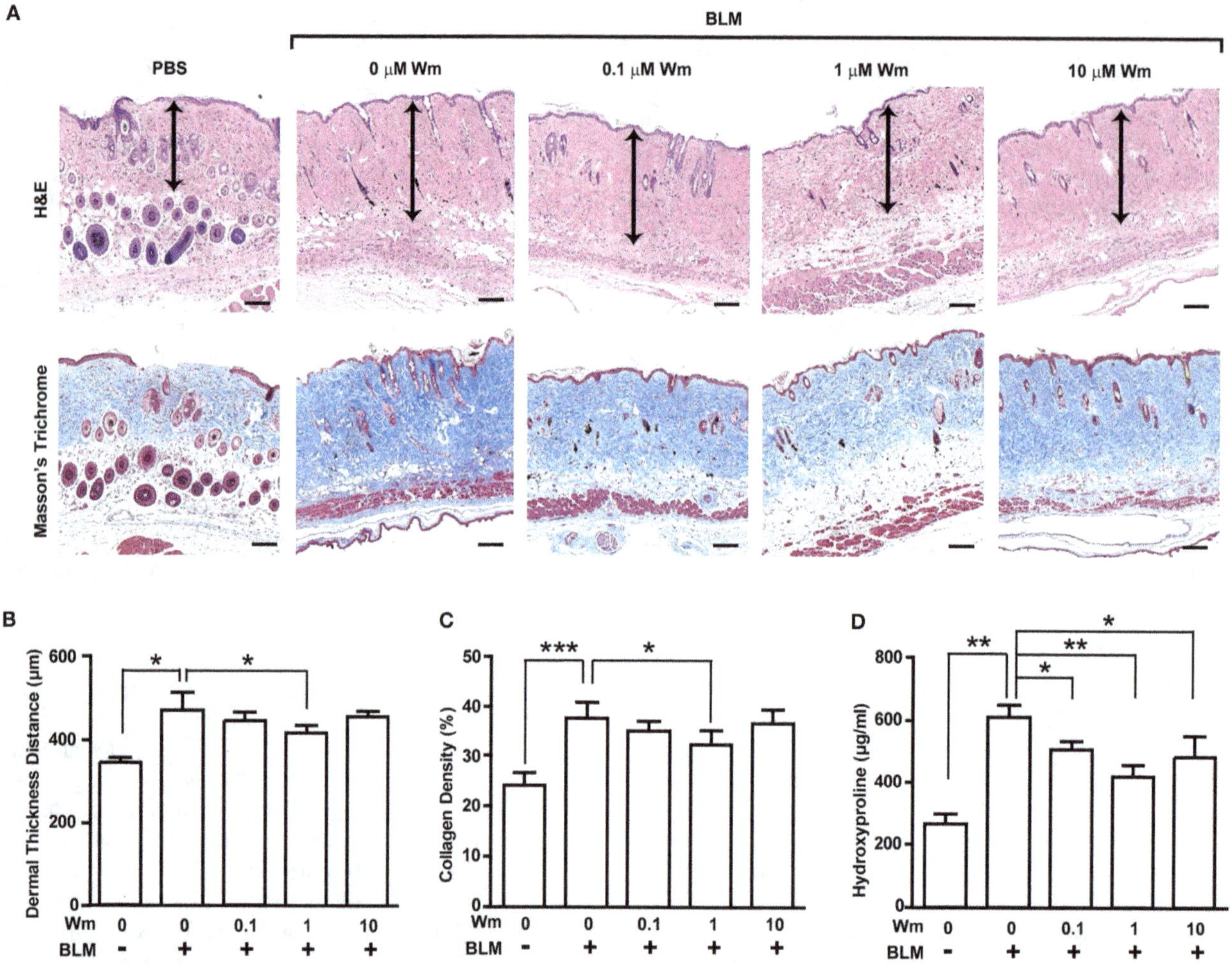

FIGURE 1 | Dose-dependent effects of WKYMVm treatment on tissue fibrosis in a scleroderma mice model. **(A)** Dose-dependent effect of WKYMVm (Wm) on BLM-induced scleroderma. The BLM-induced scleroderma mice were daily treated with the increasing dose of Wm for additional 3 weeks, and skin sections were stained using H&E and Masson's Trichrome staining kits. Dermal layer between the epidermal-dermal junction and the dermal-fat junction was indicated with an arrow on H&E-stained sections. Dermal thickness **(B)** and collagen density **(C)** were quantified from the H&E and Masson's Trichrome data, respectively. **(D)** Effect of Wm on the BLM-induced increase of hydroxyproline content in skin. The levels of hydroxyproline in skin specimens were determined as described in Materials and Methods section. The data are shown as the mean ± SD ($n = 8$ per groups). $^{*}p < 0.05$, $^{**}p < 0.01$, $^{***}p < 0.001$.

dermal thickness, collagen deposition, and myofibroblast differentiation in scleroderma skin.

WKYMVm Treatment Reduces Inflammation in BLM-Induced Scleroderma

Infiltration of inflammatory cells, including macrophages, and chronic inflammation have been reported to induce fibrotic disease (3). To explore the effect of WKYMVm on scleroderma-associated infiltration and activation of inflammatory cells, we assessed the levels of macrophage infiltration into the skin in the BLM-induced scleroderma model. The number of CD68-positive macrophages increased in the BLM-induced scleroderma skin compared with that in PBS-treated control specimens; however, this effect was suppressed by WKYMVm treatment (**Figures 4A–E**). In fibrotic disease, remodeling/profibrotic (M2) macrophages, which express CD163 or Arginase-I, have been implicated in pulmonary fibrosis disease (3, 9). The numbers of $CD68^{+}$ macrophages, $CD68^{+}NOS2^{+}$ inflammatory M1 macrophages, and $CD68^{+}$Arginase-1^{+} M2 macrophages in skin were increased within 1 week after subcutaneous administration of BLM with earlier increase of M1 type than M2 type macrophages (**Figure S4**). Therefore, we quantified the numbers of M2 macrophages, which include $CD68^{+}CD163^{+}$ or $CD68^{+}$Arginase-I^{+} populations, and M1 macrophages including $CD68^{+}NOS2^{+}$ and $CD68^{+}TLR2^{+}$ populations in scleroderma skin. The numbers of $CD68^{+}CD163^{+}$ or $CD68^{+}$Arginase-I^{+} cells were greatly increased in BLM-induced skin, and the BLM-induced increase of M2 macrophage populations was considerably attenuated by WKYMVm treatment for additional 3 weeks (**Figures 4A,B,F**). Moreover, the numbers of M1 macrophages including $CD68^{+}NOS2^{+}$ and $CD68^{+}TLR2^{+}$ populations increased in BLM-induced scleroderma skin;

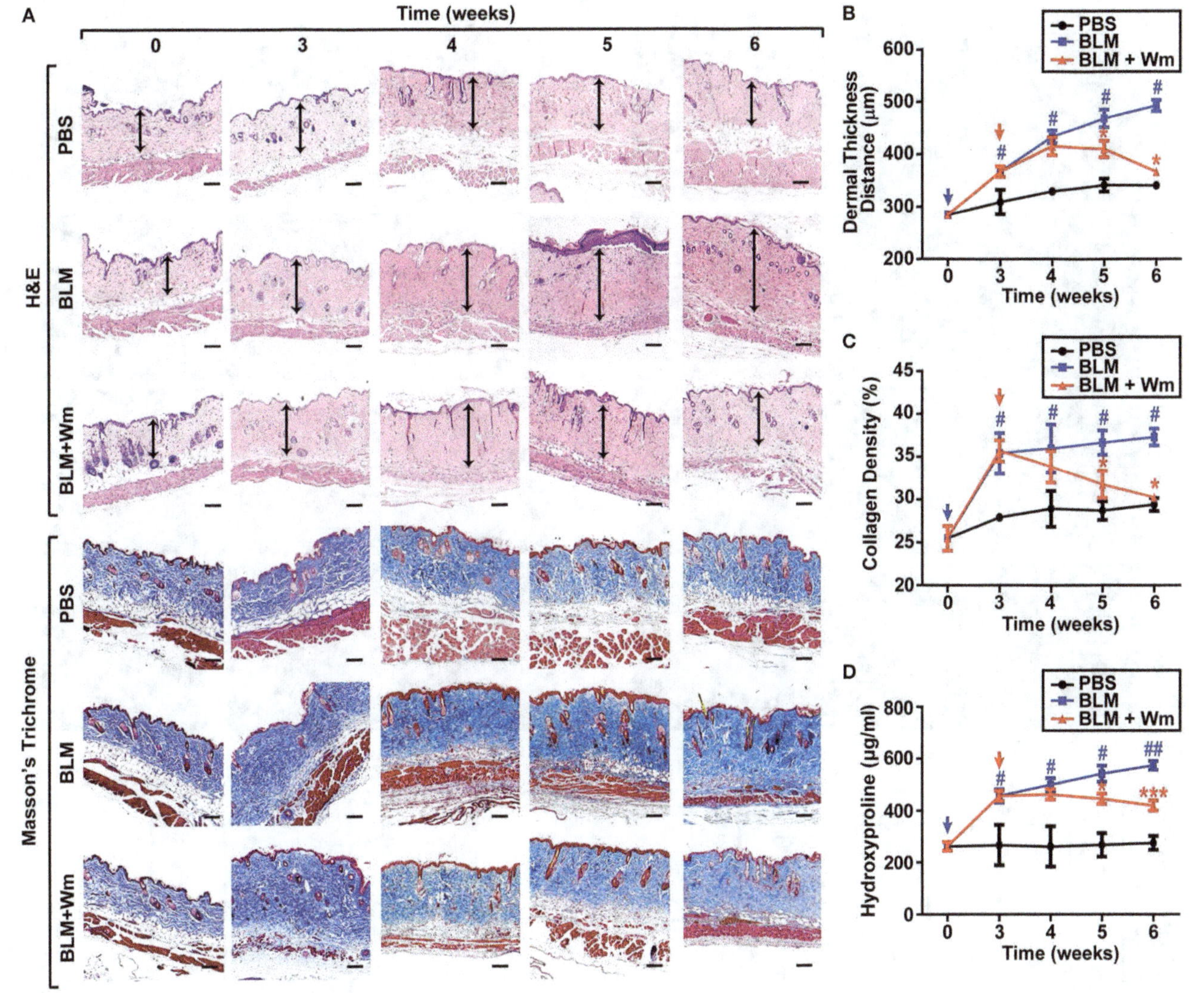

FIGURE 2 | Time-dependent effects of WKYMVm treatment on tissue fibrosis in scleroderma mice model. **(A)** Time dependence of WKYMVm-induced repair of scleroderma. The BLM-induced scleroderma mice were treated without (BLM) or with 1 μM Wm (BLM + Wm) for the indicated time periods. The mock-treated (PBS) and the scleroderma (BLM or BLM + Wm) skin specimens were stained using H&E and Masson's Trichrome staining kits. Dermal layer between the epidermal-dermal junction and the dermal-fat junction was indicated with an arrow on H&E-stained sections. Dermal thickness **(B)** and collagen density **(C)** were quantified from the H&E and Masson's Trichrome staining data, respectively. **(D)** The effects of Wm on the levels of hydroxyproline content in skin specimens were determined. Data are shown as the mean ± SD ($n = 8$). $^{\#}p < 0.05$, $^{\#\#}p < 0.01$ vs. PBS; $^{*}p < 0.05$, $^{***}p < 0.001$ vs. BLM.

however, the BLM-induced increase of M1 macrophage ($CD68^{+}NOS2^{+}$ and $CD68^{+}TLR2^{+}$) populations was not significantly affected by WKYMVm treatment (**Figures 4C,D,G**). WKYMVm treatment time-dependently decrease the number of M2 macrophages but not M1 macrophages (**Figure S5**).

The Role of Fpr2 in WKYMVm-Induced Alleviation of Scleroderma Fibrosis

To clarify the role of Fpr2 in WKYMVm-induced alleviation of scleroderma, we examined the therapeutic effects of WKYMVm on BLM-induced scleroderma in Fpr2 knockout mice. In contrast to the WKYMVm-induced decrease of fibrotic area in the scleroderma model of wild-type mice, WKYMVM treatment did not alleviate the BLM-induced dermal thickness in Fpr2 knockout mice (**Figures 5A,B**). Moreover, the BLM-induced deposition of thick collagen fibers in the dermal tissues was significantly reduced by WKYMVm treatment in wild type mice but not in Fpr2 knockout mice (**Figures 5A,C**). Consistently, the increased level of hydroxyproline in the BLM-induced scleroderma skin was not affected by WKYMVm treatment in Fpr2 KO mice, in contrast to significant decrease of hydroxyproline content in the BLM-treated skin of wild type mice (**Figure 5D**).

In order to confirm these results, we next explored the role of Fpr2 in WKYMVm-induced regulation of myofibroblast differentiation using Fpr2 knockout mice. In contrast to the

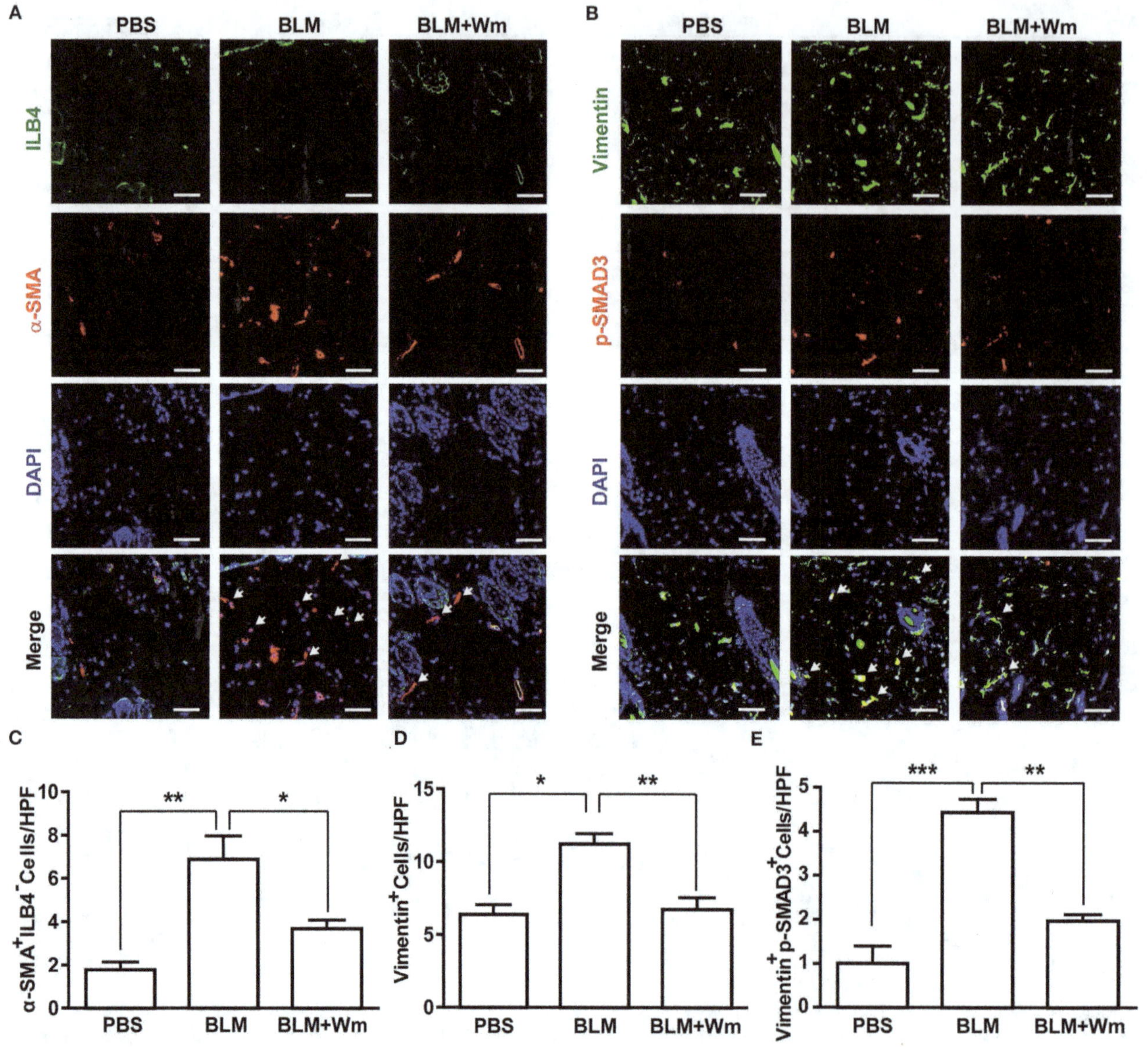

FIGURE 3 | Effects of WKYMVm treatment on myofibroblast differentiation in scleroderma. **(A)** WKYMVm-induced inhibition of myofibroblast differentiation in scleroderma. The BLM-induced scleroderma mice were treated with or without 1 μM Wm for 3 weeks, and the mock-treated (PBS) and the scleroderma (BLM or BLM + Wm) skin specimens were immunostained with antibodies against α-SMA and ILB-4. **(B)** The skin specimens were stained with antibodies against Vimentin and phospho-SMAD3. Scale bar = 50 μm. The numbers of α-SMA$^+$ILB-4$^-$ **(C)**, Vimentin$^+$ **(D)**, and Vimentin$^+$phospho-SMAD3$^+$ **(E)** cells were quantified under a high-power field. Data represent mean ± SD (*n* = 8 per group). **p* < 0.05, ***p* < 0.01, ****p* < 0.001.

WKYMVm-induced decrease of α-SMA$^+$ILB4$^-$ myofibroblasts in BLM-induced scleroderma skin of wild type mice, WKYMVm treatment had no significant effect on the number of α-SMA$^+$ILB4$^-$ myofibroblasts in the BLM-induced scleroderma skin of Fpr2 KO mice (**Figures 6A,C**). Furthermore, WKYMVm treatment did not reduce the numbers of Vimentin$^+$ or Vimentin$^+$p-SMAD3$^+$ myofibroblasts in the scleroderma skin of Fpr2 KO mice, in contrast to the significant inhibition of those in the scleroderma skin of wild type mice (**Figures 6B,D,E**). These results suggest that Fpr2 mediates WKYMVm-induced reduction of myofibroblast differentiation in scleroderma.

The Role of Fpr2 in WKYMVm-Induced Immune Resolution in Scleroderma Mice

To explore the role of Fpr2 in WKYMVm-induced alleviation of inflammatory responses in scleroderma mice, we next quantified the number of CD68-positive macrophages in Fpr2 knockout mice. In contrast to the WKYMVm-induced inhibition of CD68-positive macrophage infiltration in the scleroderma skin of wild type mice, WKYMVm treatment had no significant impact on BLM-induced infiltration of macrophages in Fpr2 KO mice (**Figures 7A–E**). Moreover, WKYMVm treatment did not reduce the numbers of CD68$^+$CD163$^+$ or CD68$^+$Arginase-I$^+$ M2

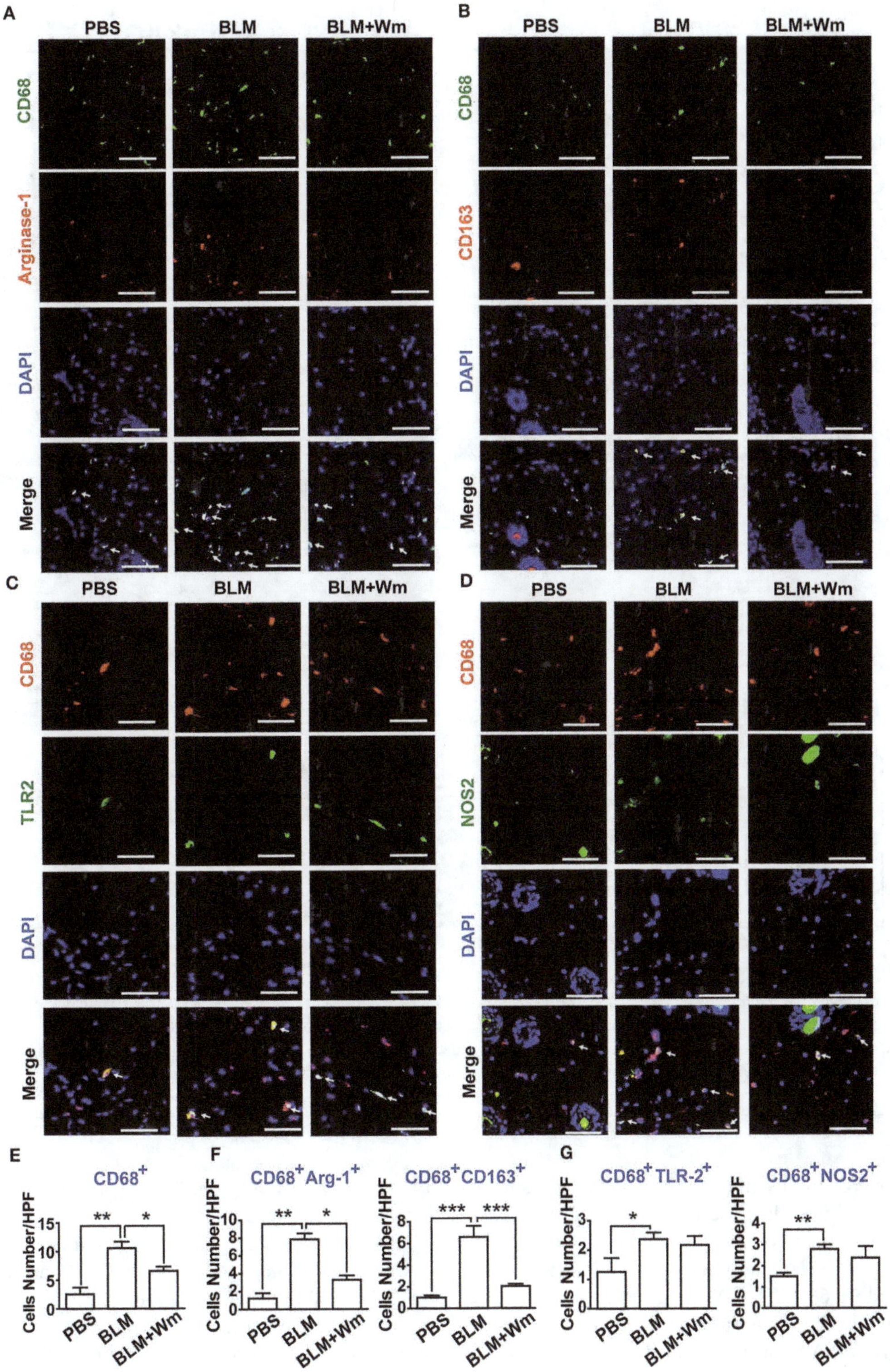

FIGURE 4 | Effects of WKYMVm treatment on macrophage polarization and inflammation in scleroderma. The BLM-induced scleroderma mice were treated with or without Wm for 3 weeks. The mock-treated (PBS) and scleroderma (BLM or BLM+Wm) skin specimens were stained with anti-CD68 antibody together with anti-Arginase-1 **(A)**, anti-CD163 **(B)**, anti-TLR2 **(C)**, or NOS2 **(D)** antibodies. Nuclei was stained with DAPI, and overlaid images are shown. Scale bar = 50 μm. The numbers of $CD68^+$ macrophages **(E)**, M2 type macrophages (**F**: $CD68^+$Arginse-1^+ and $CD68^+CD163^+$ cells), M1 type macrophages (**G**: $CD68^+TLR2^+$ and $CD68^+NOS2^+$ cells) were counted under high-power field. Data represent mean ± SD ($n = 8$ per group). $^*p < 0.05$, $^{**}p < 0.01$, $^{***}p < 0.001$.

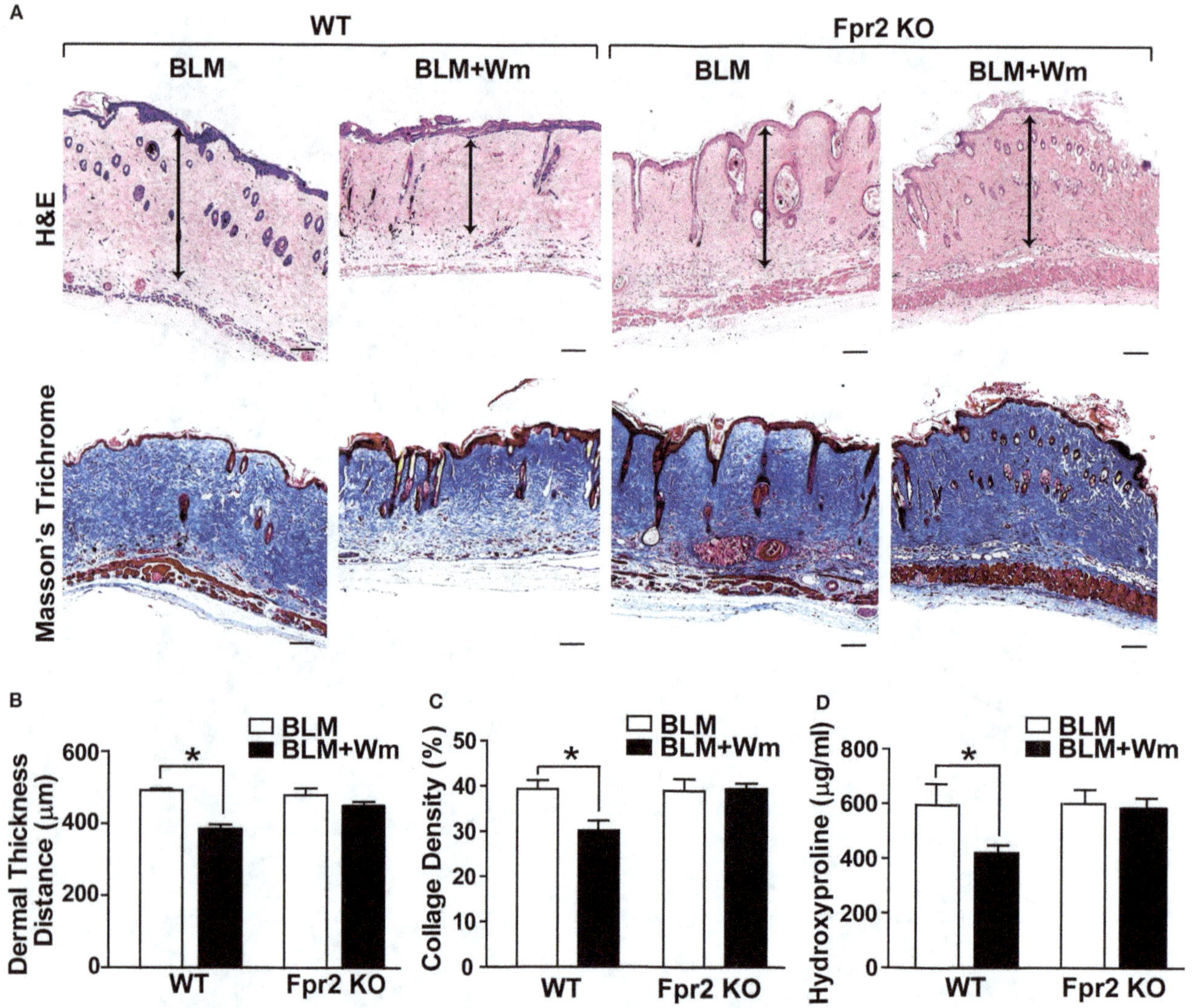

FIGURE 5 | The role of Fpr2 in WKYMVm-induced alleviation of dermal fibrosis in scleroderma. **(A)** Wild type and Fpr2 KO mice were daily injected with BLM for 3 weeks, followed by co-administration of BLM with or without 1 μM Wm for additional 3 weeks. Skin specimens of BLM-induced scleroderma mice were stained with H&E and Masson's trichrome stain. Scale bar = 100 μm. Dermal thickness **(B)** and collagen density **(C)** were quantified from the H&E and Masson's Trichrome data, respectively. **(D)** The levels of hydroxyproline content in skin specimens were determined by using a hydroxyproline assay kit. Data are shown as the mean ± SD (n = 8). $^{*}p < 0.05$.

macrophages in scleroderma skin of Fpr2 KO mice, in contrast to the WKYMVm-induced decrease of M2 macrophage levels in that of wild type mice (**Figure 7F**). Whereas, WKYMVm treatment had no significant impact on the numbers of the $CD68^{+}NOS2^{+}$ and $CD68^{+}TLR2^{+}$ M1 macrophages in not only wild type mice but also Fpr2 knockout mice (**Figure 7G**). These results suggest that WKYMVm-induced activation of Fpr2 led to inhibition of macrophage activation and decrease of M2 macrophages in scleroderma skin.

To explore the immune resolution effect of FPR activation, we measured the levels of inflammatory cytokines in the serum of BLM-induced scleroderma mice. BLM-induced scleroderma mice exhibited increased serum levels of TNF-α and INF-γ, and WKYMVm treatment alleviated the BLM-induced increase of TNF-α and INF-γ (**Figures 8A,B**). Consistently, BLM treatment increased the mRNA level of INF-γ in scleroderma tissues, and WKYMVm treatment reduced BLM-induced increase of INF-γ mRNA levels (**Figure S2B**). The WKYMVm-induced reduction of TNF-α and INF-γ levels was observed in the serum of BLM-induced scleroderma model of wild type mice, but not in Fpr2 knockout mice (**Figures 8C,D**). These results indicate that Fpr2 plays a key role in WKYMVm-induced immune resolution in scleroderma.

DISCUSSION

In this study, we showed that WKYMVm-induced activation of Fpr2 reduced the skin fibrosis which is associated with

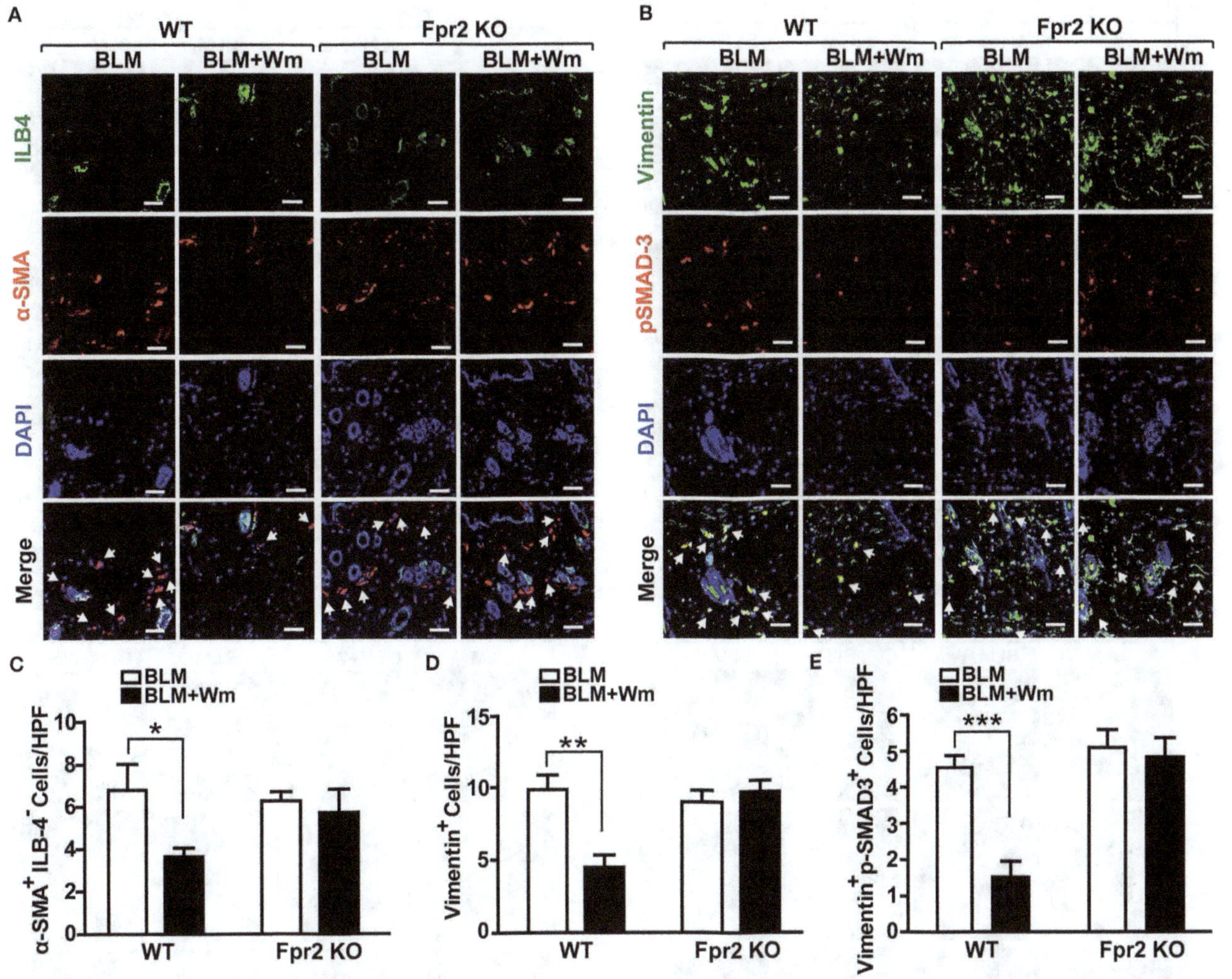

FIGURE 6 | The role of Fpr2 activation in the myofibroblast differentiation associated with scleroderma. **(A)** The BLM-induced scleroderma model of wild type and Fpr2 KO mice were daily injected with or without Wm for 3 weeks, followed by staining of the skin specimens with antibodies against α-SMA and ILB-4. **(B)** The skin specimens were stained with antibodies against Vimentin and phospho-SMAD3. Scale bar = 50 μm. The numbers of α-SMA$^+$ILB-4$^-$ **(C)**, Vimentin$^+$ **(D)**, and Vimentin$^+$phospho-SMAD3$^+$ **(E)** cells were quantified under a high-power field. Data are shown as mean ± SD ($n = 8$ per group). $^*p < 0.05$, $^{**}p < 0.01$, $^{***}p < 0.001$.

BLM-induced scleroderma. Intradermal injection of WKYMVm decreased dermal thickness and collagen deposition in the scleroderma skin of wild type mice, whereas this therapeutic effect was completely abrogated in Fpr2 knockout mice. Fpr2 in mouse has been reported to be activated by not only WKYMVm, but also various structurally diverse ligands, including annexin A1, LL37, lipoxins, and resolvins (21). In accordance with the present study, several reports have suggested that Fpr2 activation leads to alleviation of tissue fibrosis associated with chronic inflammation. Lipoxin was shown to exhibit pro-resolution effect on inflammation and inhibit growth factor-induced fibroblast proliferation and collagen synthesis (22). Moreover, 17®-resolvin D1 ameliorated BLM-induced pulmonary fibrosis by attenuating alveolar infiltration of neutrophils and inflammatory responses (23). These results support the findings of the present study, suggesting the therapeutic role of Fpr2 activation in the treatment of scleroderma.

The pro-resolving effects of Fpr2 ligands include limiting leukocyte trafficking and activation *in vitro* and *in vivo* (24) as well as stimulating efferocytosis (25), granulocyte apoptosis (26), and leukocyte egress (27). One of the downstream Fpr2 signaling events involved in the pro-resolving effects is the suppression of calcium-sensing kinase calcium-calmodulin-dependent protein kinase and subsequent inhibition of p38 mitogen-activated protein kinase (MAPK) phosphorylation in murine bone marrow-derived cells (28, 29). Another possible mechanism associated with the Fpr2-mediated immune resolution is receptor desensitization, which plays a key role in the regulation of G protein-coupled receptor signaling and trafficking (30). Recent studies have demonstrated that FPR2 agonists, lipoxin A4 and some of ureidopropanamide

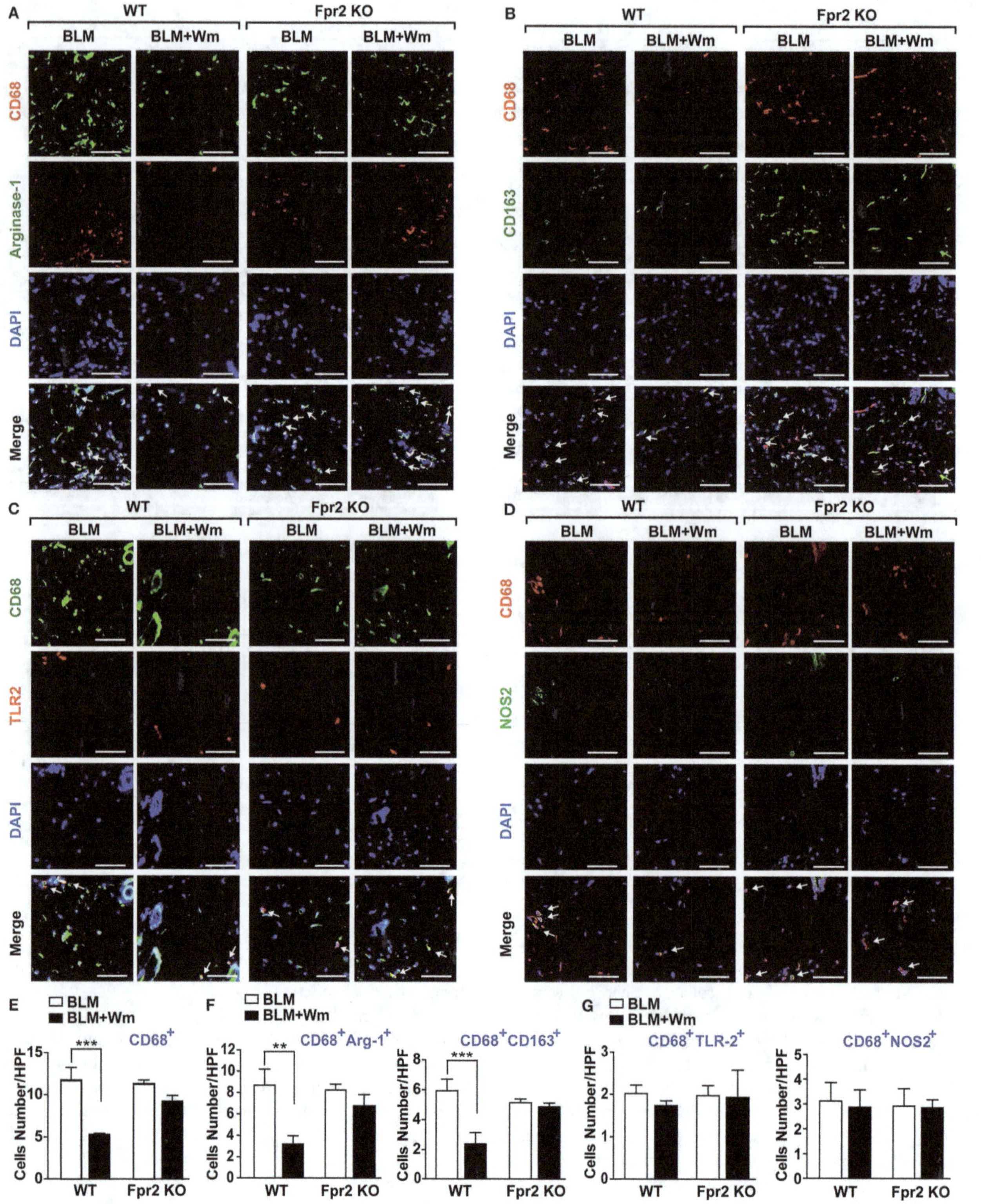

FIGURE 7 | The role of Fpr2 in WKYMVm-induced decrease of M2 macrophages in scleroderma skin. The BLM-induced scleroderma skin of wild type and Fpr2 KO mice were injected with or without Wm for 3 weeks, followed by staining with anti-CD68 antibody together with anti-Arginase-1 **(A)**, anti-CD163 **(B)**, anti-TLR2 **(C)**, or NOS2 **(D)** antibodies. Nuclei was stained with DAPI and overlaid images are shown. Scale bar = 50 µm. The numbers of $CD68^+$ macrophages **(E)**, M2 type macrophages (**F**: $CD68^+$ $Arginse\text{-}1^+$ and $CD68^+CD163^+$ cells), M1 type macrophages (**G**: $CD68^+TLR2^+$ and $CD68^+NOS2^+$ cells) were counted under high-power field. Data represent mean ± SD ($n = 8$ per group). $^{**}p < 0.01$, $^{***}p < 0.001$.

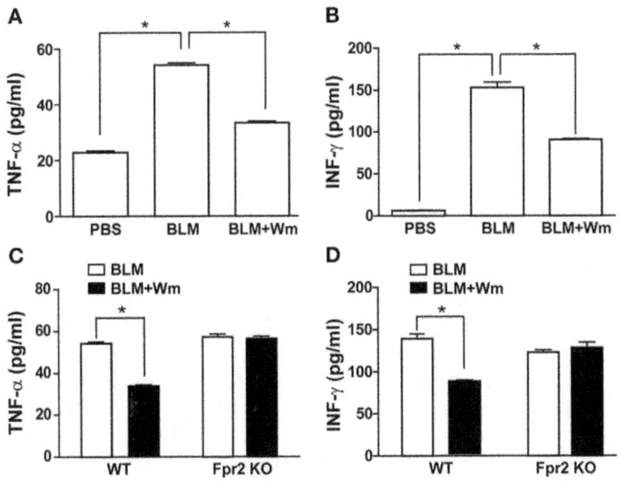

FIGURE 8 | The role of Fpr2 in WKYMVm-induced immune resolution in scleroderma. **(A,B)** Wm-induced inhibition of systemic inflammation in scleroderma. The BLM-induced scleroderma mice model were treated with or without Wm for 3 weeks, and the serum levels of TNF-α **(A)** and INF-γ **(B)** in the mock-treated (PBS) and the scleroderma mice (BLM or BLM+Wm) were determined by ELISA assay. **(C,D)** The role of Fpr2 in Wm-induced suppression of systemic inflammation in scleroderma. The BLM-induced scleroderma model of wild type and Fpr2 KO mice were daily injected with or without Wm for 3 weeks, and the serum levels of TNF-α **(C)**, and INF-γ **(D)** in the scleroderma mice were quantified by ELISA analysis. Data represent mean ± SD ($n = 8$ per group). $^{*}p < 0.05$.

derivatives, induced FPR2 internalization and desensitization (25, 31). Moreover, it has been reported that compound 43, a non-peptidyl agonist for mouse Fprl and Fpr2, inhibited neutrophil migration in mice by inducing cross-desensitization of CXCR2, a chemoattractant receptor (32). In addition, some FPR2 agonists including WKYMVm have been reported to induce cross-desensitization of CCR5 and CXCR4 (33, 34). Therefore, it is likely that inhibition of inflammatory signaling and desensitization of chemoattractant receptors may be play a key role in the WKYMVm-induced resolution of chronic inflammation.

Systemic scleroderma is a chronic autoimmune disease that causes systemic inflammation. In this study, we showed that BLM-induced scleroderma stimulated infiltration of CD68-positive macrophages into scleroderma skin, and the serum levels of the inflammatory cytokines, TNF-α and INF-γ, were up-regulated in the scleroderma model; however, WKYMVm treatment attenuated these effects. Accumulating evidence suggests that activation of FPR2 led to alleviation of chronic inflammatory diseases (35). In dextran sodium sulfate-treated ulcerative colitis animal model, WKYMVm administration alleviated mucosa destruction and shortened colon by decreasing production of interleukin-23, a pro-inflammatory cytokine, and TGF-β1 (36). WKYMVm treatment prevented the development of Thl and Th17 cell responses and inhibited the production of inflammatory cytokines (37). Moreover, WKYMVm treatment attenuated hyperoxia-induced lung injury and lung inflammation in newborn mice (38). WKYMVm treatment decreased the numbers of inflammatory cells including CD68-positive macrophages and the levels of inflammatory cytokines in the lungs of hyperoxic mice. These results suggest that WKYMVm-induced activation of Fpr2 attenuates chronic inflammation and concomitant production of inflammatory cytokines.

It has been shown that WKYMVm treatment increases the expression of Fpr2 in scleroderma fibroblasts and upregulation of Fpr2 in scleroderma fibroblasts fosters the switch to myofibroblasts (13, 14). However, lipoxin A4 has been shown to inhibit TGF-β1-dependent profibrotic activity in human lung myofibroblasts (39). Furthermore, lipoxin A4 inhibited the proliferation of human lung fibroblasts induced by connective tissue growth factor (40). In our study, WKYMVm treatment led to decreased production of myofibroblasts positive for α-SMA, Vimentin, and phospho-SMAD3 through an Fpr2-dependent mechanism in the scleroderma model. However, WKYMVm treatment did not directly affect TGF-β1-induced differentiation of fibroblasts to α-SMA-positive myofibroblasts, suggesting that WKYMVm-induced activation of Fpr2 indirectly alleviates myofibroblast differentiation in the BLM-induced scleroderma model. Macrophage-derived TGF-β stimulates myofibroblasts to produce various extracellular matrix proteins and inhibitors of metalloproteases that are involved in the degradation of matrix proteins (41). Several drugs, such as tamibarotene, glycyrrhizin, and paquinimod have been reported to ameliorate BLM-induced dermal fibrosis and infiltration of macrophages by suppressing M2 polarization of macrophages in BLM-induced scleroderma model (7, 8, 42, 43). In this study, we demonstrated that WKYMVm treatment reduced the number of $CD68^{+}CD163^{+}$ or $CD68^{+}$Arginase-I^{+} M2 macrophages in the scleroderma tissues through Fpr2-dependent mechanism. These results suggest that Fpr2 activation alleviates scleroderma by inhibiting M2 macrophage polarization and systemic levels of inflammatory cytokines in scleroderma.

In conclusion, the present study demonstrates that WKYMVm-induced Fpr2 activation relieves fibrosis by inhibiting fibroblast activation, macrophage infiltration and generation of M2 type macrophages, and inflammatory cytokine expression in BLM-induced scleroderma model. These results suggest that Fpr2 ligands including WKYMVm can be useful in the treatment of patients with scleroderma.

ETHICS STATEMENT

All animal experiments were performed according to protocols approved by the Institutional Animal Care and Use Committee of Pusan National University Institutional Animal Use and Care Committee.

AUTHOR CONTRIBUTIONS

GP and JK designed the experiments and wrote the manuscript. GP, YK, TL, and SK performed the experiments. H-CK and MK analyzed data.

ACKNOWLEDGMENTS

We thank Prof. Yoe Sik Bae and Dr. Eun Kyoung Do for technical assistance and discussion.

REFERENCES

1. Varga J, Abraham D. Systemic sclerosis: a prototypic multisystem fibrotic disorder. *J Clin Invest.* (2007) 117:557–67. doi: 10.1172/JCI31139
2. Bhattacharyya S, Wei J, Varga J. Understanding fibrosis in systemic sclerosis: shifting paradigms, emerging opportunities. *Nat Rev Rheumatol.* (2011) 8:42–54. doi: 10.1038/nrrheum.2011.149
3. Fuschiotti P. Current perspectives on the immunopathogenesis of systemic sclerosis. *Immunotargets Ther.* (2016) 5:21–35. doi: 10.2147/ITT.S82037
4. Brown M, O'Reilly S. The immunopathogenesis of fibrosis in systemic sclerosis. *Clin Exp Immunol.* (2019) 195:310–21. doi: 10.1111/cei.13238
5. Mosser DM, Edwards JP. Exploring the full spectrum of macrophage activation. *Nat Rev Immunol.* (2008) 8:958–69. doi: 10.1038/nri2448
6. Shapouri-Moghaddam A, Mohammadian S, Vazini H, Taghadosi M, Esmaeili SA, Mardani F, et al. Macrophage plasticity, polarization, and function in health and disease. *J Cell Physiol.* (2018) 233:6425–40. doi: 10.1002/jcp.26429
7. Higashi-Kuwata N, Makino T, Inoue Y, Takeya M, Ihn H. Alternatively activated macrophages (M2 macrophages) in the skin of patient with localized scleroderma. *Exp Dermatol.* (2009) 18:727–9. doi: 10.1111/j.1600-0625.2008.00828.x
8. Toyama T, Asano Y, Akamata K, Noda S, Taniguchi T, Takahashi T, et al. Tamibarotene ameliorates bleomycin-induced dermal fibrosis by modulating phenotypes of fibroblasts, endothelial cells, and immune cells. *J Invest Dermatol.* (2016) 136:387–98. doi: 10.1016/j.jid.2015.10.058
9. Wermuth PJ, Jimenez SA. The significance of macrophage polarization subtypes for animal models of tissue fibrosis and human fibrotic diseases. *Clin Transl Med.* (2015) 4:2. doi: 10.1186/s40169-015-0047-4
10. Le Y, Murphy PM, Wang JM. Formyl-peptide receptors revisited. *Trends Immunol.* (2002) 23:541–8. doi: 10.1016/S1471-4906(02)02316-5
11. VanCompernolle SE, Clark KL, Rummel KA, Todd SC. Expression and function of formyl peptide receptors on human fibroblast cells. *J Immunol.* (2003) 171:2050–6. doi: 10.4049/jimmunol.171.4.2050
12. Ye RD, Boulay F, Wang JM, Dahlgren C, Gerard C, Parmentier M, et al. International union of basic and clinical pharmacology. LXXIII. nomenclature for the formyl peptide receptor (FPR) family. *Pharmacol Rev.* (2009) 61:119–61. doi: 10.1124/pr.109.001578
13. Rossi FW, Montuori N. FPRs: linking innate immune system and fibrosis. *Oncotarget.* (2015) 6:18736–7. doi: 10.18632/oncotarget.4915
14. Rossi FW, Napolitano F, Pesapane A, Mascolo M, Staibano S, Matucci-Cerinic M, et al. Upregulation of the N-formyl peptide receptors in scleroderma fibroblasts fosters the switch to myofibroblasts. *J Immunol.* (2015) 194:5161–73. doi: 10.4049/jimmunol.1402819
15. Ammitzboll T, Serup J. Collagen metabolites in urine in localized scleroderma (morphoea). *Acta Derm Venereol.* (1984) 64:534–7.
16. Hinz B, Phan SH, Thannickal VJ, Prunotto M, Desmouliere A, Varga J, et al. Recent developments in myofibroblast biology: paradigms for connective tissue remodeling. *Am J Pathol.* (2012) 180:1340–55. doi: 10.1016/j.ajpath.2012.02.004
17. Matthijs Blankesteijn W. Has the search for a marker of activated fibroblasts finally come to an end? *J Mol Cell Cardiol.* (2015) 88:120–3. doi: 10.1016/j.yjmcc.2015.10.005
18. Biernacka A, Dobaczewski M, Frangogiannis NG. TGF-beta signaling in fibrosis. *Growth Factors.* (2011) 29:196–202. doi: 10.3109/08977194.2011.595714
19. Jinnin M. Mechanisms of skin fibrosis in systemic sclerosis. *J Dermatol.* (2010) 37:11–25. doi: 10.1111/j.1346-8138.2009.00738.x
20. Lafyatis R. Transforming growth factor beta–at the centre of systemic sclerosis. *Nat Rev Rheumatol.* (2014) 10:706–19. doi: 10.1038/nrrheum.2014.137
21. Cattaneo F, Parisi M, Ammendola R. Distinct signaling cascades elicited by different formyl peptide receptor 2 (FPR2) agonists. *Int J Mol Sci.* (2013) 14:7193–230. doi: 10.3390/ijms14047193
22. Kowal-Bielecka O, Kowal K, Distler O, Gay S. Mechanisms of disease: leukotrienes and lipoxins in scleroderma lung disease–insights and potential therapeutic implications. *Nat Clin Pract Rheumatol.* (2007) 3:43–51. doi: 10.1038/ncprheum0375
23. Yatomi M, Hisada T, Ishizuka T, Koga Y, Ono A, Kamide Y, et al. 17(R)-resolvin D1 ameliorates bleomycin-induced pulmonary fibrosis in mice. *Physiol Rep.* (2015) 3:e12628. doi: 10.14814/phy2.12628
24. Hachicha M, Pouliot M, Petasis NA, Serhan CN. Lipoxin (LX)A4 and aspirin-triggered 15-epi-LXA4 inhibit tumor necrosis factor 1alpha-initiated neutrophil responses and trafficking: regulators of a cytokine-chemokine axis. *J Exp Med.* (1999) 189:1923–30. doi: 10.1084/jem.189.12.1923
25. Maderna P, Cottell DC, Toivonen T, Dufton N, Dalli J, Perretti M, et al. FPR2/ALX receptor expression and internalization are critical for lipoxin A4 and annexin-derived peptide-stimulated phagocytosis. *FASEB J.* (2010) 24:4240–9. doi: 10.1096/fj.10-159913
26. Barnig C, Cernadas M, Dutile S, Liu X, Perrella MA, Kazani S, et al. Lipoxin A4 regulates natural killer cell and type 2 innate lymphoid cell activation in asthma. *Sci Transl Med.* (2013) 5:174ra26. doi: 10.1126/scitranslmed.3004812
27. van Gils JM, Derby MC, Fernandes LR, Ramkhelawon B, Ray TD, Rayner KJ, et al. The neuroimmune guidance cue netrin-1 promotes atherosclerosis by inhibiting the emigration of macrophages from plaques. *Nat Immunol.* (2012) 13:136–43. doi: 10.1038/ni.2205
28. Petri MH, Thul S, Andonova T, Lindquist-Liljeqvist M, Jin H, Skenteris NT, et al. Resolution of inflammation through the lipoxin and ALX/FPR2 receptor pathway protects against abdominal aortic aneurysms. *JACC Basic Transl Sci.* (2018) 3:719–27. doi: 10.1016/j.jacbts.2018.08.005
29. Fredman G, Ozcan L, Spolitu S, Hellmann J, Spite M, Backs J, et al. Resolvin D1 limits 5-lipoxygenase nuclear localization and leukotriene B4 synthesis by inhibiting a calcium-activated kinase pathway. *Proc Natl Acad Sci USA.* (2014) 111:14530–5. doi: 10.1073/pnas.1410851111
30. Kelly E, Bailey CP, Henderson G. Agonist-selective mechanisms of GPCR desensitization. *Br J Pharmacol.* (2008) 153(Suppl 1):S379–88. doi: 10.1038/sj.bjp.0707604
31. Stama ML, Lacivita E, Kirpotina LN, Niso M, Perrone R, Schepetkin IA, et al. Functional N-formyl peptide receptor 2 (FPR2) antagonists based on the ureidopropanamide scaffold have potential to protect against inflammation-associated oxidative stress. *ChemMedChem.* (2017) 12:1839–47. doi: 10.1002/cmdc.201700429
32. Sogawa Y, Ohyama T, Maeda H, Hirahara K. Inhibition of neutrophil migration in mice by mouse formyl peptide receptors 1 and 2 dual agonist: indication of cross-desensitization *in vivo*. *Immunology.* (2011) 132:441–50. doi: 10.1111/j.1365-2567.2010.03367.x
33. Deng X, Ueda H, Su SB, Gong W, Dunlop NM, Gao JL, et al. A synthetic peptide derived from human immunodeficiency virus type 1 gp120 downregulates the expression and function of chemokine receptors CCR5 and CXCR4 in monocytes by activating the 7-transmembrane G-protein-coupled receptor FPRL1/LXA4R. *Blood.* (1999) 94:1165–73.
34. Li BQ, Wetzel MA, Mikovits JA, Henderson EE, Rogers TJ, Gong W, et al. The synthetic peptide WKYMVm attenuates the function of the chemokine receptors CCR5 and CXCR4 through activation of formyl peptide receptor-like 1. *Blood.* (2001) 97:2941–7. doi: 10.1182/blood.V97.10.2941

35. Satish M, Gunasekar P, Agrawal DK. Pro-inflammatory and pro-resolving mechanisms in the immunopathology of arteriovenous fistula maturation. *Expert Rev Cardiovasc Ther.* (2019) 17:369–76. doi: 10.1080/14779072.2019.1612745
36. Kim SD, Kwon S, Lee SK, Kook M, Lee HY, Song KD, et al. The immune-stimulating peptide WKYMVm has therapeutic effects against ulcerative colitis. *Exp Mol Med.* (2013) 45:e40. doi: 10.1038/emm.2013.77
37. Tae YM, Park HT, Moon HG, Kim YS, Jeon SG, Roh TY, et al. Airway activation of formyl peptide receptors inhibits Th1 and Th17 cell responses via inhibition of mediator release from immune and inflammatory cells and maturation of dendritic cells. *J Immunol.* (2012) 188:1799–808. doi: 10.4049/jimmunol.1102481
38. Kim YE, Park WS, Ahn SY, Sung DK, Sung SI, Kim JH, et al. WKYMVm hexapeptide, a strong formyl peptide receptor 2 agonist, attenuates hyperoxia-induced lung injuries in newborn mice. *Sci Rep.* (2019) 9:6815. doi: 10.1038/s41598-019-43321-4
39. Roach KM, Feghali-Bostwick CA, Amrani Y, Bradding P. Lipoxin A4 Attenuates Constitutive and TGF-beta1-dependent profibrotic activity in human lung myofibroblasts. *J Immunol.* (2015) 195:2852–60. doi: 10.4049/jimmunol.1500936
40. Wu SH, Wu XH, Lu C, Dong L, Chen ZQ. Lipoxin A4 inhibits proliferation of human lung fibroblasts induced by connective tissue growth factor. *Am J Respir Cell Mol Biol.* (2006) 34:65–72. doi: 10.1165/rcmb.2005-0184OC
41. Murray PJ, Wynn TA. Protective and pathogenic functions of macrophage subsets. *Nat Rev Immunol.* (2011) 11:723–37. doi: 10.1038/nri3073
42. Stenstrom M, Nyhlen HC, Torngren M, Liberg D, Sparre B, Tuvesson H, et al. Paquinimod reduces skin fibrosis in tight skin 1 mice, an experimental model of systemic sclerosis. *J Dermatol Sci.* (2016) 83:52–9. doi: 10.1016/j.jdermsci.2016.04.006
43. Yamashita T, Asano Y, Taniguchi T, Nakamura K, Saigusa R, Miura S, et al. Glycyrrhizin ameliorates fibrosis, vasculopathy, and inflammation in animal models of systemic sclerosis. *J Invest Dermatol.* (2017) 137:631–40. doi: 10.1016/j.jid.2016.08.037

5

Therapeutic Targeting of Th17/Tc17 Cells Leads to Clinical Improvement of Lichen Planus

Farzan Solimani[1†], Robert Pollmann[1†], Thomas Schmidt[1‡], Ansgar Schmidt[2‡], Xiang Zheng[3], Rajkumar Savai[3,4], Stefan Mühlenbein[1], Julia Pickert[1], Verena Eubel[1], Christian Möbs[1], Rüdiger Eming[1] and Michael Hertl[1]*

[1] Department of Dermatology and Allergology, Philipps-Universität Marburg, Marburg, Germany, [2] Department of Pathology, Philipps-Universität Marburg, Marburg, Germany, [3] Max Planck Institute for Heart and Lung Research, Member of the German Center for Lung Research (DZL), Member of the Cardio-Pulmonary Institute (CPI), Bad Nauheim, Germany, [4] Department of Internal Medicine, Member of the DZL, Member of CPI, Justus Liebig University, Giessen, Germany

***Correspondence:** Michael Hertl hertl@med.uni-marburg.de*

† These authors have contributed equally to this work

‡ These authors have contributed equally to this work

Lichen planus (LP) is a common, chronic relapsing inflammatory disorder of the skin and mucous membranes which often poses a major therapeutic challenge due to its refractory course. Novel pathogenesis-based therapies are urgently needed. As several studies have shown that IL-17 may contribute to LP pathogenesis, we investigated whether therapeutic targeting of IL-17^{+} T cells leads to clinical improvement of mucosal and cutaneous LP lesions. A total of five patients with lichen planus were treated in a compassionate use trial with either secukinumab (anti-IL-17; 3 patients with acute and chronic recalcitrant muco-cutaneous LP), ustekinumab (anti-IL-12/IL-23; 1 patient with recalcitrant oral LP) or guselkumab (anti-IL-23; 1 patient with recalcitrant oral LP). The clinical course of the patients was assessed by the Autoimmune Bullous Skin Disorder Intensity Score (ABSIS) reflecting both extent and severity of disease and functional sequelae of oral involvement for at least 12 weeks. The inflammatory infiltrate in lesional and post-lesional skin was analyzed by immunohistochemistry before and after treatment. Furthermore, the cytokine profile of peripheral blood T cells from the treated patients was assessed by flow cytometry and/or ELISpot assay. Treatment with secukinumab induced rapid and prolonged clinical amelioration of muco-cutaneous LP. Clinical improvement was accompanied by a strong reduction of the Th1 and Th17/Tc17 cellular mucosal and cutaneous infiltrate. Moreover, long-term treatment of one patient with recalcitrant oral LP with ustekinumab led to healing of the ulcerative oral lesions and a reduction of peripheral blood and lesional IL-17^{+} T cells. Finally, treatment with guselkumab led to a marked clinical improvement in a patient with recalcitrant erosive oral LP. These findings show for the first time that therapeutic targeting of Th17/Tc17 cells leads to a pronounced clinical amelioration of mucosal and cutaneous LP and strongly suggests that IL-17-producing T cells are central to disease pathogenesis. Thus, therapeutic targeting of Th17/Tc17 cells opens new therapeutic avenues in the treatment of recalcitrant LP.

Keywords: lichen planus, IL-17, secukinumab, ustekinumab, guselkumab, T cells

INTRODUCTION

Lichen planus (LP) is a common chronic relapsing inflammatory skin disease of the mucous membranes and the skin which presents with pruritic papules and painful plaques on the skin and erosion and ulcers on the mucous membranes (1–3) while in lichen planopilaris, a follicular form of LP, the scalp can also be affected (4). Although common, the therapeutic options, particularly in mucosal LP, are rather limited due to a mostly chronic refractory course (3). Systemic immunosuppressants, such as glucocorticoids, ciclosporin, azathioprine, and methotrexate, or immunomodulators such as acitretin, help to ameliorate clinical symptoms but have considerable side effects upon long-term treatment. The inflammatory skin infiltrate of LP is characterized by a dense dermal T cell-dominated cellular infiltrate (1). At present, the target antigens of the T cellular response in LP are poorly characterized. Human papilloma virus (HPV) and hepatitis C virus have been implicated as etiologic factors in selected cases of oral LP (1). Our group has recently identified autoreactive Th1 and Th17 cell responses against bullous pemphigoid (BP) antigen 180, a well-known autoantigen of the skin, in LP patients with mucocutaneous involvement. Of note, IL-17-producing cells were present within the inflammatory skin infiltrate underneath the dermal epidermal basement membrane zone (BMZ) where apoptotic epidermal keratinocytes are typically seen in LP (5). In addition, different groups demonstrated the presence of Th17 cells and Th17-related cytokines in LP lesions (6–9). These findings strongly suggest a potential role of IL-17 cells in the LP pathogenesis and raise the question as to whether therapeutic targeting of IL-17 or IL-17-producing T cells leads to an amelioration of LP.

METHODS

Patients

Three patients with mucocutaneous LP were treated with the anti-IL-17A monoclonal antibody, secukinumab, one LP patient with recalcitrant oral LP was treated with the anti-p40 monoclonal antibody, ustekinumab, which targets the p40 subunit of both IL-23 and IL-12 and one LP patient with chronic lesions not responding to immunosuppressive treatments was treated with guselkumab, a monoclonal antibody targeting IL-23. The patients' characteristics are shown in **Table 1**. Diagnosis of LP was based on the clinical phenotype and histopathological findings. None of the studied LP patients were on systemic immunosuppressive treatment including glucocorticoids. All patients had an extensive clinical manifestation of LP with either severe widespread skin involvement (Patient 1) or chronic recalcitrant oral involvement (Patients 2–5) which did not sufficiently respond to standard medical care, i.e., topical and systemic glucocorticoids (**Table 1**).

Secukinumab, ustekinumab, and guselkumab are approved for the treatment of psoriasis and were administered according to the guidelines for psoriasis treatment (10–12) for at least 12 weeks (**Table 1**). LP skin lesions were initially treated with a short course of topical glucocorticoids for up to 7 days followed by plain emollients. Oral LP lesions were only treated with rinsing solutions containing antiseptics and local anesthetics. Off-label treatment with secukinumab, ustekinumab, and guselkumab, respectively, was covered by a compassionate use program aimed at identifying novel effective treatment options in refractory LP and did not require formal approval by the local ethics committee. The clinical course of the patients was assessed by the Autoimmune Bullous Skin Disorder Intensity Score (ABSIS) (13) which reflects both extent and severity of disease and functional sequelae of oral involvement.

Punch biopsies from lesional and post-lesional skin were obtained from patient 1–4 before and at week 12 of treatment which were fixed in paraformaldehyde, embedded in paraffin, and further processed for immunohistochemical analysis of the inflammatory infiltrate as recently described (5). Peripheral blood mononuclear cells of the patients were isolated from citrate-phosphate-dextrose-adenine (CPDA)-treated blood samples and stored in liquid nitrogen as previously described (5). The cytokine profile of peripheral blood T cells was determined by flow cytometry and/or ELISpot assay.

Immunohistochemical Analysis

Punch biopsies from lesional and post-lesional mucosa or skin were obtained from patients 1–4 before treatment and at week 12. A biopsy was further obtained at week 32 from the oral mucosa of patient four. Biopsies were fixed in paraformaldehyde, embedded in paraffin, and further processed for immunohistochemical analysis of the inflammatory infiltrate as recently described (5). Paraffin skin sections were processed by the automated IHC stainer BOND-MAX (Leica, Wetzlar, Germany) and Autostainer Plus automated immunostaining device (Dako, Hamburg, Germany), utilizing the following primary antibodies: mouse anti-human CD3, CD4, CD8 (all Novocastra, Leica, Wetzlar Germany); rabbit anti-human IL-17A, rabbit anti-human FoxP3 (both Novus, Littleton, Co, USA); rabbit anti-human T-bet, rabbit anti-human GATA-3 (both Cell Signaling Technology, Danvers, MA, USA). Secondary antibodies used were: Bond Polymer Refine Detection Kit (Leica, Wetzlar Germany; CD3, CD4, CD8); biotinylated anti-rabbit IgG, biotinylated anti-mouse IgG (Vector Laboratories; Burlingame, CA, USA; IL-17A, FoxP3, T-bet, GATA-3). Antibodies of Vector Laboratories were subsequently detected by peroxidase- or alkaline phosphatase-labeled ABC-systems (Dako). Visualization was carried out using 3,3′-diaminobenzide (DAB) or Liquid Permanent Red staining (both from Dako) as chromogenes. The T cell infiltrate of skin lesions was quantified based on microscopical images (Axiostar, Zeiss, Jena, Germany) in combination with Cell^D (Soft Imaging System, Berlin, Germany) and ImageJ software (**Figure S1**). At 100x magnification, $CD3^+$, $CD4^+$, $CD8^+$, and IL-$17A^+$ T cells were counted (200x magnification for $CD3^+$/T-bet^+ and $CD4^+$/GATA-3^+ T cells). After generating a grid (ImageJ software; area per point: 50.000 pixels^2), all stained T cells were counted in two squares (four squares for $CD3^+$/T-bet^+ and $CD4^+$/GATA-3^+ T cells) adjacent to basal membrane zone (ImageJ, cell counter; **Figure S1**) and their proportion of all infiltrating cells was determined afterwards. Moreover, with regard to IL-$17A^+$ T cells, the T cellular

TABLE 1 | Synopsis of studied lichen planus patients.

P	Sex (m/f)	Age (y)	Clinical phenotype	Disease duration	Study drug	Treatment and observation period	Previous treatment
1	f	25	Disseminated cutaneous polygonal papules on the trunk and extremities, extensive erosions of the oral, and vaginal mucosa	3 months	Secukinumab 300 mg s.c. at weeks 0,1,2,3,4 followed by monthly treatment	12 weeks	none
2	f	56	Palmoplantar confluent polygonal papules and plaques, moderate erosions of the oral mucosa	6 months	Secukinumab 300 mg s.c. at weeks 0,1,2,3,4 followed by monthly treatment	12 weeks	Topical corticosteroids
3	f	58	Extensive erosions of the gingivae, tongue, buccal mucosa, and the palatine	7 years	Secukinumab 300 mg s.c. at weeks 0,1,2,3,4 followed by monthly treatment	48 weeks (ongoing)	Ciclosporin, systemic and topical corticosteroids, acitretin, intravenous immunoglobulins
4	f	72	Extensive erosions of the oral mucosa, pronounced painful, and recalcitrant ulcerations of the tongue and gingivae	6 years	Ustekinumab 45 mg s.c. at weeks 0 and 4 and every 3 months thereafter	48 weeks (ongoing)	Ciclosporin, systemic and topical corticosteroids, acitretin, azathioprine
5	f	72	Recalcitrant ulcerations of the tongue	5 years	Guselkumab 100 mg s.c. at weeks 0 and 4 and every 2 months thereafter	30 weeks (ongoing)	Systemic and topical corticosteroids

infiltrate adjacent to the dermal-epidermal BMZ was further analyzed on images taken at 200x magnification and after grid formation (ImageJ software; area per point: 50.000 pixels^2) counting four squares in the basal membrane zone and dermal region (ImageJ, cell counter).

Multiplex Immunohistochemistry Staining

Sections were prepared from a paraffin-embedded biopsy of the oral mucosa of patient 5 which showed the same characteristics with a lichenoid mixed $CD4^+$ and $CD8^+$ cellular infiltrate as in the other patients. This patient biopsy was chosen because it provided enough material to establish a more refined IF analysis. The Opal multiplex staining utilizes individual TSA conjugated fluorophores to detect multiple targets (Opal 7-Color Manual IHC Kit, Catalog No. NEL811001KT). Firstly, sections were deparaffinized and fixed in 10% neutral buffered formalin prior to antigen retrieval in heated AR6 buffer for 15 min (EZ Retriever microwave, BioGenex). Each section was put through three sequential rounds of staining, each including a protein block with Opal blocking buffer followed by primary antibody incubation overnight (CD4: 1:100, Abcam; CD8: 1:50, Novus Biologicals; and IL−17: 1:200, R&D) and corresponding secondary horseradish peroxidase-conjugated polymer and Opal fluorophores- CD4 (Opal 620), CD8 (Opal 690), and IL17 (Opal 540). Additionally, DAPI was applied as a nuclear marker. To visualize the location of CD4 and CD8 cells (with IL-17 positive or negative), phenotyping maps were generated based on the aforementioned markers and inform machine-learning algorithms. Furthermore, to create classic pathology views, simulated IHC staining images indicating CD4, CD8, and IL17 expression were generated.

Blood Cell Isolation

Peripheral blood mononuclear cells of the patients were isolated from citrate-phosphate-dextrose-adenine (CPDA)-treated blood samples and stored in liquid nitrogen as previously described (5).

Flow Cytometric Analysis of Peripheral Blood Lymphocyte Subsets

After thawing, cells were cultured overnight in RPMI-1640 in RPMI-1640 supplemented with 100 U/ml penicillin, 100 µg/ml streptomycin and 2 mM L-glutamine (all Capricorn, Ebsdorfergrund, Germany) and 10% FCS (Merck Millipore, Berlin, Germany). For detection of leukocyte subsets, cells were stained with the following antibodies: mouse anti-human CD45-AlexaFluor700 (2D1), mouse anti-human CD4-BrilliantViolet510 (RPA-T4; both BioLegend, San Diego, CA, USA), mouse anti-human CD3-PE (UCHT1), mouse anti-human CD8-FITC (SK1), mouse anti-human CD19-PerCP-Cy5.5 (HIB19), mouse anti-human CD14-APC (M5E2; all BD Biosciences, Heidelberg, Germany).

For cytokine detection, cells were stimulated *ex vivo* with 5 ng/mL phorbol myristate acetate (PMA; Promega, Fitchburg, MA, USA) and 500 ng/mL ionomycin (Calbiochem, Billerica, MA, USA) for 5 h at 37°C with addition of GolgiStop (BD Biosciences, Heidelberg, Germany) to block cytokine secretion. Subsequently, cell surface markers were stained using the following antibodies: mouse anti-human CD45-AlexaFluor700 (2D1; BioLegend, San Diego, CA, USA), mouse anti-human CD3-PE-Cy5.5 (SK7; ThermoFisherScientific, Langenselbold, Germany), mouse anti-human CD8-FITC (SK1; BD Biosciences, Heidelberg).

Intracellular cytokines were detected using mouse anti-human IFN-γ-AlexaFluor647 (B27), mouse anti-human IL-21-PE (3A3-N2.1), mouse anti-human IL-17A-AlexaFluor647 (N49-653; all BD Biosciences, Heidelberg, Germany). Cells were acquired on a BD LSRFortessa (BD Biosciences, Heidelberg, Germany) and cell doublets were discriminated by FSC-H/FSC-A plots (**Figures S2, S3**). Dead cells were excluded from analysis using Zombie NIR staining (BioLegend, San Diego, CA, USA). Data was analyzed by BD FACSDiva Software 8.0.2 (BD Biosciences, Heidelberg, Germany).

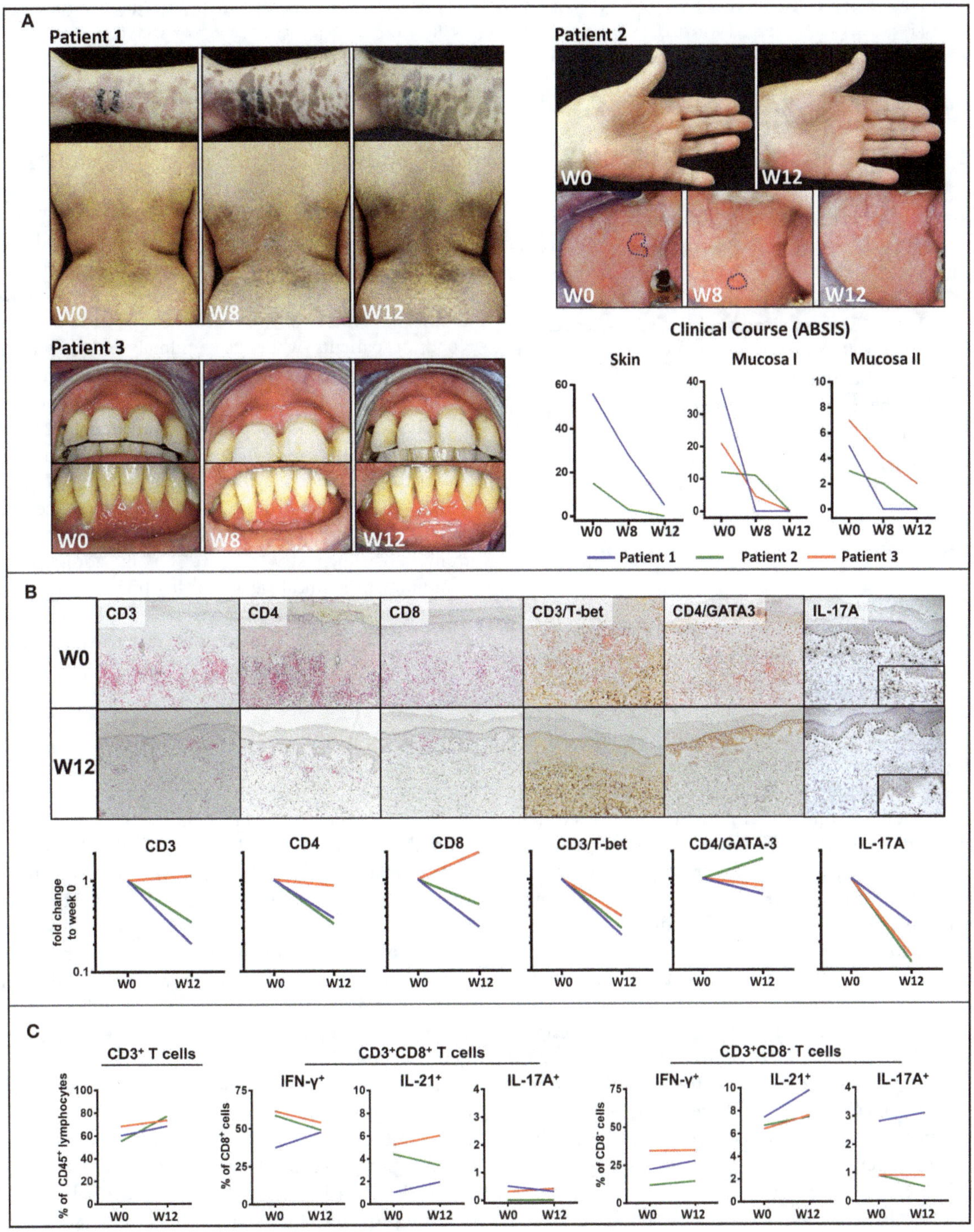

FIGURE 1 | Clinical and immunological response to treatment with the anti-IL-17 monoclonal antibody, secukinumab, in mucocutaneous lichen planus (LP). **(A)** Clinical appearance of three LP patients before (week 0; W0) and on treatment (W8, W12) with secukinumab. Patients 1 and 2 presented with muco-cutanous lesions while patient three had a recalcitrant LP of the oral mucosa unresponsive to systemic immunosuppressive treatment. Blockade of IL-17A led to a shift from erythematous inflammatory to hyperpigmented post-inflammatory skin lesions and an almost complete disappearance of the mucosal lesions by W12. Clinical course was assessed by the Autoimmune Bullous Skin Disorder Intensity Score (ABSIS) showing a marked decrease of cutaneous lesions (ABSIS Skin), mucosal lesions (ABSIS Mucosa I), and substantial improvement of the patients' ability to eat defined foods of increasing consistency without pain and/or bleeding (ABSIS Mucosa II). **(B)** Immunohistochemical analysis of the inflammatory skin infiltrate before (W0) and after 12 weeks (W12) of treatment (representative images of patient 1 are shown). Markers as below: CD3/CD4/CD8 (liquid permanent red), T-bet/GATA3/IL-17 (3,3′ diaminobenzide brown). The dermal, band-like $CD4^{+}$ and $CD8^{+}$ T cellular infiltrate was strongly reduced at W12 of secukinumab treatment compared to W0. Of note, blockade of IL-17A led to a marked decrease of both IL-$17A^{+}$ and $CD4^{+}$/T-bet^{+}

(Continued)

FIGURE 1 | (Th1) cells in the LP lesions (see **Figure S1** in the supplement for description of image quantification). **(C)** Flow cytometric analysis of peripheral blood CD8$^+$ and CD4$^+$ (defined as CD8$^-$) T cells in the three LP patients before (W0) and at W12 of treatment. In contrast to skin lesions, the number of CD3$^+$, IFNγ^+ (Th1), and IL-17A$^+$ peripheral blood T cells remained largely unaffected by blockade of IL-17A. Notably, peripheral blood IL-21$^+$ T cells were increased in all the three LP patients (see **Figure S2** and **Table S1** in the supplement for gating strategy and raw data).

Enzyme-Linked Immunospot (ELISpot) Assay of Peripheral Blood Lymphocytes

ELISpot assays were performed as previously described (5). IFNγ-, IL-5- and IL-17A- positive spots were detected according to the manufacturers' instructions (Human IFNγ-ELISpot, Human IL-5-ELISpot, Becton Dickinson, Franklin Lakes, NJ, USA; Human IL-17A ELISpot Ready-Set-Go, eBioscience, San Diego, CA, USA). PBMC were seeded at 1×10^5 – 5×10^5 cells per well on the ELISpot plates and developed plates were finally analyzed by the ELISpot plate reader A.EL.VIS (A.EL.VIS, Hanover, Germany). For data analysis, the spots of the non-stimulated controls (mean) were subtracted from the spots (mean) of the cultures with antigen (all in duplicate).

RESULTS

Two patients with extensive cutaneous LP and oral lesions (Patient 1 and 2), respectively, showed rapid clinical improvement on treatment with secukinumab which became apparent by a shift from inflammatory erythematous to post-inflammatory hyperpigmented skin lesions and a regression of oral lesions within 12 weeks (**Figure 1A**). Moreover, the patient with recalcitrant LP of both the oral mucosa and the tongue (Patient 3) experienced resolution of buccal lesions and lasting improvement of the recalcitrant ulcerative lesions of the tongue upon treatment with secukinumab (**Figure 1A**). Eventually, lesions of both upper and lower gingiva fully resolved upon long-term follow-up after 48 weeks (**Figure S4A**). Clinical improvement was reflected by a substantial decrease of ABSIS Skin and ABSIS Mucosa I scores as well as an improvement of functional sequelae of oral involvement (ABSIS Mucosa II). Within 12 weeks, there was a marked reduction of the CD4$^+$ and CD8$^+$ T cellular skin infiltrate within LP lesions, in particular of Th1 (CD3$^+$Tbet$^+$) cells (**Figure 1B**). IL-17A$^+$ T cells, which initially lined up along the dermal-epidermal BMZ, were only sparsely found after 12 weeks of secukinumab treatment (**Figure 1B**). In contrast, secukinumab did not induce major alterations of peripheral blood T cell subsets except for an increase of CD4$^+$IL-21$^+$ T cells (**Figure 1C**).

Treatment with the anti-p40 monoclonal antibody, ustekinumab of a patient with recalcitrant ulcerative oral LP (Patient 4) led to dramatic clinical improvement within 12 weeks (**Figure 2A**). The buccal lesions fully resolved and the number and size of lesions of the tongue were markedly reduced which was also reflected by improved ABSIS Mucosa I and II scores. The inflammatory cutaneous T cell infiltrate which was mainly composed of Th1 (CD3$^+$T-bet$^+$) and IL-17A$^+$ T cells markedly (Th1) or completely (IL-17A$^+$) resolved within 12 weeks of ustekinumab treatment (**Figure 2B**). On long term follow up, the ulcerative lesions of the tongue and mucosal lesions of the oral region completely fully resolved by week 48 (**Figure S4B**). In contrast to secukinumab, treatment with ustekinumab resulted in a strong reduction of peripheral blood IL-17A$^+$ as well as IL-21$^+$ T cells (**Figure 2C**). Overall, secukinumab and ustekinumab treatment had no major impact on other peripheral blood leukocyte subsets (**Figure S5**). Noteworthy, secukinumab did not inhibit the number of IL-17-producing T cells in the peripheral blood of patients while ustekinumab induced a continuous decline of IL-17-secreting T cells during treatment (**Figure S6**). Moreover, treatment of a patient with recalcitrant erosive and ulcerative LP of the tongue with the anti-IL-23 monoclonal antibody guselkumab (Patient 5) led to a constant amelioration of oral erosions which fully resolved by week 30 (**Figure 3A**).

To further determine the cellular source of IL-17A in the lesional skin of LP, we performed multiplex immunohistochemistry (**Figure 3C**) in addition to regular immunohistochemical analysis in this patient (**Figure 3B**). We here identified several positive Il-17$^+$ T cells within both, the CD4$^+$ and CD8$^+$ T cell infiltrate, in support of a mixed Th17/Tc17 infiltrate in LP lesions (**Figure 3C**).

DISCUSSION

We here show for the first time that therapeutic targeting of Th17/Tc17 cells either by blocking IL-17A with the monoclonal antibody, secukinumab, or by inhibiting the Th17/Tc17 axis with ustekinumab (anti-IL-12/IL-23) or with guselkumab (anti-IL-23) leads to a marked and prolonged improvement of mucosal and cutaneous lesions in LP. This finding is a major therapeutic advance in LP which often shows a chronic, refractory course and has a major impact on the patients' quality of life (1). Blockade of IL-17 and inhibition of Th17/Tc17 cell expansion was equally effective in reducing mucosal and cutaneous LP lesions. Thus, Th17/Tc17 cells and T cell-derived IL-17A are presumably important for disease induction and probably also for the perpetuation of the inflammatory response in LP. The concept that Th17/Tc17 cells are the major source of IL-17 in LP is supported by the finding that (1) CD4$^+$/IL-17$^+$ and CD8$^+$/IL17$^+$ cells line up along the dermal-epidermal BMZ in close proximity to apoptotic epidermal keratinocytes (5), a hallmark of LP, (2) neutrophils are virtually absent in LP, and (3) $\gamma\delta$-T cells have been only occasionally and inconsistently described in LP skin lesions and lesion-derived T cell lines (14, 15). However, other cell populations that can produce IL-17 (e.g., NK cells, NKT cells, and $\gamma\delta$ T cells), which were not analyzed in this study, may also be a source of IL-17. However, using multiplex immunohistochemistry we mainly observed CD4$^+$ or CD8$^+$ IL-17A-producing T cells pointing toward an implication of Th17 and Tc17 in LP pathogenesis (**Figure 3C**). Thus, based on these findings, we here specifically addressed the potential role of

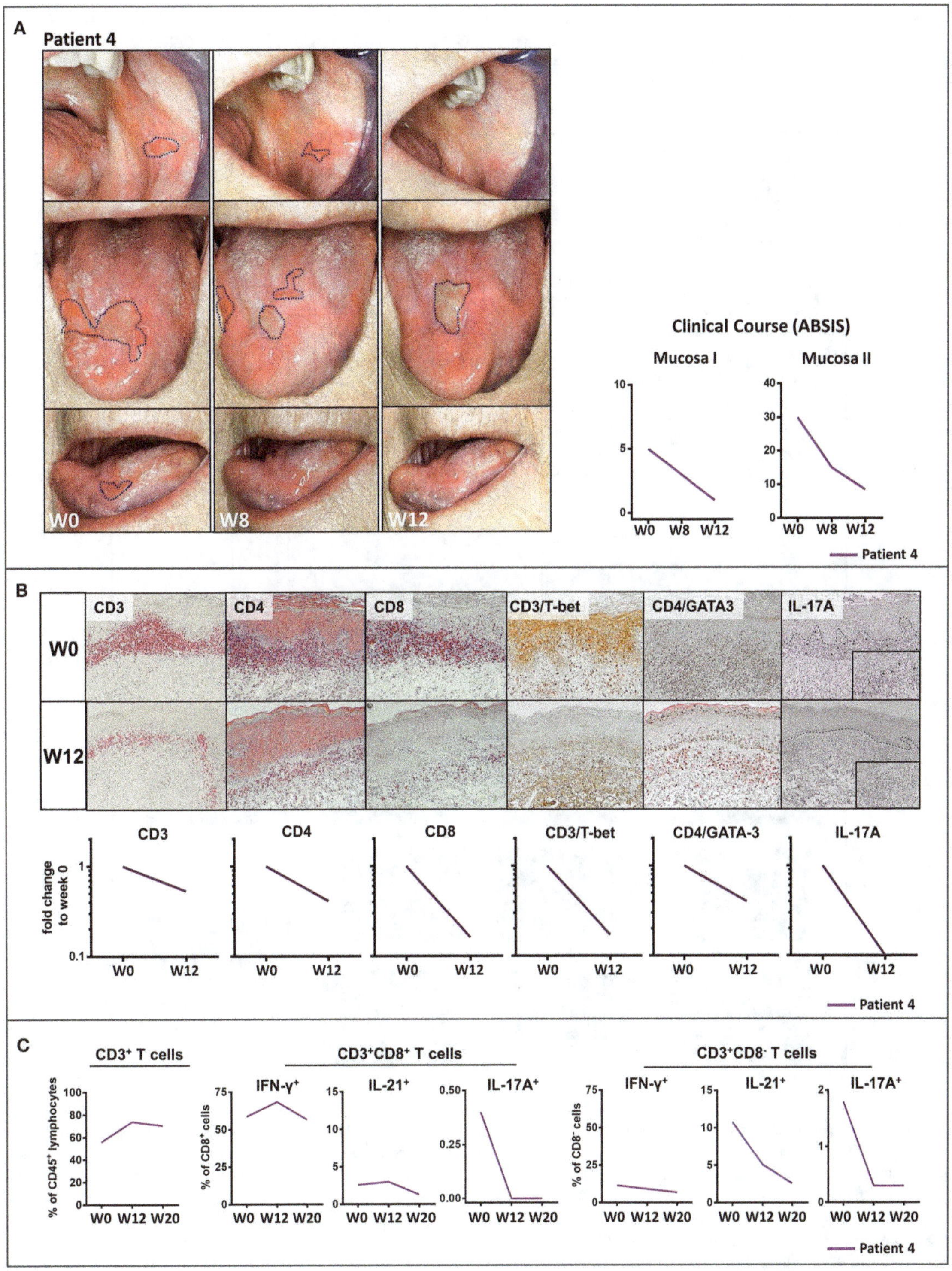

FIGURE 2 | Clinical and immunological response to treatment with the anti- IL-12/IL-23 monoclonal antibody, ustekinumab, patient 4 with recalcitrant oral lichen planus (OLP). **(A)** Clinical appearance before (week 0, W0) and at W8 and W12 of treatment with ustekinumab showing a striking clinical improvement of mucosal lesions by W8 and W12. The clinical course was characterized by a marked reduction of mucosal lesions (ABSIS Mucosa I) and a substantial improvement of the patient's ability to eat defined foods of different consistency without pain and/or bleeding (ABSIS Mucosa II). **(B)** Immunohistochemical analysis of inflammatory mucosal infiltrate before (W0) and at W12 of treatment with ustekinumab. Markers as below: CD3/CD4/CD8 (liquid permanent red), T-bet/GATA3/IL-17 (3,3' diaminobenzide brown). At W12, IL-17A$^+$ cells were completely absent and the CD4$^+$T-bet$^+$ (Th1) cell infiltrate was strongly diminished (see **Figure S1** for

(Continued)

FIGURE 2 | description of image quantification). **(C)** Flow cytometric analysis of peripheral blood $CD8^+$ and $CD4^+$ (defined as $CD8^-$) T cells before (W0) and at W12 and W20 of ustekinumab treatment. While peripheral blood $CD3^+$ T cells were not impaired, blockade of IL-12/IL-23 led to a strong decrease of peripheral blood IL-$17A^+$ and IL-21^+ T cells (see **Figure S3** and **Table S1** in the supplement for gating strategy and raw data).

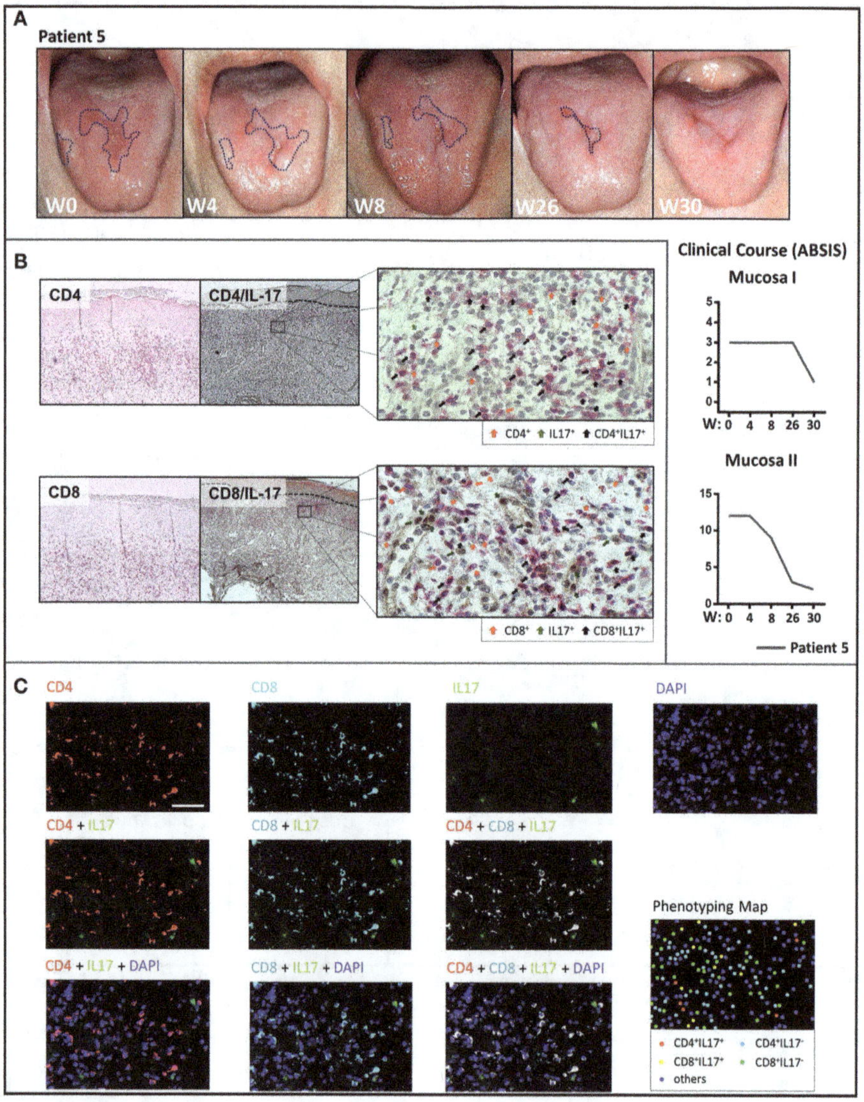

FIGURE 3 | Clinical response of oral lichen planus to treatment with guselkumab and phenotypical analysis of the T cell infiltrate by immunohistochemistry and multiplex immunohistochemistry. **(A)** Clinical appearance of the oral mucosa with marked ulcerative lesions (dotted blue line) of patient 5 on treatment with guselkumab before treatment at week 0 (W0) and at W4, W8, W26, and W30 with the clinical course assessed by ABSIS score. There is a complete resolution of the ulcerative lesions of the tongue by W30. **(B)** Immunohistochemical staining for CD4, CD8, and IL-17 before treatment with guselkumab. Single staining with $CD4^+$, $CD8^+$ (red), and IL-17 (green) as well as double positive-staining of $CD4^+$ or $CD8^+$ T cells with IL-17 (black) are highlighted by arrows. **(C)** Multiplexed immunohistochemistry images of skin lesions showing each of the individual markers in the composite image after spectral unmixing. Markers are as below: CD4 (Opal 620, pseudocoloured red), CD8 (Opal 690, pseudocoloured cyan), IL−17 (Opal 540, pseudocoloured green), and DAPI as a nuclear marker (blue) (upper row), Multiplexed immunohistochemistry images of CD4 or/and CD8 staining merged with IL-17 (middle row). Multiplexed immunohistochemistry images of CD4 or/and CD8 along with IL-17 merged with DAPI (lower row). The cell phenotyping map identifies $CD4^+IL17^+$ cells (red dots), $CD8^+IL17^+$ cells (yellow dots), $CD4^+IL17^-$ cells (cyan dots), $CD8^+IL17^-$ cells (green dots), and other cells (blue dots).

$IL17^+$ T cells in LP pathogenesis and the impact of therapeutic targeting of Th17/Tc17 cells.

Secukinumab, ustekinumab, and guselkumab were chosen for compassionate use in the studied patients with extensive or recalcitrant LP because they are licensed for the treatment of the Th17-associated inflammatory disorders, psoriasis vulgaris, psoriatic arthritis and Crohn's disease (16, 17). Th17 blockade also holds promise in the treatment of multiple sclerosis and rheumatoid arthritis (18), which are also strongly linked to a Th17-dependent pathogenesis.

A pathogenetic role of IL17 in LP had been previously suggested by several independent studies based on the detection of elevated serum concentrations of IL-17 and increased numbers of peripheral and lesional Th17 cells in patients with mucocutaneous and oral LP (7–9). Furthermore, the Th17-derived cytokines, IL-21, IL-22, and IL-23 were found to be upregulated in LP lesions (6, 7) Furthermore, also serum levels of IL17A seem to be upregulated in patients with LP (19). Recently, we showed that patients with LP have autoreactive peripheral blood Th17 cell responses against bullous pemphigoid (BP) 180, the autoantigen of BP (5). BP is considered as a mainly Th2-driven, IgG-mediated autoimmune disorder against the hemidesmosomal component, BP180, and presents with a Th2-dominated inflammatory skin infiltrate. In contrast, patients with LP showed a pronounced Th1/Th17-dominated infiltrate in LP lesions and peripheral blood autoreactive Th1/Th17 cells (5).

Th17 cells are characterized by the expression of the transcription factor, RORγt, and secretion of the signature cytokine IL-17A and other Th17-derived cytokines such as IL-17F, IL-21, and IL-22 (20). Based on the cellular and immunological context, Th17 cells display a great degree of plasticity (20, 21). Under non-pathogenic conditions, Th17 contribute to proper epithelial barrier function and the defense of fungal (Candida) or bacterial (staphylococci) pathogens (20, 22). Under pro-inflammatory conditions, Th17 cells can trans-differentiate into anti-inflammatory T regulatory type 1 (Tr1) cells in the intestine (23) whereas in experimental models of inflammatory bowel disease and multiple sclerosis, Th17 cells have been shown to also promote pro-inflammatory pathogenic immune responses by gaining IFN-γ and/or GM-CSF production (20, 24). Moreover, Th17 cell-derived IL-17 induces, in concert with IL-6 and TGF-β, a positive feedback loop that further drives Th17 cell expansion (25). Of note, pathogenic Th17 and presumably also Tc17 cells can rapidly transform into IFN-γ-secreting non-classical Th1 cells (26–28). Thus, the Th1-dominated T cellular infiltrate in LP may be at least partly Th17/Tc17 cell-derived which is supported by the marked decrease not only of Th17 but also Th1 cells in LP lesions after IL-17A blockade by secukinumab (**Figure 1B**). Blockade of IL-17 may prevent the transformation of pathogenic Th17 cell-derived non-classical Th1 cells. Accordingly, direct blockade of the Th17/Tc17 cell-axis with ustekinumab (anti-IL-12/IL-23) in a patient with refractory oral LP was not only linked to the disappearance of Th17 cells in LP lesions but also to a marked reduction of the lesional Th1 infiltrate (**Figure 2B**). IL-23 has been described as one of the key drivers of pro-inflammatory pathogenic Th17 cells mainly via induction of the B lymphocyte-induced maturation protein 1 (BLIMP1) (29, 30). Treatment with ustekinumab and guselkumab might therefore be more effective than secukinumab in suppressing Th17/Tc17 and, consecutively, Th1 cells in LP. In fact, in experimental Th17 cell-driven colitis blockade of IL-23 was shown to be superior in down-regulating inflammation than inhibition of soluble IL-17 (31).

Our observations strongly suggest that IL-17 is a critical cytokine in the immune pathogenesis of LP and thus represents a major therapeutic target. Under inflammatory conditions, IL-17 induces chemokine release from various cell types of the skin, including endothelial cells, macrophages, and keratinocytes leading to tissue remodeling and the recruitment of pro-inflammatory effector cells in the skin (32, 33). In LP, IL-17 release in the skin could facilitate initiation of a pro-inflammatory cascade leading to recruitment of T cells which are critical in the pathogenesis of LP. The fact that IL-17 blockade with secukinumab did not show systemic suppressive effect on peripheral Th17/Tc17 cells (**Figure 1C**) while suppressing the T cellular skin infiltrate further supports a pathogenic role of IL-17 in LP lesions. Instead, there was an increase of IL-17-secreting peripheral blood T cells in two patients (**Figure S6**) and a slight increase of peripheral blood $CD4^+$ T cells producing IL-21 (**Figure 1C**), an essential inducer of IL-17 secretion which is presumably a compensatory mechanism for loss of secreted IL-17. In contrast, ustekinumab treatment led to a marked reduction not only of peripheral blood Th17/Tc17 cells but also of Th1 cells (**Figure 2C**).

In summary, we demonstrate for the first time that therapeutic targeting of Th17/Tc17 cells in LP either by blocking IL17A with the anti-IL-17 monoclonal antibody, secukinumab, or by inhibiting the Th17/Tc17 axis with ustekinumab (anti-IL-12/IL-23) or guselkumab (anti-IL-23), leads to a dramatic and prolonged improvement of mucosal and cutaneous lesions in five patients with recalcitrant LP. Our observations strongly suggest a crucial role Th17/Tc17 cells in LP pathogenesis and provides novel therapeutic targets for therapeutic control of this chronic refractory skin disorder.

ETHICS STATEMENT

Compassionate use of specific drugs are warranted in Germany for treatment of up to three patients who have not shown sufficient responses of their disease to approved drugs or with contraindications to treatment with a approved drug. This was the case in the described patients with muco-cutaneous lichen planus. Prior to treatment of the patients with either secukinumab, ustekinumab, or guselkumab. The head of the local ethics committee at Marburg University confirmed that compassionate treatment of these patients with secukinumab, ustekinumab, or guselkumab did not require formal approval by the ethics committee as long as treatment was restricted to a total of three patients for each drug. The patients were explained in detail why we considered compassionate use of these drugs in their situation and they fully approved of this. This entire process was thoroughly documented in the patients' charts.

AUTHOR CONTRIBUTIONS

MH, FS, RP, and TS: study concept and design. XZ and RS: multiplexed immunohistochemistry staining and analysis. RP, FS, and MH: drafting of the manuscript. RP: statistical analysis. AS, SM, JP, VE, and CM: administrative, technical, or material support. MH: study supervision. All authors: acquisition, analysis, and interpretation of data and critical revision of the manuscript for important intellectual content.

ACKNOWLEDGMENTS

We thank the patients for participating in the compassionate use trial with secukinumab, ustekinumab, and guselkumab. We are grateful to Manuel Schulze-Dasbeck, Elke Hermann, and Viktoria Wischmann for excellent technical assistance. We thank Dr. Magdalena Huber for critical reading of the manuscript and helpful discussions.

REFERENCES

1. Le Cleach L, Chosidow O. Clinical practice. Lichen planus. *N Engl J Med.* (2012) 366:723–32. doi: 10.1056/NEJMcp1103641
2. Lehman JS, Tollefson MM, Gibson LE. Lichen planus. *Int J Dermatol.* (2009) 48:682–94. doi: 10.1111/j.1365-4632.2009.04062.x
3. Wagner G, Rose C, Sachse MM. Clinical variants of lichen planus. *J Dtsch Dermatol Ges.* (2013) 11:309–19. doi: 10.1111/ddg.12031
4. Meinhard J, Stroux A, Lünnemann L, Vogt A, Blume-Peytavi U. Lichen planopilaris: epidemiology and prevalence of subtypes - a retrospective analysis in 104 patients. *J Dtsch Dermatol Ges.* (2014) 12:229–35; 229–36. doi: 10.1111/ddg.12264
5. Schmidt T, Solimani F, Pollmann R, Stein R, Schmidt A, Stulberg I, et al. TH1/TH17 cell recognition of desmoglein 3 and bullous pemphigoid antigen 180 in patients with lichen planus. *J Allergy Clin Immunol.* (2018) 142:669–72.e7. doi: 10.1016/j.jaci.2018.02.044
6. Lu R, Zeng X, Han Q, Lin M, Long L, Dan H, et al. Overexpression and selectively regulatory roles of IL-23/IL-17 axis in the lesions of oral lichen planus. *Mediat Inflamm.* (2014) 2014:701094. doi: 10.1155/2014/701094
7. Piccinni M-P, Lombardelli L, Logiodice F, Tesi D, Kullolli O, Biagiotti R, et al. Potential pathogenetic role of Th17, Th0, and Th2 cells in erosive and reticular oral lichen planus. *Oral Dis.* (2014) 20:212–8. doi: 10.1111/odi.12094
8. Shaker O, Hassan AS. Possible role of interleukin-17 in the pathogenesis of lichen planus. *Br J Dermatol.* (2012) 166:1367–8. doi: 10.1111/j.1365-2133.2011.10793.x
9. Wang H, Han Q, Luo Z, Xu C, Liu J, Dan H, et al. Oral lichen planus may enhance the expression of Th17-associated cytokines in local lesions of chronic periodontitis. *Clin Oral Investig.* (2014) 18:1647–54. doi: 10.1007/s00784-013-1131-z
10. Nast A, Gisondi P, Ormerod AD, Saiag P, Smith C, Spuls PI, et al. European S3-Guidelines on the systemic treatment of psoriasis vulgaris–Update 2015–Short version–EDF in cooperation with EADV and IPC. *J Eur Acad Dermatol Venereol.* (2015) 29:2277–94. doi: 10.1111/jdv.13354
11. Nast A, Spuls PI, van der Kraaij G, Gisondi P, Paul C, Ormerod AD, et al. European S3-Guideline on the systemic treatment of psoriasis vulgaris—Update Apremilast and Secukinumab—EDF in cooperation with EADV and IPC. *J Eur Acad Dermatol Venereol.* (2017) 31:1951–63. doi: 10.1111/jdv.14454
12. Terui T, Kobayashi S, Okubo Y, Murakami M, Hirose K, Kubo H. Efficacy and safety of Guselkumab, an anti-interleukin 23 monoclonal antibody, for palmoplantar pustulosis: a randomized clinical trial. *JAMA Dermatol.* (2018) 154:309–16. doi: 10.1001/jamadermatol.2017.5937
13. Pfütze M, Niedermeier A, Hertl M, Eming R. Introducing a novel autoimmune bullous skin disorder intensity score (ABSIS) in pemphigus. *Eur J Dermatol.* (2007) 17:4–11. doi: 10.1684/ejd.2007.0090
14. Alaibac M, Morris J, Yu R, Chu AC. T lymphocytes bearing the gamma delta T-cell receptor: a study in normal human skin and pathological skin conditions. *Br J Dermatol.* (1992) 127:458–62. doi: 10.1111/j.1365-2133.1992.tb14840.x
15. Gadenne AS, Strucke R, Dunn D, Wagner M, Bleicher P, Bigby M. T-cell lines derived from lesional skin of lichen planus patients contain a distinctive population of T-cell receptor gamma delta-bearing cells. *J Invest Dermatol.* (1994) 103:347–51. doi: 10.1111/1523-1747.ep12394904
16. Feagan BG, Sandborn WJ, Gasink C, Jacobstein D, Lang Y, Friedman JR, et al. Ustekinumab as induction and maintenance therapy for Crohn's disease. *N Engl J Med.* (2016) 375:1946–60. doi: 10.1056/NEJMoa1602773
17. Langley RG, Elewski BE, Lebwohl M, Reich K, Griffiths CE, Papp K, et al. Secukinumab in plaque psoriasis–results of two phase 3 trials. *N Engl J Med.* (2014) 371:326–38. doi: 10.1056/NEJMoa1314258
18. Kotake S, Nanke Y, Yago T, Kawamoto M, Kobashigawa T, Yamanaka H. Elevated ratio of Th17 cell-derived Th1 cells (CD161(+)Th1 Cells) to CD161(+)Th17 cells in peripheral blood of early-onset rheumatoid arthritis patients. *Biomed Res Int.* (2016) 2016:4186027. doi: 10.1155/2016/4186027
19. Gueiros LA, Arão T, Souza T, Vieira CL, Gomez RS, Almeida OP, et al. IL17A polymorphism and elevated IL17A serum levels are associated with oral lichen planus. *Oral Dis.* (2018) 24:377–83. doi: 10.1111/odi.12718
20. Stockinger B, Omenetti S. The dichotomous nature of T helper 17 cells. *Nat Rev Immunol.* (2017) 17:535–44. doi: 10.1038/nri.2017.50
21. Ghoreschi K, Laurence A, Yang X-P, Tato CM, McGeachy MJ, Konkel JE, et al. Generation of pathogenic T(H)17 cells in the absence of TGF-β signalling. *Nature.* (2010) 467:967–71. doi: 10.1038/nature09447
22. Eyerich K, Dimartino V, Cavani A. IL-17 and IL-22 in immunity: driving protection and pathology. *Eur J Immunol.* (2017) 47:607–14. doi: 10.1002/eji.201646723
23. Gagliani N, Amezcua Vesely MC, Iseppon A, Brockmann L, Xu H, Palm NW, et al. Th17 cells transdifferentiate into regulatory T cells during resolution of inflammation. *Nature.* (2015) 523:221–5. doi: 10.1038/nature14452
24. Feng T, Qin H, Wang L, Benveniste EN, Elson CO, Cong Y. Th17 cells induce colitis and promote Th1 cell responses through IL-17 induction of innate IL-12 and IL-23 production. *J Immunol.* (2011) 186:6313–8. doi: 10.4049/jimmunol.1001454
25. Ogura H, Murakami M, Okuyama Y, Tsuruoka M, Kitabayashi C, Kanamoto M, et al. Interleukin-17 promotes autoimmunity by triggering a positive-feedback loop via interleukin-6 induction. *Immunity.* (2008) 29:628–36. doi: 10.1016/j.immuni.2008.07.018
26. Cosmi L, Liotta F, Maggi E, Romagnani S, Annunziato F. Th17 and non-classic Th1 cells in chronic inflammatory disorders: two sides of the same coin. *Int Arch Allergy Immunol.* (2014) 164:171–7. doi: 10.1159/000363502
27. Harbour SN, Maynard CL, Zindl CL, Schoeb TR, Weaver CT. Th17 cells give rise to Th1 cells that are required for the pathogenesis of colitis. *Proc Natl Acad Sci USA.* (2015) 112:7061–6. doi: 10.1073/pnas.1415675112
28. Maggi L, Santarlasci V, Capone M, Rossi MC, Querci V, Mazzoni A, et al. Distinctive features of classic and nonclassic (Th17 derived) human Th1 cells. *Eur J Immunol.* (2012) 42:3180–8. doi: 10.1002/eji.201242648
29. Langrish CL, Chen Y, Blumenschein WM, Mattson J, Basham B, Sedgwick JD, et al. IL-23 drives a pathogenic T cell population that induces autoimmune inflammation. *J Exp Med.* (2005) 201:233–40. doi: 10.1084/jem.20041257
30. McGeachy MJ, Chen Y, Tato CM, Laurence A, Joyce-Shaikh B, Blumenschein WM, et al. The interleukin 23 receptor is essential for the terminal differentiation of interleukin 17-producing effector T helper cells *in vivo*. *Nat Immunol.* (2009) 10:314–24. doi: 10.1038/ni.1698
31. Wang R, Hasnain SZ, Tong H, Das I, Che-Hao Chen A, Oancea I, et al. Neutralizing IL-23 is superior to blocking IL-17 in suppressing intestinal inflammation in a spontaneous murine colitis model. *Inflamm Bowel Dis.* (2015) 21:973–84. doi: 10.1097/MIB.0000000000000353

32. Hirota K, Duarte JH, Veldhoen M, Hornsby E, Li Y, Cua DJ, et al. Fate mapping of IL-17-producing T cells in inflammatory responses. *Nat Immunol.* (2011) 12:255–63. doi: 10.1038/ni.1993
33. Veldhoen M. Interleukin 17 is a chief orchestrator of immunity. *Nat Immunol.* (2017) 18:612–21. doi: 10.1038/ni.3742

6

The Diagnosis and Blistering Mechanisms of Mucous Membrane Pemphigoid

Mayumi Kamaguchi[1,2] *and Hiroaki Iwata*[1*]

[1] *Department of Dermatology, Hokkaido University Graduate School of Medicine, Sapporo, Japan,* [2] *Department of Oral Diagnosis and Medicine, Hokkaido University Graduate School of Dental Medicine, Sapporo, Japan*

Correspondence:
Hiroaki Iwata
hiroaki.iwata@med.hokudai.ac.jp

Mucous membrane pemphigoid (MMP) is a mucous membrane-dominated autoimmune subepithelial blistering disease that is caused by autoantibodies against various autoantigens in basement membrane zone (BMZ) proteins, including collagen XVII (COL17). Clinicians face diagnostic problems in detecting circulating antibodies and targeted antigens in MMP. The diagnostic difficulties are mainly attributed to the low titers of MMP autoantibodies in sera and to heterogeneous autoantigens. Additionally, no unanimous diagnostic criteria have been drawn for MMP, which can result in delayed diagnoses or misdiagnoses. This review aims to integrate and present currently available data to clarify diagnostic strategies and to present diagnostic criteria for MMP. The ultimate blistering mechanism in MMP has not been elucidated, and such mechanism is especially obscure in COL17-type MMP. In bullous pemphigoid (BP), which is the most common autoimmune subepidermal blistering disease, some patients show oral lesion as well as predominant skin lesions. However, there is no fundamental explanation for the onset of oral lesions in BP. This article summarizes innovative research perspectives on the pathogenesis of oral lesions in pemphigoid. Finally, we propose a potential pathogenesis for COL17-type MMP.

Keywords: mucous membrane pemphigoid, type XVII collagen, direct immunofluorescence, collagen IV, C-terminas, steric hindrance

INTRODUCTION

Mucous membrane pemphigoid (MMP) refers to mucous membrane-dominated autoimmune subepithelial blistering diseases (1–4). MMP is caused by autoantibodies against various autoantigens in the basement membrane zone (BMZ), including collagen XVII (COL17, also called BP180) (5), BP230 (6), laminin 332 (7–9), integrin α6/β4 (10–12), and collagen VII (COL7) (13, 14). Of these, the C-terminus of COL17 and laminin 332 are thought to be major autoantigens for MMP. Autoantibodies against Integrinα 6/β4 are associated with the occurrence of ocular lesions (15). Clinically, the most common site of involvement in MMP is the oral mucosa (80–90%). Also involved are the ocular mucosa (50%), the skin (20%), the genital mucosa (15%), the anal mucosa (10%), and the pharynx, esophagus and larynx (<10%) (16). In the oral cavity, the gingiva is most commonly affected (70% of oral MMP cases), followed by the buccal mucosa (60%), the palate (27%), and the tongue and lips (13%) (17).

MMP is relatively difficult to diagnose clinically, for several reasons that are documented in the next section. One reason is that the titer of autoantibodies is lower in MMP than in bullous pemphigoid (BP) (18, 19), which is the most common autoimmune skin blistering disease (2).

Therefore, circulating autoantibodies are detected less frequently in MMP than in BP (17), which leads to challenges in diagnosing MMP.

The pathogenesis of MMP has been poorly understood to date. As for the mechanism of blister formation in autoimmune blistering disorders, the direct inhibition of protein–protein binding by autoantibodies in pemphigus (steric hindrance) (20, 21) and/or Fc-mediated complement and inflammatory cell activation in pemphigoid, including in epidermolysis bullosa acquisita, have been reported (22, 23). However, the mechanism of blister formation on the oral mucosa in pemphigoid remains undiscovered. Histologically, MMP patients tend to have fewer inflammatory findings than BP patients do (24). This may indicate differences in blistering mechanisms between MMP and BP.

This article focuses on diagnostic tips for improving the clinical diagnosis of MMP and proposes a possible pathomechanism for oral mucosa-specific blister formation that is related to less severe inflammatory mechanisms.

ISSUES IN DIAGNOSING MMP

To diagnose MMP, we perform several tests, including histological and immunological analyses. Histologically, the formation of junctional separations at the BMZ is observed in specimens from lesional mucosa (25, 26). However, histopathological examination is not always performed, particularly when the lesions are limited to the eyes due to the hesitation about performing conjunctival biopsies and the concern about scar formation. In addition, such examination does not always reveal subepithelial blisters, because of tissue destruction (27). Immunologically, the deposition of IgG autoantibodies and C3, or sometimes of IgA autoantibodies, at the BMZ can be detected by direct immunofluorescence (DIF) of lesional or perilesional samples (1, 28). To identify circulating autoantibodies to the BMZ, indirect immunofluorescence (IIF) with normal human skin as the substrate is usually performed, but autoantibodies are detected in only 17–53% of MMP cases (5, 17, 18, 29). According to the latest data from our hospital, in 22% (8/36) of cases, MMP autoantibodies (IgG) are detected by IIF with normal human skin. 1 M NaCl-split skin IIF (ssIIF) is more sensitive than IIF. The staining of ssIIF with MMP sera produces linear IgG deposits in 58–82% of MMP cases on either the epidermal or the dermal side of the BMZ (17, 30, 31). Even though ssIIF might be helpful to differentiate autoantigens located on the epidermal side of the BMZ from those located on the dermal side of the BMZ by causing separation at the level of the lamina lucida, it does not definitively identify the autoantigens. Immunoblotting using epidermal or dermal extracts and recombinant antigenic polypeptides is useful for identifying specific targeted autoantigens, although the techniques are not commonly available in routine examinations. Enzyme-linked immunosorbent assays (ELISAs) are widely used to detect autoantibodies directing specific autoantigens (32, 33). Approximately 85–96% of autoantibodies in BP are detected by commercially available COL17-NC16A ELISA or chemiluminescence enzyme immunoassay (CLEIA) systems (33–36). However, the antigens targeted by commercially available ELISA/CLEIA systems are limited to the certain domains on BMZ proteins, such as COL17 (NC16A), BP230 (N/C-terminus), and COL7 (NC1/NC2) (37). Due to the low titer and the heterogeneity of MMP autoantibodies, only 30–52% of the autoantibodies in COL17-type MMP may be recognized using COL17 NC16A ELISA/CLEIA (17, 38, 39). Because of these problems, a certain share of MMP patients may not be diagnosed and treated.

Abbreviations: MMP, mucous membrane pemphigoid; BMZ, basement membrane zone; COL17, collagen XVII; COL7, collagen VII; BP, bullous pemphigoid; DIF, direct immunofluorescence; IIF, indirect immunofluorescence; ssIIF, 1 M NaCl-split skin IIF; ELISA, enzyme-linked immunosorbent assays; NC, non-collagenous; CLEIA, chemiluminescence enzyme immunoassay; DPP-4i, dipeptidyl peptidase-4 inhibitor; COL4, collagen IV.

Diagnostic Points for MMP

Structure-Maintaining Biopsy Technique for Hematoxylin and Eosin (H&E) Staining

Inadequate biopsy techniques and improper tissue handing can easily lead to the loss of the oral mucosal epithelia in samples from MMP patients. The destruction of oral mucosal tissue makes a diagnosis difficult. Endo et al. presented a "stab-and-roll" biopsy technique to maintain the gingival epithelia in desquamative gingivitis (40). This technique is designed to keep the epithelium from detaching from the biopsy specimen by reducing lateral forces during the procedure. In 52 patients with desquamative gingivitis, the epithelium was maintained in 12 of the 13 patients with MMP using this technique.

Tissue-Bound Immunoglobulin and Complement

In cases that are difficult to diagnose, DIF using the patient's tissue is a valuable test for diagnosing MMP. Shimanovich et al. showed that multiple and repeated biopsies increase the sensitivity of DIF (41). At the first workup, 69% (36/52) of patients who underwent only 1 biopsy were found to be positive, whereas 85% (22/26) of patients who underwent biopsies from more than 1 site were positive. Overall, 95% (74/78) showed positive results in DIF after repeated biopsies. The same group demonstrated that immunohistochemistry for C3d or C4d is helpful in screening for cases of suspected MMP when paraffin-embedded tissue is available (42). Linear deposits of C3d or C4d were detected in 53% (18/34) or 59% (20/34) of patients, respectively. We also reported that DIF samples taken from non-lesional buccal mucosa by punch biopsy contribute to the diagnosis of MMP (27). In 7 MMP with gingiva-dominant oral lesions, tissue-bound antibodies were detected in all cases. The buccal mucosa is easy to access, and punch biopsies provide well-maintained BMZ structures.

Detection of Autoantibodies

Laminin 332-Type MMP

Goletz et al. established a specific IIF assay using laminin 332-expressing human HEK293 cells for the detection of anti-laminin 332 autoantibodies (43). Using BIOCHIP® mosaics, the laminin 332 heterotrimer recognized 77% (72/93) of the anti-laminin 332 MMP sera. Several studies developed ELISA systems to detect autoantibodies against laminin 332. Bernard et al. presented a novel ELISA that uses purified laminin 332 from SCC25 cells and detected autoantibodies in 20.1% of MMP patients (44). Chiorean et al. showed that the results of an ELISA using purified or recombinant human laminin 332 correlated closely with those of immunoblotting in 36 MMP cases (45).

COL17-Type MMP

Ali et al. demonstrated that salivary IgG and IgA antibodies against COL17-NC16A are equal to serum in diagnostic value (39). 45% (29/64) of whole saliva samples and 53% (33/64) of serum samples were positive for IgG and/or IgA antibodies by COL17-NC16A ELISA. However, 50–70% of MMP autoantibodies were found to mainly react with the C-terminus of COL17 instead of with the COL17-NC16A domain (5, 6, 46). Immunoassays for the detection of autoantibodies against the entire extra domain of COL17 need to be provided. Schmidt et al. proposed an IF assay that uses Sf21 insect cells expressing full-length COL17 (47). The novel assay detected 84% (6/7) of circulating autoantibodies in MMP sera. Recently Izumi et al. established a novel ELISA system using full-length human COL17 recombinant protein (full-length COL17 ELISA) (48). With the full-length COL17 ELISA, 9 of 12 MMP cases (75%) showed positivity, whereas with the conventional COL17-NC16A ELISA and BP230 ELISA, 4 of 12 sera (42%), and 3 of 12 sera (25%) showed positivity, respectively. We reported on another unique concept that helped to overcome the difficulty of detecting MMP autoantibodies. IIF is usually performed using normal human skin, even though MMP mainly involves the mucosa and not the skin. We performed IIF tests using normal human oral mucosa (18). In 20 MMP sera and 20 BP sera, the sensitivities were compared by IIF using skin and mucosa. 85% (17/20) of the MMP sera reacted to mucosa, and 35% (7/20) to skin. Immunoblotting using normal human epidermal keratinocytes (skin keratinocytes) and normal human oral mucosal keratinocyte lysates was able to detect autoantibodies. Skin and mucosal keratinocyte lysates reacted to a 180-kDa protein corresponding to COL17 in 10% (2/20) and 55% (11/20) of MMP sera, respectively.

Mucosal substrates (normal oral mucosa and normal oral mucosal keratinocytes) are beneficial for detecting autoantibodies and identifying autoantigens in MMP. However, it is more difficult to obtain oral mucosa than skin. To overcome this drawback, we attempted to immortalize the oral mucosal keratinocytes by using E6/E7 proteins of HPV (49). Cell lysates of immortalized mucosal keratinocytes effectively identified MMP autoantigens in 60% (18/30) of MMP sera.

For the sensitive detection of COL17-NC16A-specific IgG, Emtenani et al. reported that normal human skin was superior to monkey esophagus. The monkey esophagus was able to detect only 17% (2/12) of COL17-NC16A antibodies, whereas skin detected 100% (12/12) of the antibodies (50). Together with the low homology of COL17-NC16A between human and monkey esophagus, these pieces of evidence suggest that the expression of COL17 protein differs by anatomical location, such as skin vs. mucosa. The use of suitable specimens for IIF from specific sites may contribute to the sensitive detection of autoantibodies in pemphigoid.

Proposed Diagnostic Strategies

The diagnostic criteria for MMP remain unclear. The lack of commonly recognized diagnostic criteria can result in delayed diagnoses or misdiagnoses. The international consensus has documented that the clinical findings of mucosa-dominant lesions and DIF detecting tissue-bound IgG, IgA, and/or C3 are essential for the diagnosis (1). Several studies have followed this criteria (41, 44, 51). We also fundamentally agree with the criteria and have introduced it in our studies. However, in pure ocular pemphigoid, up to 20% of cases are negative in DIF (52, 53).Therefore, serological analyses detecting circulating autoantibodies and histological examinations are included in the diagnostic criteria in some studies (39, 52, 54, 55). To clarify MMP diagnosis, we here propose diagnostic criteria based on current knowledge. We emphasize the significance of serological analyses, especially in cases of DIF negativity (**Figure 1**). The diagnosis of MMP is confirmed when clinical criteria and DIF findings are fulfilled. In DIF-negative or DIF-unavailable (not performed) cases, at least one serological or histological finding is needed.

THE EVIDENCE OF BLISTERING MECHANISMS FOR ORAL LESIONS IN PEMPHIGOID

Clinical Evidence of Mucosal Lesions in Pemphigoid

Several pieces of evidence demonstrate associations between mucosal lesions and certain clinical features in pemphigoid. Kridin et al. reported that BP patients with normal eosinophil counts present mucous lesions more frequently than those with elevated eosinophil counts (56). In some patients with oral involvement, the administration of a dipeptidyl peptidase-4 inhibitor (DPP-4i) is associated with BP onset (57). An association between MMP and the intake of DDP-4i was also reported (58). Furthermore, a certain HLA allele (HLA-DQB1*03:01) is associated with MMP occurrence (59–63). HLA-DQB1*03:01 is also related to a high risk of DDP-4i-associated BP (59). Hofmann et al. demonstrated that 56% of BP patients with mucosal involvement showed IgG reactivity against both the COL17-NC16A and C-terminus regions of COL17 (64). Clape et al. revealed that the absence of anti-BP230 autoantibodies was associated with the presence of mucosal lesions in BP (65).

Experimental Evidence of MMP *in vivo* and *in vitro*

In addition to the previous studies on mechanisms of blister formation in BP, several lines of evidence that partly explain the MMP pathogenesis have been demonstrated.

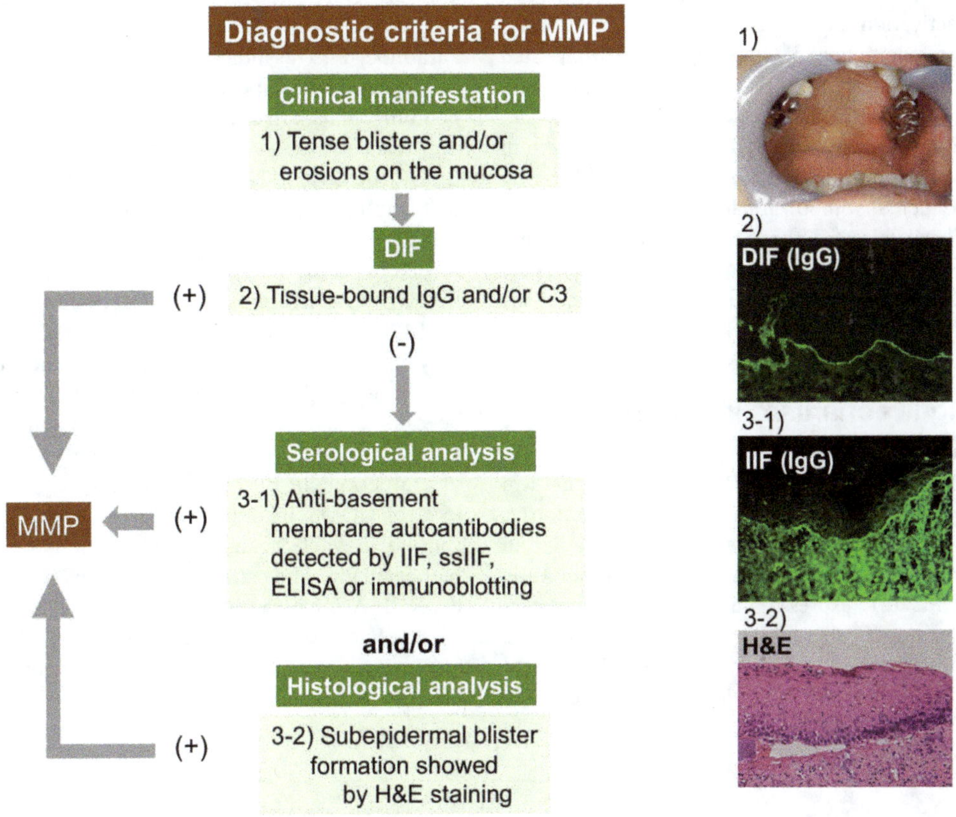

FIGURE 1 | Diagnostic strategy for MMP. The diagnosis of MMP is confirmed by clinical features and positive DIF results. In DIF-negative or DIF-unavailable cases, at least one serological or histological finding is needed. DIF, direct immunofluorescence; IIF, indirect immunofluorescence; ELISA, enzyme-linked immunosorbent assay; H&E, hematoxylin and eosin staining.

Laminin 332-Type MMP

In 2017, Heppe et al. established a mouse model in which injected rabbit anti-laminin 332 IgG antibodies caused subepidermal blisters to develop in the ears, eyes and oral cavity of adult C57BL/6 mice (66). In this model, the clinical manifestations are Fc receptor-dependent and complement-dependent, similar to those of previous BP mouse models. Meanwhile, Lazarova et al. showed that injections with rabbit anti-human laminin 332 IgG or Fab fragments induced subepithelial blisters in the skin of neonatal BALB/c mice (67, 68). In this antibody-transfer model, C5-deficient or mast cell-deficient mice also exhibited subepidermal blisters on the skin (67). The same group established a human skin graft model that uses SCID mice (69). They noted that the injection of purified IgG from MMP patients or anti-human laminin 332 IgG resulted in non-inflammatory subepidermal blisters on the skin. These models from the latter group might define the pathomechanisms in MMP; however, the models lack predominant mucosal involvement.

COL17-Type MMP

Although experimental mouse models for laminin 332-type MMP have been established, *in vivo* studies on COL17-type MMP have not made progress. In previous studies of COL17-targeted mouse models for BP, oral lesions were not addressed and there was a lack of description, both clinically and histologically (70–73).

For the pathogenesis of COL17-type MMP *in vitro*, Imanishi et al. reported that some MMP IgGs targeting the C-terminus of COL17 showed the internalization of COL17 in both oral keratinocytes and DJM-1 cells (74), which are cells from a squamous cell carcinoma cell line (75). In contrast, other MMP IgGs against the C-terminus did not induce the internalization of COL17 thoroughly. The autoantibody-induced endocytosis of COL17 is thought to play an important role in pemphigoid blister formation (76, 77). However, it remains unclear why some MMP IgGs targeting the C-terminus of COL17 show the internalization of COL17.

POTENTIAL BLISTERING MECHANISMS IN THE ORAL MUCOSA IN PEMPHIGOID

Even though COL17 is a major targeted antigen both in BP and MMP, the predominantly involved organs differ between these two diseases. The blister mechanisms in autoimmune subepidermal blistering diseases are complicated, but they are strongly associated with various factors, such as complement activation and inflammatory cell infiltrates (78, 79). In contrast, several lines of evidence have been reported regarding complement-independent blister formation in BP (80). Anti-COL17-NC16A antibodies induce the internalization and depletion of COL17 and lead to inadequate adhesion strength in keratinocytes (76). COL17 depletion is important for blistering along the lamina lucida without inflammation. We noticed that no research has addressed the pathomechanisms of oral lesions in both BP and MMP. Before addressing the possible pathogenesis of MMP, we first focus on blister formation in the oral mucosa in BP.

The Blistering Mechanism in the Oral Mucosa in BP

Recently, we gained new insight into the blister mechanism of oral lesions (81). We showed that COL17 expression is approximately 30–50% higher in mucosal keratinocytes than in skin keratinocytes, as confirmed by qPCR and immunoblotting analysis. This higher COL17 expression in mucosal keratinocytes is associated with stronger cell adhesion in such keratinocytes. The cell adhesion strength was found to be 50% higher for mucosal keratinocytes than skin keratinocytes. Furthermore, anti-COL17-NC16A antibodies induce significantly greater COL17 depletion in skin keratinocytes than in mucosal keratinocytes. This indicates that the higher expression of COL17 in mucosa may compensate for the COL17 depletion induced by pemphigoid IgG. In other words, the predominant skin blistering may relate to the residual amount of COL17 after BP-IgG induces COL17 depletion. This is similar to the blistering mechanism in pemphigus, in which desmoglein 1 and 3 compensate for each other in the oral mucosa and the skin. Potential blister formation in BP is initiated by the binding of autoantibodies to COL17, which leads to the internalization and depletion of COL17 from the plasma membrane. The depletion of COL17 may impair hemidesmosome formation and weaken the strength of adhesion to the basement membrane. Finally, separations may be caused by mechanical stress or inflammation induced via the Fc fragment of the pathogenic IgG. The lower frequency of oral lesions in BP may be attributed to the high expression level of COL17 in oral mucosa (**Figure 2A**). Additionally, we showed that IgG against the C-terminus of COL17 may have pathogenicity. The pathogenicity of IgG against regions outside the NC16A domain remains controversial *in vivo* and *in vitro* (74, 82, 83). In our study, however, COL17 depletion was significantly enhanced by stimulation with a combination of IgGs against the NC16A domain and the C-terminus (**Figure 2A**). This evidence

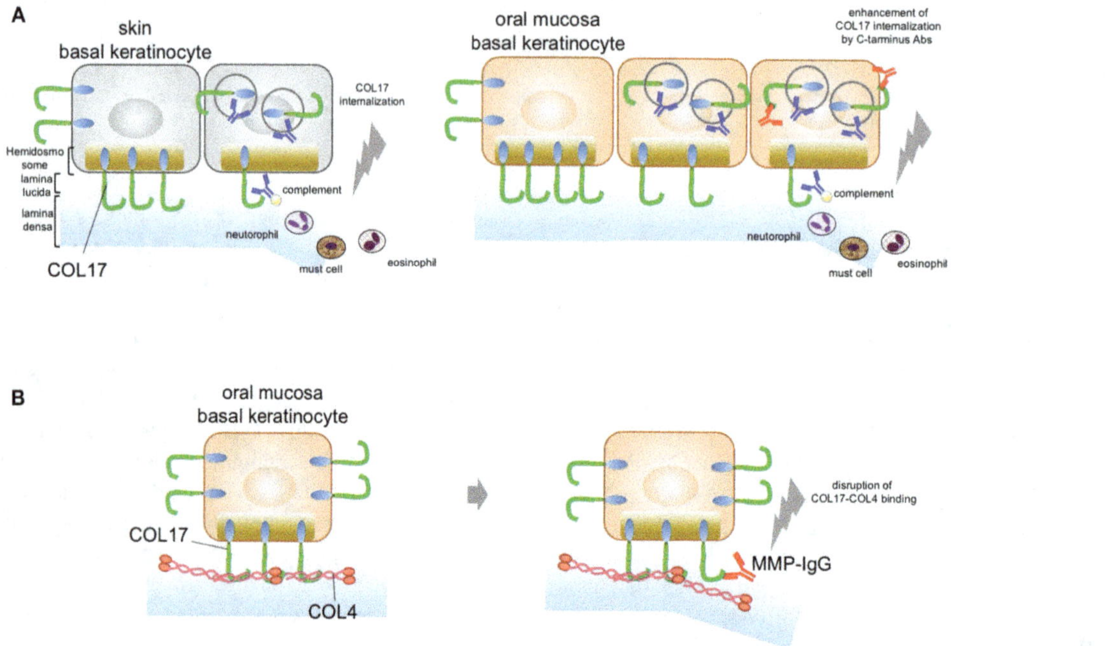

FIGURE 2 | Potential blistering mechanisms in oral mucosa. **(A)** The oral mucosal blistering in BP. COL17 molecules are located in both the hemidesmosomal and the non-hemidesmosomal plasma membranes. In the skin, autoantibodies targeting COL17-NC16A lead to the internalization of non-hemidesmosomal COL17 and result in COL17 depletion. The internalization and depletion of COL17 disturb the supply of hemidesmosomal COL17 and impair hemidesmosome formation. Eventually, intra-lamina lucida separation is caused by mechanical stress, complement activation, and/or inflammatory cell infiltration. This is mainly observed in the skin; therefore, the blisters predominantly occur in the skin (left panel). In the oral mucosa, autoantibodies targeting the C-terminus of COL17 enhance COL17 depletion induced by autoantibodies targeting COL17-NC16A. The blister formation in oral mucosa may be a result of the enhancement of COL17 depletion induced by autoantibodies targeting the C-terminus of COL17 in BP patients (right panel). **(B)** The predominant oral mucosal blistering in MMP. The direct binding of COL17 to COL4 is disrupted by IgG against the C-terminus in the oral mucosa. Autoantibodies in MMP targeting the C-terminus of COL17 inhibit the protein–protein interaction in the oral mucosa and reduce hemidesmosomal adhesion without the internalization of COL17.

suggests that BP patients with IgG targeting not only the NC16A domain but also the C-terminus may show blisters in the skin and the mucosa. To support this, several studies demonstrated an association between autoantibodies to the C-terminus and mucosal lesions in BP (64, 84). Autoantibodies targeting the C-terminus are potentially pathogenic in certain cases of BP.

MMP-Specific Blister Mechanism Without Inflammation

Histologically, MMP patients have less severe inflammatory findings than BP patients do. The blistering mechanism of MMP may differ from that of BP. We recently found direct binding between collagen IV (COL4) and COL17 in skin and oral keratinocytes (24). Interestingly, this COL4–COL17 binding is disrupted by IgG against the C-terminus in oral keratinocytes. Furthermore, several MMP IgGs that target the C-terminus of COL17 were found to inhibit COL4–COL17 binding and to result in the reduction of hemidesmosomal adhesion (**Figure 2B**). That is, MMP-IgGs may directly disrupt COL4-COL17 binding and result in separation at the BMZ without inflammation.

As for the potential blistering mechanism of laminin 332-type MMP, Fc-dependent, and complement-dependent mechanisms have been revealed by using laminin 332-type mouse models. However, laminin 332 interacts with other BMZ molecules, including COL17. Given our latest concept of MMP-specific blister formation, anti-laminin 332 antibodies may disrupt the molecular interactions of laminin 332, resulting in the predominance of mucosal blister formation in laminin 332-type MMP.

CONCLUSION

As highlighted in this review, we propose disease-specific diagnostic strategies for MMP. The pathogenesis of COL17-type MMP is distinct from that of BP and is more closely related to less inflammatory blister mechanisms due to the inhibition of COL4–COL17 binding or COL17 depletion.

ETHICS STATEMENT

The studies were conducted in accordance with the Helsinki Guidelines and were approved by the Ethics Committee of Hokkaido University.

AUTHOR CONTRIBUTIONS

All authors listed have made a substantial, direct and intellectual contribution to the work, and approved it for publication.

REFERENCES

1. Chan LS, Ahmed AR, Anhalt GJ, Bernauer W, Cooper KD, Elder MJ, et al. The first international consensus on mucous membrane pemphigoid: definition, diagnostic criteria, pathogenic factors, medical treatment, and prognostic indicators. *Arch Dermatol.* (2002) 138:370–9. doi: 10.1001/archderm.138.3.370
2. Schmidt E, Zillikens D. Pemphigoid diseases. *Lancet* (2013) 381:320–32. doi: 10.1016/S0140-6736(12)61140-4
3. Murrell DF, Marinovic B, Caux F, Prost C, Ahmed R, Wozniak K, et al. Definitions and outcome measures for mucous membrane pemphigoid: recommendations of an international panel of experts. *J Am Acad Dermatol.* (2015) 72:168–74. doi: 10.1016/j.jaad.2014.08.024
4. Di Zenzo G, Carrozzo M, Chan LS. Urban legend series: mucous membrane pemphigoid. *Oral Dis.* (2014) 20:35–54. doi: 10.1111/odi.12193
5. Schmidt E, Skrobek C, Kromminga A, Hashimoto T, Messer G, Bröcker EB, et al. Cicatricial pemphigoid: IgA and IgG autoantibodies target epitopes on both intra- and extracellular domains of bullous pemphigoid antigen 180. *Br J Dermatol.* (2001) 145:778–83. doi: 10.1046/j.1365-2133.2001.04471.x
6. Balding SD, Prost C, Diaz LA, Bernard P, Bedane C, Aberdam D, et al. Cicatricial pemphigoid autoantibodies react with multiple sites on the BP180 extracellular domain. *J Invest Dermatol.* (1996) 106:141–6. doi: 10.1111/1523-1747.ep12329728
7. Domloge-Hultsch N, Gammon WR, Briggaman RA, Gil SG, Carter WG, Yancey KB. Epiligrin, the major human keratinocyte integrin ligand, is a target in both an acquired autoimmune and an inherited subepidermal blistering skin disease. *J Clin Invest.* (1992) 90:1628–33. doi: 10.1172/JCI116033
8. Kirtschig G, Marinkovich MP, Burgeson RE, Yancey KB. Anti-basement membrane autoantibodies in patients with anti-epiligrin cicatricial pemphigoid bind the α subunit of laminin 5. *J Invest Dermatol.* (1995) 105:543–8. doi: 10.1111/1523-1747.ep12323431
9. Natsuga K, Nishie W, Shinkuma S, Moriuchi R, Shibata M, Nishimura M, et al. Circulating IgA and IgE autoantibodies in antilaminin-332 mucous membrane pemphigoid. *Br J Dermatol.* (2010) 162:513–7. doi: 10.1111/j.1365-2133.2009.09508.x
10. Tyagi S, Bhol K, Natarajan K, Livir-Rallatos C, Foster CS, Ahmed AR. Ocular cicatricial pemphigoid antigen: partial sequence and biochemical characterization. *Proc Natl Acad Sci USA.* (1996) 93:14714–9. doi: 10.1073/pnas.93.25.14714
11. Bhol KC, Dans MJ, Simmons RK, Foster CS, Giancotti FG, Ahmed AR. The autoantibodies to alpha 6 beta 4 integrin of patients affected by ocular cicatricial pemphigoid recognize predominantly epitopes within the large cytoplasmic domain of human beta 4. *J Immunol.* (2000) 165:2824–9. doi: 10.4049/jimmunol.165.5.2824
12. Rashid KA, Gürcan HM, Ahmed AR. Antigen specificity in subsets of mucous membrane pemphigoid. *J Invest Dermatol.* (2006) 126:2631–6. doi: 10.1038/sj.jid.5700465
13. Cozzani E, Di Zenzo G, Calabresi V, Carrozzo M, Burlando M, Longanesi L, et al. Autoantibody profile of a cohort of 78 Italian patients with mucous membrane pemphigoid: correlation between reactivity profile and clinical involvement. *Acta Derm Venerol.* (2016) 96:768–73. doi: 10.2340/00015555-2311
14. Bieber K, Koga H, Nishie W. *In vitro* and *in vivo* models to investigate the pathomechanisms and novel treatments for pemphigoid diseases. *Exp Dermatol.* (2017) 26:1163–70. doi: 10.1111/exd.13415
15. Li X, Qian H, Sogame R, Hirako Y, Tsuruta D, Ishii N, et al. Integrin β4 is a major target antigen in pure ocular mucous membrane pemphigoid. *Eur J Dermatol.* (2016) 26:247–53. doi: 10.1684/ejd.2016.2772
16. Amber KT, Murrell DF, Schmidt E, Joly P, Borradori L. Autoimmune subepidermal bullous diseases of the skin and mucosae: clinical features, diagnosis, and management. *Clin Rev Allergy Immunol.* (2017) 381:320–6. doi: 10.1007/s12016-017-8633-4
17. Hayakawa T, Furumura M, Fukano H, Li X, Ishii N, Hamada T, et al. Diagnosis of oral mucous membrane pemphigoid by means of combined serologic testing. *Oral Surg Oral Med Oral Pathol Oral Radiol.* (2014) 117:483–96. doi: 10.1016/j.oooo.2013.12.402
18. Kamaguchi M, Iwata H, Ujiie H, Izumi K, Natsuga K, Nishie W, et al. Oral mucosa is a useful substrate for detecting autoantibodies of mucous membrane pemphigoid. *Br J Dermatol.* (2017) 178:e119–21. doi: 10.1111/bjd.15925

19. Taylor J, McMillan R, Shephard M, Setterfield J, Ahmed R, Carrozzo M, et al. World Workshop on oral medicine VI: a systematic review of the treatment of mucous membrane pemphigoid. *Oral Surg Oral Med Oral Pathol Oral Radiol.* (2015) 120:161–71.e20. doi: 10.1016/j.oooo.2015.01.024
20. Tsunoda K, Ota T, Aoki M, Yamada T, Nagai T, Nakagawa T, et al. Induction of pemphigus phenotype by a mouse monoclonal antibody against the amino-terminal adhesive interface of desmoglein 3. *J Immunol.* (2003) 170:2170–8. doi: 10.4049/jimmunol.170.4.2170
21. Ishii K, Harada R, Matsuo I, Shirakata Y, Hashimoto K, Amagai M. *In vitro* keratinocyte dissociation assay for evaluation of the pathogenicity of anti-desmoglein 3 IgG autoantibodies in pemphigus vulgaris. *J Invest Dermatol.* (2005) 124:939–46. doi: 10.1111/j.0022-202X.2005.23714.x
22. Iwata H, Bieber K, Hirose M, Ludwig RJ. Animal models to investigate pathomechanisms and evaluate novel treatments for autoimmune bullous dermatoses. *Curr Pharm Des.* (2015) 21:2422–39. doi: 10.2174/1381612821666150316122502
23. Ludwig RJ, Vanhoorelbeke K, Leypoldt F, Kaya Z, Bieber K, McLachlan SM, et al. Mechanisms of autoantibody-induced pathology. *Front Immunol.* (2017) 8:603. doi: 10.3389/fimmu.2017.00603
24. Kamaguchi M, Iwata H, Nishie W, Toyonaga E, Ujiie H, Natsuga K, et al. The direct binding of collagen XVII and collagen IV is disrupted by pemphigoid autoantibodies. *Lab Invest.* (2018) 99:48–57. doi: 10.1038/s41374-018-0113-9
25. Scully C, Muzio Lo L. Oral mucosal diseases: mucous membrane pemphigoid. *Br J Oral Maxillofac Surg.* (2008) 46:358–66. doi: 10.1016/j.bjoms.2007.07.200
26. Rose C, Schmidt E, Kerstan A, Thoma-Uszynski S, Wesselmann U, Käsbohrer U, et al. Histopathology of anti-laminin 5 mucous membrane pemphigoid. *J Am Acad Dermatol.* (2009) 61:433–40. doi: 10.1016/j.jaad.2009.02.012
27. Kamaguchi M, Iwata H, Ujiie I, Ujiie H, Sato J, Kitagawa Y, et al. Direct immunofluorescence using non-lesional buccal mucosa in mucous membrane pemphigoid. *Front Med.* (2018) 5:20. doi: 10.3389/fmed.2018.00020
28. Benoit S, Scheurlen M, Goebeler M, Stoevesandt J. Structured diagnostic approach and risk assessment in mucous membrane pemphigoid with oesophageal involvement. *Acta Derm Venerol.* (2018) 98:660–6. doi: 10.2340/00015555-2938
29. Carrozzo M, Cozzani E, Broccoletti R, Carbone M, Pentenero M, Arduino P, et al. Analysis of antigens targeted by circulating IgG and IgA antibodies in patients with mucous membrane pemphigoid predominantly affecting the oral cavity. *J Periodontol.* (2004) 75:1302–8. doi: 10.1902/jop.2004.75.10.1302
30. Sarret Y, Hall R, Cobo LM, Thivolet J, Patton DL, Woodley DT. Salt-split human skin substrate for the immunofluorescent screening of serum from patients with cicatricial pemphigoid and a new method of immunoprecipitation with IgA antibodies. *J Am Acad Dermatol.* (1991) 24:952–8. doi: 10.1016/0190-9622(91)70152-R
31. Gammon WR, Fine JD, Forbes M, Briggaman RA. Immunofluorescence on split skin for the detection and differentiation of basement membrane zone autoantibodies. *J Am Acad Dermatol.* (1992) 27:79–87. doi: 10.1016/0190-9622(92)70161-8
32. Zillikens D, Mascaro JM, Rose PA, Liu Z, Ewing SM, Caux F, et al. A highly sensitive enzyme-linked immunosorbent assay for the detection of circulating anti-BP180 autoantibodies in patients with bullous pemphigoid. *J Invest Dermatol.* (1997) 109:679–83. doi: 10.1111/1523-1747.ep12338088
33. Kobayashi M, Amagai M, Kuroda-Kinoshita K, Hashimoto T, Shirakata Y, Hashimoto K, et al. BP180 ELISA using bacterial recombinant NC16a protein as a diagnostic and monitoring tool for bullous pemphigoid. *J Dermatol Sci.* (2002) 30:224–32. doi: 10.1016/S0923-1811(02)00109-3
34. Sakuma-Oyama Y, Powell AM, Oyama N, Albert S, Bhogal BS, Black MM. Evaluation of a BP180-NC16a enzyme-linked immunosorbent assay in the initial diagnosis of bullous pemphigoid. *Br J Dermatol.* (2004) 151:126–31. doi: 10.1111/j.1365-2133.2004.06082.x
35. Sitaru C, Dähnrich C, Probst C, Komorowski L, Blöcker I, Schmidt E, et al. Enzyme-linked immunosorbent assay using multimers of the 16th non-collagenous domain of the BP180 antigen for sensitive and specific detection of pemphigoid autoantibodies. *Exp Dermatol.* (2007) 16:770–7. doi: 10.1111/j.1600-0625.2007.00592.x
36. Fujio Y, Kojima K, Hashiguchi M, Wakui M, Murata M, Amagai M, et al. Validation of chemiluminescent enzyme immunoassay in detection of autoantibodies in pemphigus and pemphigoid. *J Dermatol Sci.* (2017) 85:208–15. doi: 10.1016/j.jdermsci.2016.12.007
37. Horváth ON, Varga R, Kaneda M, Schmidt E, Ruzicka T, Sárdy M. Diagnostic performance of the "MESACUP anti-Skin profile TEST." *Eur J Dermatol.* (2016) 26:56–63. doi: 10.1684/ejd.2015.2692
38. Izumi K, Nishie W, Mai Y, Wada M, Natsuga K, Ujiie H, et al. Autoantibody profile differentiates between inflammatory and non-inflammatory bullous pemphigoid. *J Invest Dermatol.* (2016) 136:2201–10. doi: 10.1016/j.jid.2016.06.622
39. Ali S, Kelly C, Challacombe SJ, Donaldson AN, Dart JK, Gleeson M, et al. Salivary IgA and IgG antibodies to bullous pemphigoid 180 noncollagenous domain 16a as diagnostic biomarkers in mucous membrane pemphigoid. *Br J Dermatol.* (2016) 174:1022–9. doi: 10.1111/bjd.14351
40. Endo H, Rees TD, Allen EP, Kuyama K, Aoki S, Yamamoto H, et al. A stab-and-roll biopsy technique to maintain gingival epithelium for desquamative gingivitis. *J Periodontol.* (2014) 85:802–9. doi: 10.1902/jop.2014.130428
41. Shimanovich I, Nitz JM, Zillikens D. Multiple and repeated sampling increases the sensitivity of direct immunofluorescence testing for the diagnosis of mucous membrane pemphigoid. *J Am Acad Dermatol.* (2017) 77:700–3. doi: 10.1016/j.jaad.2017.05.016
42. Shimanovich I, Nitz JM, Witte M, Zillikens D, Rose C. Immunohistochemical diagnosis of mucous membrane pemphigoid. *J Oral Pathol Med.* (2018) 47:613–9. doi: 10.1111/jop.12732
43. Goletz S, Probst C, Komorowski L, Schlumberger W, Fechner K, van Beek N, et al. Sensitive and specific assay for the serological diagnosis of anti-laminin 332 mucous membrane pemphigoid. *Br J Dermatol.* (2018) 180:149–56. doi: 10.1111/bjd.17202
44. Bernard P, Antonicelli F, Bedane C, Joly P, Le Roux-Villet C, Duvert-Lehembre S, et al. Prevalence and clinical significance of anti-laminin 332 autoantibodies detected by a novel enzyme-linked immunosorbent assay in mucous membrane pemphigoid. *JAMA Dermatol.* (2013) 149:533–40. doi: 10.1001/jamadermatol.2013.1434
45. Chiorean R, Danescu S, Virtic O, Mustafa MB, Baican A, Lischka A, et al. Molecular diagnosis of anti-laminin 332 (epiligrin) mucous membrane pemphigoid. *Orphanet J Rare Dis.* (2018) 13:111. doi: 10.1186/s13023-018-0855-x
46. Nie Z, Hashimoto T. IgA antibodies of cicatricial pemphigoid sera specifically react with C-terminus of BP180. *J Invest Dermatol.* (1999) 112:254–5. doi: 10.1046/j.1523-1747.1999.00501.x
47. Schmidt E, Kromminga A, Mimietz S, Leinfelder U, Sitaru C, Bröcker EB, et al. A highly sensitive and simple assay for the detection of circulating autoantibodies against full-length bullous pemphigoid antigen 180. *J Autoimmun.* (2002) 18:299–309. doi: 10.1006/jaut.2002.0589
48. Izumi K, Nishie W, Mai Y, Ujiie H, Iwata H, Natsuga K, et al. Detection of mucous membrane pemphigoid autoantibodies by full-length BP180 enzyme-linked immunosorbent assay. *J Dermatol Sci.* (2017) 88:247–8. doi: 10.1016/j.jdermsci.2017.07.005
49. Kamaguchi M, Iwata H, Miyauchi T, Ujiie H, Ujiie I, Nomura T, et al. The identification of autoantigens in mucous membrane pemphigoid using immortalized oral mucosal keratinocytes. *J Oral Pathol Med.* (2018) 48:60–7. doi: 10.1111/jop.12780
50. Emtenani S, Yuan H, Lin C, Pan M, Hundt JE, Schmidt E, et al. Normal human skin is superior to monkey esophagus substrate for detection of circulating BP180-NC16A-specific immunoglobulin G antibodies in bullous pemphigoid. *Br J Dermatol.* (2018). doi: 10.1111/bjd.17313. [Epub ahead of print].
51. Ong HS, Setterfield JF, Minassian DC, Dart JK. Mucous membrane pemphigoid with ocular involvement: the clinical phenotype and its relationship to direct immunofluorescence findings. *Ophthalmology* (2018) 125:496–504. doi: 10.1016/j.ophtha.2017.10.004
52. Thorne JE, Anhalt GJ, Jabs DA. Mucous membrane pemphigoid and pseudopemphigoid. *Ophthalmology* (2004) 111:45–52. doi: 10.1016/j.ophtha.2003.03.001
53. Bernauer W, Elder MJ, Leonard JN, Wright P, Dart JK. The value of biopsies in the evaluation of chronic progressive conjunctival cicatrisation. *Graefes Arch Clin Exp Ophthalmol.* (1994) 232:533–7. doi: 10.1007/BF00181996
54. Helander SD, Rogers RS. The sensitivity and specificity of direct immunofluorescence testing in disorders of mucous membranes. *J Am Acad Dermatol.* (1994) 30:65–75. doi: 10.1016/S0190-9622(94)70010-9

55. Setterfield J, Shirlaw PJ, Kerr-Muir M, Neill S, Bhogal BS, Morgan P, et al. Mucous membrane pemphigoid: a dual circulating antibody response with IgG and IgA signifies a more severe and persistent disease. *Br J Dermatol.* (1998) 138:602–10. doi: 10.1046/j.1365-2133.1998.02168.x
56. Kridin K. Peripheral eosinophilia in bullous pemphigoid: prevalence and influence on the clinical manifestation. *Br J Dermatol.* (2018) 179:1141–7. doi: 10.1111/bjd.16679
57. Mendonça FMI, Martín-Gutierrez FJ, Ríos-Martín JJ, Camacho-Martinez F. Three cases of bullous pemphigoid associated with dipeptidyl peptidase-4 inhibitors - one due to linagliptin. *Dermatology* (2016) 232:249–53. doi: 10.1159/000443330
58. Gaudin O, Seta V, Alexandre M, Bohelay G, Aucouturier F, Mignot-Grootenboer S, et al. Gliptin accountability in mucous membrane pemphigoid induction in 24 out of 313 patients. *Front Immunol.* (2018) 9:1030. doi: 10.3389/fimmu.2018.01030
59. Ujiie H, Muramatsu K, Mushiroda T, Ozeki T, Miyoshi H, Iwata H, et al. HLA-DQB1*03:01 as a biomarker for genetic susceptibility to bullous pemphigoid induced by DPP-4 inhibitors. *J Invest Dermatol.* (2017) 138:1201–4. doi: 10.1016/j.jid.2017.11.023
60. Ahmed AR, Foster S, Zaltas M, Notani G, Awdeh Z, Alper CA, et al. Association of DQw7 (DQB1*0301) with ocular cicatricial pemphigoid. *Proc Natl Acad Sci USA.* (1991) 88:11579–82. doi: 10.1073/pnas.88.24.11579
61. Setterfield J, Theron J, Vaughan RW, Welsh KI, Mallon E, Wojnarowska F, et al. Mucous membrane pemphigoid: HLA-DQB1*0301 is associated with all clinical sites of involvement and may be linked to antibasement membrane IgG production. *Br J Dermatol.* (2001) 145:406–14. doi: 10.1046/j.1365-2133.2001.04380.x
62. Oyama N, Setterfield JF, Powell AM, Sakuma-Oyama Y, Albert S, Bhogal BS, et al. Bullous pemphigoid antigen II (BP180) and its soluble extracellular domains are major autoantigens in mucous membrane pemphigoid: the pathogenic relevance to HLA class II alleles and disease severity. *Br J Dermatol.* (2006) 154:90–8. doi: 10.1111/j.1365-2133.2005.06998.x
63. Hübner F, Setterfield J, Recke A, Zillikens D, Schmidt E, Dart J, et al. HLA alleles in British Caucasians with mucous membrane pemphigoid. *Eye* (2018) 32:1540–1. doi: 10.1038/s41433-018-0092-5
64. Hofmann S, Thoma-Uszynski S, Hunziker T, Bernard P, Koebnick C, Stauber A, et al. Severity and phenotype of bullous pemphigoid relate to autoantibody profile against the NH2- and COOH-terminal regions of the BP180 ectodomain. *J Invest Dermatol.* (2002) 119:1065–73. doi: 10.1046/j.1523-1747.2002.19529.x
65. Clapé A, Muller C, Gatouillat G, Le Jan S, Barbe C, Pham BN, et al. Mucosal involvement in bullous pemphigoid is mostly associated with disease severity and to absence of anti-BP230 autoantibody. *Front Immunol.* (2018) 9:479. doi: 10.3389/fimmu.2018.00479
66. Heppe EN, Tofern S, Schulze FS, Ishiko A, Shimizu A, Sina C, et al. Experimental laminin 332 mucous membrane pemphigoid critically involves C5aR1 and reflects clinical and immunopathological characteristics of the human disease. *J Invest Dermatol.* (2017) 137:1709–18 doi: 10.1016/j.jid.2017.03.037
67. Lazarova Z, Yee C, Darling T, Briggaman RA, Yancey KB. Passive transfer of anti-laminin 5 antibodies induces subepidermal blisters in neonatal mice. *J Clin Invest.* (1996) 98:1509–18. doi: 10.1172/JCI118942
68. Lazarova Z, Hsu R, Briggaman RA, Yancey KB. Fab fragments directed against laminin 5 induce subepidermal blisters in neonatal mice. *Clin Immunol.* (2000) 95:26–32. doi: 10.1006/clim.2000.4845
69. Lazarova Z, Hsu R, Yee C, Yancey KB. Human anti-laminin 5 autoantibodies induce subepidermal blisters in an experimental human skin graft model. *J Invest Dermatol.* (2000) 114:178–84. doi: 10.1046/j.1523-1747.2000.00829.x
70. Liu Z, Diaz LA, Troy JL, Taylor AF, Emery DJ, Fairley JA, et al. A passive transfer model of the organ-specific autoimmune disease, bullous pemphigoid, using antibodies generated against the hemidesmosomal antigen, BP180. *J Clin Invest.* (1993) 92:2480–8. doi: 10.1172/JCI116856
71. Nishie W, Sawamura D, Goto M, Ito K, Shibaki A, McMillan JR, et al. Humanization of autoantigen. *Nat Med.* (2007) 13:378–83. doi: 10.1038/nm1496
72. Ujiie H, Shibaki A, Nishie W, Sawamura D, Wang G, Tateishi Y, et al. A novel active mouse model for bullous pemphigoid targeting humanized pathogenic antigen. *J Immunol.* (2010) 184:2166–74. doi: 10.4049/jimmunol.0903101
73. Schulze FS, Beckmann T, Nimmerjahn F, Ishiko A, Collin M, Köhl J, et al. Fcγ receptors III and IV mediate tissue destruction in a novel adult mouse model of bullous pemphigoid. *Am J Pathol.* (2014) 184:2185–96. doi: 10.1016/j.ajpath.2014.05.007
74. Imanishi A, Imanishi H, Hiroyasu S, Ozawa T, Koga H, Ishii N, et al. Anti-BP180-type mucous membrane pemphigoid immunoglobulin G shows heterogeneity of internalization of BP180/collagen XVII into keratinocyte cytoplasm. *Med Mol Morphol.* (2015) 49:89–97. doi: 10.1007/s00795-015-0128-x
75. Kitajima Y, Inoue S, Yaoita H. Effects of pemphigus antibody on the regeneration of cell-cell contact in keratinocyte cultures grown in low to normal Ca++ concentration. *J Invest Dermatol.* (1987) 89:167–71. doi: 10.1111/1523-1747.ep12470554
76. Iwata H, Kamio N, Aoyama Y, Yamamoto Y, Hirako Y, Owaribe K, et al. IgG from patients with bullous pemphigoid depletes cultured keratinocytes of the 180-kDa bullous pemphigoid antigen (Type XVII collagen) and weakens cell attachment. *J Invest Dermatol.* (2009) 129:919–26. doi: 10.1038/jid.2008.305
77. Iwata H, Kitajima Y. Bullous pemphigoid: role of complement and mechanisms for blister formation within the lamina lucida. *Exp Dermatol.* (2013) 22:381–5. doi: 10.1111/exd.12146
78. Liu Z, Giudice GJ, Swartz SJ, Fairley JA, Till GO, Troy JL, et al. The role of complement in experimental bullous pemphigoid. *J Clin Invest.* (1995) 95:1539–44. doi: 10.1172/JCI117826
79. Liu Z, Giudice GJ, Zhou X, Swartz SJ, Troy JL, Fairley JA, et al. A major role for neutrophils in experimental bullous pemphigoid. *J Clin Invest.* (1997) 100:1256–63. doi: 10.1172/JCI119639
80. Iwata H, Ujiie H. Complement-independent blistering mechanisms in bullous pemphigoid. *Exp Dermatol.* (2017) 26:1235–9. doi: 10.1111/exd.13367
81. Kamaguchi M, Iwata H, Ujiie H, Natsuga K, Nishie W, Kitagawa Y, et al. High expression of collagen XVII compensates for its depletion induced by pemphigoid IgG in the oral mucosa. *J Invest Dermatol.* (2018) 138:1707–15. doi: 10.1016/j.jid.2018.03.002
82. Wada M, Nishie W, Ujiie H, Izumi K, Iwata H, Natsuga K, et al. Epitope-dependent pathogenicity of antibodies targeting a major bullous pemphigoid autoantigen collagen XVII/BP180. *J Invest Dermatol.* (2016) 136:938–46. doi: 10.1016/j.jid.2015.11.030
83. Imafuku K, Iwata H, Kamaguchi M, Izumi K, Natsuga K, Ujiie H, et al. Autoantibodies of non-inflammatory bullous pemphigoid hardly deplete type XVII collagen of keratinocytes. *Exp Dermatol.* (2017) 381:320. doi: 10.1111/exd.13331
84. Di Zenzo G, Grosso F, Terracina M, Mariotti F, De Pità O, Owaribe K, et al. Characterization of the anti-BP180 autoantibody reactivity profile and epitope mapping in bullous pemphigoid patients. *J Invest Dermatol.* (2004) 122:103–10. doi: 10.1046/j.0022-202X.2003.22126.x

7

Identification of Autoreactive B Cell Subpopulations in Peripheral Blood of Autoimmune Patients with Pemphigus Vulgaris

Robert Pollmann[1], Elias Walter[2], Thomas Schmidt[1], Jens Waschke[2], Michael Hertl[1], Christian Möbs[1] and Rüdiger Eming[1]*

[1] *Department of Dermatology and Allergology, Philipps-Universität Marburg, Marburg, Germany,* [2] *Institute of Anatomy and Cell Biology, Ludwig-Maximilians-Universität München, Munich, Germany*

Correspondence:
Rüdiger Eming
eming@med.uni-marburg.de

Pemphigus vulgaris (PV) is a rare blistering disease caused by IgG autoantibodies against the epidermal adhesion molecules desmoglein (Dsg)3 and Dsg1 providing a well-characterized paradigm of an antibody-mediated organ-specific autoimmune disease. In PV patients who have achieved clinical remission after B cell-depleting therapy, relapses often coincide with a reoccurrence of B cells and Dsg-specific autoantibodies. Here, we analyzed Dsg3-specific B cell subpopulations (i.e., total $CD19^+$ B cells, $CD19^+CD27^-$ B cells, $CD19^+CD27^+$ memory B cells, and $CD19^+CD27^{hi}CD38^{hi}$ plasmablasts) in peripheral blood of both PV patients ($n = 14$) at different stages of disease and healthy individuals ($n = 14$) by flow cytometry using fluorescently labeled recombinant human Dsg3 protein. Applying this approach, Dsg3-specific B cells could be detected at low frequencies (0.11–0.53% of $CD19^+$ B cells) and numbers of Dsg3-specific memory B cells were significantly increased in PV patients in clinical remission receiving minimal immunosuppressive therapy. Finally, we confirmed *in vitro* that Dsg3-reactive memory B cells were able to produce anti-Dsg3 IgG autoantibodies upon *ex vivo* activation. Thus, monitoring of Dsg3-specific B cells in PV is of particular interest to further characterize the immunopathogenesis of PV.

Keywords: autoimmunity, pemphigus vulgaris, desmoglein 3, B cells, flow cytometry

INTRODUCTION

Pemphigus vulgaris (PV) is an autoimmune disease characterized by chronic and progressive erosive lesions of the mucosa, and blister formation at the suprabasilar layer of the skin caused by IgG autoantibodies (auto-ab) against adhesion molecules of the epidermis (1–3). The desmosomal cadherin desmoglein (Dsg)3 is the major autoantigen of PV with mucosal-dominant type while in patients with mucocutaneous PV, i.e., affecting mucosa and skin, auto-ab against Dsg1 are additionally found (4, 5). In the majority of PV patients, anti-Dsg IgG auto-ab correlate with disease activity (6, 7) and are therefore regularly used in routine diagnostics (8). The pathogenic relevance of auto-ab against Dsg3 has been shown in several *in vitro* and *in vivo* models by causing loss of keratinocyte cohesion (9–12), whereas a synergistic effect with other non-desmoglein autoantibodies is currently discussed (13, 14). Based on the well-described pathogenesis, the characterized autoantigens and the fact that Dsg-reactive IgG auto-ab are sufficient to cause blisters,

PV is considered as a paradigm of an antibody-mediated organ-specific autoimmune disease. Moreover, PV serves as a model disease for the characterization of autoimmune mechanisms that finally lead to the generation of autoantigen-specific antibodies (15).

The B cell-depleting monoclonal anti-CD20 antibody rituximab leads to a marked decrease of Dsg3 auto-ab-titers paralleled by a fast clinical remission in the majority of PV patients (16–18), underlining the crucial role of continuous auto-ab production in PV by Dsg3-specific B cells, plasmablasts, and plasma cells.

Although the majority of patients achieve clinical remission after rituximab treatment, clinical relapses occur frequently in PV patients on long-term follow-up with reoccurrence of B cells and Dsg3 auto-ab in peripheral blood (19). This data suggests that Dsg3-specific B cells reappear at a certain time point during remission providing the base for a potential disease relapse. However, whether clinical relapses result from either Dsg3-specific B cells that have not been completely depleted by therapy or by *de novo* generated autoreactive B cells has not yet been fully elucidated. Genetic characterization of anti-Dsg3-IgG produced by B cells from PV patients indicates that patients with recurrent disease maintain a limited set of autoreactive Dsg3-specific B cell clones that persist over time (20). In contrast, using proteomic analysis of serum auto-ab, a recent study revealed a much more polyclonal and diverse pool of IgG auto-ab in PV (21).

To further examine the persistence of autoreactive peripheral blood B cells in pemphigus, we sought to characterize Dsg3-specific B cell subpopulations (i.e., mature naïve, memory, and plasmablasts) in PV patients at different stages of disease utilizing fluorescently labeled recombinant human Dsg3 (Dsg3-AF647) like it has been previously demonstrated for other antigens like tetanus toxin (22, 23). Our results show that (1) Dsg3-specific B cells can be detected at low frequencies in peripheral blood of pemphigus patients, (2) Dsg3-specific memory B cells were significantly increased especially in remitting patients receiving minimal therapy, and (3) isolated Dsg3-specific memory B cells from a PV patient secreted anti-Dsg3 IgG after *in vitro* stimulation. Thus, B cell monitoring with Dsg3-AF647 provides a novel and highly specific tool to investigate the persistence and distribution of autoreactive B cells in PV during the disease course.

RESULTS

AF647-Labeled Dsg3 Detects Dsg3-Specific B Cell Clones

In this study we aimed at detecting Dsg3-specific B cells by flow cytometry using fluorescently labeled recombinant Dsg3-AF647 for staining of Dsg3-specific B cell receptors (BCR) as schematically shown in **Figure 1A**. The fluorescence labeling of recombinant Dsg3 did not functionally impair the interactions between Dsg3-AF647 and Dsg3 compared to homophilic binding of recombinant unlabeled human Dsg3 protein as determined by atomic force microscopy (AFM; **Figure 1B**). Furthermore, binding of Dsg3-AF647 to Dsg3 was reduced to the same extent compared to unlabeled Dsg3 after adding the monoclonal Dsg3-specific antibody AK23 (24) demonstrating the specificity of this interaction (**Figure 1B**). To test whether Dsg3-AF647 is capable of binding to Dsg3-specific B cells, the specificity of Dsg3-AF647 staining was evaluated by means of the monoclonal mouse B cell hybridoma (BCH) clone 2C10 producing anti-Dsg3 IgG together with the non-Dsg3-specific BCH clone 1F12 (**Figure 1C**). Production of anti-Dsg3 IgG by 2C10 was confirmed by ELISA with human Dsg3 protein (**Figure 1D**). Both BCH clones expressed surface IgG indicating the presence of a functional BCR (**Figure 1C**). However, only IgG^+ cells from clone 2C10 showed a strong positive signal upon incubation with Dsg3-AF647 while no specific staining was observed with the control clone 1F12. Binding of Dsg3-AF647 to clone 2C10 was almost completely blocked by preincubation with unlabeled Dsg3 protein (**Figure 1C**). Of note, the mean fluorescence intensity of Dsg3-AF647 strongly correlated with surface IgG in clone 2C10 (**Figure 1E**) suggesting a BCR-dependent binding of Dsg3-AF647 to 2C10. In addition, fluorescently labeled human collagen VII (ColVII; noncollagenous domain 1, NC1 (1)) protein which is structurally not related to Dsg3 served as negative control and showed no specific staining in neither of the two BCH cell clones (**Supplementary Figure 1B**). Finally, we analyzed the sensitivity of Dsg3-AF647 staining by titrating the Dsg3-reactive clone 2C10 with bulk 1F12 cells followed by incubation with Dsg3-AF647 since in peripheral blood of PV patients Dsg3-specific B cells are expected at a low frequency. Our results revealed that Dsg3-specific B cells could be detected within a pool of non-Dsg3-reactive BCH at frequencies of even <1% (**Figure 1F**).

Dsg3-Specific B Cells Mainly Appear in the Memory B Cell Pool in PV Patients

Analysis of human Dsg3-specific B cell subpopulations (total $CD19^+$ B cells, $CD19^+CD27^-$ B cells, $CD19^+CD27^+$ memory B cells, and $CD19^+CD27^{hi}CD38^{hi}$ plasmablasts) was performed in peripheral blood of 14 clinically well-defined PV patients in either complete or partial clinical remission, or with relapsing disease (**Supplementary Tables 1, 2**). Individuals with no detectable anti-Dsg3 IgG auto-ab (**Supplementary Figure 2**) served as healthy control (HC) to determine any potential non-specific staining of Dsg3-AF647 in peripheral blood cells. Since a minor background staining with both Dsg3-AF647 and fluorescently labeled ColVII could also be observed in peripheral blood mononuclear cells of HC, only B cells with a high Dsg3-AF647 signal were considered to be Dsg3-specific (**Supplementary Figure 3** for gating scheme). Specificity of Dsg3-AF647 staining in human peripheral blood was also indicated by a high Dsg3-AF647 signal that was only observed in $CD19^+$ B cells but not in the $CD19^-$ population (**Figure 2A**).

Dsg3-specific B cells were present in PV patients (0.11–0.53% of $CD19^+$ B cells) at higher frequencies compared to HC (0.09–0.22% of $CD19^+$ B cells; **Figure 2B**). The increase in $Dsg3^+$ total $CD19^+$ B cells was presumably due to the significantly

Abbreviations: AF647, Alexa Fluor 647; AFM, atomic force microscopy; auto-ab, autoantibodies; BCH, B cell hybridoma; BCR, B cell receptor; COLVII, type VII collagen; Dsg, desmoglein; HC, healthy controls; PV, pemphigus vulgaris.

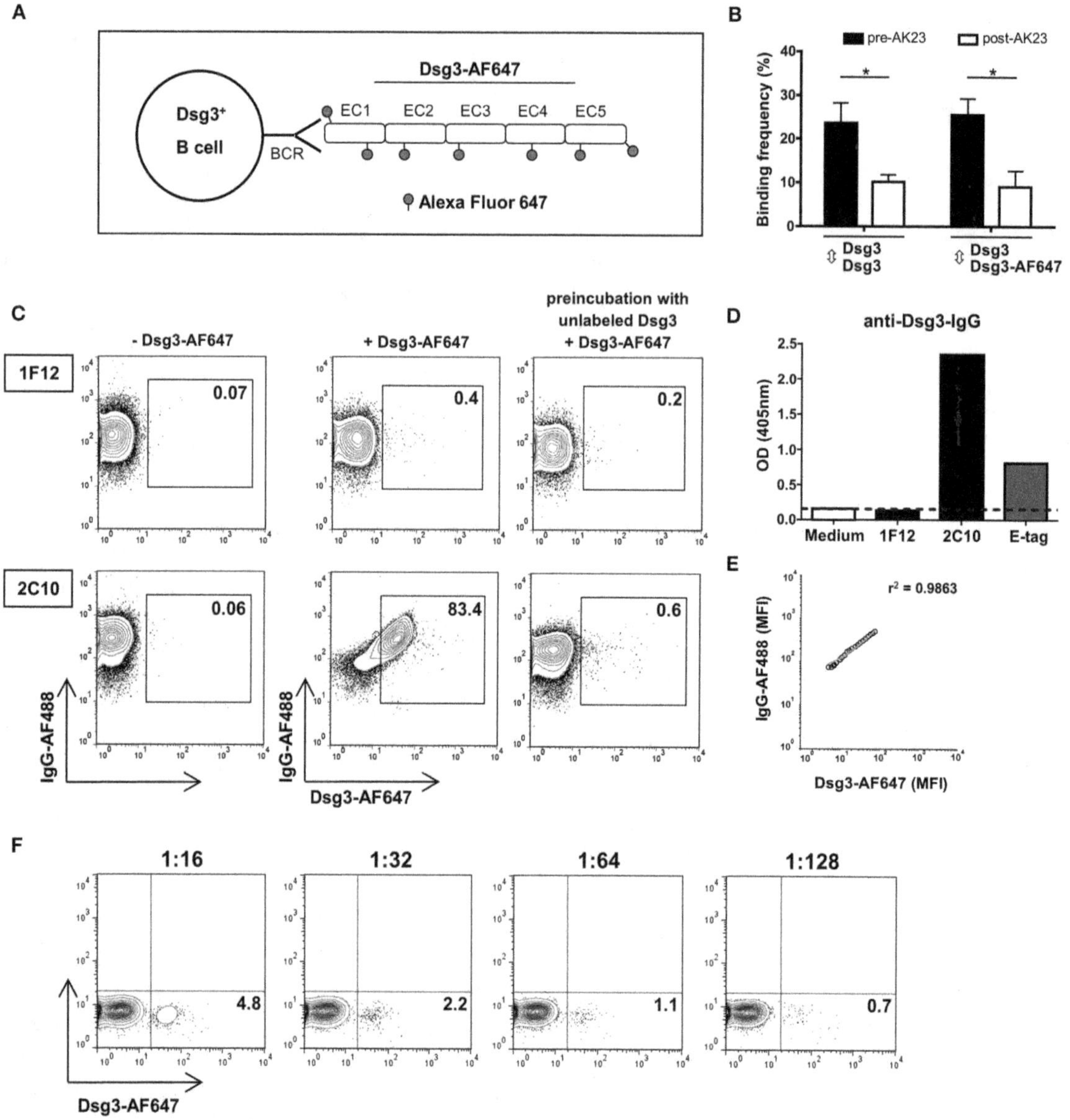

FIGURE 1 | Detection of Dsg3-specific B cell hybridoma (BCH) using fluorescently labeled Dsg3. **(A)** Schematic drawing: the recombinant human extracellular domain (EC1-EC5) of Dsg3 was labeled with the fluorescent dye Alexa Fluor 647 (Dsg3-AF647) and was used for staining of Dsg3-specifc B cell receptors (BCR). **(B)** Binding of Dsg3-AF647 to Dsg3 ± addition of the monoclonal Dsg3-specific antibody AK23 was evaluated with atomic force microscopy. Cumulative data from 3 individual measurements with five replicates for each condition are presented as mean + SD. Statistical analysis was performed by multiple *t*-tests followed by Šidák correction. Differences between groups were considered statistically significant at *p*-values of <0.05 indicated as *. **(C)** Binding efficacy of Dsg3-AF647 to Dsg3-specific BCR was determined by staining of a Dsg3-specific BCH (2C10) and an unrelated BCH (1F12) together with anti-IgG antibody. Binding of Dsg3-AF647 was blocked by preincubation with unlabeled Dsg3. FACS plots shown are representative of three individual experiments. **(D)** Specificity of monoclonal BCH cells for Dsg3 was tested by ELISA. Anti-E-Tag served as positive and culture medium as negative control. **(E)** Correlation of mean fluorescence intensity (MFI) of Dsg3-AF647 with surface IgG. **(F)** Titration of Dsg3-specific BCH (2C10) cells in unrelated 1F12 cells in a calculated ratio of 1:16 (6.25%), 1:32 (3.13%), 1:64 (1.56%), and 1:128 (0.78%) representative of three individual experiments.

higher number of Dsg3-specific $CD19^+CD27^+$ memory B cells in PV patients. On the other hand, the frequency of Dsg3-specific $CD19^+CD27^-$ B cells (including mature naïve and $CD27^-$ memory B cells) did not differ between PV patients and HC ($p = 0.3$; see **Supplementary Figure 3**) for representative FACS plots). Dsg3-specific $CD19^+CD27^{hi}CD38^{hi}$ plasmablasts were only scarcely detected in peripheral blood of PV patients and HC, respectively. To determine whether Dsg3-specific memory B cells in patients with PV are capable of producing anti-Dsg3 IgG, we sorted $CD19^+CD27^+$Dsg3-$AF647^+$ cells from a PV patient in clinical remission with persistent anti-Dsg3 IgG titers. We could demonstrate that *in vitro* stimulation of sorted

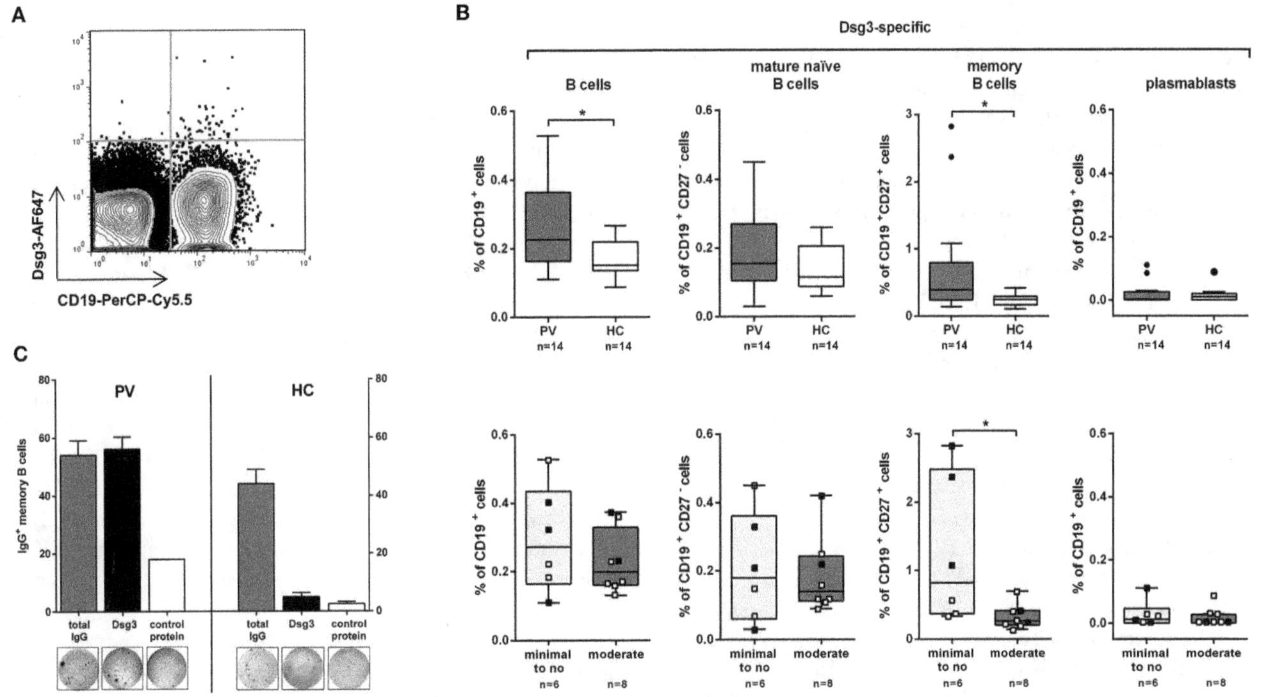

FIGURE 2 | Dsg3-specific memory B cells are increased in remitting PV patients on minimal therapy. **(A)** Representative FACS plot showing staining for $CD19^+Dsg3\text{-}AF647^+$ B cells in one PV patient. **(B)** On the upper row: Dsg3-specific B cell populations (total $CD19^+$, $CD19^+CD27^-$ mature naïve, $CD19^+CD27^+$ memory, and $CD19^+CD27^{hi}CD38^{hi}$ plasmablasts) were analyzed in PV patients ($n = 14$) and healthy controls (HC; $n = 14$). On the lower row: PV patients were further subdivided based on their systemic treatment into *minimal to no* ($n = 6$) and *moderate* therapy ($n = 8$) showing highest numbers of Dsg3-specific $CD19^+CD27^+$ memory B cells on minimal therapy. ■: after Rituximab treatment; □: no Rituximab treatment. **(C)** $CD19^+CD27^+Dsg3\text{-}AF647^+$ cells were isolated from peripheral blood of a PV patient and a healthy control by FACS sorting and stimulated with R848 and IL-2 to induce plasma cell differentiation. Dsg3-IgG-secreting and total IgG-secreting B cells were subsequently detected using ELISpot by seeding 250 cells per well on ELISpot plates coated either with recombinant human Dsg3 or human collagen VII as control protein. Statistical analysis was performed with two-tailed nonparametric Mann-Whitney-U-Test. Differences between groups were considered statistically significant at p-values of <0.05 indicated as *.

$CD19^+CD27^+Dsg3\text{-}AF647^+$ cells with toll-like receptor agonist R848 and interleukin-2 (IL-2) leads to plasma cell differentiation (according to Pinna et al. (25)) and that Dsg3-specific IgG-producing B cells were detected to a similar extent as IgG secreting cells in PV by ELISpot assay (**Figure 2C**). In contrast, although sorted $Dsg3\text{-}AF647^+$ memory B cells from HC showed a marked IgG production, the majority of these cells did not possess the capacity to produce anti-Dsg3 IgG (**Figure 2C**).

Remitting PV Patients Show the Highest Number of Dsg3-Specific Memory B Cells

As some of the PV patients received systemic treatment (systemic corticosteroids, other adjuvant immunosuppressives, B cell depletion) they were subdivided into two groups with *minimal to no* therapy (including 6 remitting patients) or *moderate* therapy (including 8 patients with relapsing disease or partial remission; **Supplementary Table 1**). Interestingly, Dsg3-specific memory B cells were only increased in remitting PV patients receiving *minimal* therapy. On *moderate* treatment Dsg3-specific B cells were hardly detected similar to HC (**Figure 2B**). Here we could show that systemic immunosuppressive treatment seems to have an impact on the frequency of circulating autoreactive B cells in PV. Of note, in the group of remitting PV patients the highest numbers of Dsg3-specific memory B cells exceeding the levels observed in HC were particularly detected in patients who underwent previous B cell depletion (Patient 4, 8, 13 in **Supplementary Table 1**) suggesting a reconstitution of autoreactive memory B cells upon anti-CD20 antibody treatment (**Supplementary Figure 4**).

DISCUSSION

In this study, we demonstrate by use of fluorescently labeled Dsg3 protein the detection of low-frequent Dsg3-specific autoreactive B cells in peripheral blood of PV patients. Flow cytometric analysis of B cell subpopulations with Dsg3-AF647 revealed significantly higher numbers of Dsg3-specific B cells in PV patients compared to HC, particularly within the memory B cell compartment.

Our present findings are in line with Nishifuji et al. (26) who detected circulating Dsg3-specific memory B cells in PV patients but not in HC using ELISpot analysis with a general low frequency (6.3–84.0 cells per 10^5 PBMC). This is similar to our study where we found low-frequent Dsg3-specific B cells in PV patients (0.11–0.53% of $CD19^+$ B cells) even though the acquired percentages can only be compared to a limited extent due to the different assays used. In the work by Nishifuji et al., Dsg3-specific B cells spontaneously producing anti-Dsg3 IgG were exclusively observed in patients with the highest disease activity while Dsg3-specific memory B cells could only be detected after *in vitro* stimulation in a group of nine out of 14 patients (26). Of note, this group included patients with low or no disease activity pointing toward a persistence of Dsg3-specific memory B cells in patients in complete or partial remission which we could also observe in our study as Dsg3-specific $CD19^+CD27^+$ memory B cells were significantly increased in PV patients compared to HC. Since the generation of $CD27^+$ memory B cells is thought to be induced in germinal centers and requires collaboration with T follicular helper (Tfh) cells (27), the presence of autoreactive memory B cells in PV patients points toward a defective Tfh cell tolerance checkpoint within the germinal center response in pemphigus as recently suggested by our group (28).

Most interestingly, the highest numbers of Dsg3-specific memory B cells were observed in 3 PV patients ~2 years after treatment with Rituximab (22–27 months; patient 4, 8, and 13; **Supplementary Table 1**), while increasing Dsg3-specific memory B cells could not be observed in a PV patient (patient 6) who experienced a relapse 35 months after rituximab (**Supplementary Figure 4**). Since disease relapses after rituximab treatment do often occur at a time point starting from 1 year after treatment (18, 19) this observation may point toward an ongoing reconstitution of autoreactive memory B cells. Those memory B cells would initially not produce autoantibodies however, upon immune activation with Dsg3 and other trigger factors, they possess the capability to rapidly differentiate into autoantibody-secreting plasma cells, hence providing the base for a potential disease relapse.

However, Dsg3-specific plasmablasts, representing antibody-secreting cells, were only scarcely detected in our study despite high anti-Dsg3 IgG titers in individual patients. This might be explained by their reduced expression of surface immunoglobulin which limits the capability for detecting these cells using fluorescently labeled Dsg3 (29). Furthermore, due to the restriction to peripheral blood for analysis of Dsg3-specific B cells we were not able to identify autoreactive plasma cells residing within the niches of lymphoid tissues or bone marrow that might account for the continuous secretion of autoreactive autoantibodies in PV. Nonetheless, clonal analysis of autoreactive B cells in PV showed that Dsg3-specific B cells in peripheral blood can persist in PV patients for many years during active disease, clinical remission or even after B cell-depleting therapy indicating the suitability of peripheral blood for monitoring autoreactive B cell responses (20). Whether these B cells are newly generated or persistent cells that were not completely removed by immunosuppressive therapy is still under investigation. Recent results showed that autoreactive B cells could persist in patients with PV but also in patients with lupus erythematosus (SLE) and to a much lower frequency in healthy individuals (30, 31).

In general, anti-Dsg3 IgG is found at a very low prevalence in healthy individuals (32), thus the low frequency of Dsg3-specific B cells in HC is suggestive of IgM^+ B cells producing non-pathogenic, potentially cross-reactive natural IgM antibodies (33, 34). However, the observed signal for Dsg3-AF647 in HC may also be in part due to unspecific binding of the fluorescently labeled protein to B cells. Hence, inclusion of unspecific staining in samples from patients and controls was minimized to the best possible extent as only B cells with a very high Dsg3-AF647 signal were considered to be Dsg3-specific (**Figure 2A**).

To summarize, the present identification of peripheral blood Dsg3-reactive B cells in peripheral blood of PV patients provides further insights into the autoimmune B cell repertoire in PV. Monitoring of Dsg3-specific peripheral B cells with a special focus on Dsg3-specific $CD19^+CD27^+$ memory B cells might be a predictive tool to determine the effectiveness of therapeutic interventions in patients with PV. Particularly as recent studies suggest that clinical remission in PV upon therapy is associated with an increase of IL-10-secreting B cells downregulating B cell activation (18, 35), the extended flow cytometric analysis of Dsg3-specific IL-10-producing B cells in PV patients at different disease stages can provide further insights into the individual progression of disease.

MATERIALS AND METHODS

Human Subjects

Peripheral blood from 14 PV patients (**Supplementary Table 1**) as well as 14 HC with no signs of autoimmune skin inflammation and no serum anti-Dsg3 IgG (**Supplementary Figure 2**) was drawn into citrate-phospate-dextrose-adenine (CPDA) anticoagulant. Each study participant gave written informed consent before inclusion in the study, which was approved by the Ethics Committee of the Medical Faculty of the Philipps-Universität, Marburg (Az. 20/14). The study was conducted in accordance with the Declaration of Helsinski.

Fluorescent Labeling of Recombinant Human Dsg3

Recombinant human Dsg3 (extracellular domain, aa 1-566), produced in the baculovirus expression system (36, 37), was fluorescently labeled using the AlexaFluor647 Labeling kit (Thermo Fisher Scientific, Schwerte, Germany) according to the manufacturers' protocol.

Detection of Dsg3-Specific B Cells

Peripheral blood mononuclear cells (PBMC) were isolated from peripheral blood using Lymphocyte Separation Medium (Capricorn, Ebsdorfergrund, Germany). Mouse BCH clones were cultured in RPMI-1640 supplemented with 100 U/ml penicillin, 100 μg/ml streptomycin, and 2 mM L-glutamine (all Capricorn) and 10% FCS (Merck Millipore, Berlin, Germany). PBMC were washed twice with PBS + 1% FCS and 1×10^6 cells per sample were subsequently stained with Dsg3-AF647 together with mouse anti-human CD19-PerCP-Cy5.5 (HIB19), mouse anti-human CD27-PE (M-T271), mouse anti-human CD38-FITC (HIT2) and the respective isotype controls (all BD Biosciences, Heidelberg, Germany) or with goat anti-mouse IgG-AF488 (A-11029; Thermo Fisher Scientific, Waltham, MA, USA) for mouse

BCH clones. After incubation for 20 min at 4°C cells were washed twice with PBS + 1% FCS and a minimum of 2.5×10^5 PBMC or 0.5×10^5 BCH per sample were acquired on a FACS Calibur (BD Biosciences). In a subset of experiments, sorting of cells was performed using FACS Aria III (BD Biosciences). Data analysis was performed using FlowJo 7.6 (TreeStar Inc., Ashland, USA).

ELISpot Assay

Dsg3-specific B cells ($CD19^+CD27^+Dsg3\text{-}AF647^+$) were isolated from PBMC by FACS sorting. 2×10^3 cells were seeded in 96-well U-bottom microplates and cultured in RPMI-1640 +100 U/ml penicillin, +100 µg/ml streptomycin, +2 mM L-glutamine +10% FCS together with 2.5 µg/ml R848 (Mabtech AB, Nacka Strand, Sweden), and 1,000 U/ml human recombinant IL-2 (Roche, Mannheim, Germany) as previously described (25). After 5 days, cells were seeded at 250 cells/well in duplicates on an ELISpot plate coated with recombinant human Dsg3 or collagen VII and incubated for 20 h at 37°C in a humidified atmosphere containing 5% CO_2. Detection of Dsg3-specific IgG^+ spots was performed according to the manufacturer's protocol (Mabtech AB) and spots were counted automatically with an ELISpot plate reader (A.EL.VIS, Hanover, Germany).

Atomic Force Microscopy

Cell-free AFM measurements were performed on a NanoWizard 3 AFM (JPK-Instruments, Berlin, Germany) as previously described (38) (see **Supplementary Material** for detailed description).

Detection of Anti-Dsg IgG

The presence of IgG auto-ab against Dsg1 or Dsg3 in blood of PV patients and HC was evaluated by anti-Dsg1- and anti-Dsg3-ELISA (Euroimmun, Lübeck, Germany) according to the manufacturer's protocol.

Statistical Analysis

Statistical analysis was performed using GraphPad Prism 6.02 (GraphPad Software Inc., La Jolla, USA). Cumulative data are displayed as box plots with median. For group comparisons two-tailed nonparametric Mann-Whitney-U-Test was applied. Data from AFM experiments were statistically evaluated by multiple *t*-tests followed by Šidák correction. Differences between the groups were considered as statistically significant at p values <0.05.

ETHICS STATEMENT

Each study participant gave written informed consent before inclusion in the study, which was approved by the Ethics Committee of the Medical Faculty of the Philipps-Universität, Marburg (Az. 20/14). The study was conducted in accordance with the Declaration of Helsinki.

AUTHOR CONTRIBUTIONS

RP performed the experiments, analyzed the data, and wrote the manuscript. EW performed and analyzed the AFM experiments. TS, JW, MH, and CM participated to the study design, contributed to the manuscript, and supervised the study. RE conceived the study, recruited pemphigus patients, and revised the manuscript.

REFERENCES

1. Pollmann R, Schmidt T, Eming R, Hertl M. Pemphigus: a comprehensive review on pathogenesis, clinical presentation and novel therapeutic approaches. *Clin Rev Allergy Immunol.* (2018) 54:1–25. doi: 10.1007/s12016-017-8662-z
2. Spindler V, Waschke J. Pemphigus-A disease of desmosome dysfunction caused by multiple mechanisms. *Front Immunol.* (2018) 9:136. doi: 10.3389/fimmu.2018.00136
3. Bystryn J-C, Rudolph JL. Pemphigus. *Lancet.* (2005) 366:61–73. doi: 10.1016/S0140-6736(05)66829-8
4. Amagai M, Klaus-Kovtun V, Stanley JR. Autoantibodies against a novel epithelial cadherin in pemphigus vulgaris, a disease of cell adhesion. *Cell.* (1991) 67:869–77. doi: 10.1016/0092-8674(91)90360-B
5. Amagai M, Tsunoda K, Zillikens D, Nagai T, Nishikawa T. The clinical phenotype of pemphigus is defined by the anti-desmoglein autoantibody profile. *J Am Acad Dermatol.* (1999) 40:167–70. doi: 10.1016/S0190-9622(99)70183-0
6. Harman KE, Seed PT, Gratian MJ, Bhogal BS, Challacombe SJ, Black MM. The severity of cutaneous and oral pemphigus is related to desmoglein 1 and 3 antibody levels. *Br J Dermatol.* (2001) 144:775–80. doi: 10.1046/j.1365-2133.2001.04132.x
7. Schmidt E, Dähnrich C, Rosemann A, Probst C, Komorowski L, Saschenbrecker S, et al. Novel ELISA systems for antibodies to desmoglein 1 and 3: correlation of disease activity with serum autoantibody levels in individual pemphigus patients. *Exp Dermatol.* (2010) 19:458–63. doi: 10.1111/j.1600-0625.2010.01069.x
8. Witte M, Zillikens D, Schmidt E. Diagnosis of autoimmune blistering diseases. *Front Med.* (2018) 5:296. doi: 10.3389/fmed.2018.00296
9. Hofrichter M, Dworschak J, Emtenani S, Langenhan J, Weiß F, Komorowski L, et al. Immunoadsorption of desmoglein-3-specific IgG abolishes the blister-inducing capacity of pemphigus vulgaris IgG in neonatal mice. *Front Immunol.* (2018) 9:1935. doi: 10.3389/fimmu.2018.01935
10. Amagai M, Hashimoto T, Shimizu N, Nishikawa T. Absorption of pathogenic autoantibodies by the extracellular domain of pemphigus vulgaris antigen. (Dsg3) produced by baculovirus. *J Clin Invest.* (1994) 94:59–67. doi: 10.1172/JCI117349
11. Ludwig RJ, Vanhoorelbeke K, Leypoldt F, Kaya Z, Bieber K, McLachlan SM, et al. Mechanisms of autoantibody-induced pathology. *Front Immunol.* (2017) 8:603. doi: 10.3389/fimmu.2017.00603
12. Koch PJ, Mahoney MG, Ishikawa H, Pulkkinen L, Uitto J, Shultz L, et al. Targeted disruption of the pemphigus vulgaris antigen. (desmoglein 3) gene in mice causes loss of keratinocyte cell adhesion with a phenotype similar to pemphigus vulgaris. *J Cell Biol.* (1997) 137:1091–102. doi: 10.1083/jcb.137.5.1091

13. Amber KT, Valdebran M, Grando SA. Non-desmoglein antibodies in patients with pemphigus vulgaris. *Front Immunol.* (2018) 9:1190. doi: 10.3389/fimmu.2018.01190
14. Sinha AA, Sajda T. The evolving story of autoantibodies in pemphigus vulgaris: development of the "super compensation hypothesis". *Front Med* (2018) 5:218. doi: 10.3389/fmed.2018.00218
15. Hertl M, Veldman C. Pemphigus—paradigm of autoantibody-mediated autoimmunity. *Skin Pharmacol Appl Skin Physiol.* (2001) 14:408–18. doi: 10.1159/000056375
16. Joly P, Mouquet H, Roujeau J-C, D'Incan M, Gilbert D, Jacquot S, et al. A single cycle of rituximab for the treatment of severe pemphigus. *N Engl J Med.* (2007) 357:545–52. doi: 10.1056/NEJMoa067752
17. Eming R, Nagel A, Wolff-Franke S, Podstawa E, Debus D, Hertl M. Rituximab exerts a dual effect in pemphigus vulgaris. *J Invest Dermatol.* (2008) 128:2850–8. doi: 10.1038/jid.2008.172
18. Colliou N, Picard D, Caillot F, Calbo S, Le Corre S, Lim A, et al. Long-term remissions of severe pemphigus after rituximab therapy are associated with prolonged failure of desmoglein B cell response. *Sci Transl Med.* (2013) 5:175ra30. doi: 10.1126/scitranslmed.3005166
19. Ahmed AR, Shetty S. A comprehensive analysis of treatment outcomes in patients with pemphigus vulgaris treated with rituximab. *Autoimmun Rev* (2015) 14:323–31. doi: 10.1016/j.autrev.2014.12.002
20. Hammers CM, Chen J, Lin C, Kacir S, Siegel DL, Payne AS, et al. Persistence of anti-desmoglein 3 IgG(+) B-cell clones in pemphigus patients over years. *Invest Dermatol.* (2015) 135:742–9. doi: 10.1038/jid.2014.291
21. Chen J, Zheng Q, Hammers CM, Ellebrecht CT, Mukherjee EM, Tang H-Y, et al. Proteomic analysis of pemphigus autoantibodies indicates a larger, more diverse, and more dynamic repertoire than determined by B cell genetics. *Cell Rep.* (2017) 18:237–47. doi: 10.1016/j.celrep.2016.12.013
22. Frölich D, Giesecke C, Mei HE, Reiter K, Daridon C, Lipsky PE, et al. Secondary immunization generates clonally related antigen-specific plasma cells and memory B cells. *J Immunol.* (2010) 185:3103–10. doi: 10.4049/jimmunol.1000911
23. Odendahl M, Mei H, Hoyer BF, Jacobi AM, Hansen A, Muehlinghaus G, et al. Generation of migratory antigen-specific plasma blasts and mobilization of resident plasma cells in a secondary immune response. *Blood.* (2005) 105:1614–21. doi: 10.1182/blood-2004-07-2507
24. Tsunoda K, Ota T, Aoki M, Yamada T, Nagai T, Nakagawa T, et al. Induction of pemphigus phenotype by a mouse monoclonal antibody against the amino-terminal adhesive interface of desmoglein 3. *J Immunol.* (2003) 170:2170–8. doi: 10.4049/jimmunol.170.4.2170
25. Pinna D, Corti D, Jarrossay D, Sallusto F, Lanzavecchia A. Clonal dissection of the human memory B-cell repertoire following infection and vaccination. *Eur J Immunol.* (2009) 39:1260–70. doi: 10.1002/eji.200839129
26. Nishifuji K, Amagai M, Kuwana M, Iwasaki T, Nishikawa T. Detection of antigen-specific B cells in patients with pemphigus vulgaris by enzyme-linked immunospot assay: requirement of T cell collaboration for autoantibody production. *J Invest Dermatol.* (2000) 114:88–94. doi: 10.1046/j.1523-1747.2000.00840.x
27. Crotty S. T follicular helper cell differentiation, function, and roles in disease. *Immunity.* (2014) 41:529–42. doi: 10.1016/j.immuni.2014.10.004
28. Hennerici T, Pollmann R, Schmidt T, Seipelt M, Tackenberg B, Möbs C, et al. Increased frequency of T follicular helper cells and elevated interleukin-27 plasma levels in patients with pemphigus. *PLoS ONE.* (2016) 11:e0148919. doi: 10.1371/journal.pone.0148919
29. Perez-Andres M, Paiva B, Nieto WG, Caraux A, Schmitz A, Almeida J, et al. Human peripheral blood B-cell compartments: a crossroad in B-cell traffic. *Cytometry B Clin Cytom.* (2010) 78(suppl. 1):S47–60. doi: 10.1002/cyto.b.20547
30. Mietzner B, Tsuiji M, Scheid J, Velinzon K, Tiller T, Abraham K, et al. Autoreactive IgG memory antibodies in patients with systemic lupus erythematosus arise from nonreactive and polyreactive precursors. *Proc Natl Acad Sci USA.* (2008) 105:9727–32. doi: 10.1073/pnas.0803644105
31. Tiller T, Tsuiji M, Yurasov S, Velinzon K, Nussenzweig MC, Wardemann H. Autoreactivity in human IgG+ memory B cells. *Immunity.* (2007) 26:205–13. doi: 10.1016/j.immuni.2007.01.009
32. Prüßmann W, Prüßmann J, Koga H, Recke A, Iwata H, Juhl D, et al. Prevalence of pemphigus and pemphigoid autoantibodies in the general population. *Orphanet J Rare Dis.* (2015) 10:63. doi: 10.1186/s13023-015-0278-x
33. Lobo PI. Role of natural autoantibodies and natural IgM anti-leucocyte autoantibodies in health and disease. *Front Immunol.* (2016) 7:198. doi: 10.3389/fimmu.2016.00198
34. Wardemann H, Yurasov S, Schaefer A, Young JW, Meffre E, Nussenzweig MC. Predominant autoantibody production by early human B cell precursors. *Science.* (2003) 301:1374–7. doi: 10.1126/science.1086907
35. Kabuto M, Fujimoto N, Tanaka T. Increase of interleukin-10-producing B cells associated with long-term remission after i.v. immunoglobulin treatment for pemphigus. *J Dermatol.* (2016) 43:815–8. doi: 10.1111/1346-8138.13295
36. Müller R, Svoboda V, Wenzel E, Gebert S, Hunzelmann N, Müller H-H, et al. IgG reactivity against non-conformational NH-terminal epitopes of the desmoglein 3 ectodomain relates to clinical activity and phenotype of pemphigus vulgaris. *Exp Dermatol.* (2006) 15:606–14. doi: 10.1111/j.1600-0625.2006.00451.x
37. Müller R, Dahler C, Möbs C, Wenzel E, Eming R, Messer G, et al. T and B cells target identical regions of the non-collagenous domain 1 of type VII collagen in epidermolysis bullosa acquisita. *Clin Immunol.* (2010) 135:99–107. doi: 10.1016/j.clim.2009.12.010
38. Vielmuth F, Hartlieb E, Kugelmann D, Waschke J, Spindler V. Atomic force microscopy identifies regions of distinct desmoglein 3 adhesive properties on living keratinocytes. *Nanomedicine.* (2015) 11:511–20. doi: 10.1016/j.nano.2014.10.006

8

Checkpoint Inhibition May Trigger the Rare Variant of Anti-LAD-1 IgG-Positive, Anti-BP180 NC16A IgG-Negative Bullous Pemphigoid

Christian D. Sadik†, Ewan A. Langan†, Victoria Grätz, Detlef Zillikens and Patrick Terheyden*

Department of Dermatology, Allergy, and Venereology, University of Lübeck, Lübeck, Germany

Correspondence:
Christian D. Sadik
christian.sadik@uksh.de

† These authors have contributed equally to this work

Bullous pemphigoid (BP) is an autoimmune blistering skin disease characterized by an autoimmune response to type XVII collagen (BP180). The generation of anti-BP180-NC16A IgG autoantibodies is considered to be central to the pathogenesis of BP, in part due to the close correlation between serum concentration and disease activity. However, ~60% of BP patients also generate IgG autoantibodies against LAD-1, the soluble 120 kDa ectodomain of BP180. Whilst the pathogenic significance of anti-LAD-1 IgG remains unclear, it may be sufficient to precipitate the development of BP, even in the absence of anti-BP180-NC16A IgG, based on several case reports in Japanese patients. There is increasing recognition that immune-checkpoint inhibitors may trigger and/or exacerbate BP as an immune-related adverse event (irAE). Until now, all of these cases have been associated with the induction of anti-BP180-NC16A IgG. Here, we report the case of a female Caucasian patient who developed BP during treatment with the programmed cell death protein 1 (PD-1) inhibitor nivolumab. Intriguingly, the patient exclusively generated anti-LAD-1 IgG, suggesting that anti-LAD-1 IgG was responsible for the development of her autoimmune blistering dermatosis. This is the first such case documented in a non-Japanese patient, thus, lending further support to the pathogenic relevance of anti-LAD-1 IgG in BP.

Keywords: checkpoint inhibitors, bullous pemphigoid, LAD-1, skin inflammation, melanoma, nivolumab

INTRODUCTION

Nivolumab, an immune checkpoint inhibitor, is an IgG_4 antibody which antagonizes the programmed cell death protein 1 (PD-1) receptor (1) and was licensed by the FDA in 2014 for the treatment of metastatic melanoma (1). It has subsequently been approved for the treatment of a wide variety of malignant tumors, including small and non-small cell lung cancer, head and neck cancer, urothelial tract cancer, Hodgkin's lymphoma, hepatocellular, and renal cell carcinoma (2). As with other checkpoint inhibitors, the major side-effects are termed "immune-related adverse events" (irAEs) and present with organ-specific tissue inflammation (1). In fact, up to 42% of patients receiving nivolumab develop cutaneous irAEs (1), ranging from itch to maculopapular, lichenoid, eczematous, granulomatous, or erythema multiforme-like skin changes (3, 4).

There is now increasing evidence that checkpoint inhibition can also result, in rare cases, in the development of blistering skin diseases; clinically and immunopathologically indistinguishable from bullous pemphigoid (BP) (5–14) and associated with the development of tense blisters and erosions on erythematous skin. Histologically, these lesions are characterized by subepidermal clefts and immunofluorescence reveals linear deposition of IgG and C3 at the dermal-epidermal junction (DEJ). In most cases, circulating IgG autoantibodies, directed to the NC16A domain of the hemidesmosomal protein BP180 (type XVII collagen), are detectable in the serum. The presence of these antibodies supports the clinical observation that checkpoint inhibitors can trigger BP.

The immunodominant autoantigen in spontaneous BP is BP180-NC16A with anti-BP180-NC16A IgG detectable in the serum of ~90% of patients with BP (15–17). In addition, 60–70% of patients with BP also produce IgG autoantibodies against the intracellular hemidesmosomal plaque protein BP230 (15). Approximately 60% of these patients also generate antibodies targeting the 120 kDa soluble ectodomain (LAD-1) of BP180 (18, 19), but the significance of these antibodies in the aetiopathogenesis of BP remains uncertain (20).

Interestingly, evidence from Japanese patients suggests that BP may develop in the presence of anti-LAD-1 IgG antibodies alone (21–24). Here, we present a case of BP which developed during treatment with nivolumab, in which anti-LAD-1 IgG antibodies alone were detectable. To our knowledge, this is the first case of checkpoint inhibitor-induced BP in a Caucasian associated with the production of anti-LAD-1 but absence of anti-BP180 NC16A IgG antibodies.

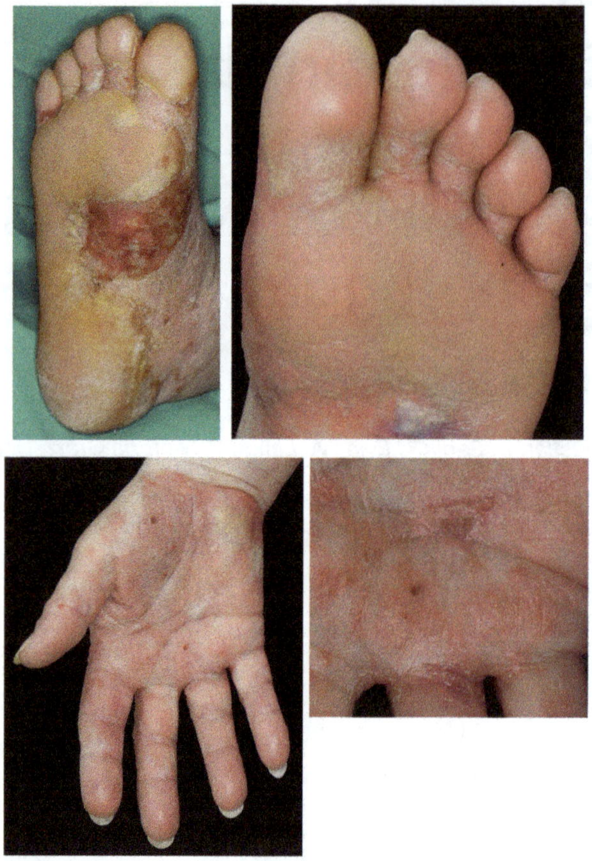

FIGURE 1 | Initial clinical presentation of the cutaneous irAE with vesicles and pustules on the volar skin and the soles.

CASE PRESENTATION

In 2009, a 69-year-old female was diagnosed with a superficial spreading melanoma (Clark level IV; 0.83 mm Breslow thickness; pT1b N3b M1a) of the right lower leg. The melanoma was surgically removed with a 1 cm safety margin. Six years later, in May 2015, the patient developed a subcutaneous in-transit metastasis on her right upper leg. The lesion was surgically excised and simultaneously a complete right inguinal lymph node dissection was performed. In October 2015, new inguinal, para-aortal, and iliac lymph node metastases, as well as new in-transit metastases, were radiologically detected. An immunotherapy with nivolumab (3 mg/kg) every 2 weeks was initiated based on the extent of the loco-regional disease. There was a rapid clinical response, with CT imaging evidencing a regression of the lymph node metastases by early February 2016 and only residual metastases remaining by April 2016.

Prior to the diagnosis of melanoma, the patient had been otherwise fit with no significant co-morbidities. After 11 cycles of nivolumab, the patient developed thyroid peroxidase (TPO) autoantibodies, heralding the development of an immune-mediated thyroiditis which ultimately required substitution therapy with thyroxine. Concurrently, the patient developed small vesicles and pustules on the medial aspects of her palms and soles (**Figure 1**). Despite the application of topical corticosteroids (methylprednisolone cream) both the number and size of these lesions increased (**Figure 2A**). The patient also developed lichenoid papules and plaques on the legs and buttocks (**Figure 2B**). Given the clinical suspicion of an autoimmune blistering disorder, a diagnostic work-up including skin biopsies and serological testing was completed. Direct immunofluorescence (IF) microscopy of perilesional skin demonstrated linear, n-serrated disposition of IgG antibodies and C3 along the DEJ. There was no deposition of IgA autoantibodies.

In line with these findings, serum IgG antibodies were detected by indirect IF microscopy on both monkey esophagus and human salt-split skin (**Figure 3A**). IgA autoantibodies were not detectable. IgG was specifically deposited at the epidermal basement membrane zone on monkey esophagus and on the epidermal side of salt-split skin at a titer of 1:80. Interestingly, serum analysis for anti-BP180-NC16A and anti-BP230 IgG was negative using commercially available ELISA kits (EUROIMMUN, Lübeck, Germany). Therefore, the serum was subsequently examined for the presence of anti-LAD-1 IgG antibodies by immunoblot, using concentrated supernatant of cultured keratinocytes as the antigen, and revealed the presence of autoantibodies in the serum (**Figure 3B**).

Histopathologically, lesional skin exhibited a moderate, predominantly lymphohistiocytic dermal. Taken together, the

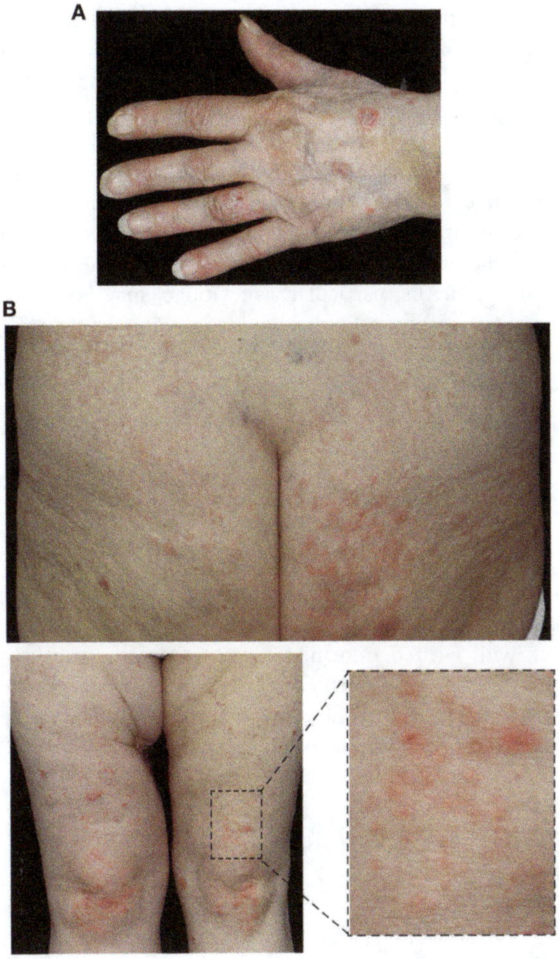

FIGURE 2 | Progression of skin lesions with **(A)** blisters and erosions affecting the lower arms and dorsal hands and **(B)** lichenoid papules on the buttocks and thighs.

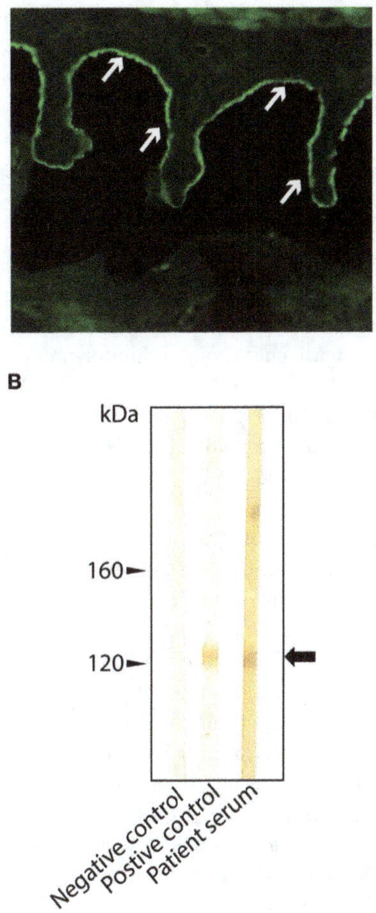

FIGURE 3 | Routine laboratory diagnostic with **(A)** deposition of IgG (indicated by arrows) at the epidermal side of human split skin, and **(B)** detection of anti-LAD IgG autoantibodies by immunoblot on concentrated supernatant of cultured keratinocytes. The arrow indicates the signal identified as LAD-1.

clinical presentation and laboratory findings were consistent with the diagnosis of BP. The immune checkpoint therapy was discontinued after a total of 15 treatment cycles. Combined systemic (oral prednisolone, 50 mg per day; dapsone, 125 mg per day) and topical treatment (clobetasol propionate, twice daily on the entire integument) was initiated. The patient responded slowly to treatment with new blister formation ceasing after 4 weeks of treatment. The lichenoid papules also resolved slowly. The patient continued to suffer from severe pruritus, particularly on the feet, and developed vitiligo.

DISCUSSION

Cutaneous irAEs are the most common side effects of checkpoint inhibitors and can present with a range of skin manifestations; most frequently a non-specific dermatitis. However, our case suggests that in addition to increasing T-lymphocyte activation, the use of checkpoint inhibitors may also be associated with the development of highly specific, B cell-driven autoimmune responses. In fact, the growing number of case reports describing the emergence of anti-BP180 NC16A IgG autoantibodies in patients undergoing checkpoint therapy, the antibody most commonly responsible for the development of autoimmune blistering skin disease, supports this hypothesis. In our patient, however, the administration of nivolumab was associated with the induction of anti-LAD-1 IgG and the emergence of skin changes clinically and immunopathologically indistinguishable from BP. Anti-BP180 NC16A IgG was not detectable and neither was anti-BP230 IgG. With respect to the latter, we must draw our conclusions with the caveat that the ELISA kit used to determine anti-B230 IgG levels can only detect antibodies directed to the C-terminal end of the protein. Hence, we cannot exclude that antibodies against other epitopes of BP230 were generated in our patient and might have contributed to the eruption of BP.

Therefore, given that cutaneous irAEs may initially present with widespread pruritus and non-specific skin changes, patients should be closely monitored for the development of widespread urticarial, eczematous, and blistering skin lesions. Indeed, there should be a high index of suspicion that such patients have begun to develop, or will go on to develop, immunotherapy mediated-BP. Consequently, there should be a low threshold for obtaining a skin biopsy in patients with skin changes, particularly blistering lesions during checkpoint therapy, to determine whether linear deposition of IgG at the DEJ is present. Secondly, in addition to circulating anti-BP180 NC16A IgG antibodies, the presence of anti-LAD-1 IgG autoantibodies should also be determined.

Our case illustrates that merely determining circulating anti-BP180 NC16A IgG levels may not be sufficient to reliably diagnose checkpoint inhibitor mediated BP. Currently, whether some patients with checkpoint inhibitor-induced BP produce both anti-BP180 NC16A IgG and anti-LAD-1 IgG, as reported for a subset of spontaneous BP, is unknown. In this case, the determination of both anti-BP180 NC16A IgG and anti-LAD-1 IgG levels for diagnostic and disease monitoring purposes would be necessary.

Understanding the mechanisms through which checkpoint inhibitors induce BP may shed new light on the pathogenesis of spontaneous BP. For instance, our case supports the notion that anti-LAD-1 IgG alone is sufficient to induce skin blisters and erosions of significant severity. Intriguingly, most recently, a retrospective study in Japanese BP patients found that among those cases of BP, serologically negative for anti-BP180 NC16A IgG, 71% were positive for anti-LAD-1 IgG (17). This suggests that anti-LAD-1 IgG may be pathogenically more significant and more common than previously recognized. In line with previous studies, reporting that cases of BP missing anti-BP180 NC16A IgG autoantibodies tend to exhibit a lower degree of severity with respect to skin inflammation (25), in our case inflammation was on the milder than the average BP patient both on the clinical and the histopathological level.

As a consequence, anti-LAD-1 IgG should be assayed more frequently in the diagnostic workup of suspected cases of BP, particularly in the context of treatment with immune checkpoint inhibitors and when anti-BP180 NC16A IgG autoantibodies are not detectable.

Future studies should examine the extent to which the production of specific antibodies in BP (anti-BP180 NC16A IgG and/or anti-LAD-1 IgG) may actually affect treatment response, because there is first evidence that the emergence of cutaneous irAEs, particularly of vitiligo, may be associated with a better response to checkpoint inhibitor treatment (26). Furthermore, PD-1 activation may actually present a novel therapeutic strategy to suppress flares of BP, which could be investigated in future studies.

ETHICS STATEMENT

This study was carried out in accordance with the recommendations of the Ethics committee of the University of Lübeck with written informed consent from the subject. The subject gave written informed consent in accordance with the Declaration of Helsinki. The protocol was approved by the Ethics committee of the University of Lübeck.

AUTHOR CONTRIBUTIONS

CS, EL, VG, DZ, and PT analyzed and compiled the case. CS, EL, and PT wrote the manuscript. DZ edited the manuscript.

REFERENCES

1. Callahan MK, Postow MA, Wolchok JD. Targeting T cell co-receptors for cancer therapy. *Immunity.* (2016) 44:1069–78. doi: 10.1016/j.immuni.2016.04.023
2. Ribas A, Wolchok JD. Cancer immunotherapy using checkpoint blockade. *Science.* (2018) 359:1350–5. doi: 10.1126/science.aar4060
3. Sibaud V. Dermatologic reactions to immune checkpoint inhibitors: skin toxicities and immunotherapy. *Am J Clin Dermatol.* (2018) 19:345–61. doi: 10.1007/s40257-017-0336-3
4. Tetzlaff MT, Jazaeri AA, Torres-Cabala CA, Korivi BR, Landon GA, Nagarajan P, et al. Erythema nodosum-like panniculitis mimicking disease recurrence: a novel toxicity from immune checkpoint blockade therapy-Report of 2 patients. *J Cutan Pathol.* (2017) 44:1080–6. doi: 10.1111/cup.13044
5. Carlos G, Anforth R, Chou S, Clements A, Fernandez-Penas P. A case of bullous pemphigoid in a patient with metastatic melanoma treated with pembrolizumab. *Melanoma Res.* (2015) 25:265–8. doi: 10.1097/CMR.0000000000000155
6. Naidoo J, Schindler K, Querfeld C, Busam K, Cunningham J, Page DB, et al. Autoimmune bullous skin disorders with immune checkpoint inhibitors targeting PD-1 and PD-L1. *Cancer Immunol Res.* (2016) 4:383–9. doi: 10.1158/2326-6066.CIR-15-0123
7. Mochel MC, Ming ME, Imadojemu S, Gangadhar TC, Schuchter LM, Elenitsas R, et al. Cutaneous autoimmune effects in the setting of therapeutic immune checkpoint inhibition for metastatic melanoma. *J Cutan Pathol.* (2016) 43:787–91. doi: 10.1111/cup.12735
8. Parakh S, Nguyen R, Opie JM, Andrews MC. Late presentation of generalised bullous pemphigoid-like reaction in a patient treated with pembrolizumab for metastatic melanoma. *Australas J Dermatol.* (2017) 58:e109–e12. doi: 10.1111/ajd.12488
9. Hirotsu K, Chiou AS, Chiang A, Kim J, Kwong BY, Pugliese S. Localized bullous pemphigoid in a melanoma patient with dual exposure to PD-1 checkpoint inhibition and radiation therapy. *JAAD Case Rep.* (2017) 3:404–6. doi: 10.1016/j.jdcr.2017.06.004
10. Garje R, Chau JJ, Chung J, Wanat K, Zakharia Y. Acute flare of bullous pemphigus with pembrolizumab used for treatment of metastatic urothelial cancer. *J Immunother.* (2018) 41:42–4. doi: 10.1097/CJI.0000000000000191
11. Anastasopoulou A, Papaxoinis G, Diamantopoulos P, Christofidou E, Benopoulou O, Stratigos A, et al. Bullous pemphigoid-like skin lesions and overt eosinophilia in a patient with melanoma treated with nivolumab: case report and review of the literature. *J Immunother.* (2018) 41:164–7. doi: 10.1097/CJI.0000000000000210
12. Thomsen K, Diernaes J, Ollegaard TH, Spaun E, Vestergaard C. Bullous pemphigoid as an adverse reaction to pembrolizumab: two case reports. *Case Rep Dermatol.* (2018) 10:154–7. doi: 10.1159/000489661
13. Lopez AT, Geskin L. A case of nivolumab-induced bullous pemphigoid: review of dermatologic toxicity associated with programmed cell death protein-1/programmed death ligand-1 inhibitors and recommendations

for diagnosis and management. *Oncologist.* (2018) 23:1119–26. doi: 10.1634/theoncologist.2018-0128
14. Rofe O, Bar-Sela G, Keidar Z, Sezin T, Sadik CD, Bergman R. Severe bullous pemphigoid associated with pembrolizumab therapy for metastatic melanoma with complete regression. *Clin Exp Dermatol.* (2017) 42:309–12. doi: 10.1111/ced.13042
15. Schmidt E, Zillikens D. Pemphigoid diseases. *Lancet.* (2013) 381:320–32. doi: 10.1016/S0140-6736(12)61140-4
16. Liu Y, Li L, Xia Y. BP180 is critical in the autoimmunity of bullous pemphigoid. *Front Immunol.* (2017) 8:1752. doi: 10.3389/fimmu.2017.01752
17. Nakama K, Koga H, Ishii N, Ohata C, Hashimoto T, Nakama T. Clinical and immunological profiles of 14 patients with bullous pemphigoid without IgG autoantibodies to the BP180 NC16A domain. *JAMA Dermatol.* (2018) 154:347–50. doi: 10.1001/jamadermatol.2017.5465
18. Schumann H, Baetge J, Tasanen K, Wojnarowska F, Schacke H, Zillikens D, et al. The shed ectodomain of collagen XVII/BP180 is targeted by autoantibodies in different blistering skin diseases. *Am J Pathol.* (2000) 156:685–95. doi: 10.1016/S0002-9440(10)64772-4
19. Pas HH, Kloosterhuis GJ, Heeres K, van der Meer JB, Jonkman MF. Bullous pemphigoid and linear IgA dermatosis sera recognize a similar 120-kDa keratinocyte collagenous glycoprotein with antigenic cross-reactivity to BP180. *J Invest Dermatol.* (1997) 108:423–9. doi: 10.1111/1523-1747.ep12289703
20. Izumi K, Nishie W, Mai Y, Wada M, Natsuga K, Ujiie H, et al. Autoantibody profile differentiates between inflammatory and noninflammatory bullous pemphigoid. *J Invest Dermatol.* (2016) 136:2201–10. doi: 10.1016/j.jid.2016.06.622
21. Miyashita K, Iioka H, Miyagawa F, Ishii N, Hashimoto T, Asada H. A case of bullous pemphigoid with IgG antibodies against LAD-1, but not BP180 NC16a domain or BP230. *Eur J Dermatol.* (2018) 28:248–50. doi: 10.1684/ejd.2018.3229
22. Ikawa T, Tada Y, Ohnishi T, Miyagaki T, Watanabe R, Ishii N, et al. Bullous pemphigoid with immunoglobulin G anti-LAD-1 antibodies without evident erythema and eosinophil infiltration. *Acta Derm Venereol.* (2016) 96:832–3. doi: 10.2340/00015555-2400
23. Matsui K, Makino T, Takegami Y, Murayama S, Seki Y, Ishii N, et al. Bullous pemphigoid with IgG anti-LAD-1 antibodies. *Eur J Dermatol.* (2014) 24:275–6. doi: 10.1684/ejd.2014.2322
24. Tsuruta D, Nishikawa T, Yamagami J, Hashimoto T. Unilateral bullous pemphigoid without erythema and eosinophil infiltration in a hemiplegic patient. *J Dermatol.* (2012) 39:787–9. doi: 10.1111/j.1346-8138.2012.01562.x
25. Horikawa H, Kurihara Y, Funakoshi T, Umegaki-Arao N, Takahashi H, Kubo A, et al. Unique clinical and serological features of bullous pemphigoid associated with dipeptidyl peptidase-4 inhibitors. *Br J Dermatol.* (2018) 178:1462–3. doi: 10.1111/bjd.16479
26. Sanlorenzo M, Vujic I, Daud A, Algazi A, Gubens M, Luna SA, et al. Pembrolizumab cutaneous adverse events and their association with disease progression. *JAMA Dermatol.* (2015) 151:1206–12. doi: 10.1001/jamadermatol.2015.1916

9

Role of Dsg1- and Dsg3-Mediated Signaling in Pemphigus Autoantibody-Induced Loss of Keratinocyte Cohesion

Elias Walter[1]*, Franziska Vielmuth*[1]*, Marie-Therès Wanuske*[1]*, Matthias Seifert*[1]*, Robert Pollmann*[2]*, Rüdiger Eming*[2] *and Jens Waschke*[1*]

[1] *Institute of Anatomy and Cell Biology, Ludwig-Maximilians-Universität München, Munich, Germany,* [2] *Department of Dermatology and Allergology, Philipps-Universität Marburg, Marburg, Germany*

***Correspondence:**
Jens Waschke
jens.waschke@med.uni-muenchen.de

Pemphigus is an autoimmune dermatosis in which mucocutaneous blisters are induced primarily by autoantibodies against Desmoglein (Dsg) 1 and 3. Pemphigus vulgaris (PV) usually is associated with autoantibodies against Dsg3 whereas pemphigus foliaceus (PF) patients present autoantibodies against Dsg1. Several signaling pathways were proposed to cause loss of keratinocyte adhesion. However, relevance of different signaling pathways and role of Dsg1 and 3 to trigger signaling are not fully understood. Here, we show that Ca^{2+} chelation reduced PV-IgG- and PF-IgG-mediated loss of HaCaT keratinocyte cohesion whereas EGFR inhibition did not inhibit effects of PF-IgG. PV-IgG activated EGFR in a Src-dependent manner whereas both PV-IgG and PF-IgG caused Ca^{2+} influx independent of EGFR. ERK activation was Src-dependent in response to PV-IgG but not PF-IgG. To delineate the roles of Dsg isoforms to trigger signaling pathways, Dsg3- and Dsg2-deficient HaCaT keratinocyte cell lines were generated using CRISPR/Cas9. Dsg3- but not Dsg2-deficient cells were protected against PV-IgG-induced loss of cell adhesion. Ca^{2+} influx and ERK activation in response to PF-IgG were preserved in both cell lines.

Keywords: autoimmunity, pemphigus, keratinocytes, desmoglein, signaling, CRISPR/Cas9

1. INTRODUCTION

Pemphigus is an autoimmune blistering disease affecting mucous membranes and the epidermis (1). The pathogenesis of pemphigus is complex and includes genetic factors facilitating production of autoantibodies and enhancing susceptibility of keratinocytes for loss of cell adhesion (2, 3). Factors contributing to blister formation include antibodies against the desmosomal cadherins desmoglein (Dsg) 1 and 3 (1) as well as non-antibody factors such as soluble Fas ligand (4). Autoantibodies against other keratinocyte antigens are also found in patients' sera and blister fluid and may augment pathogenic effects, however, their role for blister formation is undefined at present (5, 6). Thus, it is generally accepted that antibodies against desmosomal cadherins are sufficient to cause acantholysis in pemphigus (7). Desmosomes are highly specialized adhesive contacts most abundant in tissues subjected to high mechanical stress such as the epidermis and heart muscle (8). Indeed, it was demonstrated recently that desmosomes bear mechanical load primarily when cells are exposed to external mechanical stress (9). Usually, in pemphigus vulgaris a mucosal-dominant phenotype (m-PV) is paralleled by autoantibodies against Dsg3 whereas epidermal involvement in PV (mc-PV) is in addition associated with formation of autoantibodies against Dsgl which can also be found in pemphigus foliaceus (PF) (10). The mechanisms by which antibodies against desmosomal cadherins induce loss of cell adhesion are multiple and comprise direct inhibition of Dsg3 binding as well as a large number of signaling pathways which finally interfere with desmosome turn-over (7, 11, 12). In this context, desmosomal cadherins have been proposed to serve as signaling hubs to coordinate cell adhesion with cell-specific functions such as wound-healing in keratinocytes (13, 14). However, despite the intriguing correlation between clinical phenotype and autoantibody profiles, the factors defining the different clinical phenotypes in pemphigus are poorly understood. Previously, it was reported that autoantibody profiles also correlate with different subsets of signaling pathways engaged suggesting that signaling pattern define the clinical course of the disease (15). Antibodies specific for Dsg3 such as the mouse pemphigus antibody AK23 (16) similar to m-PV-IgG was sufficient to activate p38MAPK and Src whereas Ca^{2+} influx and ERK activation were detectable only when antibodies against Dsgl were present in patients IgG fractions such as mc-PV-IgG and PF-IgG (15). Here, we further characterized the role of the different signaling mechanisms and of antibodies against Dsgl and Dsg3. We observed that signaling mechanisms such as EGFR and ERK activation or influx of Ca^{2+} not only correlated with autoantibody profiles but also were at least in part dependent on other signaling molecules such as Src. We established human keratinocyte cell lines deficient for Dsg3 and observed that in the absence of Dsg3 PV-IgG-induced loss of cell adhesion was abolished indicating that autoantibodies against Dsg3 are required for this process.

2. MATERIALS AND METHODS

2.1. Cell Culture

HaCaT (Human adult high Calcium low Temperature) keratinocytes (17) were cultured in Dulbecco's Modified Eagle Medium (DMEM) containing 10% FCS (Biochrom, Berlin, Germany), 50 U/ml penicillin and 50 mg/ml streptomycin (AppliChem, Darmstadt, Germany) in a humidified atmosphere of 5% CO_2 and 37°C. On the day cells reached confluency medium was changed and experiments were performed 24 h later.

2.2. Pemphigus Sera and IgG Purification

Patient sera were acquired from the Dermatology department of the Philipps Universität Marburg. Patients and donors gave written consent for research use. A positive vote of the Ethics Committee from the Medical Faculty of the University of Marburg was given. During disease diagnosis the phenotype was histologically and immunologically confirmed (**Table 1**). All patients presented phenotype as well as antibody profile typical clinical features. Sera of patients and healthy volunteers were purified to IgG-fractions for experimental use by protein A affinity chromatography as described previously (18). All IgG fractions including c-IgG were subjected to ELISA assays (Euroimmun, Lübeck, Germany) to determine Dsg3 and Dsgl antibody profiles. All scores below a 20 U/ml cut-off were considered as negative.

TABLE 1 | Antibody profiles of IgG-fractions determined by Dsg1 and Dsg3 ELISA and their clinical phenotypes.

	ELISA score (U/ml)		Clinical phenotype
	aDsg1	aDsg3	
c-IgG	–	–	healthy control
m-PV	–	162.93	mucosal PV
mc-PV	153.76	172.53	mucocutaneous PV
mc-PV2	101.18	106.72	mucocutaneous PV
PF	215.34	–	cutaneous PF

Cut off values are considered as 20 U/ml.

2.3. Pharmacological Mediators

Signaling pathway inhibition was accomplished using pharmacological mediators which were used at the indicated concentrations and time periods prior to treatment to assure sufficient effects (**Table 2**). Vehicle control conditions were treated with the respective DMSO concentration.

2.4. Immunostaining

Cell monolayers were grown on glass coverslips until confluency and fixed with 2% formaldehyde from paraformaldehyde for 10 min. After permeabilization of cells with 0.1% Triton X-100 in PBS for 5 min, blocking was achieved by incubation of 3% bovine serum albumin (BSA) and 1% normal goat serum (NGS) in PBS for 60 min. The following primary antibodies were incubated overnight at 4°C: anti-Dsg3 mAb (clone 5G11, Invitrogen, Carlsbad, CA, USA), anti-Dsg2 mAb (OriGene, Herford, Germany), anti-E-Cadherin mAb (BD Transduction Laboratories, Heidelberg, Germany), anti-PG mAb (Progen, Heidelberg, Germany), anti-DP mAb (NW6, kind gift from Kathleen J. Green, Northwestern University, Chicago, USA). Cy3 coupled goat anti-rabbit or goat anti-mouse secondary antibodies (Dianova, Hamburg, Germany) were used to visualize the respective protein by incubation for 1 h at room temperature. Finally, cover slips were mounted with 2% n-propyl-gallate (NPG) on glass coverslides and evaluated on a SP5.II confocal microscope equipped with a 63x NA 1.4 PL APO objective (Leica, Mannheim, Germany).

2.5. Dispase-Based Dissociation Assay

Confluent monolayers were subjected to treatment as indicated in the respective experiment. Afterwards, cells were detached from the well bottom by application of 200 μl Dispase-II solution (Sigma-Aldrich) for 20 min. Following successful detachment, 350 μl Hank's Balanced Salt Solution (HBSS) was used to substitute the enzyme. Defined mechanical shear stress was applied with an electrical pipette (Finnpipette Novus, ThermoFisher, Waltham, USA). Cell-sheet fragments correlate with loss of adhesion (19) and were counted under a binocular

TABLE 2 | Pharmacological mediators with their target molecule, concentration, pretreatment as well as commercial origin.

Inhibitor	Target	Concentration (μM)	Pre-treatment (h)	Origin
U0126	MEK 1/2	5	1	New England Biolabs, Ipswich, USA
PP2	Src-family kinases	10	1	Merck Millipore, Billerica, USA
BAPTA-AM	Intracellular Ca^{2+} chelation	200	4	Merck Millipore, Billerica, USA
Erlotinib	EGFR	2.5	1	Santa Cruz Biotechnology,Santa Cruz, USA

microscope (Stemi 508, Zeiss, Jena, Germany). Pictures were taken with a Canon EOS 600D camera (Krefeld, Germany).

2.6. Cell Lysis, Gel Electrophoresis, and Western Blotting

After reaching confluency, cell monolayers were switched to 300 μl fresh medium for 24 h. IgG fractions and mediators were incubated as indicated. The following protocol was performed as described previously (15). In short, cell lysates were separated into a soluble cytosolic and insoluble cytoskeletal bound fraction by incubation of triton extraction buffer (0.5% Triton X-100, 50 mmol/l MES, 25 mmol/l EGTA, 5 mmol/l $MgCl_2$, pH 6.8, 0.1% of each Pepstatin, Aprotinin and Leupeptin, 1% PMSF) for 15 min on ice under gentle shaking. Cells were harvested with a cell scraper and the insoluble pellet was sedimented by centrifugation for 10 min at 4°C as well as 14,000 rcf. Supernatants were collected and the pellet was resuspended in SDS lysis buffer (25 mM Hepes, 2 mM EDTA, 25 mM NaF, 1% SDS, pH 7.6, complete Protease Inhibitors). Protein amount was determined with a commercial Pierce BCA Protein Assay Kit and lysates were subjected to Western blot analysis with a standard wet blotting protocol on nitrocellulose membranes (Life Technologies, Carlsbad, USA). Membranes were blocked by 5% bovine serum albumin (BSA) in Tris-buffered saline with 0.05% Tween (TBS-T) for 1 h at room temperature and following primary antibodies were used overnight at 4°C in blocking solution: phospho-EGF Receptor mAb (Tyr845) (Cell Signaling Technologies, Danvers, USA), EGF Receptor mAb (CST), phospho-p44/42 MAPK mAb (CST), p44/42 MAPK mAb (CST), GAPDH (Santa Cruz, Heidelberg, Germany), Desmoplakin I/II (H-300) (Santa Cruz), α-Tubulin (Abcam, Cambridge, UK), Dsg3 pAb (Biozol, Eching, Germany), PG (Progen, Heidelberg, Germany), E-Cad (BD Transduction), Dsg2 (OriGene, Herford, Germany), Desmocollin (Dsc) 3 (Progen). Horseradish-peroxidase coupled secondary antibodies (Dianova, Hamburg, Germany) from the respective species were used in TBS-T for 1 h at room temperature and visualized by a self-made ECL solution on a FluorchemE (Protein Simple, San Jose, USA) developer. Every analyzed signaling protein was exclusively localized in the soluble fraction. Therefore, only this fraction is shown in most figures.

2.7. Ratiometric Intracellular Ca^{2+} Measurements

Fura-2AM (ThermoFisher) was used to determine the intracellular Ca^{2+} concentration in real time. Cells were therefore grown in an 8-Well μ-slide (Ibidi, Martinsried, Germany) until confluency. Mediators were used before the Fura-2AM dye was applied and were also present during dye loading. A mix of 1 μM Fura-2AM and 0.02% Pluronic (ThermoFisher) was applied for 20 min in measurement buffer (140 mM NaCl, 3.6 mM KCl, 2.6 mM $CaCl_2(H_2O)_2$, 0.5 mM $NaH_2PO_4(H_2O)_2$, 2 mM $NaHCO_3$, HEPES and 5 mM D+ Glucose) at 37°C to facilitate transfer of the dye into cells. After replacing the solution with fresh measurement buffer cells were measured with MetaFluor (Moleculardevices, San Jóse, USA) on an Axio Observer A1 (Zeiss, Jena, Germany) with a Polychrome V (Till Photonics, Planegg, Germany), a CoolSNAP-Hq2 digital camera (Photometrics, Tucson, USA) and a Fura-2 filter set.

2.8. Atomic Force Microscopy

AFM data were acquired using a NanoWizard® 3 AFM (JPK-Instruments, Berlin, Germany) mounted on an inverted optical microscope (Carl Zeiss, Jena, Germany), which allowed the selection of the scanning area by visualizing the cells with a 63x objective. The pyramidal-shaped D-Tip of Si_3N_4 MLCT cantilevers (Bruker, Mannheim, Germany) with a nominal spring constant of 0.03 N/m and tip radius of 20 nm were used for all experiments. Cantilevers were functionalized with recombinant Dsg3-Fc (at a concentration of 0.15mg/ml) using a flexible heterobifunctional acetal-polyethylenglycol (PEG) linker (Gruber Lab, Institute of Biophysics, Linz, Austria) following a well-established protocol (20). Force-distance curves were sampled in force-mapping mode in which a picture is composed of single pixels, each containing the information of one force-distance curve. To measure Dsg3 single molecule interactions HaCaT cells were measured in DMEM containing 1.8 mM Ca^{2+} at 37°C after incubation with the respective conditions. As pathogenic aDsg3 Abs directly interfere with Dsg3 interactions (21, 22) AFM cantilevers were removed during Ab incubation and residual antibodies in the medium were vigorously cleared before reintroducing the AFM tip to avoid antibody binding to the scanning tip. Force maps were acquired at small areas along cell borders (5 × 2.5 μm) at a resolution of 50 × 25 pixels each. The setpoint was set to 0.2 nN to avoid damage of the cells during measurements. Further, a Z-length of 1.5 μm, a pulling speed of 10 μm/s and a resting contact time of 0.1 s were applied throughout all measurements.

2.9. CRISPR/Cas9 Mediated Gene Editing

Dsg3 and Dsg2 HaCaT knock out cell lines were generated utilizing the CRISPR/Cas9 mediated gene editing system. HaCaT keratinocytes were therefore purchased freshly and used at passage 32. Two expression vectors encoding *Streptococcus pyogenes* Cas9 coupled to green fluorescent protein (GFP) (pCMV-Cas9-GFP) with different target sites for each protein of interest were purchased (Sigma-Aldrich, St. Louis, USA) and chosen to specifically induce a double strand break at the beginning of the protein resulting in non-homologous end joining (NHEJ) repairs as indicated in **Figure 4** (Target ID: Dsg2: HS0000249131, HS0000249134; Dsg3: HS0000249170, HS0000249174). The plasmid was transiently introduced into cells using Lipofectamin-2000 in Opti-MEM as instructed by the manual (ThermoFisher). Sub cloning was initiated after an expression period of 24 h by sorting single GFP-positive cells into five 96-well plates by a FACSAria III (BD Transduction) cell sorting unit for each transfection. The medium was renewed every third day for a time span of 4 weeks and wells were inspected for monoclonal cultures every week followed by individual expansion to a bigger culture dish on demand. Eventually, around 40 different monoclonal clones for each target site could be evaluated for the absence of either Dsg3 or Dsg2 by immunoblot as well as immunostaining. Afterwards, genomic DNA was extracted using a standard Phenol-Chloroform DNA extraction protocol and send for Sanger sequencing with an area of 500 base pairs flanking both ends of the target site (Eurofins, Ebersberg, Germany). Results were aligned to the known DNA sequence and alleles separated by hand in case of heterozygous mutations.

2.10. Analysis and Statistics

Images and figures were processed using Photoshop CC (Adobe Creative Cloud, Adobe, San Jóse, USA). The blot analysis function in ImageJ (Wayne Rasband, https://imagej.nih.gov/ij) was used to quantify protein density in immunoblots and graphs were generated in Graphpad Prism (GraphPad Software, San Diego, USA). Each n represents an independent experiment. Statistical Analysis was performed in Prism using either paired one-way ANOVA corrected by Dunett's test for multiple comparisons or paired two-way ANOVA corrected by Fisher's LSD test for experiments with separate factors as indicated in the figure legends. Statistical significance was assumed at $p \leq 0.05$. Bar diagrams are presented as mean ± standard error.

3. RESULTS

3.1. Relevance of Ca^{2+} and EGFR Signaling for Pemphigus Autoantibody-Induced Loss of Cell Adhesion

The relevance of signaling pathways during the pathogenesis of pemphigus is widely accepted (7). Recently, we reported pemphigus phenotype-specific differences in the roles of signaling pathways for loss of adhesion in HaCaT as well as primary normal human epidermal keratinocytes (NHEK) (15). In this study, we observed that Ca^{2+} influx was associated with autoantibodies against Dsg1 in patients' IgG. Others have reported that epidermal growth factor receptor (EGFR) is activated by AK23, a murine pathogenic Dsg3-specific antibody (16, 23). Therefore, we investigated the relevance of Ca^{2+} influx and EGFR signaling for loss of keratinocyte adhesion in response to IgG fractions containing different profiles of aDsg1 and aDsg3 antibodies from patients suffering from m-PV, mc-PV and PF in dispase-based dissociation assays. First, Fura measurements were performed to evaluate the efficiency of BAPTA-AM. Therefore, HaCaT keratinocytes were treated for 4 h with BAPTA-AM at different concentrations. A concentration of 200 μM BAPTA-AM was suited best to block PF-IgG induced Ca^{2+}-influx (**Figure 1A**). In Dispase assays this concentration was effective to reduce loss of cell cohesion by approximately 40% in all conditions compared to conditions incubated with autoantibodies alone (**Figure 1B**). Inhibition of EGFR using Erlotinib, a specific EGFR tyrosine kinase inhibitor, reduced loss of adhesion only in response to IgG fractions containing autoantibodies targeting Dsg3, specifically in response to m-PV-IgG and mc-PV-IgG but not to PF-IgG (**Figure 1C**).

3.2. Time Dependency of Pemphigus-IgG Mediated EGFR and ERK Activation

Ca^{2+} influx is known to occur within 60 s after application of antibodies (24, 25), which is also supported by data from this study (**Figure 3C**). Next, we determined the kinetics of autoantibody-induced activation of EGFR in comparison to ERK, which we previously observed to correlate with autoantibodies against Dsg1 (15). HaCaT cells were incubated with the different IgG fractions for 5 min, 30 min as well as for 60 min. Afterwards, cell lysates were subjected to Triton fractionation and Western blotting to determine the phosphorylation of EGFR at the Src-dependent site Y845 as well as of ERK. Of note, a marked EGFR activation was detectable after 30 and 60 min but only showed a significant increase when cells were incubated with m-PV-IgG for 30 min in the soluble pool (**Figure 2A**). In contrast, ERK activation in response to PF-IgG was observed at all time-points but significant only after 30 and 60 min also in the soluble fraction (**Figure 2B**). Mc-PV-IgG-induced activation of ERK was significant after 30 min. From these experiments we concluded that for the following experiments studying the interdependence of signaling pathways, 30 min would be most suitable.

3.3. Interdependency of Signaling Pathways Involved in Pemphigus Autoantibody-Induced Loss of Cell Adhesion

We tested the dependency of EGFR and ERK activation on each other as well as on Src and Ca^{2+} influx after 30 min of autoantibody incubation (**Figures 3A,B**). In addition to Erlotinib and BAPTA-AM, PP2, a Src family kinase inhibitor, and U0126, an inhibitor of MEK upstream of ERK, were applied in parallel to the different IgG fractions. In absence of inhibitors and BAPTA-AM, m-PV-IgG and mc-PV significantly enhanced EGFR phosphorylation (**Figure 3A**). Activation was abolished when PP2 or Erlotinib were added. Chelation of Ca^{2+} enhanced the variability of EGFR phosphorylation, which was not significantly different to experiments using control IgG. Interestingly, after inhibition of MEK using U0126, PF-IgG-induced EGFR phosphorylation was increased

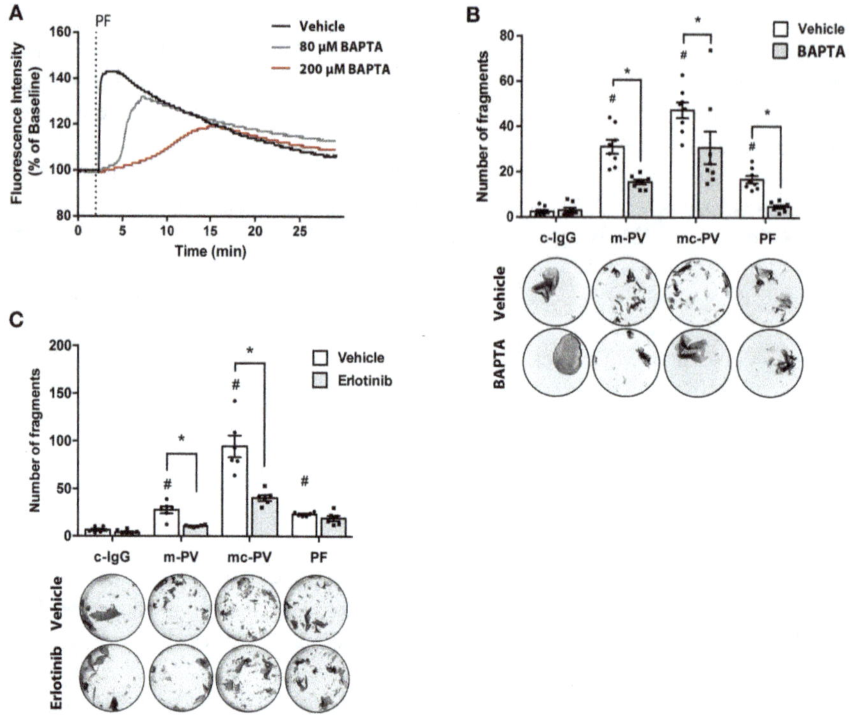

FIGURE 1 | Relevance of EGFR and Ca^{2+} signaling for pemphigus autoantibody-induced loss of cell adhesion. **(A)** Fura measurements of HaCaT cells pretreated with 80 μM as well as 200 μM BAPTA-AM for 4 h to determine Ca^{2+} chelation efficiency after PF-IgG treatment ($n = 4$, representative graph). HaCaT keratinocytes were subjected to dispase assays following incubation with different IgG fractions in presence or absence of pharmacological inhibitors to evaluate the relevance of Ca^{2+} influx as well as the EGFR signaling pathway for loss of keratinocyte adhesion. **(B)** Fragment numbers revealed reduced loss of adhesion under all conditions after chelation of intracellular Ca^{2+} by BAPTA ($n = 8$, two-way ANOVA, $\#p \leq 0.05$ vs. vehicle c-IgG, $^*p \leq 0.05$) **(C)** Inhibition of EGFR by Erlotinib for 1 h followed by addition of IgG fractions for 2 h revealed a decrease of fragments in monolayers treated with m-PV-IgG as well as mc-PV-IgG but not PF-IgG ($n = 6$, two-way ANOVA, $\#p \leq 0.05$ vs. vehicle c-IgG, $^*p \leq 0.05$).

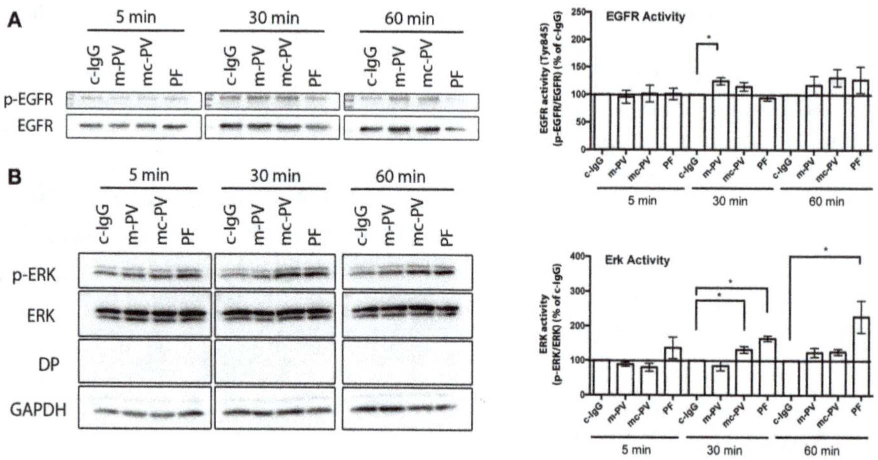

FIGURE 2 | Time course of pemphigus IgG-mediated EGFR and ERK activation. Confluent HaCaT cell monolayers were incubated with different IgG fractions for 5 min, 30 min as well as 60 min to evaluate activation due to phosphorylation of **(A)** EGFR and **(B)** ERK in immunoblots. EGFR was activated after 30 min by IgG fractions containing antibodies against Dsg3 ($n \geq 7$, $^*p \leq 0.05$, one-way ANOVA, normalized to respective c-IgG). ERK was activated only when antibodies targeting Dsg1 were present ($n \geq 7$, $^*p \leq 0.05$, one-way ANOVA, normalized to respective c-IgG).

whereas PV-IgG-induced activation was not. ERK activation was significant following incubation with mc-PV-IgG or PF-IgG but not m-PV-IgG (**Figure 3B**). Moreover, Erlotinib, PP2 and U0126 prevented mc-PV-IgG-induced ERK activation whereas ERK phosphorylation in response to PF-IgG was blunted by Erlotinib only. After chelation of Ca^{2+}, PV-IgG-induced ERK

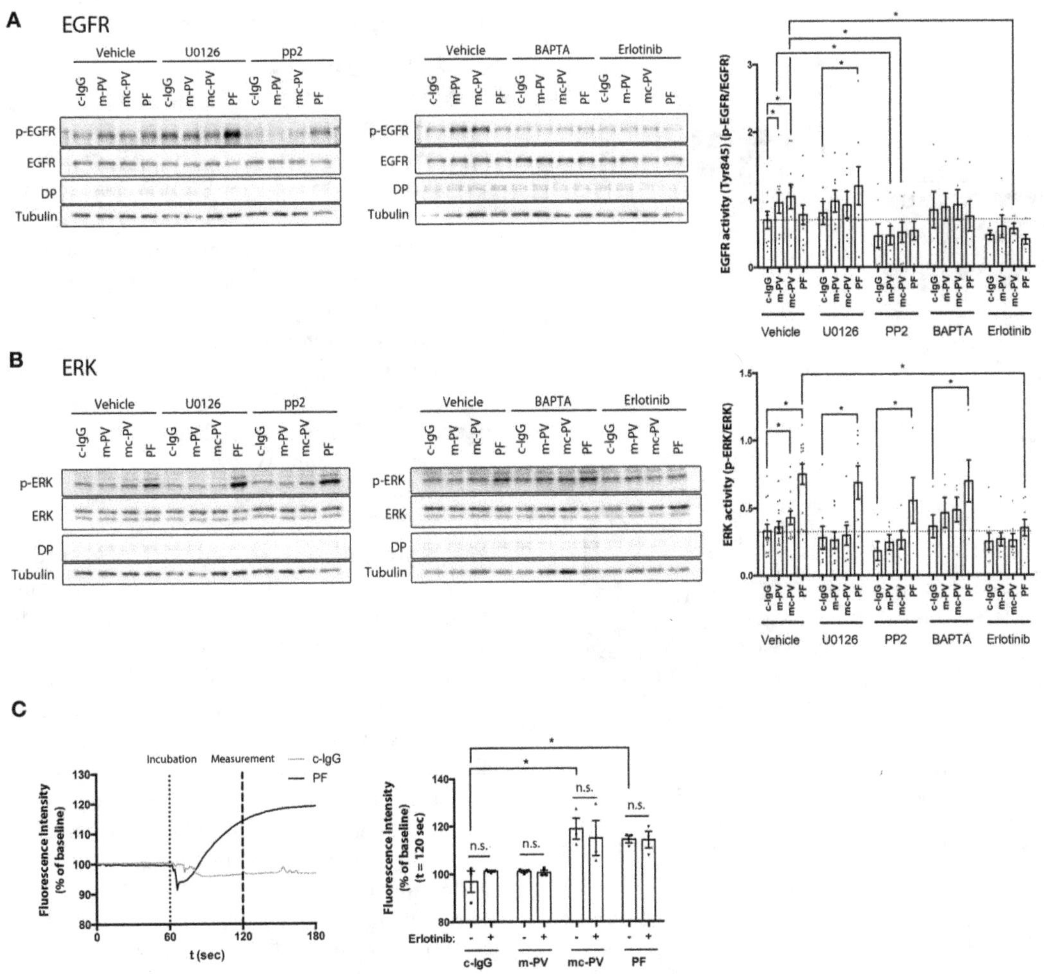

FIGURE 3 | Interdependency of signaling pathways activated by pemphigus autoantibodies. Immunoblots of cell monolayers pretreated with either pharmacological inhibitors for 1 h or BAPTA-AM for 4 h followed by IgG fractions for 30 min. **(A)** EGFR activity was reduced after Src inhibition by PP2 ($n \geq 6$, $^*p \leq 0.05$, two-way ANOVA) **(B)** After inhibition of EGFR by Erlotinib, ERK phosphorylation was significantly reduced in cells treated with PF-IgG. ($n \geq 6$, $p \leq 0.05$, two-way ANOVA) **(C)** Ca^{2+} influx was measured by Fura-2 ratiometric fluorescence imaging and found to be independent of EGFR ($n = 3$, $^*p \leq 0.05$, two-way ANOVA) Representative graph with experimental setup on the left and analysis at t = 120 s on the right. Dotted line indicates application of the respective IgG fraction.

activation was variable but not significant, whereas PF-IgG-induced ERK activation was significant. Ca^{2+} influx has been recognized down-stream of EGFR activation (26). Therefore, we employed Fura-2 ratiometric measurements after application of autoantibodies in presence or absence of Erlotinib. A baseline was established for 60 s in HaCaT keratinocytes, followed by application of either c-IgG, m-PV, mc-PV or PF for another 120 s. Intracellular Ca^{2+} concentrations were evaluated 60 s after addition of IgG fractions. Both, mc-PV-IgG and PF-IgG but not m-PV-IgG were effective to induce a transient Ca^{2+} influx which was not affected by inhibition of EGFR by Erlotinib (**Figure 3C**). Taken together, these results indicate that PV-IgG-induced activation of both EGFR and ERK are Src- and EGFR kinase-dependent whereas PF-IgG-induced ERK activation is completely independent of Src, MEK and Ca^{2+}. Moreover, mc-PV-IgG- and PF-IgG-induced Ca^{2+} influx appears not to be related to EGFR signaling.

3.4. EGFR Activation Reduces Binding Frequency but Not Binding Strength of Dsg3 Interactions on Living HaCaT Keratinocytes

The mechanism by which EGFR activation reduces desmosome adhesion in pemphigus is not fully understood. It was shown previously that stimulation of EGFR by EGF reduced Dsg2 binding frequency on DLD1 enterocytes (27). Thus, we hypothesized that Dsg3 in keratinocytes may also be regulated by EGFR and evaluated Dsg3 single molecule binding properties at cell borders of living HaCaT cells before and after stimulation with EGF by atomic force microscopy (AFM). EGFR activation reduced Dsg3 binding frequency on keratinocytes significantly from 7.67 to 3.20% in a Src-dependent manner because inhibition by PP2 restored Dsg3 binding frequency to 8.48% (**Figure 4A**). The unbinding force remained unchanged at a median of

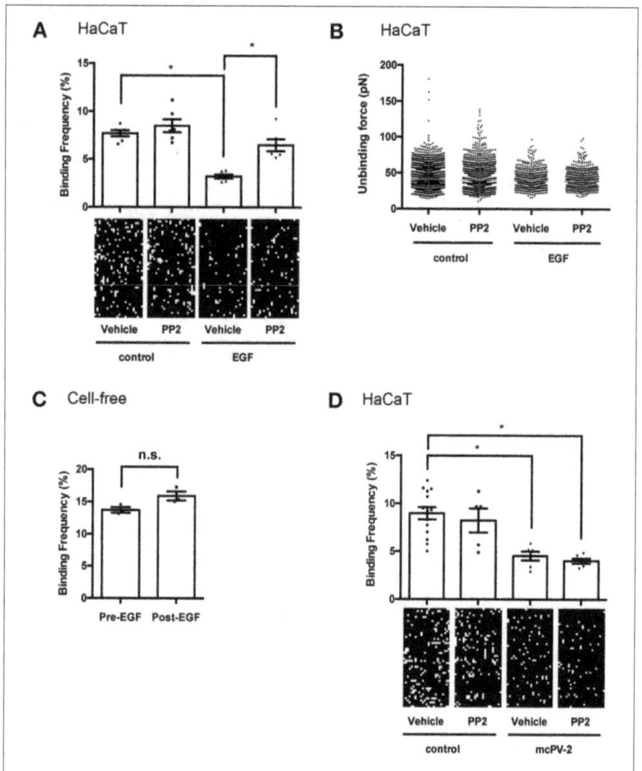

FIGURE 4 | EGFR activation reduces binding frequency of Dsg3 interactions on living HaCaT keratinocytes. **(A)** Atomic force microscopy (AFM) adhesion measurements on cell borders of living HaCaT keratinocytes using a Dsg3 Fc-functionalized tip and 1 h incubation of EGF with representative force maps. A reduction in binding frequency is observable in a Src-dependent manner, ($n = 3$ with two separate cell borders per experiment, one-way ANOVA, $^*p \leq 0.05$) whereas **(B)** binding forces remained unaffected. **(C)** Cell-free AFM measurements on Dsg3 Fc-functionalized mica sheets prove that reduction in binding frequency is not induced by direct inhibition ($n = 3$, *t*-test, $^*p \leq 0.05$) **(D)** Binding frequency was reduced in HaCaT cells treated for 1 h with mc-PV2-IgG independently of Src ($n \geq 3$, with two separate cell borders per experiment, one-way ANOVA, $^*p \leq 0.05$).

around 40 pN (**Figure 4B**). To prove that the reduction in binding frequency is mediated by cellular processes and direct inhibition of Dsg3 by EGF, cell-free measurements using mica sheets functionalized with Dsg3-Fc were performed. Homophilic Dsg3 interactions were determined before as well as after EGF incubation for 1 h yielding similar results indicating that cellular mechanisms are required for reduction of Dsg3 binding (**Figure 4C**). Lastly, PP2 was used together with mc-PV2-IgG to evaluate if Src inhibition modulates PV-IgG-mediated direct inhibition of Dsg3 interactions. Indeed, mc-PV2-IgG reduced Dsg3 binding from 8.89 to 4.53% which in line with previous studies and most likely caused by antibody-induced steric hindrance (28, 29). However, loss of Dsg3 binding was not affected by PP2 (**Figure 4D**). Taken together, these results demonstrate that, on the molecular level, EGFR via Src regulates Dsg3 adhesion but inhibition of this mechanism does not interfere with autoantibody-induced direct inhibition.

3.5. Role of Dsg3 for Pemphigus Autoantibody-Induced Loss of Keratinocyte Adhesion

To delineate the role of Dsg3 for pemphigus autoantibody-induced signaling and loss of keratinocyte adhesion, HaCaT cell lines lacking either Dsg3 (ΔDsg3) or Dsg2 (ΔDsg2) were generated using the CRISPR/Cas9 gene editing technology. Generating Dsg1-deficient cells was not successful (unpublished observation). After expansion of monoclonal cultures, Sanger sequencing revealed one clone deficient for either Dsg2 or Dsg3. The Dsg3-deficient cell line presented a heterozygous deletion of 34 base pairs (bp) in one and 2 bp in a second allele in Exon 5. The cell line lacking Dsg2 presented a homozygous deletion of 4 bp in Exon 5. All genetic alterations resulted in a frameshift (**Figure 5A**). Deficiencies of Dsg2 or Dsg3 were validated by immunostaining and Western blot analyses (**Figures 5B,C**). Thereby, significant increase of Dsg2 was detectable in cells missing Dsg3 and Dsg3 was up-regulated in Dsg2-deficient keratinocytes. In contrast, protein levels and localization of plakoglobin (PG), desmoplakin (DP) or E-cadherin (E-Cad) remained unaltered in both lines. Interestingly, Dsg1 levels also remained unchanged in both cell lines. Next, Dsg-deficient cell lines were subjected to dispase-based dissociation assays. Baseline adhesion of keratinocytes lacking Dsg3 but not of cells missing Dsg2 was slightly reduced when compared to wild-type cells, which is in line with previous studies were both proteins were depleted by siRNA (30) (**Figure 5D**). Adhesion was still reduced after incubation of both PV-IgG fractions for 24 h in cells lacking Dsg2 but not in keratinocytes deficient for Dsg3, highlighting the importance of autoantibodies targeting Dsg3 for loss of cell adhesion in PV. PF-IgG on the other hand was still able to reduce adhesion significantly in Dsg3 deficient HaCaT cells (**Figure 5E**).

3.6. Dsg3-Dependence of Autoantibody-Induced Signaling

Lastly, ERK activity and Ca^{2+} influx were studied in keratinocytes deficient for either Dsg3 or Dsg2. Cell monolayers were incubated for 30 min with the respective IgG fractions and ERK phosphorylation was evaluated in immunoblots. Comparable to WT keratinocytes, PF-IgG significantly activated ERK in Dsg3- and Dsg2-deficient cells whereas PV-IgG-induced ERK phosphorylation was not consistent (**Figures 6A,B**). Additionally, PF-IgG mediated Ca^{2+} influx was evaluated by ratiometric Fura-2 imaging. A transient increase of intracellular Ca^{2+} was observed in all cell lines without major differences (**Figure 6C**). These results indicate that Dsg3 and Dsg2 are not required for activation of ERK and influx of Ca^{2+}, at least in response to PF-IgG.

4. DISCUSSION

This study demonstrates that IgG-induced signaling mechanisms in keratinocytes correlate with different autoantibody profiles in PV and PF. PV-IgG but not PF-IgG activated EGFR in a Src-dependent manner suggesting that Dsg1 is not required for

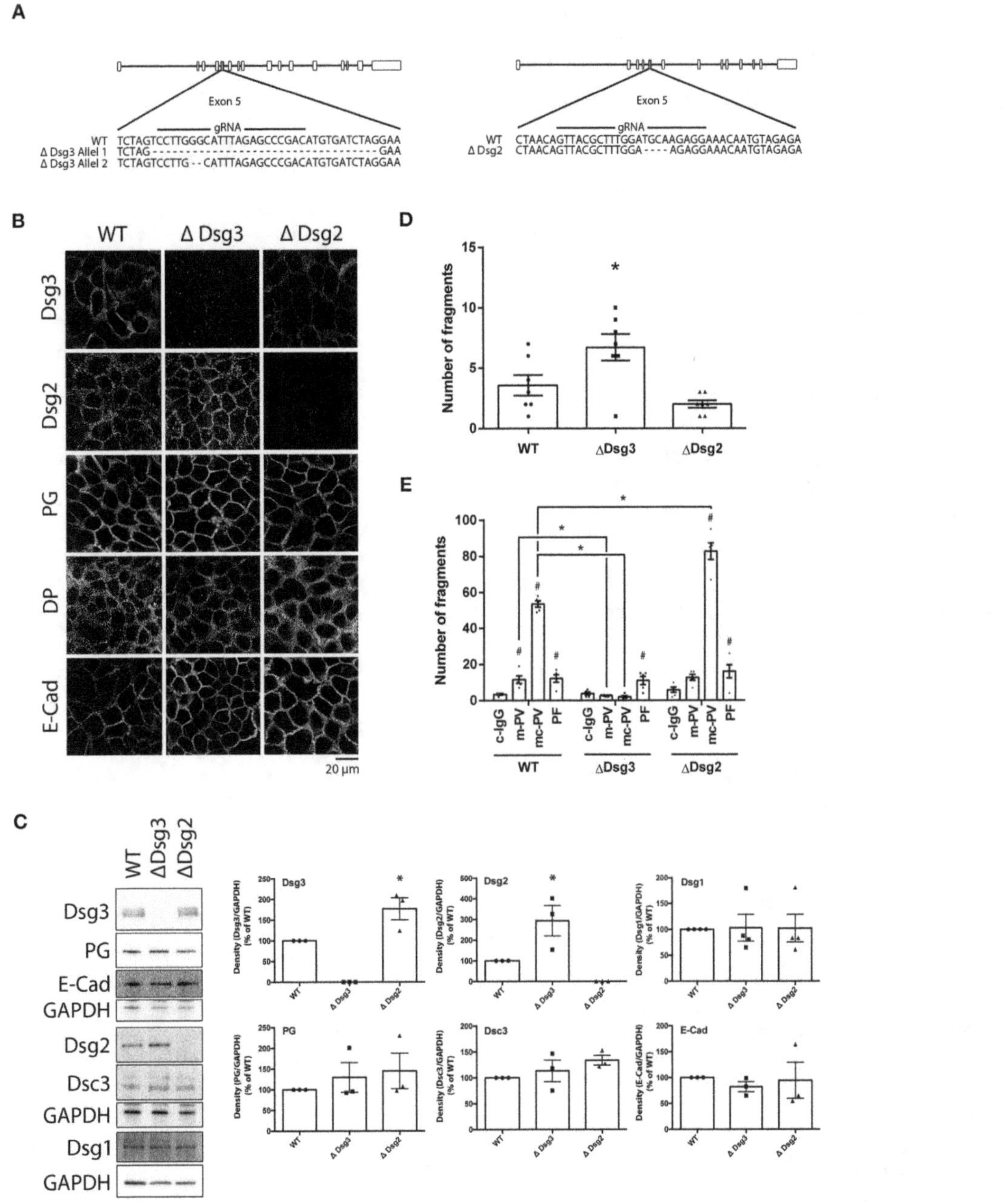

FIGURE 5 | Genetic deletion of Dsg3 and Dsg2 using CRISPR/Cas9 in HaCaT keratinocytes. **(A)** Schematic of sequencing results after inducing a DSB with NHEJ repair in Exon 5 of either Dsg3 or Dsg2 using CRISPR/Cas9. **(B)** Cell line characterization by immunostaining of desmosomal proteins ($n = 3$). **(C)** Cell line characterization by immunoblot with representative images on the left and densitometric quantification on the right ($n = 3$, one-way ANOVA, $^*p \leq 0.05$ vs. WT). **(D)** Dispase assay of WT and Dsg-deficient cell lines under baseline treatment. ($n = 7$, one-way ANOVA, $^*p \leq 0.05$ vs. WT) **(E)** Cell lines incubated with IgG fractions for 24 h and subjected to Dispase assays ($n = 5$, two-way ANOVA, $\#p \leq 0.05$ vs. respective c-IgG, $^*p \leq 0.05$ vs. WT).

EGFR activation. On the other hand, both PV-IgG and PF-IgG activated ERK and induced Ca^{2+} influx when antibodies targeting Dsg1 were present. In Dsg3-deficient keratinocytes, in which PV-IgG-induced loss of cell adhesion was abolished, ERK activation and Ca^{2+} influx were preserved in response to PF-IgG. These results indicate that these signaling pathways were indeed independent from Dsg3, but were in the absence of Dsg3, at least when induced by mc-PV, not able to reduce adhesion (**Figure 7**). Nevertheless, because inhibition of EGFR strongly reduced loss of cell adhesion in response to PV-IgG but not PF-IgG and Ca^{2+} chelation significantly reduced effects of both PV-IgG and PF-IgG, we conclude that both Dsg3- and Dsg1-dependent signaling mechanisms contribute to loss of keratinocyte adhesion in pemphigus.

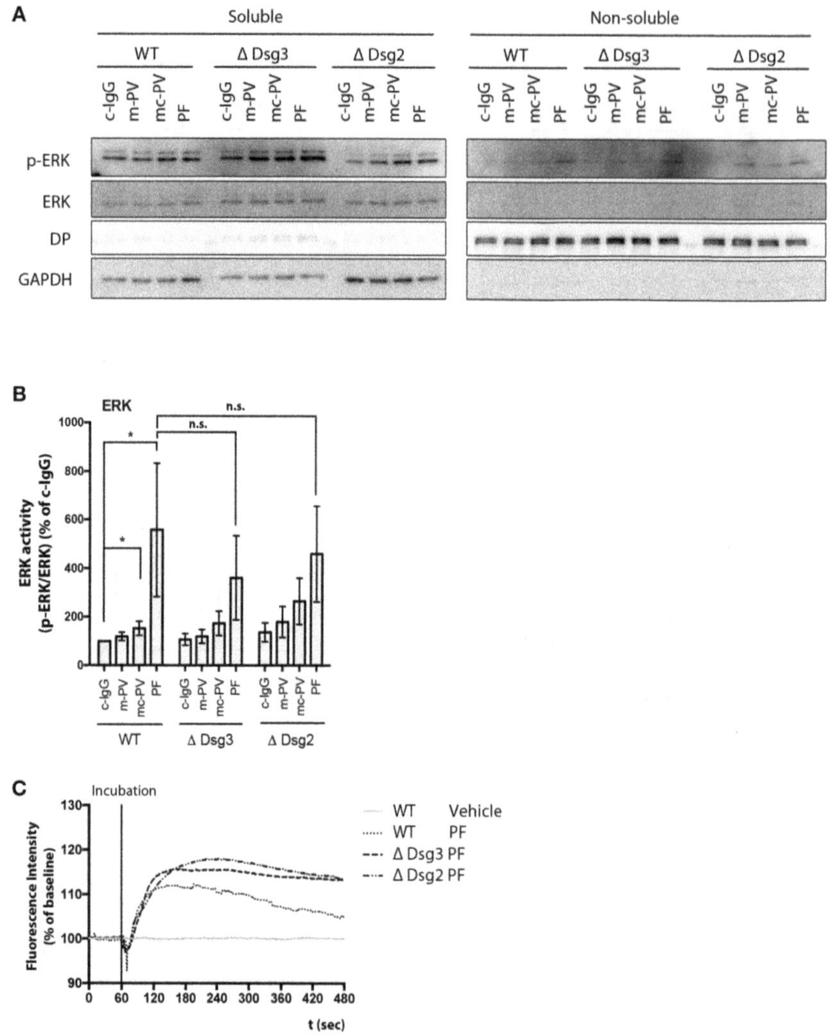

FIGURE 6 | Signaling pathway modulation by pemphigus IgG fractions in Dsg-deficient cell lines. Analysis of ERK activation after 30 min application of IgG fractions by immunoblot in Dsg3- and Dsg2-deficient cell lines. **(A)** Representative immunoblot and **(B)** densitometric analysis ($n = 9$, two-way ANOVA, $^*p \leq 0.05$). **(C)** Representativ graph of Fura-2 ratiometric Ca^{2+} imaging reveals a PF-IgG mediated Ca^{2+} influx in all cell lines used ($n = 3$).

4.1. Role of Signaling Pathways for Loss of Cell Adhesion in Pemphigus

It is generally accepted that loss of keratinocyte adhesion in pemphigus is mediated via both direct inhibition of Dsg3 binding and several signaling mechanisms (7). Amongst the plethora of signaling events implicated in pemphigus pathogenesis, p38MAPK, EGFR, Src and PKC have been suggested to be central for regulation of desmosome turn-over (5, 31). Indeed, inhibition of these pathways was protective in PV mouse models *in vivo* and human epidermis *ex vivo* (32–37). Activation of EGFR in response to PV-IgG was shown after 30-60 min *in vitro* (38, 39) and by AK23 after 120 min *in vivo* (23). This is in line with results shown here in which EGFR was significantly activated after 30 min. We found that EGFR activation in response to PV-IgG was blocked by Ca^{2+} chelation when compared to c-IgG, indicating that EGFR activation is dependent on Ca^{2+}. Moreover, we demonstrated that PV-IgG-induced EGFR activation is Src-dependent, which is in line with a previous report (39). Similarly, EGFR activation in response to PV-IgG has been reported downstream of p38MAPK (40). Other studies showed that Src is downstream of EGFR signaling (41). This discrepancy may be explained by different mechanisms to activate EGFR. Similar to our study using PV-IgG, it was shown for AK23 in mice that EGFR was phosphorylated at Y845 after 2 h, which is typically a site for Src-mediated trans-activation (23). However, phosphorylation at the ligand-mediated activation site Y1173 was observed after 24 h as well. Since EGFR family ligands such as EGF and betacellulin are upregulated upon PV-IgG incubation (41), it is possible that both canonical ligand-mediated and more rapid Src-induced transactivation of EGFR occur. In a previous study, in contrast to EGF, loss of cell adhesion and Dsg3- and Dsg1-mediated binding in response to PV-IgG were

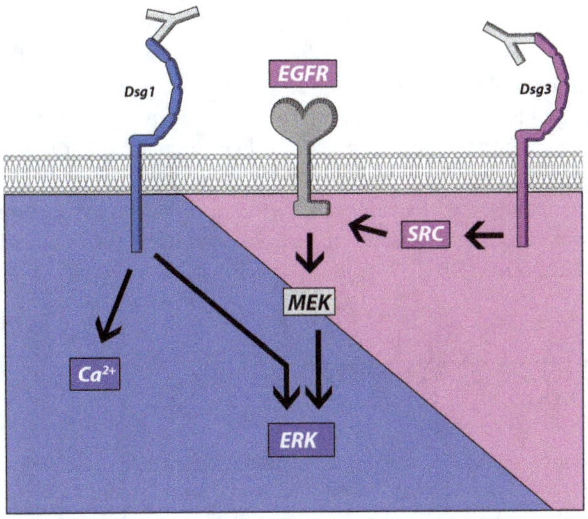

FIGURE 7 | Schematic of signaling pathways activated by pemphigus autoantibodies directed against Dsg1 and Dsg3. Src and EGFR activation is associated with antibodies targeting Dsg3 whereas autoantibody fractions against Dsg1 induce ERK activation and Ca^{2+} influx.

not blocked by inhibitors of EGFR or Src (28). Moreover, EGFR phosphorylation at Y1173 and Y845 was induced by EGF but not by four different PV-IgG fractions. However, EGFR activation was tested after 60 min only and meanwhile efficacy of EGFR inhibitors to block autoantibody-induced skin blistering was reported to be strictly dose-dependent (34). Therefore, based on the latter study, a role of EGFR for PV-IgG-induced loss of keratinocyte adhesion cannot be ruled out. Nevertheless, these data suggest that not in all PV patients EGFR and Src contribute to skin blistering.

It is not entirely clear how EGFR regulates desmosomal adhesion. EGFR may reduce cell adhesion together with ADAMs via shedding of Dsg isoforms and inhibition of desmosome assembly as has been shown for Dsg2 (42, 43). In line with this, AFM revealed that EGF similar to PV-IgG reduced Dsg3 binding frequency. However, EGF- but not PV-IgG-induced loss of Dsg3 binding was Src-dependent. Since PV-IgG cause direct inhibition of Dsg3 binding on the molecular level, it is plausible that Src inhibition cannot override this effect as shown previously for p38MAPK (28, 29). Nevertheless, these data indicate that EGFR via Src can contribute to loss of Dsg3 adhesion similar as shown before for Dsg2 in enterocytes (27). Alternatively, EGFR may activate ERK, which is activated in response to PV-IgG and PF-IgG (15, 38), Here, we showed that ERK activation by mc-PV-IgG was significant after 30 min and was dependent on EGFR and Src. In contrast, PF-IgG-induced ERK activation was detected after 30 min and after 60 min but was independent of Src and MEK and not paralleled by EGFR activation. Nevertheless, EGFR inhibition blunted PF-IgG-induced ERK activation indicating that baseline EGF activity was required. Taken together, these data suggest that PF-IgG and mc-PV-IgG activated ERK by different mechanisms.

Besides the functional interplay of EGFR, Src and ERK, we further characterized the role of Ca^{2+} for autoantibody-induced loss of keratinocyte adhesion. As the first signaling mechanism demonstrated to be activated by pemphigus autoantibodies (24), Ca^{2+} influx was shown to be induced within 10-80 sec and shown to trigger PKC activation (25, 44). However, so far it remained unclear whether Ca^{2+} contributes to loss of adhesion. The data presented here, which show that Ca^{2+} chelation reduces loss of cell cohesion in response to all pemphigus autoantibodies, would be in line with this hypothesis. Moreover, mc-PV-IgG- but not PF-IgG-induced ERK activation was blocked by Ca^{2+} chelation, suggesting that for ERK activation Ca^{2+} influx is not absolutely required, at least when induced by PF-IgG.

4.2. Function of Dsg1 and Dsg3 to Trigger Signaling and Loss of Cell Cohesion in Pemphigus

In contrast to Dsg1, pemphigus autoantibodies against Dsg3 directly interfere with Dsg interaction (15, 18, 28), which alone is not sufficient to cause loss of keratinocyte adhesion (29). This suggests that signaling is important for loss of keratinocyte adhesion in pemphigus and regulation of signaling pathways downstream of autoantibodies may differ and might be responsible to induce different clinical phenotypes in pemphigus. Some signaling pathways such as p38MAPK, which has been shown to inhibit the small GTPase RhoA in keratinocytes, were found to be activated by both PV-IgG and PF-IgG and contribute to blistering and desmosome alterations in mouse and human epidermis (15, 32, 37, 45–47). In contrast, other signaling pathways correlate with autoantibody profiles against Dsg1 and Dsg3. We demonstrate that both Ca^{2+} influx and ERK activation were observed in the presence of autoantibodies targeting Dsg1 only (mc-PV-IgG and PF-IgG), which is in line with previous observations (15). In contrast, Src-dependent EGFR activation was found in response to PV-IgG containing antibodies against Dsg3. To clarify the role of Dsg3 in this context, we established Dsg3-deficient HaCaT cells by CRISPR/Cas9 mediated gene editing. We found that ERK activation and Ca^{2+} influx in response to PF-IgG were preserved in both cells lines whereas ERK activation induced by mc-PV-IgG was blunted. These data suggest that Ca^{2+} influx and ERK activation are mediated by antibodies not targeting Dsg3, which may include antibodies against Dsg1, whereas EGFR via Src is activated by antibodies not targeting Dsg1 which may comprise antibodies against Dsg3 (**Figure 7**). In line with this, in a previous study we found that AK23, which is specific for Dsg3, did not induce Ca^{2+} influx in human keratinocytes (15). Nevertheless, since siRNA-mediated depletion of Dsg1 and Dsg3 was not sufficient to significantly reduce PV-IgG-mediated EGFR and Src activation, it is possible that autoantibodies against other targets are involved in this process as well (39). These may include antibodies against Dsc3, M3 muscarinic acetylcholine receptor, Secretory Pathway Ca^{2+} ATPase (SPCA)1, Human Thyroid Peroxidase (TPO), Thyroglobulin (Tg) or others (11, 48). In this scenario, it is not entirely clear how PF-IgG induces ERK activation. ERK was activated independent of Src and MEK indicating that PF-IgG regulates ERK signaling by other mechanisms (**Figure 7**). It was shown that Dsg1 binds to Erbin to suppress EGFR-induced

ERK activation via Erbin-mediated sequestration of SHOC2 to allow epidermal differentiation (49, 50). Therefore, it is possible that antibodies against Dsg1 may be required to disinhibit ERK activation which is in line with our observation that baseline EGFR activity is required for PF-IgG-induced ERK activation.

4.3. Antibodies Targeting Dsg3 Contribute to Loss of Cell Cohesion in Pemphigus

Dsg1 appears to be more critical for epidermal integrity compared to Dsg3 because Dsg3-deficient mice develop mild skin lesions, which spontaneously heal, whereas Dsg1-deficient mice completely lose superficial epidermal layers during birth and die within 24 h (51, 52). However, Dsg3-specific antibodies were effective to cause skin blistering in mice (53) whereas in patients as well as in human epidermis *ex vivo* antibodies against Dsg3 alone usually are not sufficient to cause skin blisters (1, 37). Nevertheless, in non-lesional skin of m-PV patients Dsg3 distribution was altered but on the ultrastructural level size and number of desmosomes remained normal, whereas in skin lesions and experiments using autoantibodies from mc-PV and PF patients desmosome size and keratin insertion were reduced as well (37, 54–56). These observations indicate that autoantibodies against Dsg3 may contribute to loss of keratinocyte adhesion. In line with this, it was demonstrated recently that immune-adsorption of autoantibodies targeting Dsg3 and Dsg1 abolished PV-IgG-induced blistering whereas Dsg3-specific antibodies alone were sufficient to induce blisters in mice (57). Therefore, it is important to characterize the role and mechanisms of autoantibodies targeting Dsg3 in pemphigus. We observed that Ca^{2+} influx and ERK activation were preserved in Dsg3-deficient cells but not sufficient to cause md-PV-IgG mediated loss of keratinocyte cohesion. Since Dsg2 was up-regulated in Dsg3-deficient cells we cannot rule out completely that enhanced expression contributed to out-balance pathogenic effects of autoantibodies. Nevertheless, we conclude that autoantibodies in m-PV, which include antibodies targeting Dsg3, may interfere with desmosome turn-over via direct inhibition of Dsg3 binding and several signaling pathways such as Src, EGFR and p38MAPK and thereby sensitize desmosomes for autoantibodies against Dsg1 and other antigens which together induce an mc-PV phenotype. This would also provide further explanation to why epidermal blistering in PV occurs in supra-basal rather than in the superficial epidermis as in patients suffering from PF.

ETHICS STATEMENT

Patients gave written informed consent for research use of their blood sera. It was additionally approved by the Ethics Committee of the University of Marburg Medical Faculty.

AUTHOR CONTRIBUTIONS

EW, M-TW, and MS performed and analyzed experiments. FV performed and analyzed AFM data. RP and RE provided patient sera. EW and JW analyzed and interpretated the data, designed the study and wrote the manuscript.

ACKNOWLEDGMENTS

We thank Martina Hitzenbichler, Thomas Korbica and Silke Gotschy for their excellent technical assistance.

REFERENCES

1. Kasperkiewicz M, Ellebrecht CT, Takahashi H, Yamagami J, Zillikens D, Payne AS, et al. Pemphigus. *Nat Rev Dis Primers.* (2017) 3:17026. doi: 10.1038/nrdp.2017.26
2. Vodo D, Sarig O, Sprecher E. The genetics of pemphigus vulgaris. *Front Med (Lausanne).* (2018) 5:226. doi: 10.3389/fmed.2018.00226
3. Sajda T, Hazelton J, Patel M, Seiffert-Sinha K, Steinman L, Robinson W, et al. Multiplexed autoantigen microarrays identify HLA as a key driver of anti-desmoglein and -non-desmoglein reactivities in pemphigus. *Proc Natl Acad Sci USA.* (2016) 113:1859–64. doi: 10.1073/pnas.1525448113
4. Lotti R, Shu E, Petrachi T, Marconi A, Palazzo E, Quadri M, et al. Soluble fas ligand is essential for blister formation in pemphigus. *Front Immunol.* (2018) 9:370. doi: 10.3389/fimmu.2018.00370
5. Sinha AA, Sajda T. The evolving story of autoantibodies in pemphigus vulgaris: development of the "super compensation hypothesis". *Front Med (Lausanne).* (2018) 5:218. doi: 10.3389/fmed.2018.00218
6. Amber KT, Valdebran M, Grando SA. Non-desmoglein antibodies in patients with pemphigus vulgaris. *Front Immunol.* (2018) 9:1190. doi: 10.3389/fimmu.2018.01190
7. Spindler V, Eming R, Schmidt E, Amagai M, Grando S, Jonkman MF, et al. Mechanisms causing loss of keratinocyte cohesion in pemphigus. *J Invest Dermatol.* (2018) 138:32–7. doi: 10.1016/j.jid.2017.06.022
8. Waschke J. The desmosome and pemphigus. *Histochem Cell Biol.* (2008) 130:21–54. doi: 10.1007/s00418-008-0420-0
9. Price AJ, Cost AL, Ungewiss H, Waschke J, Dunn AR, Grashoff C. Mechanical loading of desmosomes depends on the magnitude and orientation of external stress. *Nat Commun.* (2018) 9:5284. doi: 10.1038/s41467-018-07523-0
10. Pollmann R, Schmidt T, Eming R, Hertl M. Pemphigus: a comprehensive review on pathogenesis, clinical presentation and novel therapeutic approaches. *Clin Rev Allergy Immunol.* (2018) 54:1–25. doi: 10.1007/s12016-017-8662-z
11. Sajda T, Sinha AA. Autoantibody signaling in pemphigus vulgaris: development of an integrated model. *Front Immunol.* (2018) 9:692. doi: 10.3389/fimmu.2018.00692
12. Stahley SN, Kowalczyk AP. Desmosomes in acquired disease. *Cell Tissue Res.* (2015) 360:439–56. doi: 10.1007/s00441-015-2155-2
13. Waschke J, Spindler V. Desmosomes and extradesmosomal adhesive signaling contacts in pemphigus. *Med Res Rev.* (2014) 34:1127–45. doi: 10.1002/med.21310
14. Waschke J. Desmogleins as signaling hubs regulating cell cohesion and tissue/organ function in skin and heart-EFEM lecture 2018. *Ann Anat.* (2018). doi: 10.1016/j.aanat.2018.11.006. [Epub ahead of print].

15. Walter E, Vielmuth F, Rotkopf L, Sardy M, Horvath ON, Goebeler M, et al. Different signaling patterns contribute to loss of keratinocyte cohesion dependent on autoantibody profile in pemphigus. *Sci Rep.* (2017) 7:3579. doi: 10.1038/s41598-017-03697-7
16. Tsunoda K, Ota T, Aoki M, Yamada T, Nagai T, Nakagawa T, et al. Induction of pemphigus phenotype by a mouse monoclonal antibody against the amino-terminal adhesive interface of desmoglein 3. *J Immunol.* (2003) 170:2170. doi: 10.4049/jimmunol.170.4.2170
17. Boukamp P, Petrussevska RT, Breitkreutz D, Hornung J, Markham A, Fusenig NE. Normal keratinization in a spontaneously immortalized aneuploid human keratinocyte cell line. *J Cell Biol.* (1988) 106:761–71. doi: 10.1083/jcb.106.3.761
18. Waschke J, Bruggeman P, Baumgartner W, Zillikens D, Drenckhahn D. Pemphigus foliaceus IgG causes dissociation of desmoglein 1-containing junctions without blocking desmoglein 1 transinteraction. *J Clin invest.* (2005) 115:3157–65. doi: 10.1172/JCI23475
19. Ishii K, Harada R, Matsuo I, Shirakata Y, Hashimoto K, Amagai M. *In vitro* keratinocyte dissociation assay for evaluation of the pathogenicity of anti-desmoglein 3 IgG autoantibodies in pemphigus vulgaris. *J Invest Dermatol.* (2005) 124:939–46. doi: 10.1111/j.0022-202X.2005.23714.x
20. Ebner A, Wildling L, Kamruzzahan ASM, Rankl C, Wruss J, Hahn CD, et al. A new, simple method for linking of antibodies to atomic force microscopy tips. *Bioconjug Chem.* (2007) 18:1176–84. doi: 10.1021/bc070030s
21. Vielmuth F, Walter E, Fuchs M, Radeva MY, Buechau F, Magin TM, et al. Keratins regulate p38MAPK-dependent desmoglein binding properties in pemphigus. *Front Immunol.* (2018) 9:528. doi: 10.3389/fimmu.2018.00528
22. Vielmuth F, Waschke J, Spindler V. Loss of desmoglein binding Is not sufficient for keratinocyte dissociation in pemphigus. *J Invest Dermatol.* (2015) 135:3068–77. doi: 10.1038/jid.2015.324
23. Schulze K, Galichet A, Sayar BS, Scothern A, Howald D, Zymann H, et al. An adult passive transfer mouse model to study desmoglein 3 signaling in pemphigus vulgaris. *J Invest Dermatol.* (2012) 132:346–55. doi: 10.1038/jid.2011.299
24. Seishima M, Esaki C, Osada K, Mori S, Hashimoto T, Kitajima Y. Pemphigus IgG, but not bullous pemphigoid IgG, causes a transient increase in intracellular calcium and inositol 1,4,5-triphosphate in DJM-1 cells, a squamous cell carcinoma line. *J Invest Dermatol.* (1995) 104:33–7. doi: 10.1111/1523-1747.ep12613469
25. Memar O, Christensen B, Rajaraman S, Goldblum R, Tyring SK, Brysk MM, et al. Induction of blister-causing antibodies by a recombinant full-length, but not the extracellular, domain of the pemphigus vulgaris antigen (desmoglein 3). *J Immunol.* (1996) 157:3171–7.
26. Tinhofer I, Maly K, Dietl P, Hochholdinger F, Mayr S, Obermeier A, et al. Differential Ca^{2+} signaling induced by activation of the epidermal growth factor and nerve growth factor receptors. *J Biol Chem.* (1996) 271:30505–9. doi: 10.1074/jbc.271.48.30505
27. Ungewiss H, Rotzer V, Meir M, Fey C, Diefenbacher M, Schlegel N, et al. Dsg2 via Src-mediated transactivation shapes EGFR signaling towards cell adhesion. *Cell Mol Life Sci.* (2018) 75:4251–68. doi: 10.1007/s00018-018-2869-x
28. Heupel WM, Zillikens D, Drenckhahn D, Waschke J. Pemphigus vulgaris IgG directly inhibit desmoglein 3-mediated transinteraction. *J Immunol.* (2008) 181:1825–34. doi: 10.4049/jimmunol.181.3.1825
29. Vielmuth F, Hartlieb E, Kugelmann D, Waschke J, Spindler V. Atomic force microscopy identifies regions of distinct desmoglein 3 adhesive properties on living keratinocytes. *Nanomedicine* (2015) 11:511–20. doi: 10.1016/j.nano.2014.10.006
30. Hartlieb E, Rötzer V, Radeva M, Spindler V, Waschke J. Desmoglein 2 compensates for desmoglein 3 but does not control cell adhesion via regulation of p38 mitogen-activated protein kinase in keratinocytes. *J Biol Chem.* (2014) 289:17043–53. doi: 10.1074/jbc.M113.489336
31. Spindler V, Waschke J. Pemphigus-A disease of desmosome dysfunction caused by multiple mechanism. *Front Immunol.* (2018) 9:136. doi: 10.3389/fimmu.2018.00136
32. Berkowitz P, Hu P, Warren S, Liu Z, Diaz LA, Rubenstein DS. p38MAPK inhibition prevents disease in pemphigus vulgaris mice. *Proc Natl Acad Sci USA.* (2006) 103:12855–60. doi: 10.1073/pnas.0602973103
33. Espana A, Modol T, Gil MP, Lopez-Zabalza MJ. Neural nitric oxide synthase participates in pemphigus vulgaris acantholysis through upregulation of *Rous sarcoma*, mammalian target of rapamycin and focal adhesion kinase. *Exp Dermatol.* (2013) 22:125–30. doi: 10.1111/exd.12088
34. Sayar BS, Ruegg S, Schmidt E, Sibilia M, Siffert M, Suter MM, et al. EGFR inhibitors erlotinib and lapatinib ameliorate epidermal blistering in pemphigus vulgaris in a non-linear, V-shaped relationship. *Exp Dermatol.* (2014) 23:33–8. doi: 10.1111/exd.12290
35. Sanchez-Carpintero I, Espana A, Pelacho B, Lopez Moratalla N, Rubenstein DS, Diaz LA, et al. *In vivo* blockade of pemphigus vulgaris acantholysis by inhibition of intracellular signal transduction cascades. *Br J Dermatol.* (2004) 151:565–70. doi: 10.1111/j.1365-2133.2004.06147.x
36. Spindler V, Endlich A, Hartlieb E, Vielmuth F, Schmidt E, Waschke J. The extent of desmoglein 3 depletion in pemphigus vulgaris is dependent on Ca^2+-induced differentiation: a role in suprabasal epidermal skin splitting? *Am J Pathol.* (2011) 179:1905–16. doi: 10.1016/j.ajpath.2011.06.043
37. Egu DT, Walter E, Spindler V, Waschke J. Inhibition of p38MAPK signalling prevents epidermal blistering and alterations of desmosome structure induced by pemphigus autoantibodies in human epidermis. *Br J Dermatol.* (2017) 177:1612–8. doi: 10.1111/bjd.15721
38. Frusic-Zlotkin M, Raichenberg D, Wang X, David M, Michel B, Milner Y. Apoptotic mechanism in pemphigus autoimmunoglobulins-induced acantholysis–possible involvement of the EGF receptor. *Autoimmunity.* (2006) 39:563–75. doi: 10.1080/08916930600971836
39. Chernyavsky AI, Arredondo J, Kitajima Y, Sato-Nagai M, Grando SA. Desmoglein versus non-desmoglein signaling in pemphigus acantholysis: characterization of novel signaling pathways downstream of pemphigus vulgaris antigens. *J Biol Chem.* (2007) 282:13804–12. doi: 10.1074/jbc.M611365200
40. Bektas M, Jolly PS, Berkowitz P, Amagai M, Rubenstein DS. A pathophysiologic role for epidermal growth factor receptor in pemphigus acantholysis. *J Biol Chem.* (2013) 288:9447–56. doi: 10.1074/jbc.M112.438010
41. Pretel M, Espana A, Marquina M, Pelacho B, Lopez-Picazo JM, Lopez-Zabalza MJ. An imbalance in Akt/mTOR is involved in the apoptotic and acantholytic processes in a mouse model of pemphigus vulgaris. *Exp Dermatol.* (2009) 18:771–80. doi: 10.1111/j.1600-0625.2009.00893.x
42. Lorch JH, Klessner J, Park JK, Getsios S, Wu YL, Stack MS, et al. Epidermal growth factor receptor inhibition promotes desmosome assembly and strengthens intercellular adhesion in squamous cell carcinoma cells. *J Biol Chem.* (2004) 279:37191–200. doi: 10.1074/jbc.M405123200
43. Klessner JL, Desai BV, Amargo EV, Getsios S, Green KJ. EGFR and ADAMs cooperate to regulate shedding and endocytic trafficking of the desmosomal cadherin desmoglein 2. *Mol Biol Cell.* (2009) 20:328–37. doi: 10.1091/mbc.e08-04-0356
44. Osada K, Seishima M, Kitajima Y. Pemphigus IgG activates and translocates protein kinase C from the cytosol to the particulate/cytoskeleton fractions in human keratinocytes. *J Invest Dermatol.* (1997) 108:482–7. doi: 10.1111/1523-1747.ep12289726
45. Berkowitz P, Chua M, Liu Z, Diaz La, Rubenstein DS. Autoantibodies in the autoimmune disease pemphigus foliaceus induce blistering via p38 mitogen-activated protein kinase-dependent signaling in the skin. *Am J Pathol.* (2008) 173:1628–36. doi: 10.2353/ajpath.2008.080391
46. Waschke J, Spindler V, Bruggeman P, Zillikens D, Schmidt G, Drenckhahn D. Inhibition of Rho A activity causes pemphigus skin blistering. *J Cell Biol.* (2006) 175:721–7. doi: 10.1083/jcb.200605125
47. Yoshidaa K, Ishiia K, Shimizu A, Yokouchi M, Amagai M, Shiraishi K, et al. Non-pathogenic pemphigus foliaceus (PF) IgG acts synergistically with a directly pathogenic PF IgG to increase blistering by p38MAPK-dependent desmoglein 1 clustering. *J Dermatol Sci.* 2016 85:197–207. doi: 10.1016/j.jdermsci.2016.12.010
48. Chernyavsky A, Amber KT, Agnoletti AF, Wang C, Grando SA. Synergy among non-desmoglein antibodies contributes to the immunopathology of desmoglein antibody–negative pemphigus vulgaris. *J Biol Chem.* (2019) 1:jbc.RA118.006743. doi: 10.1074/jbc.RA118.006743
49. Getsios S, Simpson CL, Kojima SI, Harmon R, Sheu LJ, Dusek RL, et al. Desmoglein 1-dependent suppression of EGFR signaling promotes epidermal differentiation and morphogenesis. *J Cell Biol.* 185:1243–58. doi: 10.1083/jcb.200809044
50. Harmon RM, Simpson CL, Johnson JL, Koetsier JL, Dubash AD, Najor

NA, et al. Desmoglein-1/erbin interaction suppresses erk activation to support epidermal differentiation. *J Clin Invest.* (2013) 123:1556–70. doi: 10.1172/JCI65220

51. Rötzer V, Hartlieb E, Winkler J, Walter E, Schlipp A, Sardy M, et al. Desmoglein 3-dependent signaling regulates keratinocyte migration and wound healing. *J Invest Dermatol.* (2015) 136:301–10. doi: 10.1038/jid.2015.380
52. Kugelmann D, Radeva MY, Spindler V, Waschke J. Dsg1 deficiency causes lethal skin blistering. *J Invest Dermatol.* (2019). doi: 10.1016/j.jid.2019.01.002. [Epub ahead of print].
53. Spindler V, Rotzer V, Dehner C, Kempf B, Gliem M, Radeva M, et al. Peptide-mediated desmoglein 3 crosslinking prevents pemphigus vulgaris autoantibody-induced skin blistering. *J Clin Invest.* (2013) 123:800–11. doi: 10.1172/JCI60139
54. Oktarina DAM, Van Der Wier G, Diercks GFH, Jonkman MF, Pas HH. IgG-induced clustering of desmogleins 1 and 3 in skin of patients with pemphigus fits with the desmoglein nonassembly depletion hypothesis. *Br J Dermatol.* (2011) 165:552–62. doi: 10.1111/j.1365-2133.2011.10463.x
55. Van Der Wier G, Pas HH, Kramer D, Diercks GFH, Jonkman MF. Smaller desmosomes are seen in the skin of pemphigus patients with anti-desmoglein 1 antibodies but not in patients with anti-desmoglein 3 antibodies. *J Invest Dermatol.* (2014) 134:2287–90. doi: 10.1038/jid.2014.140
56. Van Der Wier G, Jonkman MF, Pas HH, Diercks GFH. Ultrastructure of acantholysis in pemphigus foliaceus re-examined from the current perspective. *Br J Dermatol.* (2012) 167:1265–71. doi: 10.1111/j.1365-2133.2012.11173.x
57. Hofrichter M, Dworschak J, Emtenani S, Langenhan J, Weiß F, Komorowski L, et al. Immunoadsorption of desmoglein-3-specific IgG abolishes the blister-inducing capacity of pemphigus vulgaris IgG in neonatal mice. *Front Immunol.* (2018) 9:1935. doi: 10.3389/fimmu.2018.01935

10

New Insights into the Pathogenesis of Bullous Pemphigoid

Giovanni Genovese [1,2], Giovanni Di Zenzo [3], Emanuele Cozzani [4], Emilio Berti [1,2], Massimo Cugno [2,5] and Angelo Valerio Marzano [1,2]*

[1] Dermatology Unit, Fondazione IRCCS Ca' Granda Ospedale Maggiore Policlinico, Milan, Italy, [2] Department of Physiopathology and Transplantation, Università degli Studi di Milano, Milan, Italy, [3] Molecular and Cell Biology Laboratory, Istituto Dermopatico dell'Immacolata (IDI) IRCCS, Rome, Italy, [4] DISSAL Section of Dermatology, Università degli Studi di Genova, Genoa, Italy, [5] Internal Medicine Unit, Fondazione IRCCS Ca' Granda Ospedale Maggiore Policlinico, Milan, Italy

***Correspondence:**
Angelo Valerio Marzano
angelo.marzano@unimi.it

There are several lines of evidence indicating that the physiopathological bases of bullous pemphigoid (BP), the most common subepidermal autoimmune bullous disease, are hallmarked by the production of autoantibodies directed against the hemidesmosomal anchoring proteins BP180 and BP230. In contrast to the robustness of the latter assumption, the multifaceted complexity of upstream and downstream mechanisms implied in the pathogenesis of BP remains an area of intense speculation. So far, an imbalance between T regulatory cells and autoreactive T helper (Th) cells has been regarded as the main pathogenic factor triggering the autoimmune response in BP patients. However, the contributory role of signaling pathways fostering the B cell stimulation, such as Toll-like receptor activation, as well as that of ancillary inflammatory mechanisms responsible for blister formation, such as Th17 axis stimulation and the activation of the coagulation cascade, are still a matter of debate. In the same way, the pathomechanisms implied in the loss of dermal-epidermal adhesion secondary to autoantibodies binding are not fully understood. Herein, we review in detail the current concepts and controversies on the complex pathogenesis of BP, shedding light on the most recent theories emerging from the literature.

Keywords: bullous pemphigoid, pathogenesis, autoantibodies, autoimmunity, skin, autoimmune blistering diseases

INTRODUCTION

Bullous pemphigoid (BP), the most common autoimmune bullous disease, typically presents with generalized crops of tense, pruritic cutaneous blisters and mostly affects the elderly (1). In up to 20% of cases, BP may initially exhibit a non-bullous phase characterized by eczematous, excoriated, urticaria-like or nodular lesions, which may last weeks, months, or occasionally remain the sole clinical manifestation (2). Together with mucous membrane pemphigoid, pemphigoid gestationis, linear immunoglobulin (Ig) A bullous dermatosis (LABD), anti-laminin $\gamma 1$ pemphigoid, and epidermolysis bullosa acquisita (EBA), BP is encompassed in the heterogeneous group of subepithelial autoimmune bullous disorders (1). Indeed, the histopathological assessment of a recent blister generally reveals a dermal-epidermal split associated with a dermal inflammatory infiltrate mainly consisting of lymphocytes and eosinophils (3). In BP, blisters are caused by autoantibodies of the IgG class directed against two structural components of the hemidesmosome, a multiprotein complex of the dermal-epidermal junction providing structural adhesion between basal keratinocytes and dermal extracellular matrix; these antigens are BP180, a transmembrane glycoprotein consisting of a globular cytoplasmic N-terminal domain, a short transmembrane stretch and a large extracellular C-terminal domain containing 15 collagenous repeats (4–7), and BP230, a protein of the hemidesmosomal inner plaque with a central rod domain flanked by globular end domains (4, 5). In addition to IgG also IgE autoantibodies are involved in disease pathogenesis and could be detected in the skin and/or serum of BP patients by means of immunofluorescence studies, immunoblot/immunoprecipitation and enzyme-linked immunoassay (ELISA) analyses (8). Whilst the crucial role of these autoantibodies in triggering the inflammatory cascade is fully acknowledged (9), many ancillary mechanisms involved in the complex etiology of BP need to be elucidated yet (10). In this regard, the development of animal models, which include the transfer of autoantibodies to experimental animals, the adoptive transfer of autoantigen-specific B lymphocytes to immunodeficient mice and immunization-induced models, greatly contributed to dissect these pathogenic aspects (11). This review provides a breakdown of the most recent studies on the pathogenic mechanisms involved in BP.

ESTABLISHED STATUS OF KNOWLEDGE ON BULLOUS PEMPHIGOID PATHOGENESIS

It has been recognized that a combination of genetic predisposing factors, such as class II HLA (e.g., HLA-DQβ1*0301) (12), and environmental influences, such as UV radiation, traumas, and drugs, may contribute to the loss of immune tolerance toward the above-mentioned antigens of the dermal-epidermal junction (13). As shown in **Figure 1**, it has also been suggested that the imbalance between autoreactive T helper (Th) and T regulatory (T_{reg}) cells (14, 15) as well as a T cell-independent activation of toll-like receptor (TLR) system (16) may induce B cell stimulation, with consequent BP autoantibody secretion. In parallel, the Th17 pathway activation appeared to maintain the inflammatory cascade started by humoral hyperactivation, by triggering Th2 response, recruiting neutrophils and eosinophils and stimulating the release of proinflammatory cytokines and proteolytic enzymes (14, 17).

While the role of IgA or IgM is still elusive and their deposits did not seem to affect the disease course (18), the role of IgE is controversial. Some authors demonstrated that their deposits along the basement membrane zone (BMZ) or their serum levels correlated to specific BP clinical features, namely more infiltrated lesions, such as urticarial plaques (18–20) or nodules (21), while other ones observed no association between circulating anti-BP180 IgE antibodies and a non-bullous urticaria-like presentation (21, 22). Furthermore, serum anti-BP180 IgE levels were shown to reflect disease activity throughout the course of the disease (21, 22), even if it has been suggested that it might not happen in the early phases of medication (23). However, on direct immunofluorescence studies IgG are usually predominant. Mihai et al. (24) showed that IgG1 and IgG4 were the most frequent IgG subtypes found in BP along the dermal-epidermal junction. By means of a cryosection assay, the same authors proved also that IgG1 promoted blister formation through complement fixation, whereas IgG4, which cannot fix the complement, activated leucocytes and induced dermal-epidermal separation with a lower pathogenic potential as compared to IgG1 (24).

BP180 is the main BP autoantigen and IgG and/or IgE against this antigen may be detected in most patients (8). The immunodominant non-collagenous region 16A (NC16A) of the BP180 ectodomain is extensively accepted to be the main target for BP autoantibodies. However, also domains of BP180 outside of NC16A, such as the C-terminal domain of BP180 and a 120-kDa fragment of BP180 known as LAD-1, may be recognized (25–27). The IgG directed against BP180 domains other than NC16A seemed to be responsible of less inflammatory manifestations (28) due to the fact that they hardly induce any BP180 depletion respect to anti-BP180-NC16A IgG in experimental studies (29). Moreover, IgG reactivity with extracellular but not intracellular epitopes of BP180 paralleled the severity of the disease course (25) and higher levels of anti-BP180 IgG were associated with increased 1-year mortality (30). The pathogenic role of IgG anti-BP180 has been validated by the following remarks: (i) the induction of BP-like lesions in mice in which anti-BP180-NC16A antibodies had been passively transferred (31); (ii) the onset of BP-like bullae and a human disease phenotype in BP180-knockout mice rescued by the human ortholog after being injected with IgG from BP patients (32); (iii) the direct correlation of anti-BP180-NC16A antibody titers to disease activity (33, 34). Anti-BP180 IgE antibodies showed also pathogenic features; indeed, the pathogenicity of anti-BP180 IgE antibodies has been demonstrated via an IgE hybridoma to LABD97, a component of the shed ectodomain of BP180, which was injected in severe combined immunodeficiency (SCID) mice with engrafted human skin, with consequent development in the skin grafts of eosinophil infiltration and histological subepidermal blisters resembling those of BP (35). Furthermore, the injection of total IgE isolated from two BP patients sera into human skin grafted onto athymic nude mice induced erythematous plaques reminiscent of those clinically seen in BP (36). Antibodies of the IgG class reacting against BP230, combined or not with anti-BP180 antibodies, are usually found in a smaller proportion of BP patients (37). Although the actual pathogenic role of anti-BP230 autoantibodies has been initially debated (38, 39), it has been more recently well-documented (40, 41) and IgG reactivity with intracellular epitopes of BP230 has been shown to correlate to BP severity (25).

The pathogenic mechanisms cooperating in the blister formation secondary to BP autoantibody binding to their targets are complex and may be subdivided into complement-dependent and complement-independent ones. Indeed, IgG1 have been demonstrated to start the inflammatory complement cascade leading to the recruitment of neutrophils and eosinophils in BP, and, consequently, to release of proteolytic enzymes in an experimental mouse model of BP (42). In addition to complement-mediated mechanisms, more and more evidence emerges that also complement-independent pathways play a fundamental role in BP pathogenesis. It has been postulated that there may be a direct influence of autoantibodies in adhesion functions of autoantigens. Indeed, Iwata et al. (43) disclosed that

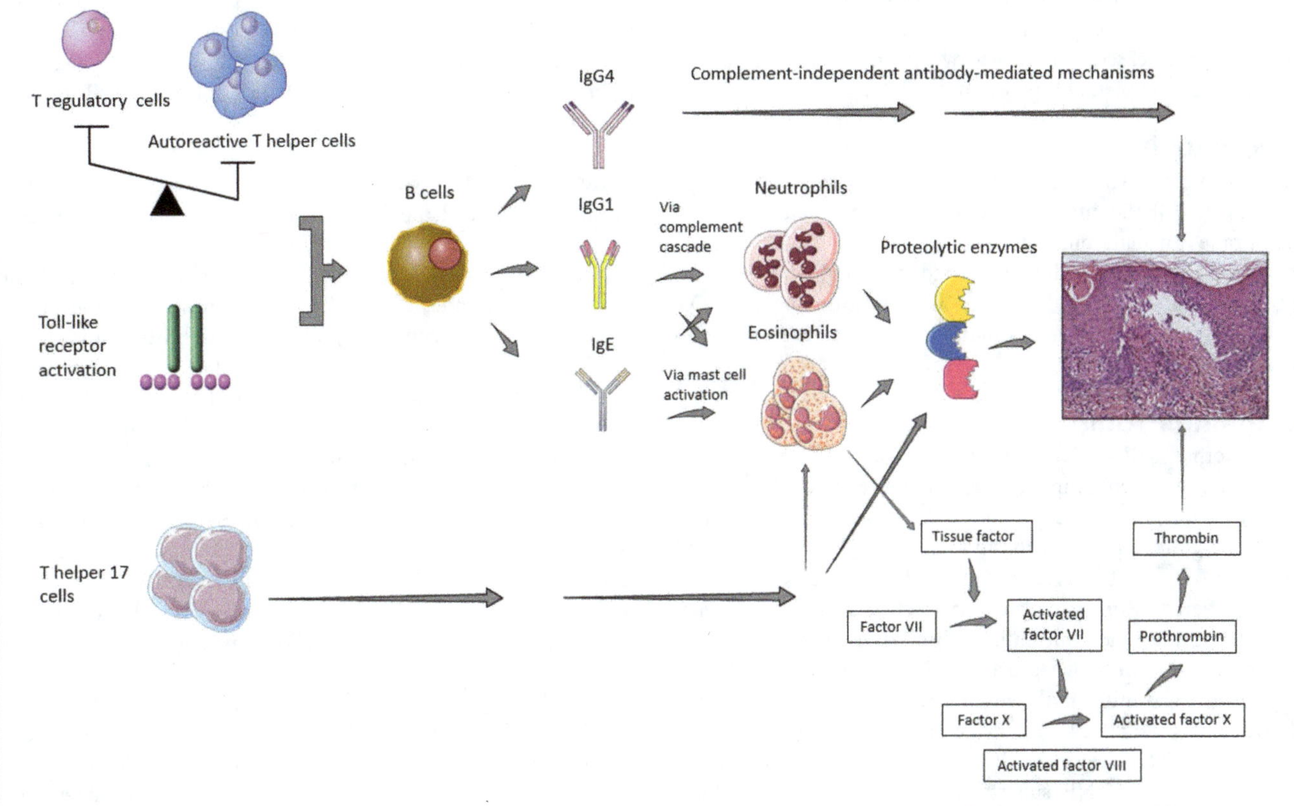

FIGURE 1 | Representative figure of the main pathogenic pathways implied in blister formation in patients with bullous pemphigoid.

serum IgG from BP patients could deplete cultured keratinocytes of BP180 and decrease cell adhesion to the bottom of the culture plate, thus suggesting that hemidesmosomes had an insufficient adhesive function due to a reduced hemidesmosomal BP180 content. Furthermore, Ujiie et al. showed that passive transfer of BP autoantibodies caused BP180 depletion in lesional skin independently by complement deposition in neonatal C3-deficient BP180-humanized mice (44). The role of IgG4 in inducing the blister formation without complement cascade intervention has been supported by Dainichi et al., who reported two cases of IgG4-positive BP without complement activation (45). Mast cells also have been proposed to contribute to BP development and the presence of IgE autoantibodies especially in patients with urticarial lesions provided indirect support to the idea that IgE autoantibodies contribute to tissue damage and to certain distinct clinical features, most likely by triggering mast cell and basophil histamine release (19). Moreover, anti-BP180 IgG (46) and IgE (47) autoantibodies have been demonstrated to elicit the internalization of BP180 also through pinocytic mechanisms.

BLISTER FORMATION MECHANISMS: UPDATE AND NEW THEORIES

Complement Cascade

The role of classical and, to a lesser extent, alternative pathways of the complement cascade in BP blister formation is fully acknowledged (48). The strength of this assumption based mainly on *in vitro* and *ex vivo* experimental models has been recently reinforced by an observational study on a large cohort of BP patients ($n = 301$) showing complement deposits in 83.1% of skin biopsies (49). These authors proved also that complement deposition was related to clinical and serological disease activity. Similarly, Chiorean et al. (50) strengthened the relevance of complement activation in BP pathogenesis by substantiating that complement activation by autoantibodies *ex vivo* as measured by the complement-fixation assay in serum correlated to disease activity. Furthermore, Kasprick et al. (51) recently assessed the impact of a mouse monoclonal IgG2 antibody inhibiting the activation of complement component 1s (C1s), a classic complement pathway-specific serine protease, on the classic complement pathway inhibition. Using cryosections of human skin incubated with serum of BP patients and a complement source leading to complement deposition along the BMZ of skin section, the authors confirmed that this monoclonal antibody was able to block the classic complement pathway activation in this model, thus providing favorable data for further studies on anti-complement monoclonal antibodies in BP patients. On the other hand, complement-dependent mechanisms may trigger independent ones in the blister formation process. Indeed, in a recent knock-out mice and pharmacological inhibition study (52), the activated fifth component of complement (C5a) along with its receptor 1 (C5aR1) appeared to be involved in the early phase of the disease, while C5a receptor 2 (C5aR2) seemed to be protective. Thus, as soon as the inflammatory process has completely developed, reactive oxygen species (ROS) and proteases are released, particularly by neutrophils and mast cells, regardless of complement involvement (45).

Pinocytosis

In accordance with the hypothesis that anti-BP180 IgG may induce BP180 internalization from the keratinocyte cell membrane through pinocytosis (44), Tie et al. (53) showed that human keratinocytes incubated with BP IgG display dysfunctional mitochondria, increased production of ROS, and intercellular vesicle formation, leading eventually to keratinocyte detachment.

Cytokine Profile

Unlike other skin inflammatory diseases, the key cytokines orchestrating the inflammatory cell recruitment in BP lesional skin have not yet been fully elucidated. However, a recent study (17) highlighted the central role of interleukin (IL)-17A, showing that mRNA levels of IL-17A were upregulated in perilesional skin of BP patients. Moreover, using cryosection of normal human skin and in mice, the same authors showed that inhibiting IL-17 with anti-IL-17 antibodies prevented BP180 IgG-induced blister formation. In addition, in the antibody transfer mouse BP model, IL-17A levels paralleled disease severity (17). Furthermore, the contribute of TNF-related weak inducer of apoptosis (TWEAK), a member of the TNF superfamily, and TWEAK/Fibroblast growth factor-inducible 14 (Fn14) interaction in inducing blister formation in BP has been investigated by Liu et al., who showed that TWEAK serum levels correlated inversely to BP180 expression and cellular adherence. Moreover, TWEAK activation resulted to trigger inflammation via extracellular signal–regulated kinases (ERK) and nuclear factor kappa-light-chain-enhancer of activated B cells (NF-κB) pathways (54).

IgE, Eosinophils, and Mast Cells

Eosinophilic lesional infiltrates and peripheral eosinophilia are well-known features of BP (55–57). High levels of cytotoxic proteins stored in the secretory granules, such as eosinophil cationic protein and major basic protein, as well as a Th2 milieu associated with augmented levels of IL-4, IL-5, and IL-13, the main cytokines involved in eosinophil biology, are usually seen both in lesional skin and serum of BP patients (55, 58). In addition, eosinophils have been recognized also as a major source of IL-31, a cytokine playing a significant role in itch-related inflammation, in BP (59). The release of matrix metalloproteinase-9 (MMP-9) and the production of ROS have been found to be one of the main events depending on eosinophil involvement (56, 60). In addition, eosinophils have been hypothesized to have a strict relationship with anti-BP180 IgE autoantibodies, whose pathogenic role in BP has increasingly recognized in recent years (61, 62). Lin et al. recently proved that eosinophils are crucial for IgE-mediated blister formation, showing that binding of anti-BP180-NC16A IgE to basal keratinocytes induced eosinophil recruitment in a humanized high-affinity IgE receptor (FcεRI) mouse model of BP (63). Moreover, the interplay between FcεRI, that have been observed to be highly expressed on eosinophils in BP patients (64), and anti-BP180 IgE resulted essential in eosinophil degranulation and consequent blister formation (63). Conceivably, FcεRI plays a fundamental role also in activation of mast cell-induced inflammation in BP lesional skin (65).

Coagulation Cascade

Eosinophils have also been demonstrated to be the main source of tissue factor (TF), an initiator of blood coagulation, in BP, representing an important link with the activation of the coagulation cascade, an ancillary mechanism contributing to blister formation. Moreover, plasma and blister fluid F1+2 prothrombin fragments (F1+2) and D-dimer levels paralleled blood and tissue eosinophilia. In turn, TF fostered the early trans-endothelial migration of eosinophils (66) and increased skin expression of adhesins and matrix metalloproteinases (67). Furthermore, blister fluid levels of eosinophilic cationic protein, a protein released during degranulation of eosinophils, positively correlated to both F1+2 and D-dimer levels (68). These findings, in conjunction with the higher expression of TF in skin biopsies of BP patients as compared to healthy controls (69, 70), outline the role of coagulation cascade in BP pathogenesis.

Regulatory T- and B-Cell Dysfunction

The essential role of T_{reg} cells in preventing the spontaneous generation of BP autoantibodies has been recently demonstrated by Muramatsu et al. in a Stat6 (signal transducer and activator of transcription 6) gene knockout scurfy mouse model (40). The same authors identified autoantibodies to BP180 and BP230 in patients with immune dysregulation, polyendocrinopathy, enteropathy, X-linked (IPEX) syndrome and underlined an association between anti-BP180 antibody levels and an eczematous skin phenotype (40). Moreover, the absence of T_{reg} cells led to the appearance of histological subepidermal blisters in scurfy mice, with the production of pathogenic autoantibodies targeting BP230 (41). Consistent with these findings, Bieber et al. (71) demonstrated in pemphigoid mouse models that T_{reg} impair the migratory capabilities of myeloid cells by downregulating their expression of β_2-integrin rather than their release of ROS, thus alleviating the disease severity. In addition to T_{reg}, also B regulatory (B_{reg}) cells have been hypothesized to play a pathogenic role in BP. In fact, Liu et al. (72) showed that B_{reg} cells from BP patients had a proinflammatory cytokine profile and were defective in suppressing $CD4^+$ T cell proliferation and anti-BP180 autoantibody production, suggesting that B_{regs} play a pro-inflammatory role rather than a regulatory role in BP.

Neutrophils and Monocytes

In addition to the well-recognized role of lymphocytes and eosinophils, it is clearly established that a cross-talk among other immune cells, notably neutrophils and monocytes, contributes in BP pathophysiology. The role of monocyte/neutrophil interaction in blister formation has been recently investigated by de Graauw et al. (73), who have highlighted in an *ex vivo* BP model that monocytes enhance the capability of neutrophils to release MMP-9, thus resulting in a more pronounced pathogenic potential and dermal-epidermal splitting. In a recent study, Fang et al. (74) provided strong evidence that BP blister fluid-derived exosomes, a subtype of extracellular vesicles involved in the transmission of inflammation signaling, recruited neutrophils through the upregulation of C-X-C Motif Chemokine Ligand 8 (CXCL8).

Proteolytic Enzymes

Among proteolytic enzymes implied in blister formation, neutrophil elastase, and MMP-9 are the most studied. However, the role of other proteases, such as granzyme B is lately emerging. Although its pro-apoptotic functions in cytotoxic T lymphocyte-mediated are more well-known, Russo et al. have recently displayed that granzyme B is elevated in the context of dermal-epidermal junction of lesional BP skin and contribute to its disruption by cleaving BP180 (75).

LINKS BETWEEN BULLOUS PEMPHIGOID PATHOGENESIS AND DISEASE-RELATED COMORBIDITIES

Neurologic and Neurodegenerative Disorders

Several epidemiological studies have confirmed that patients affected by neurologic and neurodegenerative diseases, such as multiple sclerosis and Alzheimer's disease, have an increased risk of developing BP (76). Since BP180 has been described to be expressed at low levels in neuronal tissue (77), it has been argued that neurodegeneration or neuroinflammation may lead to loss of self-tolerance toward BP180 and consequent BP development. Although a certain degree of cross-reactivity between BP180 and/or BP230 brain and skin isoforms exist (78), a recent study (79) evidenced that in Alzheimer's disease and multiple sclerosis patients the autoantibodies against BP180 targeted epitopes different than those targeted in patients with BP and did not bind natively folded BP180, thus suggesting their low potential to induce BP. Future studies could investigate the role of epitope spreading phenomenon in the induction of BP (80).

Vitamin D Deficiency

A higher prevalence of vitamin D deficiency and lower 25-hydroxyvitamin D levels were found in BP patients as compared to controls by our group (81). An extended study additionally showed that 25-hydroxyvitamin D levels inversely correlated to disease severity (82). Indeed, vitamin D has been shown to have an immune regulatory function and hypovitaminosis D has been correlated to an increased risk of developing autoimmune disorders (83). Moreover, vitamin D3 has been revealed to elicit down-regulation of the BP230 gene through post-transcriptional mechanisms independently by active protein synthesis (84), while non-toxic doses of calcitriol, the hormonally active vitamin D metabolite, reduced the release of the proinflammatory cytokines IL-6 and IL-8 induced by purified human BP IgG from HaCaT cells (85). A similarly beneficial effect of calcitriol has been recently reported also in mice with experimental EBA (86).

Thrombosis

The risk of thrombosis and/or thromboembolism is augmented in BP patients (87), as witnessed by a recent multicenter cohort study showing that BP patients have a 4-fold increased risk of developing venous thromboembolism compared to the general population (88). Indeed, several studies revealed that the inflammatory response in patients with BP activated the coagulation cascade, which paralleled disease activity (66, 70, 89, 90). In particular, D-dimer and F1+2, two coagulation activation markers, have been observed to be increased in blister fluid, lesional skin and plasma (90), with F1+2 correlating to the anti-BP180 levels (89). Moreover, during remission phases, blood concentration of coagulation activation markers reverted to normal (70). Therefore, extrinsic blood coagulation pathway activation may be regarded as a contributory mechanism leading to local inflammation and blister formation in BP (79, 80, 82). Fibrinolysis resulted also inhibited in BP, chiefly due to increased plasminogen activator inhibitor type 1 (PAI-1) activity and plasma levels (91). Interestingly, the recent observation that serum levels of soluble P-selectin, a marker of platelet activation, were significantly higher in BP patients than controls led to hypothesize a role of platelets in disease pathogenesis (92).

CONCLUSION

As highlighted in this review, the pathogenesis of BP is complex, and evidence is growing that new ancillary pathomechanisms flanking the traditional ones—e.g., IgG1-mediated complement activation—may play a role in the events leading to subepithelial blister formation.

AUTHOR CONTRIBUTIONS

GG and AM designed and wrote the initial draft of the manuscript. GD, EC, EB, and MC reviewed the paper and provided critical intellectual input. All the authors approved the final version of the manuscript.

REFERENCES

1. Amber KT, Murrell DF, Schmidt E, Joly P, Borradori L. Autoimmune subepidermal bullous diseases of the skin and mucosae: clinical features, diagnosis, and management. *Clin Rev Allergy Immunol.* (2018) 54:26–51. doi: 10.1007/s12016-017-8633-4
2. Cozzani E, Gasparini G, Burlando M, Drago F, Parodi A. Atypical presentations of bullous pemphigoid: clinical and immunopathological aspects. *Autoimmun Rev.* (2015) 14:438–45. doi: 10.1016/j.autrev.2015.01.006
3. Iwata H, Kitajima Y. Bullous pemphigoid: role of complement and mechanisms for blister formation within the lamina lucida. *Exp Dermatol.* (2013) 22:381–5. doi: 10.1111/exd.12146
4. Labib RS, Anhalt GJ, Patel HP, Mutasim DF, Diaz LA. Molecular heterogeneity of the bullous pemphigoid antigens as detected by immunoblotting. *J Immunol.* (1986) 136:1231–5.

5. Amagai M, Hashimoto T, Tajima S, Inokuchi Y, Shimizu N, Saito M, et al. Partial cDNA cloning of the 230-kD mouse bullous pemphigoid antigen by use of a human monoclonal anti-basement membrane zone antibody. *J Invest Dermatol.* (1990) 95:252–9. doi: 10.1111/1523-1747.ep12484863
6. Tanaka T, Korman NJ, Shimizu H, Eady RAJ, Klaus-Kovtun V, Cehrs K, et al. Production of rabbit antibodies against carboxy-terminal epitopes encoded by bullous pemphigoid cDNA. *J Invest Dermatol.* (1990) 95:252–9. doi: 10.1111/1523-1747.ep12876200
7. Meyer LJ, Taylor TB, Kadunce DP, Zone JJ. Two groups of bullous pemphigoid antigens are identified by affinity-purified antibodies. *J Invest Dermatol.* (1990) 94:611–6. doi: 10.1111/1523-1747.ep12876194
8. Liu Y, Li L, Xia Y. BP180 is critical in the autoimmunity of bullous pemphigoid. *Front Immunol.* (2017) 8:1752. doi: 10.3389/fimmu.2017.01752
9. Goletz S, Zillikens D, Schmidt E. Structural proteins of the dermal-epidermal junction targeted by autoantibodies in pemphigoid diseases. *Exp Dermatol.* (2017) 26:1154–62. doi: 10.1111/exd.13446
10. Schmidt E, Spindler V, Eming R, Amagai M, Antonicelli F, Baines JF, et al. Meeting report of the pathogenesis of pemphigus and pemphigoid meeting in Munich, September 2016. *J Invest Dermatol.* (2017) 137:1199–203. doi: 10.1016/j.jid.2017.01.028
11. Bieber K, Koga H, Nishie W. *In vitro* and *in vivo* models to investigate the pathomechanisms and novel treatments for pemphigoid diseases. *Exp Dermatol.* (2017) 26:1163–70. doi: 10.1111/exd.13415
12. Delgado JC, Turbay D, Yunis EJ, Yunis JJ, Morton ED, Bhol K, et al. A common major histocompatibility complex class II allele HLA-DQB1* 0301 is present in clinical variants of pemphigoid. *Proc Natl Acad Sci USA.* (1996) 93:8569–71. doi: 10.1073/pnas.93.16.8569
13. Lo Schiavo A, Ruocco E, Brancaccio G, Caccavale S, Ruocco V, Wolf R. Bullous pemphigoid: etiology, pathogenesis, and inducing factors: facts and controversies. *Clin Dermatol.* (2013) 31:391–9. doi: 10.1016/j.clindermatol.2013.01.006
14. Arakawa M, Dainichi T, Ishii N, Hamada T, Karashima T, Nakama T, et al. Lesional Th17 cells and regulatory T cells in bullous pemphigoid. *Exp Dermatol.* (2011) 20:1022–4. doi: 10.1111/j.1600-0625.2011.01378.x
15. Hashimoto T, Takahashi H, Sakaguchi S. Regulatory T-cell deficiency and autoimmune skin disease: beyond the scurfy mouse and immune dysregulation, polyendocrinopathy, enteropathy, X-linked syndrome. *J Allergy Clin Immunol.* (2018) 142:1754–6. doi: 10.1016/j.jaci.2018.08.028
16. Shlomchik MJ. Activating systemic autoimmunity: B's, T's, and tolls. *Curr Opin Immunol.* (2009) 21:626–33. doi: 10.1016/j.coi.2009.08.005
17. Chakievska L, Holtsche MM, Künstner A, Goletz S, Petersen BS, Thaci D, et al. IL-17A is functionally relevant and a potential therapeutic target in bullous pemphigoid. *J Autoimmun.* (2019) 96:104–12. doi: 10.1016/j.jaut.2018.09.003
18. Moriuchi R, Nishie W, Ujiie H, Natsuga K, Shimizu H. *In vivo* analysis of IgE autoantibodies in bullous pemphigoid: a study of 100 cases. *J Dermatol Sci.* (2015) 78:21–5. doi: 10.1016/j.jdermsci.2015.01.013
19. Yayli S, Pelivani N, Beltraminelli H, Wirthmuller U, Beleznay Z, Horn M, et al. Detection of linear IgE deposits in bullous pemphigoid and mucous membrane pemphigoid: a useful clue for diagnosis. *Br J Dermatol.* (2011) 165:1133–7. doi: 10.1111/j.1365-2133.2011.10481.x
20. Cho Y-T, Liao S-L, Wang L-F, Chu C-Y. High serum anti-BP180 IgE levels correlate to prominent urticarial lesions in patients with bullous pemphigoid. *J Dermatol Sci.* (2016) 83:78–80. doi: 10.1016/j.jdermsci.2016.03.009
21. Hashimoto T, Ohzono A, Teye K, Numata S, Hiroyasu S, Tsuruta D, et al. Detection of IgE autoantibodies to BP180 and BP230 and their relationship to clinical features in bullous pemphigoid. *Br J Dermatol.* (2017) 177:141–51. doi: 10.1111/bjd.15114
22. Van Beek N, Lüttmann N, Huebner F, Recke A, Karl I, Schulze FS, et al. Correlation of serum levels of ige autoantibodies against BP180 with bullous pemphigoid disease activity. *JAMA Dermatol.* (2017) 153:30–8. doi: 10.1001/jamadermatol.2016.3357
23. Bing L, Xiping Z, Li L, Jun P, Yi-Xia W, Min Y, et al. Levels of anti-BP180 NC16A IgE do not correlate with severity of disease in the early stages of bullous pemphigoid. *Arch Dermatol Res.* (2015) 307:849–54. doi: 10.1007/s00403-015-1598-3
24. Mihai S, Chiriac MT, Herrero-González JE, Goodall M, Jefferis R, Savage COS, et al. IgG4 autoantibodies induce dermal-epidermal separation. *J Cell Mol Med.* (2007) 11:1117–28. doi: 10.1111/j.1582-4934.2007.00081.x
25. Di Zenzo G, Thoma-Uszynski S, Calabresi V, Fontao L, Hofmann SC, Lacour JP, et al. Demonstration of epitope-spreading phenomena in bullous pemphigoid: results of a prospective multicenter study. *J Invest Dermatol.* (2011) 131:2271–80. doi: 10.1038/jid.2011.180
26. Fairley JA, Bream M, Fullenkamp C, Syrbu S, Chen M, Messingham KN. Missing the target: characterization of bullous pemphigoid patients who are negative using the BP180 enzyme-linked immunosorbant assay. *J Am Acad Dermatol.* (2013) 68:395–403. doi: 10.1016/j.jaad.2012.09.012
27. Nakama K, Koga H, Ishii N, Ohata C, Hashimoto T, Nakama T. Clinical and immunological profiles of 14 patients with bullous pemphigoid without IgG autoantibodies to the BP180 NC16A domain. *JAMA Dermatol.* (2018) 154:347–50. doi: 10.1001/jamadermatol.2017.5465
28. Izumi K, Nishie W, Mai Y, Wada M, Natsuga K, Ujiie H, et al. Autoantibody profile differentiates between inflammatory and noninflammatory bullous pemphigoid. *J Invest Dermatol.* (2016) 136:2201–10. doi: 10.1016/j.jid.2016.06.622
29. Imafuku K, Iwata H, Kamaguchi M, Izumi K, Natsuga K, Ujiie H, et al. Autoantibodies of non-inflammatory bullous pemphigoid hardly deplete type XVII collagen of keratinocytes. *Exp Dermatol.* (2017) 26:1171–4. doi: 10.1111/exd.13331
30. Holtsche MM, Goletz S, van Beek N, Zillikens D, Benoit S, Harman K, et al. Prospective study in bullous pemphigoid: association of high serum anti-BP180 IgG levels with increased mortality and reduced Karnofsky score. *Br J Dermatol.* (2018) 179:918–24. doi: 10.1111/bjd.16553
31. Liu Z, Diaz LA, Troy JL, Taylor AF, Emery DJ, Fairley JA, et al. A passive transfer model of the organ-specific autoimmune disease, bullous pemphigoid, using antibodies generated against the hemidesmosomal antigen, BP180. *J Clin Invest.* (1993) 92:2480–8. doi: 10.1172/JCI116856
32. Nishie W, Sawamura D, Goto M, Ito K, Shibaki A, McMillan JR, et al. Humanization of autoantigen. *Nat Med.* (2007) 13:378–83. doi: 10.1038/nm1496
33. Haase C, Büdinger L, Borradori L, Yee C, Merk HF, Yancey K, et al. Detection of IgG autoantibodies in the sera of patients with bullous and gestational pemphigoid: ELISA studies utilizing a baculovirus-encoded form of bullous pemphigoid antigen 2. *J Invest Dermatol.* (1998) 110:282–6. doi: 10.1046/j.1523-1747.1998.00126.x
34. Schmidt E, Obe K, Bröcker E, Zillikens D. Serum levels of autoantibodies to BP180 correlate with disease activity in patients with bullous pemphigoid. *Arch Dermatol.* (2000) 136:174–8.
35. Zone JJ, Taylor T, Hull C, Schmidt L, Meyer L. IgE basement membrane zone antibodies induce eosinophil infiltration and histological blisters in engrafted human skin on SCID mice. *J Invest Dermatol.* (2007) 127:1167–74. doi: 10.1038/sj.jid.5700681
36. Fairley JA, Burnett C, Fu C, Larson D, Fleming M, Giudice G. A pathogenic role for IgE in autoimmunity: bullous pemphigoid IgE reproduces the early phase of lesion development in human skin grafted to nu/nu mice. *J Invest Dermatol.* (2007) 127:2605–11. doi: 10.1038/sj.jid.5700958
37. Ludwig RJ. Bullous pemphigoid: more than one disease? *J Eur Acad Dermatol Venereol.* (2019) 33:459–60. doi: 10.1111/jdv.15445
38. Kiss M, Husz S, Jánossy T, Marczinovits I, Molnár J, Korom I, et al. Experimental bullous pemphigoid generated in mice with an antigenic epitope of the human hemidesmosomal protein BP230. *J Autoimmun.* (2005) 24:1–10. doi: 10.1016/j.jaut.2004.09.007
39. Feldrihan V, Licarete E, Florea F, Cristea V, Popescu O, Sitaru C, et al. IgG antibodies against immunodominant C-terminal epitopes of BP230 do not induce skin blistering in mice. *Hum Immunol.* (2014) 75:354–63. doi: 10.1016/j.humimm.2014.01.005
40. Muramatsu K, Ujiie H, Kobayashi I, Nishie W, Izumi K, Ito T, et al. Regulatory T-cell dysfunction induces autoantibodies to bullous pemphigoid antigens in mice and human subjects. *J Allergy Clin Immunol.* (2018) 142:1818–30.e6. doi: 10.1016/j.jaci.2018.03.014
41. Haeberle S, Wei X, Bieber K, Goletz S, Ludwig RJ, Schmidt E, et al. Regulatory T-cell deficiency leads to pathogenic bullous pemphigoid antigen 230 autoantibody and autoimmune bullous disease. *J Allergy Clin Immunol.* (2018) 142:1831–42.e7. doi: 10.1016/j.jaci.2018.04.006
42. Liu Z, Giudice GJ, Swartz SJ, Fairley JA, Till GO, Troy JL, et al. The role of complement in experimental bullous pemphigoid. *J Clin Invest.* (1995) 95:1539–44. doi: 10.1172/JCI117826

43. Iwata H, Kamio N, Aoyama Y, Yamamoto Y, Hirako Y, Owaribe K, et al. IgG from patients with bullous pemphigoid depletes cultured keratinocytes of the 180-kDa bullous pemphigoid antigen (type XVII collagen) and weakens cell attachment. *J Invest Dermatol.* (2009) 129:919–26. doi: 10.1038/jid.2008.305
44. Ujiie H, Sasaoka T, Izumi K, Nishie W, Shinkuma S, Natsuga K, et al. Bullous pemphigoid autoantibodies directly induce blister formation without complement activation. *J Immunol.* (2014) 193:4415–28. doi: 10.4049/jimmunol.1400095
45. Dainichi T, Nishie W, Yamagami Y, Sonobe H, Ujiie H, Kaku Y, et al. Bullous pemphigoid suggestive of complement-independent blister formation with anti-BP180 IgG4 autoantibodies. *Br J Dermatol.* (2016) 175:187–90. doi: 10.1111/bjd.14411
46. Hiroyasu S, Ozawa T, Kobayashi H, Ishii M, Aoyama Y, Kitajima Y, et al. Bullous pemphigoid IgG induces BP180 internalization via a macropinocytic pathway. *Am J Pathol.* (2013) 182:828–40. doi: 10.1016/j.ajpath.2012.11.029
47. Messingham KN, Srikantha R, DeGueme AM, Fairley JA. FcR-Independent Effects of IgE and IgG autoantibodies in bullous pemphigoid. *J Immunol.* (2011) 187:553–60. doi: 10.4049/jimmunol.1001753
48. Giang J, Seelen MAJ, van Doorn MBA, Rissmann R, Prens EP, Damman J. Complement activation in inflammatory skin diseases. *Front Immunol.* (2018) 9:639. doi: 10.3389/fimmu.2018.00639
49. Romeijn TR, Jonkman MF, Knoppers C, Pas HH, Diercks GFH. Complement in bullous pemphigoid: results from a large observational study. *Br J Dermatol.* (2017) 176:517–9. doi: 10.1111/bjd.14822
50. Chiorean RM, Baican A, Mustafa MB, Lischka A, Leucuta DC, Feldrihan V, et al. Complement-activating capacity of autoantibodies correlates with disease activity in bullous pemphigoid patients. *Front Immunol.* (2018) 9:2687. doi: 10.3389/fimmu.2018.02687
51. Kasprick A, Holtsche MM, Rose EL, Hussain S, Schmidt E, Petersen F, et al. The anti-C1s antibody TNT003 prevents complement activation in the skin induced by bullous pemphigoid autoantibodies. *J Invest Dermatol.* (2018) 138:458–61. doi: 10.1016/j.jid.2017.08.030
52. Karsten CM, Beckmann T, Holtsche MM, Tillmann J, Tofern S, Schulze FS, et al. Tissue destruction in bullous pemphigoid can be complement independent and may be mitigated by C5aR2. *Front Immunol.* (2018) 9:488. doi: 10.3389/fimmu.2018.00488
53. Tie D, Da X, Natsuga K, Yamada N, Yamamoto O, Morita E. Bullous pemphigoid IgG induces cell dysfunction and enhances the motility of epidermal keratinocytes via Rac1/proteasome activation. *Front Immunol.* (2019) 10:200. doi: 10.3389/fimmu.2019.00200
54. Liu Y, Peng L, Li L, Liu C, Hu X, Xiao S, et al. TWEAK/Fn14 activation contributes to the pathogenesis of bullous pemphigoid. *J Invest Dermatol.* (2017) 137:1512–22. doi: 10.1016/j.jid.2017.03.019
55. Simon D, Borradori L, Simon HU. Eosinophils as putative therapeutic targets in bullous pemphigoid. *Exp Dermatol.* (2017) 26:1187–92. doi: 10.1111/exd.13416
56. de Graauw E, Sitaru C, Horn M, Borradori L, Yousefi S, Simon HU, et al. Evidence for a role of eosinophils in blister formation in bullous pemphigoid. *Allergy Eur J Allergy Clin Immunol.* (2017) 72:1105–13. doi: 10.1111/all.13131
57. Kridin K. Peripheral eosinophilia in bullous pemphigoid: prevalence and influence on the clinical manifestation. *Br J Dermatol.* (2018) 179:1141–7. doi: 10.1111/bjd.16679
58. Maurer M, Altrichter S, Schmetzer O, Scheffel J, Church MK, Metz M. Immunoglobulin E-mediated autoimmunity. *Front Immunol.* (2018) 9:689. doi: 10.3389/fimmu.2018.00689
59. Rüdrich U, Gehring M, Papakonstantinou E, Illerhaus A, Engmann J, Kapp A, et al. Eosinophils are a major source of interleukin-31 in bullous pemphigoid. *Acta Derm Venereol.* (2018) 98:766–71. doi: 10.2340/00015555-2951
60. Amber KT, Valdebran M, Kridin K, Grando SA. The role of eosinophils in bullous pemphigoid: a developing model of eosinophil pathogenicity in mucocutaneous disease. *Front Med.* (2018) 5:201. doi: 10.3389/fmed.2018.00201
61. Dresow SK, Sitaru C, Recke A, Oostingh GJ, Zillikens D, Gibbs BF. IgE autoantibodies against the intracellular domain of BP180. *Br J Dermatol.* (2009) 160:429–32. doi: 10.1111/j.1365-2133.2008.08858.x
62. Cozzani E, Gasparini G, Di Zenzo G, Parodi A. Immunoglobulin E and bullous pemphigoid. *Eur J Dermatol.* (2018) 28:440–8. doi: 10.1684/ejd.2018.3366
63. Lin L, Hwang BJ, Culton DA, Li N, Burette S, Koller BH, et al. Eosinophils mediate tissue injury in the autoimmune skin disease bullous pemphigoid. *J Invest Dermatol.* (2018) 138:1032–43. doi: 10.1016/j.jid.2017.11.031
64. Messingham KN, Holahan HM, Frydman AS, Fullenkamp C, Srikantha R, Fairley JA. Human eosinophils express the high affinity IgE receptor, FceRI, in bullous pemphigoid. *PLoS ONE.* (2014) 9:e107725. doi: 10.1371/journal.pone.0107725
65. Fang H, Zhang Y, Li N, Wang G, Liu Z. The autoimmune skin disease bullous pemphigoid: The role of mast cells in autoantibody-induced tissue injury. *Front Immunol.* (2018) 9:407. doi: 10.3389/fimmu.2018.00407
66. Marzano AV, Tedeschi A, Fanoni D, Bonanni E, Venegoni L, Berti E, et al. Activation of blood coagulation in bullous pemphigoid: Role of eosinophils, and local and systemic implications. *Br J Dermatol.* (2009) 160:266–72. doi: 10.1111/j.1365-2133.2008.08880.x
67. Narbutt J, Waszczykowska E, Lukamowicz J, Sysa-Jędrzejowska A, Kobos J, Zebrowska A. Disturbances of the expression of metalloproteinases and their tissue inhibitors cause destruction of the basement membrane in pemphigoid. *Polish J Pathol.* (2006) 57:71–6.
68. Tedeschi A, Marzano AV, Lorini M, Balice Y, Cugno M. Eosinophil cationic protein levels parallel coagulation activation in the blister fluid of patients with bullous pemphigoid. *J Eur Acad Dermatol Venereol.* (2015) 29:813–7. doi: 10.1111/jdv.12464
69. Zebrowska A, Wagrowska-Danilewicz M, Danilewicz M, Wieczfinska J, Pniewska E, Zebrowski M, et al. Tissue factor in dermatitis herpetiformis and bullous pemphigoid: link between immune and coagulation system in subepidermal autoimmune bullous diseases. *Mediators Inflamm.* (2015) 2015:1–9. doi: 10.1155/2015/870428
70. Cugno M, Tedeschi A, Borghi A, Bucciarelli P, Asero R, Venegoni L, et al. Activation of blood coagulation in two prototypic autoimmune skin diseases: a possible link with thrombotic risk. *PLoS ONE.* (2015) 10:e129456. doi: 10.1371/journal.pone.0129456
71. Bieber K, Sun S, Witte M, Kasprick A, Beltsiou F, Behnen M, et al. Regulatory T cells suppress inflammation and blistering in pemphigoid diseases. *Front Immunol.* (2017) 8:1628. doi: 10.3389/fimmu.2017.01628
72. Liu Z, Dang E, Li B, Qiao H, Jin L, Zhang J, et al. Dysfunction of $CD19^{+}CD24^{hi}CD27^{+}$ B regulatory cells in patients with bullous pemphigoid. *Sci Rep.* (2018) 8:703. doi: 10.1038/s41598-018-19226-z
73. de Graauw E, Sitaru C, Horn MP, Borradori L, Yousefi S, Simon D, et al. Monocytes enhance neutrophil-induced blister formation in an *ex vivo* model of bullous pemphigoid. *Allergy Eur J Allergy Clin Immunol.* (2018) 73:1119–30. doi: 10.1111/all.13376
74. Fang H, Shao S, Jiang M, Dang E, Shen S, Zhang J, et al. Proinflammatory role of blister fluid-derived exosomes in bullous pemphigoid. *J Pathol.* (2018) 245:114–25. doi: 10.1002/path.5061
75. Russo V, Klein T, Lim DJ, Solis N, Machado Y, Hiroyasu S, et al. Granzyme B is elevated in autoimmune blistering diseases and cleaves key anchoring proteins of the dermal-epidermal junction. *Sci Rep.* (2018) 8:1–11. doi: 10.1038/s41598-018-28070-0
76. Försti AK, Huilaja L, Schmidt E, Tasanen K. Neurological and psychiatric associations in bullous pemphigoid—more than skin deep? *Exp Dermatol.* (2017) 26:1228–34. doi: 10.1111/exd.13401
77. Seppänen A. Collagen XVII: a shared antigen in neurodermatological interactions? *Clin Dev Immunol.* (2013) 2013:240570. doi: 10.1155/2013/240570
78. Julio TA, Vernal S, Massaro JD, Silva MC, Donadi EA, Moriguti JC, et al. Biological predictors shared by dementia and bullous pemphigoid patients point out a cross-antigenicity between BP180/BP230 brain and skin isoforms. *Immunol Res.* (2018) 66:567–76. doi: 10.1007/s12026-018-9028-1
79. Tuusa J, Lindgren O, Tertsunen HM, Nishie W, Kokkonen N, Huilaja L, et al. BP180 autoantibodies target different epitopes in multiple sclerosis or Alzheimer's disease than in bullous pemphigoid. *J Invest Dermatol.* (2019) 139:293–9. doi: 10.1016/j.jid.2018.09.010
80. Didona D, Di Zenzo G. Humoral epitope spreading in autoimmune bullous diseases. *Front Immunol.* (2018) 9:779. doi: 10.3389/fimmu.2018.00779
81. Marzano AV, Trevisan V, Eller-Vainicher C, Cairoli E, Marchese L, Morelli V, et al. Evidence for vitamin D deficiency and increased prevalence of fractures in autoimmune bullous skin diseases. *Br J Dermatol.* (2012) 167:688–91. doi: 10.1111/j.1365-2133.2012.10982.x

82. Marzano AV, Trevisan V, Cairoli E, Eller-Vainicher C, Morelli V, Spada A, et al. Vitamin D and skeletal health in autoimmune bullous skin diseases: a case control study. *Orphanet J Rare Dis.* (2015) 10:1–7. doi: 10.1186/s13023-015-0230-0
83. Peelen E, Knippenberg S, Muris AH, Thewissen M, Smolders J, Tervaert JWC, et al. Effects of vitamin D on the peripheral adaptive immune system: a review. *Autoimmun Rev.* (2011) 10:733–43. doi: 10.1016/j.autrev.2011.05.002
84. Yamamoto C, Tamai K, Nakano H, Matsuzaki Y, Kaneko T, Sawamura D. Vitamin D3 inhibits expression of bullous pemphigoid antigen 1 through post-transcriptional mechanism without new protein synthesis. *J Dermatol Sci.* (2008) 50:155–8. doi: 10.1016/j.jdermsci.2007.12.003
85. Tukaj S, Grüner D, Tukaj C, Zillikens D, Kasperkiewicz M. Calcitriol exerts anti-inflammatory effects in keratinocytes treated with autoantibodies from a patient with bullous pemphigoid. *J Eur Acad Dermatol Venereol.* (2016) 30:288–92. doi: 10.1111/jdv.12929
86. Tukaj S, Bieber K, Witte M, Ghorbanalipoor S, Schmidt E, Zillikens D, et al. Calcitriol treatment ameliorates inflammation and blistering in mouse models of epidermolysis bullosa acquisita. *J Invest Dermatol.* (2018) 138:301–9. doi: 10.1016/j.jid.2017.09.009
87. Langan SM, Hubbard R, Fleming K, West J. A population-based study of acute medical conditions associated with bullous pemphigoid. *Br J Dermatol.* (2009) 161:1149–52. doi: 10.1111/j.1365-2133.2009.09350.x
88. Cugno M, Marzano AV, Bucciarelli P, Balice Y, Cianchini G, Quaglino P, et al. Increased risk of venous thromboembolism in patients with bullous pemphigoid. The INVENTEP (INcidence of VENous ThromboEmbolism in bullous Pemphigoid) study. *Thromb Haemost.* (2016) 115:193–9. doi: 10.1038/sj.bjc.6602945
89. Marzano AV, Tedeschi A, Spinelli D, Fanoni D, Crosti C, Cugno M. Coagulation activation in autoimmune bullous diseases. *Clin Exp Immunol.* (2009) 158:31–6. doi: 10.1111/j.1365-2249.2009.03989.x
90. Marzano AV, Tedeschi A, Berti E, Fanoni D, Crosti C, Cugno M. Activation of coagulation in bullous pemphigoid and other eosinophil-related inflammatory skin diseases. *Clin Exp Immunol.* (2011) 165:44–50. doi: 10.1111/j.1365-2249.2011.04391.x
91. Marzano AV, Tedeschi A, Polloni I, Crosti C, Cugno M. Prothrombotic state and impaired fibrinolysis in bullous pemphigoid, the most frequent autoimmune blistering disease. *Clin Exp Immunol.* (2013) 171:76–81. doi: 10.1111/j.1365-2249.2012.04674.x
92. Bieber K, Ernst AL, Tukaj S, Holtsche MM, Schmidt E, Zillikens D, et al. Analysis of serum markers of cellular immune activation in patients with bullous pemphigoid. *Exp Dermatol.* (2017) 26:1248–52. doi: 10.1111/exd.13382

11

C5a/C5aR1 Pathway is Critical for the Pathogenesis of Psoriasis

Quan-you Zheng[1,2], Shen-ju Liang[3], Feng Xu[1], Gui-qing Li[1], Na Luo[4], Shun Wu[5], You Li[5], Ming Tang[5], Yu Zhong[2], Jian Chen[1], Di Yang[1], Dao-dong Sun[2], Ke-qin Zhang[5] and Gui-lian Xu[1]*

[1] Department of Immunology, Army Medical University (Third Military Medical University), Chongqing, China, [2] Department of Urology, 958th Hospital of PLA, Army Medical University (Third Military Medical University), Chongqing, China, [3] Department of Rheumatism and Immunology, Daping Hospital, Army Medical University (Third Military Medical University), Chongqing, China, [4] Department of Dermatology, Southwest Hospital, Army Medical University (Third Military Medical University), Chongqing, China, [5] Department of Nephrology, Southwest Hospital, Army Medical University (Third Military Medical University), Chongqing, China

***Correspondence:**
Gui-lian Xu
xuguilian2004@163.com

Psoriasis is one of the most common chronic inflammatory skin diseases, affecting ~2% of the population. The lack of characterization of the pathogenesis of psoriasis has hindered efficient clinical treatment of the disease. In our study, we observed that expression of complement component 5a receptor 1(C5aR1) was significantly increased in skin lesions of both imiquimod (IMQ) and IL23-induced psoriatic mice and patients with psoriasis. C5aR1 deficiency or treatment with C5a receptor 1 antagonist (C5aR1a) in mice significantly attenuated psoriasis-like skin lesions and expression of inflammatory cytokines and chemokines. Moreover, C5aR1 deficiency significantly decreased IMQ-induced infiltration of plasmacytoid dendritic cells (pDCs), monocytes and neutrophils in psoriatic skin lesions and functions of pDCs, evidenced by the remarkable reduction in the IMQ-induced production of interferon-α (IFN-α) and tumor necrosis factor α (TNF-α), and FMS-like tyrosine kinase 3 ligand (FLT3L)-dependent pDCs differentiation. Accordingly, *in vitro* treatment with recombinant C5a accelerated pDCs migration and the differentiation of bone marrow cells into pDCs. Furthermore, biopsies of psoriatic patients showed a dramatic increase of $C5aR1^+$ pDCs infiltration in psoriatic skin lesions, compared to healthy subjects. Our results provide direct evidence that C5a/C5aR1 signaling plays a critical role in the pathogenesis of psoriasis. Inhibition of C5a/C5aR1 pathway is expected to be beneficial in the treatment of patients with psoriasis.

Keywords: complement system, C5a/C5aR1, psoriasis, inflammation, mouse models

INTRODUCTION

Psoriasis is one of the most common chronic inflammatory skin diseases, affecting ~2% of the world's population (1). Psoriatic lesions are characterized by various histological features, including epidermal hyperplasia caused by excessive proliferation of keratinocytes, termed "acanthosis;" parakeratosis caused by impaired differentiation of keratinocytes; hypervascularity; and immune cell infiltration by neutrophils, dendritic cells, T cells, and macrophages (2, 3). Although the underlying mechanism is not fully understood, increasing evidence indicates that the innate immune system plays an essential role in the development of psoriasis (4–7).

The complement system, one of the most important arms of innate immunity, comprises a series of soluble and cell surface proteins, including plasma components, specific receptors, and diverse regulators. The complement system serves as the first line defense against the foreign pathogens by applying complement activation elements acting with antibodies, phagocytes, or through the formation of the terminal membrane attack complex (MAC) (8–10). Complement component 5a (C5a), a powerful, pro-inflammatory anaphylatoxin synthesized after cleavage of complement component C5, exerts its biological action by binding to its specific receptor C5aR1, also known as CD88, expressed on macrophages, neutrophils, monocytes, keratinocytes, and human plasmacytoid dendritic cells (pDCs) (11–13). A second receptor of C5a, C5-like receptor 2 (C5L2), was identified to be a negative regulator of C5a-dependent signaling (14).

Multiple reports indicated that excessive production of C5a leads to deleterious exaggeration of of the innate and adaptive immune responses, contributing to the development of several diseases such as allograft ischemia-reperfusion injury (IRI) and sepsis (15–17). Furthermore, high levels of cleaved C5a and C5a des-Arg were exhibited in skin lesions and psoriatic scales (18–21). However, the role of C5a/C5aR1 signaling in the development and progression of psoriasis remains unclear.

Although psoriasis has not been detected in any mammalian species other than humans, there exist several mouse models that mimic certain features of the human skin disease. Imiquimod (IMQ), a synthetic agonist for toll-like receptor 7 (TLR7), is a potent immune response activator and induces psoriasis-like skin inflammation (4). Significant increase in pDCs infiltration and abundant expression of type I interferon are critical hallmarks of IMQ-induced psoriasis in animal models (22, 23). However, the role of the C5a/C5aR1 signaling pathway in pDCs function in the pathogenesis of psoriasis is unknown.

In the present study, we explored the role of the C5a/C5aR1 complement pathway in the development of psoriasis and the potential relationship between C5aR1 signaling and inflammatory cells including pDCs, monocytes and neutrophils using IMQ-induced psoriasis in mice as the model. Our results suggest that C5a/C5aR1 signaling plays a critical role in the pathogenesis of psoriasis.

MATERIALS AND METHODS

Mice and Treatment

C5aR1-deficient BALB/c mice were purchased from the Jackson Laboratory. Wild-type BALB/c mice were obtained from the animal institute of the Academy of Medical Science (Beijing, China). Animals were bred in a specific-pathogen-free facility (SPF), and female mice of 8–12 weeks were used for all experiments (Although both male and female BALB/c mice were susceptible for IMQ or IL23- induced psoriasis, the docile character of female mice is convenient to applicate IMQ evenly on the back skin of mice under non-anesthesia, we used female mice in the present study, but still with a limitation that it may not fully represent some of the behaviors of male mice since hormonal effects). Animal experiments were conducted according to the guidelines of the Institutional Animal Care and Use Committee of the Third Military Medical University.

Female mice of 8–12 weeks were treated with daily topical doses (62.5 mg) of commercially available IMQ cream (5%; Si-Chuan Med-Shine Pharmaceutical, H20030128, Chengdu, Sichuan, China). Treatment was applied to the shaved backs and ears of mice for the indicated periods of time. Mice within the control group were treated with Vaseline cream. C5aR1 peptide antagonist (24) (peptide sequence: Ac-Phe-[Orn-Pro-dCha-Trp-Arg]) (1 mg/kg, equal to 1.1 μM/kg; GL Biochem, Shanghai, China) was injected into mice via peritoneal cavity 2 h prior to IMQ application. Saline buffer (0.9%) was injected as a vehicle control.

Intradermal Injection of Interleukin 23 (IL-23)

Mice were anesthetized and PBS (20 μL), either alone or containing recombinant mouse IL-23 (500 ng; Biolegend, San Diego, CA, USA), was injected intradermally into the ears, using a 30 gauge needle, for five consecutive days. Ear thickness was measured prior to injection at day 0, and thereafter, on days following cytokine injections, using a dial thickness gauge (Jiuliang, Shanghai, China). All tests were performed blinded.

Measuring Skin Inflammation

To assess psoriatic lesion severity, an objective scoring system based onclinical Psoriasis Area and Severity Index (PASI) was used. Scaling, thickness, and erythema of the back skin were scored daily for severity on a scale from 0 to 4, where 4 represented maximum severity. Level of erythema was scored using a table of red taints, as previously described (22). Total modified PASI (mPASI) scores (0-12) were used as a measure of skin lesion severity before and after IMQ application.

Human Blood and Skin Samples

Human blood samples were collected from psoriatic patients ($n = 15$) and healthy subjects ($n = 15$). Peripheral blood mononuclear cells (PBMCs) were separated by Ficoll density gradient centrifugation (TBD Science, Tian Jin, China). Skin paraffin sections were obtained from psoriatic patients after histological confirmation ($n = 8$) and biopsies sections were only collected from patients with no exposure to topical or systemic treatment for at least 2 weeks. Healthy control skin paraffin sections were obtained from individuals undergoing plastic surgery ($n = 5$). Patient studies were approved by the Institutional Ethical Board of the Army medical university (Third Military Medical University) and written informed consent was obtained from all subjects.

Histopathological Analysis

Back or ear skin samples were collected from mice. Then, skin samples were either fixed in 4% paraformaldehyde and embedded in paraffin for hematoxylin and eosin (H&E) staining, or immersed in Tissue Tek (Leica Microsystem, Wetzlar, Germany), snap frozen in liquid nitrogen, and stored at −80°C. For immunohistochemistry assay, paraffin sections (4 μm) were incubated with rabbit anti-mouse/human C5aR1 polyclonal antibody (1:100, Abcam, Cambridge, UK) and rat anti-mouse Ki67 (1:100, SolA15, eBioscience, San Diego, CA, USA) overnight at 4°C and then incubated with horse radish peroxidase (HRP)-labeled anti-rabbit and anti-rat secondary antibodies, respectively (1:1000, Beyotime, Shanghai, China) for 60 min at room temperature. After washing in PBS, 3,3′-diaminobenzidine chromogen solution (Beyotime, Shanghai, China) was added for 2 min at room temperature. Slides were counterstained with hematoxylin and then examined via light microscope (Olympus, Tokyo, Japan). For immunofluorescence assay, cryosections were cut into 6 μm slices using a cryostat (Leica Microsystem, Wetzlar, Germany) and fixed in cold acetone for 15 min on ice (IF), slides were blocked with PBS containing 5% BSA for 60 min. Slides were incubated with antibodies for Alexa Fluor 488 labeled rat anti-mouse PDCA-1 (1:200, eBio927, eBioscience, San Diego, CA, USA) overnight at 4°C. Human skin samples paraffin sections (4 μm) were stained with rabbit anti-human/mouse C5aR1 polyclonal antibody (1:100, Abcam, Cambridge, UK) and mouse anti-human CD123 (1:100, 6H6, eBioscience, San Diego, CA, USA) at 4 °C overnight. Horse radish peroxidase (HRP) labeled secondary antibodies (1:1000, Beyotime Shanghai, China) or Dylight^{TM} 488 donkey anti-mouse IgG and Cy3^{TM} goat anti-rabbit IgG (1:200, BioLegend, San Diego, CA, USA) were incubated for 60 min at room temperature. Sections were incubated with an antibody of the same isotype as a control. Slides were counterstained with hematoxylin and then examined via light microscope (Olympus, Tokyo, Japan) or slides were stained with Hoechst 33258 (5 μg/mL; Sigma-Aldrich, St. Louis, MO, USA) for nucleus staining and visualized via confocal laser microscope (Leica Microsystem, Wetzlar, Germany).

Ki67$^+$, PDCA-1$^+$ and C5aR1$^+$CD123$^+$ cells were quantified by counting the number of positively stained cells. 5–8 viewing fields randomly selected for each skin sections were examined and expressed as a number of cells per filed (0.04 mm^2). The mentioned quantitative analysis were conducted in a bind fashion by 2 experienced persons.

Quantitative Reverse Transcription-Polymerase Chain Reaction (qRT-PCR) Analysis

Total RNA was obtained from back or ear skin samples of mice, using TRIzol reagent (Biomed, Beijing, China). cDNA was synthesized via PrimeScript^{TM} RT reagent kit (Takara, Shiga, Japan). Real-time PCR was conducted with an MxPro3000P (Agilent StrataGene, America) and SYBR® Premix Ex Taq^{TM} reagent kit (Takara, Shiga, Japan). PCR mix (25 μL) included cDNA (2 μL) and primer pairs (0.5 μmol) for the target genes or GAPDH (listed in **Table 1**). Amplification was performed according to the manufacturer's protocol, and experiments were conducted in triplicate. Gene expression was quantified by ΔΔCt method (25). Samples were normalized to GAPDH.

Bone Marrow pDCs Induction and Differentiation

Bone marrow (BM) pDCs were generated from C5aR1$^{+/+}$ and C5aR1$^{-/-}$ mice using a modified protocol previously described

TABLE 1 | PCR primer sequences.

Gene	Primer sequence
C5aR1 Forward	5-ATGGACCCCATAGATAACAGCA-3
C5aR1 Reverse	5-GAGTAGATGATAAGGGCTGCAAC-3
PDCA-1 Forward	5-TGTTCGGGGTTACCTTAGTCA-3
PDCA-1 Reverse	5-GCAGGAGTTTGCCTGTGTCT-3
GAPDH Forward	5-ACCACAGTCCATGCCATCAC-3
GAPDH Reverse	5-TCCACCACCCTGTTGCTGTA-3
IFN-α Forward	5-CCAAGTGCTGCCGTCATTTTC-3
IFN-α Reverse	5-GGCTCGCAGGGATGATTTCAA-3
IFN-γ Forward	5-ATGAACGCTACACACTGCATC-3
IFN-γ Reverse	5-CCATCCTTTTGCCAGTTCCTC-3
Krt10 Forward	5-TTTGGTGGCGGTACTATGGAG-3
Krt10 Reverse	5-CTCTCGCTGGCTTGAGTTG-3
MIP-1α Forward	5-TTCTCTGTACCATGACACTCTGC-3
MIP-lα Reverse	5-CGTGGAATCTTCCGGCTGTAG-3
MIP-2 Forward	5-CCAACCACCAGGCTACAGG-3
MIP-2 Reverse	5-GCGTCACACTCAAGCTCTG-3
TNF-α Forward	5-TCTTCTCATTCCTGCTTGTGG-3
TNF-α Reverse	5-GGTCTGGGCCATAGAACTGA-3
IL-22 Forward	5-ATGAGTTTTTCCCTTATGGGGAC-3
IL-22 Reverse	5-GCTGGAAGTTGGACACCTCAA-3
IL-I7A Forward	5-TTTAACTCCCTTGGCGCAAAA-3
IL-I7A Reverse	5-CTTTCCCTCCGCATTGACAC-3
IL-23A Forward	5-ATGCTGGATTGCAGAGCAGTA-3
IL-23A Reverse	5-ACGGGGCACATTATTTTTAGTCT-3

(26, 27). Briefly, BM cells were harvested from mouse femurs and tibias. BM cells (2 × 10^6) from C5aR1$^{+/+}$ and C5aR1$^{-/-}$ mice were seeded in 6-well plates and cultured with RPMI 1640 medium containing 10% fetal calf serum, streptomycin (100 μg/mL), penicillin (100 U/mL), 2 μM glutamine, 50 μM β-mercaptoethanol, and recombinant mouse FLT3L (200 ng/mL; eBioscience, San Diego, CA, USA). Half culture medium was replaced every 5 days. In the another experiment, BM cells from C5aR1$^{+/+}$ mice were simulated with FLT3L alone or the combination of FLT3L and recombinant mouse C5a (42 nM; Peprotech, Rocky Hill, NJ, USA), and medium group was used as the negative control. At day 10, detached cells were collected and analyzed the percentage of pDCs by FCM.

ELISA

pDCs were isolated from mouse splenocytes with EasysepTM Mouse Plasmacytoid DC Isolation Kit (Stem cell Technologies, London, UK). The purity of pDCs was routinely at least 80% (**Figure S9**). Sorted pDCs from C5aR1$^{+/+}$ and C5aR1$^{-/-}$ mice were cultured (1 × 10^5 cells) in a 96-well round-bottom plate for 24 h in the presence of IMQ (10 μg/mL) or resiquimod R848 (10 μg/mL; Sigma-Aldrich, St. Louis, MO, USA), and medium group was used as the negative control. The levels of interferon α (IFN-α) and tumor necrosis factor α (TNF-α) in culture supernatants were measured using mouse IFN-α and TNF-α ELISA kits (BioLegend, San Diego, CA, USA). C5a levels in

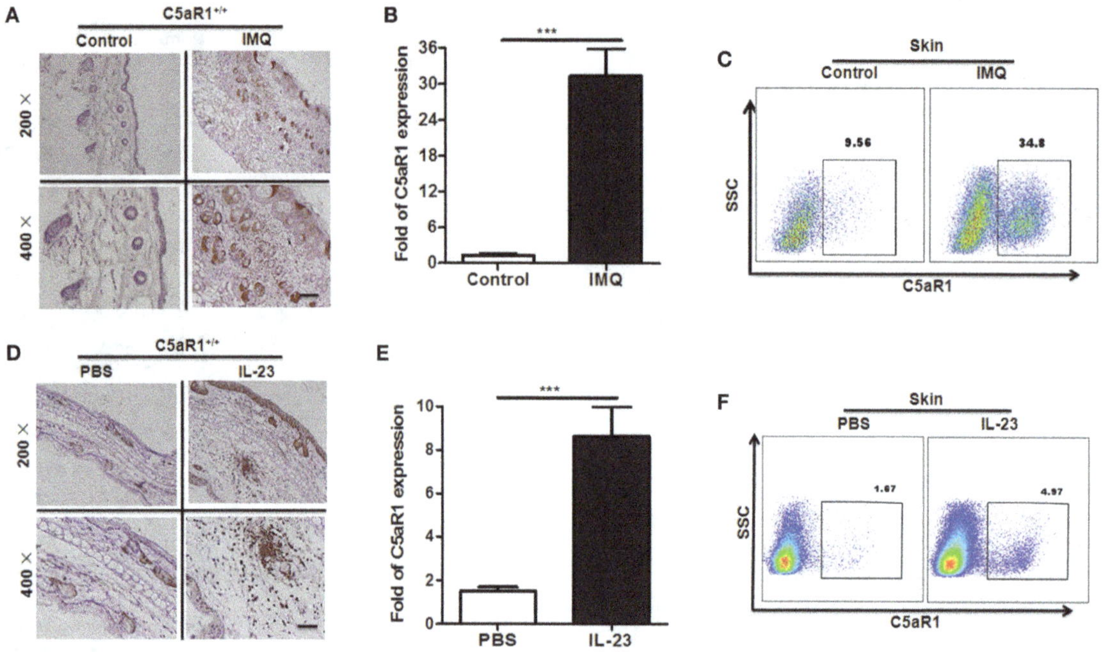

FIGURE 1 | Increased C5aR1 expression in psoriatic skin lesions in mice. To induce a psoriatic animal model, IMQ was topically applied to the shaved back of wild-type ($C5aR1^{+/+}$) mice for 6 days **(A–C)**, or the ears of wild-type ($C5aR1^{+/+}$) mice were intradermally injected with IL-23 for 5 days **(D–F)**. Samples were collected and tested for C5aR1 expression ($n = 5$/group). **(A,D)** C5aR1 expression in local skin tissues was detected by IHC. **(B,E)** C5aR1 mRNA levels in skin tissues were analyzed. **(C,F)** C5aR1 expression in infiltrated cells from skin lesions was measured by FCM. Values are presented as mean ± SEM ($n = 5$/group). Gating strategy for **(C,F)**, isotype control for **(A,D)**, and negative control of C5aR1 expression was shown in **Figure S1**. Data are representative of two independent experiments. $^{***}p < 0.001$.

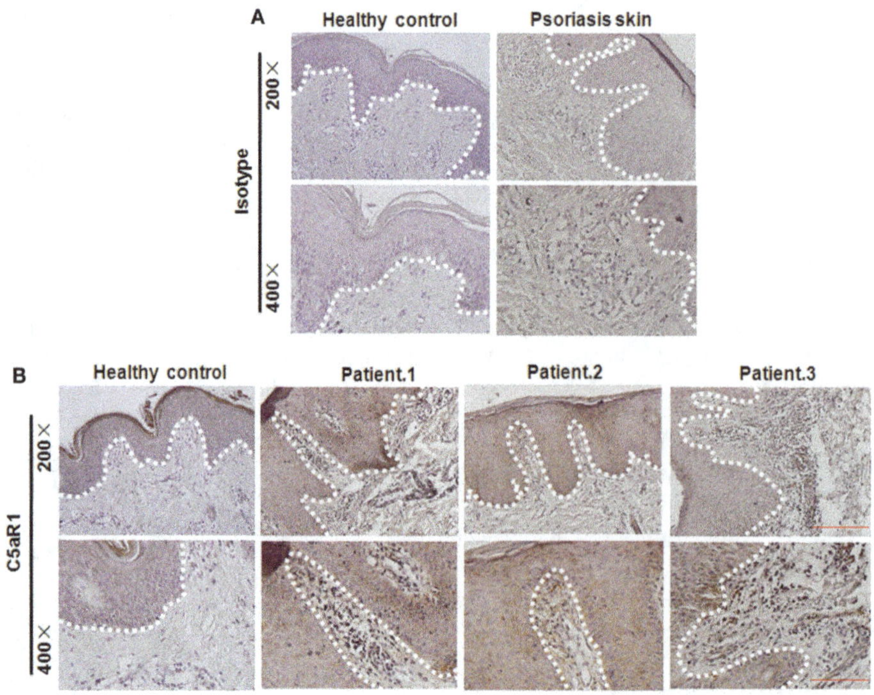

FIGURE 2 | Increased C5aR1 expression in psoriatic skin lesions in patients with psoriasis. **(A)** Isotype control and **(B)** C5aR1 expression by Immunohistochemistry. Healthy volunteer was used as healthy control ($n = 8$ for psoriasis patient; $n = 5$ for healthy volunteer). White dotted line: the location of the basal membrane.

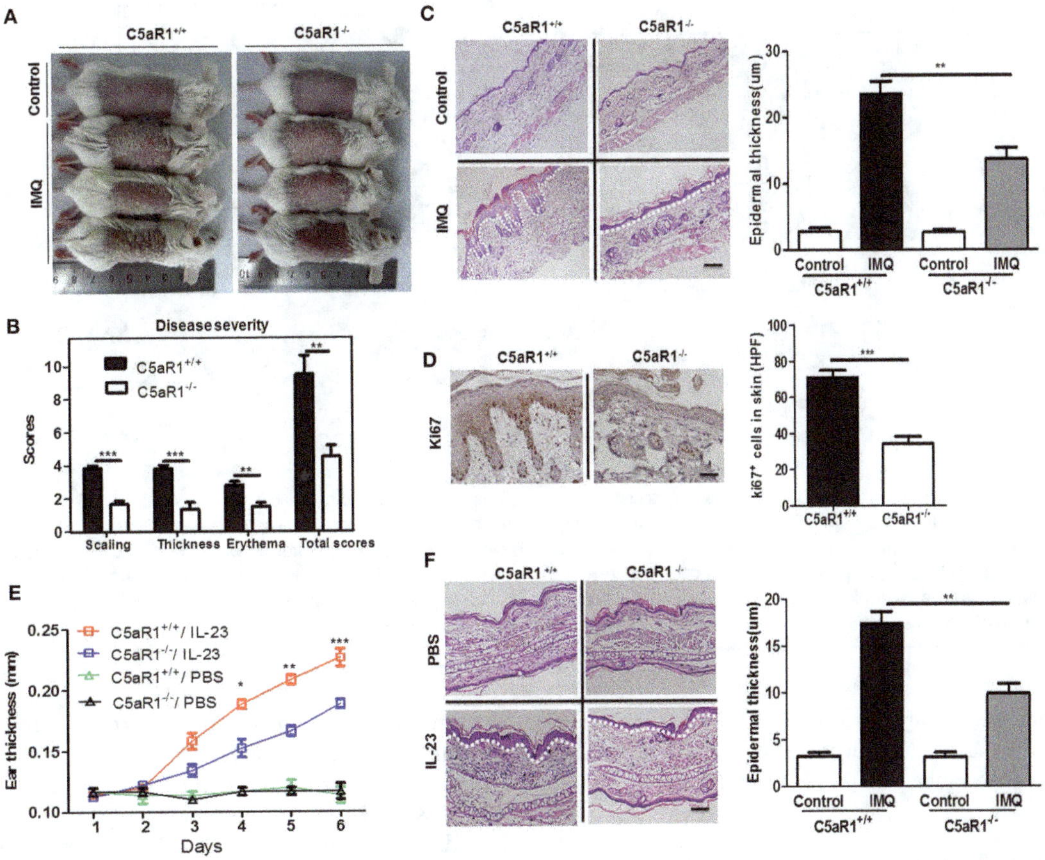

FIGURE 3 | C5aR1 deficiency reduced psoriatic skin inflammation. Wild-type (C5aR1$^{+/+}$) and C5aR1-deficient (C5aR1$^{-/-}$) mice were treated with IMQ for six consecutive days or intradermally injected with IL-23 for 5 days, skin samples were collected 24 h after the final IMQ application **(A–D)** or IL-23 injection **(E,F)**. **(A)** Macroscopic phenotype of psoriatic lesions in C5aR1$^{+/+}$ and C5aR1$^{-/-}$ mice treated with IMQ or Vaseline cream (control). **(B)** Disease severity was scored by a modified clinical Psoriasis Area and Severity Index (mPASI). The cumulative mPASI scores after 6 days treatment with IMQ were presented. **(C)** H&E staining of mice skin lesion sections. Epidermal thickness of the skin was measured. Scale bar = 20 μm. **(D)** IHC staining for Ki67 in skin lesion sections. Right: Ki67-positive cells quantification. **(E)** Ear thickness was measured following IL-23 injection. **(F)** H&E staining of ear skin lesion sections. Epidermal thickness of the ears was measured. White dotted line: the location of the basal membrane. Scale bar = 5 μm. Values are presented as mean ± SEM. Data are representative of three independent experiments and each group consisted of more than five mice. *$p < 0.05$; **$p < 0.01$; ***$p < 0.001$.

culture supernatants of the medium group and in serum of naïve C5aR1$^{+/+}$ and C5aR1$^{-/-}$ mice were measured with commercial ELISA kit from USCN (SEA388Mu, Wuhan, China), according to the manufacturer's instruction.

Flow Cytometry

The shaved back of C5aR1$^{+/+}$ and C5aR1$^{-/-}$ mice were topically applied with IMQ for indicated times or the ears of C5aR1$^{+/+}$ mice were intradermally injected with IL-23 for 5 days. Cells were isolated from psoriatic skin lesion samples. Briefly, skin samples were minced and digested in collagenase type IV (2 mg/mL; Sigma-Aldrich, St. Louis, MO, USA) and DNase I (200 U/mL; Sigma-Aldrich, St. Louis, MO, USA) for 60 min at 37°C. Cells at 1 × 10^6 cells/ml were incubated with Fc blocking for 20 min on ice and then stained with PE-labeled rat anti-mouse C5aR1 (1 μl/test, 20/70, BioLegend, San Diego, CA, USA), PerCP-Cy5.5-labeled rat anti-mouse Gr-1 (1 μl/test, RB6-8C5, Biolegend, San Diego, CA, USA), PE-Cy7-labeled rat anti- mouse CD11b (1 μl/test, CBRM1/5, BioLegend, San Diego, CA, USA), or FITC-labeled rat anti-mouse PDCA-1 (1 μl/test, eBio927, eBioscience, San Diego, CA, USA) antibodies for 25 min on ice in the dark. For bone marrow derived pDCs, cells were stained with FITC-labeled rat anti-mouse PDCA-1. For pDCs purified from mouse splenocytes, the purity was measured by FITC-labeled rat anti-mouse PDCA-1 and PE-labeled rat anti-mouse B220 (1 μl/test, RA3-6B2, Biolegend, San Diego, CA, USA). Sorted pDCs from C5aR1$^{+/+}$ mice were cultured (1 × 10^5 cells) in a 96-well round-bottom plate for 24 h in the presence of IMQ, and was stained with PE-labeled rat anti-mouse C5aR1 antibody. For human PBMCs from psoriatic patients and healthy subjects, cells were stained with PE-labeled mouse anti-human C5aR1 (1 μl/test, S5/1, BioLegend, San Diego, CA, USA) and FITC-labeled rat anti-human CD123 (1 μl/test, 6H6, eBioscience, San Diego, CA, USA). Corresponding rat or mouse isotype IgG was used as the negative control. Stained cells were assessed by flow cytometry (BD FACS Canto II, Franklin Lakes, NJ,

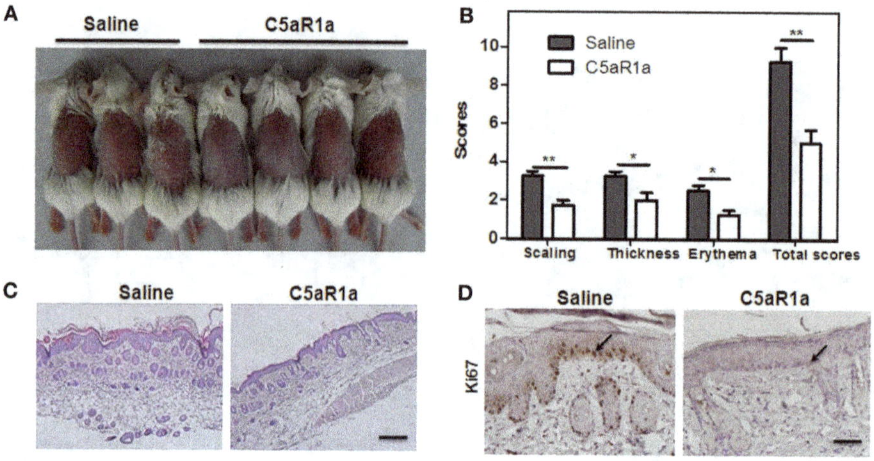

FIGURE 4 | Blockage of C5aR1 signaling with C5a receptor antagonist (C5aR1a) attenuated IMQ-induced psoriatic skin inflammation. C5aR1$^{+/+}$ mice were pre-treated with C5aRa (1 mg/kg) or 0.9% saline for 2 h prior to treatment with IMQ. After IMQ treatment for six consecutive days, digital pictures were obtained and skin samples were collected. **(A)** Phenotype of IMQ-induced psoriatic skin lesions. The left three mice were pre-treated with saline, while the right four mice were pre-treated with C5aRa. **(B)** Disease severity was scored as described (n = 5–6/group). **(C)** H&E staining of psoriatic skin lesions. Scale bar = 20 μm. **(D)** IHC staining for Ki67 in psoriatic skin lesions. Scale bar = 5 μm. Arrows indicate positively stained cells. Data are representative of at least three independent experiments and each group consisted of more than five mice. $^{*}p < 0.05$; $^{**}p < 0.01$.

USA) and data were analyzed using Flow Jo software (Tree Star, Ashland, OR, USA). The acquired cells number for each sample keeps in the range of $2 \times 10^5 \sim 1 \times 10^6$ depending on different situations.

Chemotaxis Assay

Chemotaxis migration assays were performed using 24-well transwell plates (5 μm pore size; Corning, NY 14831, USA). pDCs were purified from mouse splenocytes and seeded (1×10^6 cells) in the upper chamber and chemoattractant medium (600 μL) containing C5a (42 nM; PeproTech, Rocky Hill, NJ, USA) was added to the lower chamber. Transwell plates were incubated for 90 min at 37°C in the presence of 5% CO_2. Migrated cells in the lower chamber were collected and counted by FCM. Experiments were performed in triplicate and results were calculated as mean values of three experiments.

Statistical Analysis

Results were presented as mean ± standard error of the mean (SEM). GraphPad Prism 5.0 software (GraphPad Software, Inc., La Jolla, CA) was used for statistical analysis. The student's t-test or two-way ANOVA were used to compare samples, and $p < 0.05$ was considered statistically significant.

RESULTS

Increased C5aR1 Expression in Psoriatic Mouse Skin Lesions

Abundant levels of C5a des-Arg were extracted from psoriatic scales (19, 21). As shown in **Figures 1A–C**, C5aR1 expression was significantly increased in the local skin lesions tissues and in cells isolated from skin lesions in IMQ-induced psoriatic mice, compared to the control mice, according to immunohistochemistry (IHC), qRT-PCR, and FCM analyses. Moreover, C5aR1 expression of IMQ-treated back skin tissues in mice was predominantly on keratinocytes including the epidermis and hair follicles as wells as skin tissues infiltrating cells. Similar results were observed when mice were treated with recombinant IL-23 in ears (**Figures 1D–F**), which is another well-defined mouse model of psoriatic skin inflammation (28, 29). Consistent with the results in psoriatic mice, C5aR expression in psoriatic skin tissues from patients with psoriasis was also significantly increased, compared with that from healthy controls (**Figure 2**).

All these results suggest that C5aR1 signaling pathway is closely related to the pathogenesis of psoriasis.

C5aR1 Deficiency Reduces Severity of Psoriasis

To determine the importance of the C5aR1 signaling pathway in psoriasis, we used C5aR1-deficient mice. As shown in **Figures 3A,B**, topical application of IMQ on the shaved back of wild-type C5aR1$^{+/+}$ mice for six consecutive days induced psoriatic lesions, including erythema, scales, and crust formation, as previously reported (22). Interestingly, IMQ-induced psoriasis-like skin inflammation and total mPASI scores of C5aR1$^{-/-}$ mice were significantly less than those of C5aR1$^{+/+}$ mice (**Figures 3A,B**). Furthermore, we observed a significant decrease in the epidermal thicknesses (**Figure 3C**) and the occurrence of parakeratosis (**Figure S2**) in C5aR1$^{-/-}$ mice, compared to C5aR1$^{+/+}$ mice. Expression levels of Ki67, a marker for cells proliferation, was significantly reduced in the local skin tissues of IMQ-treated C5aR1$^{-/-}$

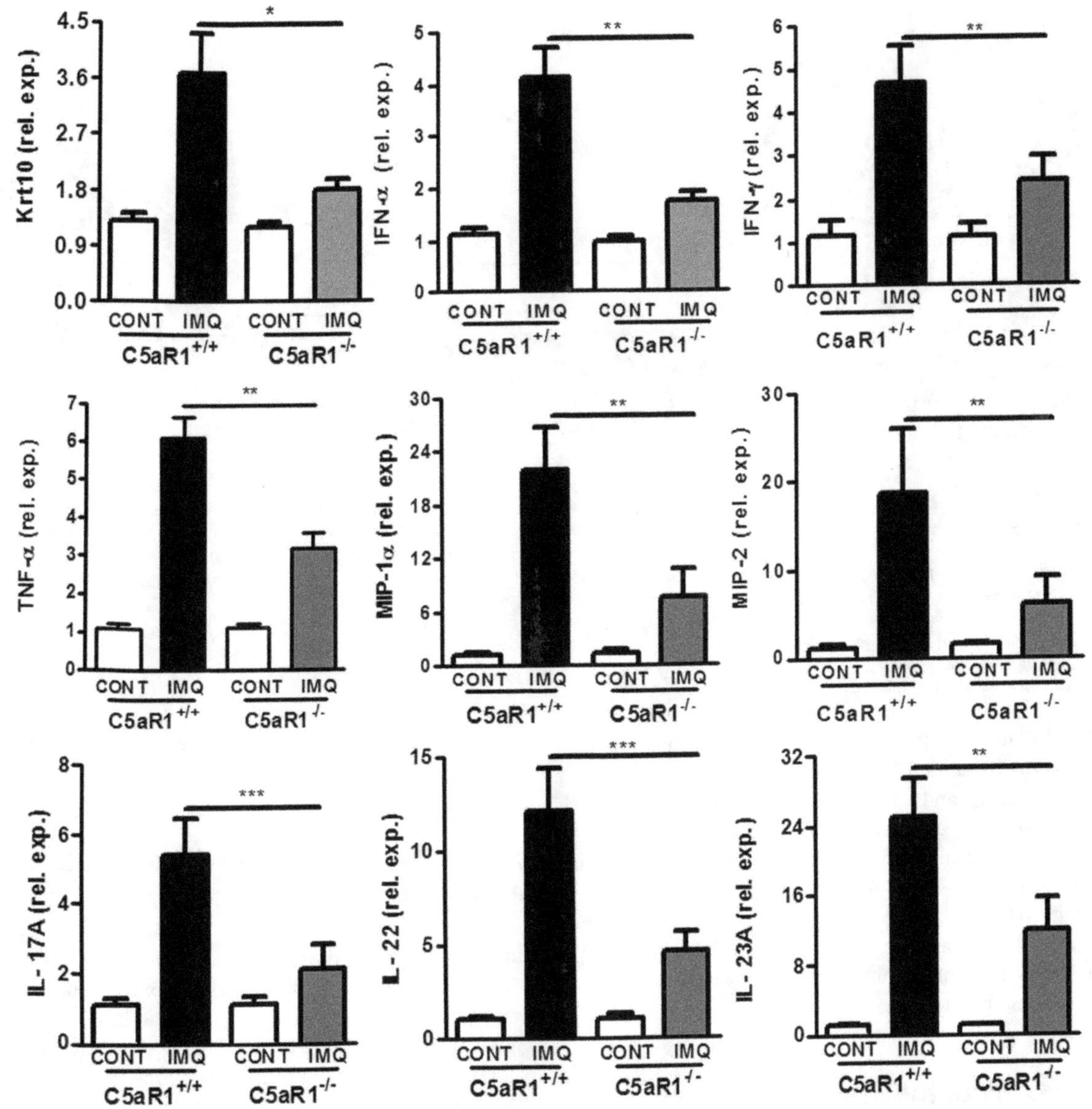

FIGURE 5 | C5aR1 deficiency attenuated inflammatory cytokines and chemokines expression of psoriatic skin lesions. IMQ was topically applied to the shaved back of C5aR1$^{+/+}$ and C5aR1$^{-/-}$ mice for six consecutive days, and back skin samples were obtained on day 7. Expression levels of the indicated genes in psoriatic skin lesions were measured by qRT-PCR ($n = 5$–6/group). Values are presented as mean ± SEM and data were obtained from at least three independent experiments. $^{*}p < 0.05$; $^{**}p < 0.01$, $^{***}p < 0.001$.

mice (**Figure 3D**). Similar attenuation effects in psoriatic development were observed in the ear skin samples of IMQ-treated and IL-23-treated C5aR1$^{-/-}$ mice (**Figure S3** and **Figures 3E,F**).

To validate the function of C5aR1 signaling in the pathogenesis of psoriasis, we inhibited the C5aR1 signaling pathway using a C5aR1 peptide antagonist (C5aR1a). As shown in **Figure 4**, C5aR1a-treated mice exhibited a significant attenuation in IMQ-induced psoriasiform skin inflammation (**Figure 4A**), total mPASI scores (**Figure 4B**), epidermal thicknesses (**Figure 4C**), and keratinocyte proliferation (**Figure 4D**).

These results clearly indicate that C5a/C5aR1 signaling is essential for the development of psoriasis.

C5aR1 Deficiency Attenuates Inflammatory Cytokines and Chemokines Expression in Psoriatic Skin Lesions

Increased expression of inflammatory cytokines and chemokines plays a critical role in the progression of IMQ-induced skin inflammation (30–34). The expression levels of keratinocyte-specific factors and inflammatory cytokines were analyzed by qRT-PCR. Compared to C5aR1$^{+/+}$ mice, skin tissues

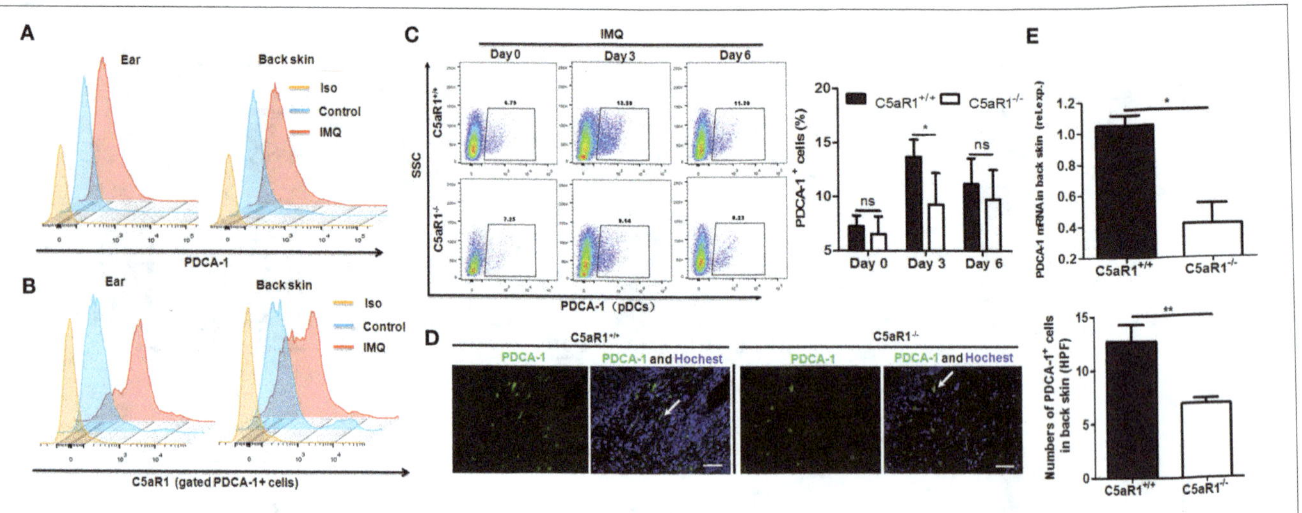

FIGURE 6 | C5aR1 deficiency reduced pDCs infiltration in psoriatic lesions. C5aR1$^{+/+}$ and C5aR1$^{-/-}$ mice were treated with IMQ (Vaseline cream treatment as a control) on the shaved ear or back skin for indicated days, and then skin samples were obtained and infiltrated cells of skin lesions were isolated. **(A)** Frequencies of pDCs (PDCA-1^{+} cells) in the infiltrated cells of psoriatic ear and back skin lesions and **(B)** C5aR1 expression on these pDCs in C5aR1$^{+/+}$ mice following 3 days IMQ application. **(C)** Frequencies of pDCs (PDCA-1^{+}) in IMQ-treated back skin of C5aR1$^{+/+}$ and C5aR1$^{-/-}$ mice were compared at indicated times. Percentages of PDCA-1^{+} pDCs is shown ($n = 5$–6). **(D)** Infiltration of pDCs (PDCA-1^{+}) on day 3 in IMQ-treated back skin tissues of C5aR1$^{+/+}$ and C5aR1$^{-/-}$ mice was measured by immunofluorescence. Arrows indicate positively stained cells. Scale bar = 5 μm. **(E)** PDCA-1 expression in IMQ-treated back skin tissues of C5aR1$^{+/+}$ and C5aR1$^{-/-}$ mice was analyzed by qRT-PCR following 3 days IMQ treatment. ($n = 5$–6/group). Gating strategy is shown in **Figure S5**. Values are presented as mean ± SEM and data were obtained from three independent experiments. $^{*}p < 0.05$; $^{**}p < 0.01$.

of C5aR1$^{-/-}$ mice exhibited a significant reduction in mRNA levels of keratin 10 (Krt10), TNF-α, IFN-α/γ, IL-17A, IL-22, IL-23A, and the chemokines of T cells and neutrophils, macrophage inflammatory protein 1α (MIP-1α) and macrophage inflammatory protein 2 (MIP-2) (**Figure 5**). Similar results were observed in mice with C5aR1 signaling blockage (**Figure S4**).

Collectively, these results demonstrate that C5aR1 deficiency impairs production of inflammatory cytokines and chemokines in IMQ-induced skin lesions.

C5aR1 Is Critical for pDCs Infiltration in Psoriatic Skin Lesions

It has been reported that IMQ induces rapid pDCs accumulation and pDCs play a crucial role in the initiation of psoriatic lesions (23, 35, 36). Consistent with previous reports, we demonstrated that IMQ treatment significantly increased infiltration of pDCs (plasmacytoid dendritic cell antigen-1 positive, PDCA-1^{+} cells) in ear and back skin lesions (**Figure 6A**). Similar results were observed in monocytes and neutrophils (**Figure S6**). Moreover, C5aR1 expression was clearly enhanced in these infiltrated skin cells (**Figure 6B** and **Figure S7**). Accordingly, C5aR1 deficiency significantly reduced these inflammatory cells accumulation and local infiltration in IMQ-treated back skin lesions at day 3 or 6 (**Figures 6C–E** and **Figure S6**).

Similar results were observed in patients with psoriasis, as the frequency of C5aR1^{+} pDCs (CD123^{+} cells) substantially increased in both local skin tissues (**Figure 7A**) and PBMCs (**Figures 7B,C**), compared to healthy individuals.

All these results indicating that C5a/C5aR1 signaling pathway is essential for early pDCs accumulation in local skin during the development of psoriasis.

C5aR1 Signaling Pathway Potentiates pDCs Function and Differentiation

To further investigate the role of C5aR1 signaling in pDCs functions, we isolated pDCs from splenocytes of C5aR1$^{+/+}$ and C5aR1$^{-/-}$ mice. It was found that C5aR1 deficiency led to a significant decrease in the IMQ and R848-induced IFN-α and TNF-α secretion (**Figure 8A**) and in the chemoattractive capacity of pDCs, as assessed by transwell migration assay (**Figure 8B**). FLT3L has been reported to induce pDCs differentiation from bone marrow cells (BMs) (26, 27). To explore the effect of C5aR1 on pDCs differentiation, BMs from C5aR1$^{+/+}$ and C5aR1$^{-/-}$ were primed with FLT3L for 10 days, and then the percentage of pDCs was determined. It was showed that the proportion of pDCs was dramatically lower in FLT3L-stimulated BMs derived from C5aR1$^{-/-}$ mice than those derived from C5aR1$^{+/+}$ mice (**Figure 8C**). In accordance, treatment of BMs with recombinant mouse C5a further increased FLT3L-dependent differentiation of pDCs *in vitro* (**Figure 8D**).

Altogether, our data demonstrate the vital role of C5a/C5aR1 signaling in pDCs differentiation and functions.

DISCUSSION

Activation of the complement system was reported during the development of psoriasis and skin lesions exhibited high levels of activated C5a fragments (18–21). In agreement with these findings, our results showed that C5aR1 expression was

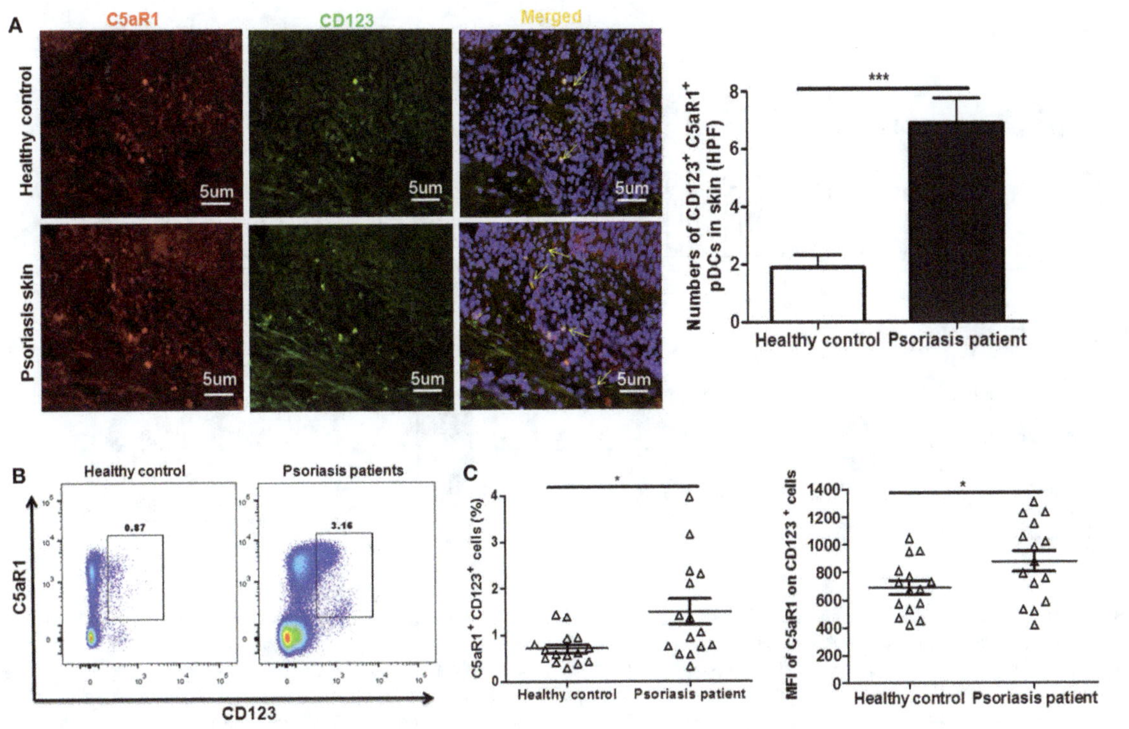

FIGURE 7 | Increased C5aR1 expression on pDCs from psoriasis patients. Skin tissues and PBMCs of psoriatic patients and healthy individuals were collected. **(A)** Immunofluorescence staining for C5aR1 expression (red) on pDCs (stained with anti-CD123) (green) in skin tissues. Nuclei (blue) were stained with Hoechst 33258. Arrows indicate cells positively stained for both C5aR1 and CD123. Scale bar = 5 μm. Right: Quantification of C5aR1^{+} CD123^{+} cells is shown. **(B)** C5aR1 expression on pDCs (CD123^{+} cells) of PBMCs from psoriatic patients and healthy individuals ($n = 15$/group). Representative FCM analyses of C5aR1^{+}CD123^{+} cells are illustrated. Gating strategy is shown in **Figure S8**. **(C)** Percentage of C5aR1^{+}CD123^{+} cells and MFI of C5aR1 expression on pDCs (CD123^{+} cells). Values are presented as mean ± SEM and data were obtained from at least two independent experiments. $^{*}p < 0.05$; $^{***}p < 0.001$.

clearly increased in keratinocytes (epidermis and hair follicles) as well as skin infiltrating cells from both psoriatic mice and patients with psoriasis. However, the role and underlying mechanisms of the complement C5a/C5aR1 signaling pathway in the pathogenesis of psoriasis remain unclear. In the present study, we reported that C5aR1 deficiency or inhibition with C5aR1a significantly reduced psoriasis-like skin inflammation, validating the importance of the C5a/C5aR1 pathway in IMQ-induced mouse psoriatic skin lesions. Furthermore, C5a/C5aR1 signaling potentiated pDCs, monocytes and neutrophils recruitment, and pDCs differentiation and functions, which suggest a possible mechanistic contribution of C5a/C5aR1 signaling in the pathogenesis of psoriasis, that requires further investigation in the future.

Multiple studies have demonstrated that IMQ-induced expression of pro-inflammatory cytokines and chemokines, specifically TNF-α, IFN-α/γ,IL-17A, IL-22, IL-23A, MIP-1α, and MIP-2, is essential for the development of psoriatic skin lesions (2, 3, 30). Our results provided evidence that C5a/C5aR1 signaling mediated development of psoriatic skin lesions, as C5aR1-deficient mice exhibited impaired expression of these genes.

Psoriasis is a chronic skin disease mediated by IFN-α- driven T cells, characterized by local accumulation of pDCs (23). pDCs are considered to be key in the development of psoriasis because of the significant production IFN-α (23). Moreover, it was previously demonstrated that TLR7 expression of pDCs was targeted by IMQ, representing an important upstream event that initiates the psoriatic skin inflammation (35, 36). However, the mechanism of regulation of pDC accumulation in psoriatic lesions is currently unknown. In our study, we showed that C5aR1 deficiency significantly reduced IMQ-induced pDCs infiltration, implicating the C5aR1 signaling pathway in pDCs infiltration in psoriasiform inflammation. Consistent with a previous study (13), we observed significantly increased C5aR1 expression in pDCs derived from PBMCs of psoriatic patients. There was a significant reduction in the production of IFN-α and TNF-α, a cytokine critical for the initiation of psoriasis, in cells treated with IMQ and R848. In addition, the chemo-attractive capacity of pDCs derived from C5aR1-deficient mice was significantly decreased. Altogether, we demonstrate that the C5a/C5aR1 pathway is critical for pDCs functions during the development of psoriasis in mice.

FLT3Lhas been shown to be an essential physiological factor for pDCs differentiation (26, 27). In the present study, C5aR1 deficiency clearly impaired FLT3L-dependent differentiation of pDCs from BMs, whereas exogenous recombinant C5a enhanced pDCs differentiation. These results suggest an

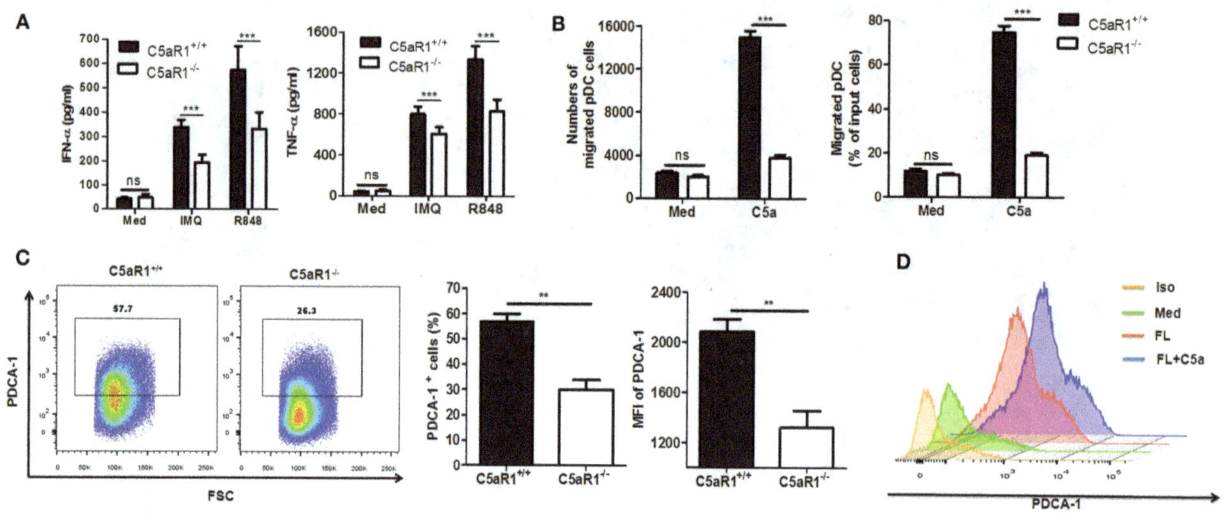

FIGURE 8 | C5aR1 deficiency impaired pDCs function and differentiation *in vitro*. **(A,B)** pDCs were isolated from splenocytes of C5aR1$^{+/+}$ and C5aR1$^{-/-}$ mice. Culture medium was used as a control. **(A)** Purified pDCs (1 × 10^6/ml) were stimulated with IMQ or R848 (10 μg/mL) *in vitro* for 24 hr. The levels of IFN-α and TNF-α in the culture supernatants were measured by ELISA. **(B)** pDCs (1 × 10^6/ml) in transwell plates were exposed to C5a (42 nM) for 90 min. Cells that migrated to the lower chamber were measured. The purity of isolated pDCs and IMQ-induced C5aR1 expression of isolated pDCs are shown in **Figure S9**. C5a levels in cultural supernatant of purified pDCs and in serum of naïve C5aR1$^{+/+}$ or C5aR1$^{-/-}$ mice are shown in **Figure S10**. **(C)** BM cells from C5aR1$^{+/+}$ and C5aR1$^{-/-}$ mice were stimulated with recombinant mouse FLT3L (200 ng/ml for 10 days and the frequency of pDCs was measured by FCM. Left, a representative FCM graph. Right, average percentages and MFIs of PDCA-1$^+$ cells. **(D)** BM cells from C5aR1$^{+/+}$ mice were stimulated with recombinant mouse FLT3L (200 ng/mL) alone or with C5a (42 nM) for 10 days, culture medium was used as a control. The frequency of pDCs was analyzed by FCM. Values are presented as mean ± SEM and data were obtained from at least three independent experiments. $^{**}p < 0.01$; $^{***}p < 0.001$.

essential role for C5aR1 signaling in FLT3L-dependent pDCs development. However, additional studies are necessary to investigate the underlying mechanisms by which C5a/C5aR1 signaling potentiates pDCs differentiation.

In conclusion, our study defined and characterized the role of C5a/C5aR1 signaling in the pathogenesis of IMQ-induced psoriatic lesions. Moreover, we demonstrated for the first time the dependency of C5a/C5aR1 signaling in pDCs differentiation and function, specifically in IMQ-induced psoriatic skin inflammation. Therefore, targeting C5a/C5aR1 interaction may prove to be a novel therapeutic approach for psoriasis.

AUTHOR CONTRIBUTIONS

QZ and GX designed the study and prepared the manuscript. QZ, FX, SW, YL, MT, and GL carried out the experiments. NL and SL collected the specimens from patients and healthy donors. QZ, GX, JC, DY, DS, YZ, and KZ analyzed data. All authors made substantial contributions toward drafting the manuscript, reviewing the final manuscript for intellectual content, and authorizing the submission. That written informed consent was obtained from the participants of this study.

SUPPLEMENTARY MATERIAL

Figure S1 | Isotype control and gating strategy of C5aR1 staining. After IMQ or IL-23 treatment, lesions skin sample of mice was collected and skin cells were isolated. **(A)** Skin single cell suspensions were stained with isotype IgG or anti-mouse C5aR1. The gating strategy is shown. **(B)** Skin paraffin sections were stained with rabbit IgG isotype antibody. **(C)** Skin paraffin sections from IMQ-treated C5aR1$^{-/-}$ were stained with rabbit isotype IgG or rabbit anti-mouse C5aR1 antibody.

Figure S2 | C5aR1 deficiency attenuated the parakeratosis of psoriatic skin in mice. The shaved back skin of C5aR1$^{+/+}$ and C5aR1$^{-/-}$ mice were topically applied with IMQ for 6 days. H&E staining of mice skin sections and one representative image analysis for parakeratosis are shown. White dotted line: the location of the basal membrane. The length of parakeratosis was measured per high-power field (HPF, 200×) from 5 to 6 mice per group. Values are presented as mean ± SEM and data were obtained from at least two independent experiments. $^{**}p < 0.01$.

Figure S3 | C5aR1 deficiency alleviated IMQ-induced psoriatic skin inflammation in ears. C5aR1$^{+/+}$ and C5aR1$^{-/-}$ ears were topically treated with IMQ (Vaseline cream treatment as a control) for six consecutive days (n = 5–6 per group). Ear skin tissues were collected. **(A)** Macroscopic phenotype of psoriasiform lesions in

C5aR1$^{+/+}$ and C5aR1$^{-/-}$ mice. **(B)** H&E staining of ear skin sections. Data represent three independent experiments.

Figure S4 | C5aR1 antagonist treatment led to a reduction in the levels of inflammatory response genes in psoriatic skin lesions. Mouse C5aR1 antagonist (1 mg/kg) or 0.9% saline was injected via intraperitoneal cavity 2 h prior to IMQ application in C5aR1$^{+/+}$ wild type mice. After six consecutive days of IMQ application, skin samples were collected and expression of inflammatory response genes were analyzed by qRT-PCR ($n = 4$–8). Values are presented as mean ± SEM and data were obtained from at least three independent experiments. $^{*}p < 0.05$; $^{**}p < 0.01$.

Figure S5 | Gating strategy of pDCs staining. After IMQ treatment for indicated days, whole-skin cells were isolated from psoriatic skin lesions samples and stained with isotype IgG or anti-mouse PDCA-1 antibody.

Figure S6 | C5aR1 deficiency led to decrease in neutrophils and monocytes infiltration of psoriatic skin lesions in mice. C5aR1$^{+/+}$ and C5aR1$^{-/-}$ mice were topically treated with IMQ for indicated days. Back skin samples were obtained. Infiltrated cells of skin lesions were isolated and the percentage of neutrophils and monocytes in the infiltrated cells was measured by FCM. **(A)** Gating strategy. **(B)** Monocytes (CD11b^{+} cells). **(C)** Neutrophils (Gr-1^{+} cells). ($n = 5$–6/group). Data were obtained from at least two independent experiments. ns, no significant, $^{*}p < 0.05$; $^{**}p < 0.01$.

Figure S7 | Increased C5aR1 expression in infiltrated skin cells in psoriatic skin lesions in mice. To induce a psoriatic animal model, IMQ was topically applied to the shaved back of wild-type (C5aR1$^{+/+}$) mice for six days. Samples were collected and cells were isolated from the skin lesions. **(A)** Gating strategy. **(B)** C5aR1 expression on pDCs (PDCA-1^{+}), monocytes (CD11b^{+}) and neutrophils (Gr-1^{+}) was assayed by FCM. ($n = 5$/group). ** $p < 0.01$.

Figure S8 | Gating strategy of CD123 and C5aR1 staining in human PBMCs. Human PBMCs were prepared as described in methods ($n = 15$/group), and then stained with isotype IgG or anti-human CD123 and C5aR1 antibodies, followed by flow cytometric analysis.

Figure S9 | The purity of isolated pDCs and IMQ-induced C5aR1 expression of isolated pDCs. pDCs were isolated from splenocytes of C5aR1$^{+/+}$ mice. **(A)** The purity of isolated pDCs (PDCA-1 positive cells) was measured by FCM. **(B)** C5aR1 expression on pDCs after IMQ stimulation for 24 h was measured by FCM.

Figure S10 | C5a levels in cultural supernatant of purified pDCs and in serum of naïve C5aR1$^{+/+}$ or C5aR1$^{-/-}$ mice. **(A)** pDCs were isolated from splenocytes of C5aR1$^{+/+}$ or C5aR1$^{-/-}$ mice and cultured in medium for 24 h. C5a levels in cell-free culture supernatant was measured by ELISA ($n = 6$/group). **(B)** C5a levels in serum from naïve C5aR1$^{+/+}$ and C5aR1$^{-/-}$ mice measured by ELISA ($n = 5$/group). Values are presented as mean ± SEM and data were obtained from at least two independent experiments.

REFERENCES

1. Boehncke WH, Schon MP. Psoriasis. *Lancet.* (2015) 386:P983–94. doi: 10.1016/S0140-6736(14)61909-7
2. Lowes MA, Suarez-Farinas M, Krueger JG. Immunology of psoriasis. *Ann Rev Immunol.* (2014) 32:227–55. doi: 10.1146/annurev-immunol-032713-120225
3. Lowes MA, Bowcock AM, Krueger JG. Pathogenesis and therapy of psoriasis. *Nature.* (2007) 445:866–73. doi: 10.1038/nature05663
4. Wagner EF, Schonthaler HB, Guinea-Viniegra J, Tschachler E. Psoriasis: what we have learned from mouse models. *Nat Rev Rheumatol.* (2010) 6:0704–14. doi: 10.1038/nrrheum.2010.157
5. Kondelkova K, Krejsek J, Borska L, Fiala Z, Hamakova K, Ettler K, et al. Membrane and soluble Toll-like receptor 2 in patients with psoriasis treated by Goeckerman therapy. *Int J Dermatol.* (2014) 53:e512–7. doi: 10.1111/ijd.12381
6. Kakeda M, Schlapbach C, Danelon G, Tang MM, Cecchinato V, Yawalkar N, et al. Innate immune cells express IL-17A/F in acute generalized exanthematous pustulosis and generalized pustular psoriasis. *Arch Dermatol Res.* (2014) 306:933–8. doi: 10.1007/s00403-014-1488-0
7. Nickoloff BJ. Skin innate immune system in psoriasis: friend or foe? *J Clin Invest.* (1999) 104:1161–4. doi: 10.1172/JCI8633
8. Walport MJ. Complement. First of two parts. *N Engl J Med.* (2001) 344:1058–66. doi: 10.1056/NEJM200104053441406
9. Carroll MC. The complement system in regulation of adaptive immunity. *Nat Immunol.* (2004) 5:981–6. doi: 10.1038/ni1113
10. Ricklin D, Hajishengallis G, Yang K, Lambris JD. Complement: a key system for immune surveillance and homeostasis. *Nat Immunol.* (2010) 11:785–97. doi: 10.1038/ni.1923
11. Fayyazi A, Sandau R, Duong LQ, Gotze O, Radzun HJ, Schweyer S, et al. C5a receptor and interleukin-6 are expressed in tissue macrophages and stimulated keratinocytes but not in pulmonary and intestinal epithelial cells. *Am J Pathol.* (1999) 154:495–501. doi: 10.1016/S0002-9440(10)65295-9
12. Peng Q, Li K, Sacks SH, Zhou W. The role of anaphylatoxins C3a and C5a in regulating innate and adaptive immune responses. *Inflamm Allergy Drug Targets.* (2009) 8:236–46. doi: 10.2174/187152809788681038
13. Gutzmer R, Kother B, Zwirner J, Dijkstra D, Purwar R, Wittmann M, et al. Human plasmacytoid dendritic cells express receptors for anaphylatoxins C3a and C5a and are chemoattracted to C3a and C5a. *J Inves Dermatol.* (2006) 126:2422–9. doi: 10.1038/sj.jid.5700416
14. Chen NJ, Mirtsos C, Suh D, Lu YC, Lin WJ, McKerlie C, et al. C5L2 is critical for the biological activities of the anaphylatoxins C5a and C3a. *Nature.* (2007) 446:203–7. doi: 10.1038/nature05559
15. Peng Q, Li K, Smyth LA, Xing G, Wang N, Meader L, et al. C3a and C5a promote renal ischemia-reperfusion injury. *J Am Soc Nephrol.* (2012) 23:1474–85. doi: 10.1681/ASN.2011111072
16. Guo RF, Ward PA. Role of C5a in inflammatory responses. *Ann Rev Immunol.* (2005) 23:821–52. doi: 10.1146/annurev.immunol.23.021704.115835
17. Ward PA. The harmful role of C5a on innate immunity in sepsis. *J Innate Immun.* (2010) 2:439–45. doi: 10.1159/000317194
18. Kapp A, Wokalek H, Schopf E. Involvement of complement in psoriasis and atopic dermatitis–measurement of C3a and C5a, C3, C4 and C1 inactivator. *Arch Dermatol Res.* (1985) 277:359–61. doi: 10.1007/BF00509233
19. Ohkohchi K, Takematsu H, Tagami H. Increased C5a anaphylatoxin in the sera of psoriatic patients and patients with inflammatory dermatoses. *J Dermatol.* (1986) 13:266–9. doi: 10.1111/j.1346-8138.1986.tb02939.x
20. Takematsu H, Ohkohchi K, Tagami H. Demonstration of anaphylatoxins C3a, C4a and C5a in the scales of psoriasis and inflammatory pustular dermatoses. *Br J Dermatol.* (1986) 114:1–6. doi: 10.1111/j.1365-2133.1986.tb02773.x
21. Bergh K, Iversen OJ, Lysvand H. Surprisingly high levels of anaphylatoxin C5a des Arg are extractable from psoriatic scales. *Arch Dermatol Res.* (1993) 285:131–4. doi: 10.1007/BF01112914
22. van der Fits L, Mourits S, Voerman JS, Kant M, Boon L, Laman JD, et al. Imiquimod-induced psoriasis-like skin inflammation in mice is mediated via the IL-23/IL-17 axis. *J Immunol.* (2009) 182:5836–45. doi: 10.4049/jimmunol.0802999
23. Nestle FO, Conrad C, Tun-Kyi A, Homey B, Gombert M, Boyman O, et al. Plasmacytoid predendritic cells initiate psoriasis through interferon-alpha production. *J Exp Med.* (2005) 202:135–43. doi: 10.1084/jem.20050500
24. Finch AM, Wong AK, Paczkowski NJ, Wadi SK, Craik DJ, Fairlie DP, et al. Low-molecular-weight peptidic and cyclic antagonists of the receptor for the complement factor C5a. *J Med Chem.* (1999) 42:1965–74. doi: 10.1021/jm9806594
25. Yuan JS, Reed A, Chen F, Stewart CN Jr. Statistical analysis of real-time PCR data. *BMC Bioinform.* (2006) 7:85. doi: 10.1186/1471-2105-7-85
26. Gilliet M, Boonstra A, Paturel C, Antonenko S, Xu XL, Trinchieri G, et al. The development of murine plasmacytoid dendritic cell precursors is differentially regulated by FLT3-ligand and granulocyte/macrophage colony-stimulating factor. *J Exp Med.* (2002) 195:953–8. doi: 10.1084/jem.20020045
27. Brawand P, Fitzpatrick DR, Greenfield BW, Brasel K, Maliszewski CR, De Smedt T. Murine plasmacytoid pre-dendritic cells generated from Flt3 ligand-supplemented bone marrow cultures are immature APCs. *J Immunol.* (2002) 169:6711–9. doi: 10.4049/jimmunol.169.12.6711

28. Lindroos J, Svensson L, Norsgaard H, Lovato P, Moller K, Hagedorn PH, et al. IL-23-mediated epidermal hyperplasia is dependent on IL-6. *J Invest Dermatol.* (2011) 131:1110–8. doi: 10.1038/jid.2010.432
29. Hedrick MN, Lonsdorf AS, Shirakawa A-K, Lee C-CR, Liao F, Singh SP, et al. CCR6 is required for IL-23–induced psoriasis-like inflammation in mice. *J Clin Invest.* (2009) 119:2317–29. doi: 10.1172/JCI37378
30. Di Cesare A, Di Meglio P, Nestle FO. The IL-23/Th17 axis in the immunopathogenesis of psoriasis. *J Invest Dermatol.* (2009) 129:1339–50. doi: 10.1038/jid.2009.59
31. Johansen C, Usher PA, Kjellerup RB, Lundsgaard D, Iversen L, Kragballe K. Characterization of the interleukin-17 isoforms and receptors in lesional psoriatic skin. *Br J Dermatol.* (2009) 160:319–24. doi: 10.1111/j.1365-2133.2008.08902.x
32. Kollipara R, Downing C, Gordon R, Tyring S. Interleukin-23 in the pathogenesis and treatment of psoriasis. *Skin Ther Lett.* (2015) 20:1–4.
33. Chiricozzi A. Pathogenic role of IL-17 in psoriasis and psoriatic arthritis. *Actas Dermosifiliogr.* (2014) 105:9–20. doi: 10.1016/S0001-7310(14)70014-6
34. Lee E, Trepicchio WL, Oestreicher JL, Pittman D, Wang F, Chamian F, et al. Increased expression of interleukin 23 p19 and p40 in lesional skin of patients with psoriasis vulgaris. *J Exp Med.* (2004) 199:125–30. doi: 10.1084/jem.20030451
35. Palamara F, Meindl S, Holcmann M, Luhrs P, Stingl G, Sibilia M. Identification and characterization of pDC-Like cells in normal mouse skin and melanomas treated with imiquimod. *J Immunol.* (2004) 173:3051–61. doi: 10.4049/jimmunol.173.5.3051
36. Gibson SJ, Lindh JM, Riter TR, Gleason RM, Rogers LM, Fuller AE, et al. Plasmacytoid dendritic cells produce cytokines and mature in response to the TLR7 agonists, imiquimod and resiquimod. *Cell Immunol.* (2002) 218:74–86. doi: 10.1016/S0008-8749(02)00517-8

12

Genetics and Omics Analysis of Autoimmune Skin Blistering Diseases

Michael Olbrich[1,2], Axel Künstner[1,2], Mareike Witte[3], Hauke Busch[1,2] and Anke Fähnrich[1,2]*

[1] Medical Systems Biology, Institute of Experimental Dermatology, University of Lübeck, Lübeck, Germany, [2] Institute of Cardiogenetics, University of Lübeck, Lübeck, Germany, [3] Department of Dermatology, University of Lübeck, Lübeck, Germany

***Correspondence:**
Anke Fähnrich
anke.faehnrich@uksh.de

Autoimmune blistering diseases (AIBDs) of the skin are characterized by autoantibodies against different intra-/extracellular structures within the epidermis and at the basement membrane zone (BMZ). Binding of the antibodies to their target antigen leads to inflammation at the respective binding site and degradation of these structures, resulting in the separation of the affected skin layers. Clinically, blistering, erythema and lesions of the skin and/or mucous membranes can be observed. Based on the localization of the autoantigen, AIBDs can be divided into pemphigus (intra-epidermal blistering diseases) and pemphigoid diseases (sub-epidermal blistering diseases), respectively. Although autoantigens have been extensively characterized, the underlying causes that trigger the diseases are still poorly understood. Besides the environment, genetic factors seem to play an important role in a predisposition to AIBDs. Here, we review currently known genetic and immunological mechanisms that contribute to the pathogenesis of AIBDs. Among the most commonly encountered genetic predispositions for AIBDs are the HLA gene region, and deleterious mutations of key genes for the immune system. Particularly, HLA class II genes such as the *HLA-DR* and *HLA-DQ* alleles have been shown to be prevalent in patients. This has prompted further epidemiological studies as well as unbiased Omics approaches on the transcriptome, microbiome, and proteome level to elucidate common and individual genetic risk factors as well as the molecular pathways that lead to the pathogenesis of AIBDs.

Keywords: autoimmune bullous diseases, autoantigens, HLA class II genes, systems medicine, genetics, transcriptomics

1. INTRODUCTION

Autoimmune blistering diseases (AIBDs) of the skin are rare, yet potentially fatal autoimmune disorders. The autoantibodies are directed against distinct molecules expressed in the epidermis and at the dermal-epidermal junction (DEJ) of skin and/or mucous membranes. Binding of these autoantibodies ultimately leads to loss of cell-cell and cell-matrix adhesion in the skin and/or mucous membranes, which results in erosions and/or blister formation (1, 2). Antigens are presented as a cleaved fragment via the major histocompatibility complex (MHC). MHC, also known as the human leukocyte antigen (HLA) region in humans, comprises a region of 7.6 megabases (Mb) on chromosome 6p21. It is the most gene-dense region of the human genome, encoding 252 expressed loci, of which 40% are thought to play a key role in the immune system (3). The HLA region is furthermore characterized by an extraordinarily high degree of polymorphisms with more than 1000 known alleles for HLA-A and -B. The HLA class I and class II gene clusters comprise the isotypes HLA-A/-B/-C as well as *HLA-DPA1*, *HLA-DPB1*, *HLA-DQA1*, *HLA-DQB1*, *HLA-DRA*, and *HLA-DRB1*), respectively. They are involved in antigen processing and presentation, and usually show highly significant associations with autoimmune diseases, representing the strongest predisposing genetic factors (3, 4).

The development of autoimmune diseases is generally multifactorial. Factors involved are a genetic predisposition, ethnicity, age, the environment, and gender. Autoimmune diseases show a prevalence and age of onset bias toward females (5, 6), which is particularly strong in systemic lupus erythematosus, Sjogren's syndrome, and autoimmune thyroiditis with females representing over 85% of all cases. In rheumatoid arthritis (RA) and multiple sclerosis, 60–75% of patients are female (5, 7). Sex-specific immune responses were also observed in mice. Female mice produced more antibodies and showed a stronger T cell activation than male mice after immunization (7–9). Yet, similar approaches in humans, in which responses to vaccination were analyzed, showed mixed results, with either no differences between males and females or an increased antibody response in females (9). It was found that females have a higher absolute number of CD4+ T lymphocytes than men (10) and produce more Th1 cytokines after vaccination. While these observations are still not completely understood, recent studies suggest that differences in the sex hormone composition, like progesterone and testosterone, may explain the differences in the immune mechanisms and autoimmune disease prevalence in females (5, 9, 11). Sex steroids may directly influence the immune system and affect components of antigen presentation, lymphocyte activation, cytokine gene expression, and/or homing of immune cells. They may also have indirect effects on corticosterone-cortisol concentrations, which are higher in females than in males. Additionally, glucocorticoids suppress the production of sex hormones and their mechanism of action in tissues (5, 11).

So far, more than 80 autoimmune diseases are known, ranging from familiar types like RA to rare forms like myasthenia gravis. Likewise, AIBDs can be subdivided into two major groups: pemphigus and pemphigoid diseases, based on the autoantigen localization. In the following sections we provide a brief description on the different AIBDs, together with their clinical manifestation and known genetic predispositions. An overview over the most common AIBDs is provided in **Table 1**.

1.1. Pemphigus Diseases

Pemphigus diseases are characterized by intraepidermal autoantibody binding. The two major pemphigus types are pemphigus vulgaris (PV) and pemphigus foliaceus (PF), accounting for 70% and 15–20% of all pemphigus cases, respectively. Rarer forms of pemphigus diseases include pemephigus herpetiformis (PH), paraneoplastic pemphigus (PNP) and IgA pemphigus (AP). The incidence of pemphigus diseases is population-dependent (36) and ranges between 0.7 and 5 per million/year. It is highest in Central Europe and the United States with an estimated range for new cases between 1 and 7 per million/year. PV is between 4- and 10-fold more common among the Jewish population as compared to other Caucasian populations (37). In contrast, PF is not particularly prevalent among the Jewish population, but endemic PF-variants have been described in South America and Tunisia (38). Another endemic form of PF, namely fogo selvagem, occurs in rural areas of Brazil with a prevalence of 3.4% on certain Amerindian link reservations and an incidence of 1–4 cases per 1,200 persons per year (38). Depending on the subtype, pemphigus antibodies are mostly directed against desmoglein 3 (Dsg3) and desmoglein 1 (Dsg1). In some cases, antibodies against other antigens, such as desmocollins (Dsc) and plakins can be found. The abundance of transmembrane glycoproteins varies with the different skin layers (cf. **Figure 1A**); Dsg1 is predominantly expressed in the upper layers, while Dsg3 is expressed in the lower layers of the epidermis (39). Degradation of these structures leads to a loss of cell-cell adhesion and formation of intra-epidermal blisters. Accordingly, this AIBD subtype is also referred to as intra-epidermal blistering disorders.

1.1.1. Pemphigus Vulgaris

PV is a pemphigus disease with autoantibodies against Dsg3 and, in some cases, additionally against Dsg1. Due to the expression of Dsg3 in the lower layers of the epidermis and in the epithelium, PV mainly affects mucous membranes. Skin involvement is determined by the presence of Dsg1 autoantibodies: In mucocutaneus PV, both Dsg1 and Dsg3 autoantibodies can be observed (40).

The age of onset is around 50–60 years. However, early and even childhood cases of PV have been reported. PV predominantly affects females (female-to-male ratio of 1.5:1) (41). Additionally, the outcome of PV may be worse in females, as a recent analysis showed that the HLA alleles *DRB1*04:02* and *DQB1*03:02* were associated with severe PV, and *DQB1*03:02* were found more frequently in female as compared to male patients (42, 43).

> Search strategy and selection criteria
>
> Literature: We searched the public literature databases PubMed, ResearchGate and Google Scholar, using the terms *AIBD*, *autoimmune blistering disorders of the skin*, *pemphigus* and *pemphigoid*. The search covered articles in English published between Jan 1, 2015, and March 31, 2019. Further publications, beyond the denoted selection criteria, were selected from the reference lists of the retrieved articles.
>
> Data repositories: The NCBI databases, particularly Gene Expression Omnibus (GEO), and European Nucleotide Archive (ENA) were searched for high-throughput data studies of the outlined phenotypes.

So far, the genetic association between PV and HLA class II genes remains the strongest and the most reported. While some of the HLA types are more population specific, others are associated with PV across different ethnicities. Several studies have found associations between PV and HLA class I alleles including *HLA-A3*, *HLA-A26*, and *HLA-B60* in the Han Chinese population; *HLA-B38*, *HLA-C12*, *HLA-B57*, and *HLA-C15* in the Brazilian population; *HLA-A10*, and *HLA-B15* in the Japanese population; *HLA-B35* and *HLA-B44* in the Turkish population; *HLA-B38* in the Jewish and Spanish population; and *HLA-B4402*,

TABLE 1 | Autoimmune skin blistering diseases: summary of targeted antigens, produced antibodies and associated genetics of common phemphigus and pemphigoid disease.

	Name	Antigen	Antibody	Genes	Cormorbidity	Source
	Pemphigus					
PV	Pemphigus Vulgaris	Dsg3, Dsg1	IgG, IgA, IgM, C3	*C3*, *HLA-DRA*, *TNF*, *IL6*, *IL6R*, *IL10*, *IL10RA*, *IL10RB*, *TAP2*, *GP9*, *DSG1-4*, *DUSP5*, *ST18*, *CD86*, *ANXA9*, *DSP*, *PPL*, *DST*, *DSC3*, *CDH1*	Hypothyroidism, IBD, T1DM, SLE, Sjörgren's Syndrome, Alopecia Areata, AITD, Juvenile Rheumatoid Arthritis, Peridontitis	(12–16)
PF	Pemphigus Foliaceus	Dsg1	IgG4	*DSG1*, *FOXP3*, *PPL*, *EVPL*, *DST*, *HLA-DRB1*, *CTLA4*		(12, 14, 16)
PH	Pemphigus Herpetiformis	Dsg1 a/o Dsg3, Dsc1, Dsc3	IgG, C3	*DSG1*, *DSG3*, *DSC1*, *DSC3*, *DST*, *C3*	Psoriasis thyroid disease, SLE, HIV, lung cancer, esophageal carcinoma, prostatic cancer, cutaneous angiosarcoma	(16–20)
PNP	Paraneoplastic Pemphigus	BP180, BP230, Dsg1-3, desmoplakin1;2, envoplakin, pectin, periplakin, A2ML1, epiplakin	IgG, C3	*COL17A1*, *DST*, *DSG1*, *DSG2*, *DSG3*, *DSP*, *EVPL*, *PLEC*, *PPL*, *EPPK1*, *A2ML1*, *C3*, *DSC1*, *DSC2*, *HLA-DRB1*	Carcinoma, Thymoma, Sarcoma, Non-Hodgkin lymphoma, Chroniclymphcytic leukemia, Castlemandisease	(12, 16, 20, 21)
AP	IgA Pemphigus	SPD type: Dsc1 IEN type: Dsg1 (1 case), unknown	IgA, IgG, C3	*DSC1*, *DSG1*, *DSG3*, *C3*	IgA gammopathy to myeloma, cancer, CD, Gluten-sensitive enteropathy (single case)	(16, 20, 22)
PE	Pemphigus Erthematosus	Dsg1, Dsg3	ANAs: Ro/La/Sm, IgG	*DSP*, *DSG1*, *DSG3*		(16, 23)
	Pemphigoid					
BP	Bullous Pemphigoid	BP180 NC16A, BP230	IgG, C3, C5, IgA, IgE	*COL17A1*, *DST*, *C3*, *C5*, *HLA-DRB1*, *HLA-DQB1*, *IL3*, *IL3RA*, *IL4*, *IL4R*, *IL5*, *IL5RA*, *IL6*, *IL6R*, *IL7*, *IL7R*, *IL8*, *IL10*, *IL10RA*, *IL10RB*, *IL15*, *IL15RA*, *TNF*, *CCL2*, *CCL5*, *CCL11*, *CCL13*, *CCL18*, *FIGF*, *ICAM1*, *DSP*, *DSG1*, *PPL*, *EVPL*, *ITGB4*, *ITGA6*	Diabetes mellitus	(16, 24–27)
PG	Pemphigoid Gestationis	BP180 NC16A, BP230	IgG	*COL17A1*, *DST*, *HLA-DRA*	Pregnancy	(12, 16, 28)

(Continued)

TABLE 1 | Continued

	Name	Antigen	Antibody	Genes	Cormorbidity	Source
EBA	Epidermolysis Bullosa Acquisita	COL7	IgG, IgA, IgM, IgE, C3(a) (1/3 of patients), C5(a)	*COL7A1, C3, C5, HLA-DRA, FCGR1A, SYK, LTB4R, LTB4R2, FLII, IL6, IL6R, RORA, PIK3CB, PIK3CG*	IBD, UC, CD, Myeloma, SLE amyloidosis, thyroiditis, multiple endocrinopathy syndrome, RA, pulmonary fibrosis, chronic lymphocytic leukemia, thyoma, diabetes	(12, 29–33)
ALP	Anti-Laminin γ1 / p200 Pemphigoid	Laminin γ1	IgG	*LAMC1*		(12, 16, 34)
LABD	Linear IgA-Dermatosis	Ladinin 1, COL7	IgA	*COL17A1, DST, LAD1, CD79A, ITGB4*		(12)
MMP	Mucus Membrane Pemphigoid	BP180, BP230, Laminin 332 (laminin-5), Laminin 311 (laminin-6), α6 and β4 Integrin	IgG, IgA, C3	*COL17A1, DST, LA-MA3, LAMB3, LAMC2, LAMB1, LAMC1, ITGB4, ITGA6, C3, CD79A, SERPINH1, CFP, TNFRSF1B*	Peridontitis	(12, 16, 35)

SPD type, Subcorneal Pustular Dermatosis type; IEN type, Intraepidermal Neutrophilic type; ANAs, Antinuclear Antibodies; IBD, Inflammatory Bowel Disease; T1DM, Type I Diabetes Mellitus; SLE, Systemic Lupus Erythematosus; AITD, Autoimmune Thyroid Disease; HIV, Human Immunodeficiency Virus; CD, Crohn's Disease; UC, Ulcerative Colitis; RA, Rheumatoid Arthritis.

HLA-C0401, and *HLA-C1502* in the Iranian population (13, 44–46), respectively. Population studies have shown an association between certain class II alleles and PV in different ethnic groups. For example, *HLA-DRB1*0402* is associated with PV in over 90% of Ashkenazi Jews, and *HLA-DQB1*0503* is associated in non-Jewish populations. Likewise, *HLA-DRB1*1404* is the most important risk factor in an Indo-Asian population. The two most common PV-associated alleles are *HLA-DQB1*0503* and *HAL-DRB1*0402*, both of which were found to be associated with the disease in the Spanish, French, Italian, Slovak, North American and Brazilian population (47). In addition, several studies have shown an association between PV and non-classic HLA class Ib alleles (*HLA-E*, *HLA-F*, and *HLA-G*). *HLA-G* polymorphisms were found to have a significant association with Jewish PV patients, while *HLA-E*, previously demonstrated to play a role in multiple autoimmune conditions, was found in association with Caucasian and Ashkenazi Jewish patients and was suggested to be involved in the disruption of immune tolerance in PV (44–46, 48).

1.1.2. Pemphigus Foliaceus

In PF, the autoantibodies are directed against Dsg1, while Dsg3 antibodies cannot be detected. Thus, PF affects only the skin, while mucosal lesions are completely absent (39, 49). Skin lesions are also more superficial than in PV, with desquamation/scaling rather than erosions involving the deeper skin layers. The average age of onset for sporadic PF is between 50 and 60 years with no reported gender bias. There are endemic forms of PF in Tunisia, Brazil, Peru and Colombia, which diverge in rate of incidence and observed sexual predisposition. For example, the Brazilian and Tunisian forms of PF present with higher incident rates (50, 51). A male prevalence is observed in Colombian PF, where about 95% of the cases are reported in males (52). The endemic subtypes in particular, indicate the role of environmental factors in their pathogenesis. The hotspot regions for endemic PF are characterized by poor living standards and hygienic conditions, low age of onset (around 20 years), and a seasonally varying incidence rate, which is highest at the end of the rainy season and lowest in dry summers.

Previous studies have shown that the DSG1 gene is polymorphic and that a coding synonymous T/C single nucleotide polymorphism at position 809 is associated with PF. To determine whether the disease occurs due to complex genetic interactions, it was tested whether MHC class II genes and DSG1 polymorphisms contribute to PF sensitivity. An analysis performed in 31 PF patients and 84 healthy controls first confirmed the previously reported common *DRB1*04* and *DRB1*14* genetic background in PF and individualized *DRB1*0102*, *DRB1*0402* and *DRB1*0406*, and *DRB1*1404* as susceptibility MHC class II alleles in French Caucasian PF patients (47, 53).

1.1.3. Pemphigus Herpetiformis

Pemphigus herpetiformis (PH), also known as mixed bullous disease, eosinophilic spongiosis in pemphigus or acantholytic herpetiform dermatitis, is considered a clinical

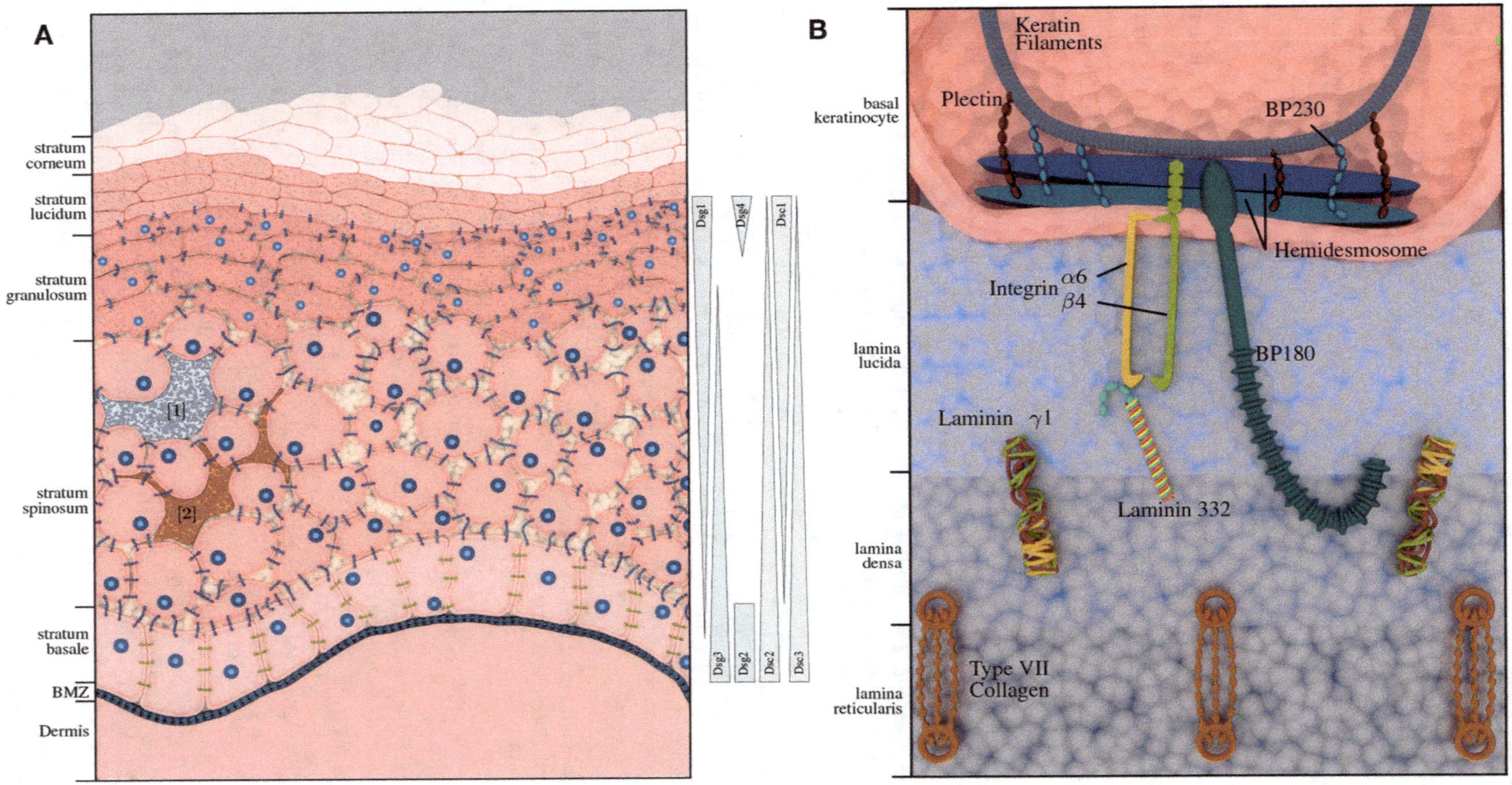

FIGURE 1 | Structural composition of human epidermis and basement membrane zone (BMZ). **(A)** Shows the composition of the human skin, including melanocytes [1] (3) and immunocompetent Langerhans cells [2] (4). The approximate distribution of pemphigus antigens within the layers of the epidermis is depicted on the right-hand side. While desmogleins 1 and 4 and desmocollin 1 are expressed in the upper layers of the epidermis; desmogleins 2 and 3 as well as desmocollin 2 and 3 are expressed in the lower layers of the epidermis. **(B)** Depicts the BMZ with its cellular adhesion proteins, connecting epidermis and dermis, which are the main autoantigens in pemphigoid diseases.

variant of pemphigus that combines the clinical features of dermatitis herpetiformis with the immunopathologic features of pemphigus. It accounts for 6–7.3% of all pemphigus patients. Clinically, PH is characterized by erythematous, itchy blisters and hive like swellings on several areas of the body. In contrast to PV and PF, the characteristic intense inflammation may not be associated with acantholysis (54, 55). Even though the phenotype closely resembles the features presented in dermatitis herpetiformis, its immunologic features conform to pemphigus (19). Autoantibodies in PH mainly target Dsg1 and, less commonly, Dsg3. Recently, several cases of PH without anti-Dsg1 or anti-Dsg3 autoantibodies have been reported with reactivity against other antigens such as desmocollin (Dsc) (56). It is currently unclear why the same autoantibodies result in a different clinical representation for PH and PF/PV. One explanation could be preferential binding to different epitopes on the same antigen molecule.

1.1.4. Paraneoplastic Pemphigus

Paraneoplastic pemphigus (PNP) is an AIBD that may be accompanied by both malignant and benign neoplasms which are often hematologic and lymphomatoid. The most frequently associated malignancies are chronic lymphocytic leukemia, B cell lymphoma, Castleman's disease, thymoma, and Waldenstrom's macroglobulinemia (21). Autoantibodies in paraneoplastic pemphigus typically target Dsg3 and proteins of the plakin family, including periplakin, envoplakin, plectin, desmoplakin 1 and 2, BP230, and the protease inhibitor alpha-2-macroglobulin-like-1 (57). The average age of onset for PNP is 51 years with no reported gender preference. Due to the association with neoplasms, PNP is hypothesized to be a side-effect of an antitumor response that cross-reacts with epithelial cells, either because the tumor is comprised of epithelial tissue or anomalously produces desmosome-like junctions (21). However, it should be considered that other pemphigus diseases may also be associated with malignancy (58).

1.1.5. IgA Pemphigus

IgA pemphigus is characterized by IgA autoantibodies against desmosomal and non-desmosomal keratinocyte cell surface components. The two major types of IgA pemphigus are subcorneal pustular dermatosis (SPD) and intraepidermal neutrophilic IgA dermatosis (IEN). The autoantigen of the SPD type was identified as Dsc1, while the antigen of the IEN type is variable (59, 60). However, in some reported cases of IEN type IgA pemphigus, IgA autoantibodies reacted with Dsg1 or Dsg3 (20, 59, 60). IgA pemphigus may be associated with monoclonal IgA gammopathy, multiple myeloma, HIV infection, Sjogren's syndrome, RA, and Crohn's disease. It is still unclear whether these diseases precede or follow IgA pemphigus. As one of the rarest AIBDs, the knowledge on IgA pemphigus is limited. No evident gender prevalence has been reported so far and the disorder may affect all age groups (22).

1.1.6. Pemphigus Erythematosus

Pemphigus erythematosus, also known as Senear-Usher syndrome, was originally described as a variant of pemphigus with features of lupus erythematosus but is today regarded as a localized form of PF and is considered an AIBD in it's own right. Autoantibodies target Dsg1, but may further target Ro, La, Sm, and double-stranded DNA antigens (23, 61). Clinically, blistering coincides with a seborrheic erythematous rash resembling the rash associated with lupus (61).

1.2. Pemphigoid Diseases

Pemphigoid diseases are characterized by autoantibodies against connective molecules at the DEJ, which is shown in **Figure 1B**. Binding of the autoantibodies leads to inflammation at the DEJ and degradation of the anchoring filaments and fibrils, resulting in sub-epidermal blistering. Accordingly, this group is also referred to as sub-epidermal blistering disorders. The most common pemphigoid diseases include bullous pemphigoid (BP), and mucous membrane pemphigoid (MMP). Other, less common types include pemphigoid gestationis (PG), epidermolysis bullosa acquisita (EBA), linear IgA dermatosis (LABD), and anti-laminin $\gamma 1$ / p200 pemphigoid.

1.2.1. Bullous Pemphigoid

Bullous pemphigoid (BP) is the most common pemphigoid disease in Central Europe, with an incidence rate of about 10–20 per million/year. It is characterized by sub-epidermal blistering accompanied by inflammatory cell infiltration in the upper dermis (62). There are two major target antigens in BP patients: Bullous Pemphigoid Antigen 2 (*BPAG2* also known as *BP180* or type XVII collagen), and the Bullous Pemphigoid Antigen 1 (*BPAG1*, also known as *BP230*), a cytoplasmic plakin protein family member that links the hemidesmosome to the keratin of intermediate filaments. *BP180* is a transmembrane glycoprotein that extends from the intracellular domain of basal keratinocytes to the lamina densa. The immunodominant region of BP180 is the noncollagenous domain 16A (NC16A). *BP230* is a 230-kDa protein with an intracellular component associated with the hemidesmosome plate belonging to the family of plakin proteins [**Figure 1B**; (63, 64)]. The major immunoglobulin class in BP is IgG. It has been shown however, that some patients also develop anti-BP180 IgA and IgE autoantibodies. In fact, most of the BP sera contain both IgG and IgA autoantibodies to *BP180* (65). Autoreactive CD4+ T lymphocytes recognize unique epitopes within the extracellular region of *BP180*. *BP180*-reactive Th cells and IgG autoantibodies recognize similar or identical epitopes clustered in distinct regions of the *BP180* ectodomain and *BP230*. Many polymorphisms of HLA-II class alleles have been identified in patients with BP in several populations, especially HLA-DQ alleles. These polymorphic HLA class II alleles are likely to occur due to changes in the active binding site on the HLA molecules for binding autoantigenic peptides. A common HLA class II allele, *HLA-DQB1*0301*, is positively associated with BP in multiple populations and also appears to be associated with distinct clinical pemphigoid variants. Computer-based models demonstrate that the *HLA-DQB1*0301* allele is capable of binding to multiple T cell epitopes within *BP230* and

BP180 for BP and $\alpha 6$ integrin, and $\beta 4$ integrin for MMP. Binding leads to the activation of antigen specific T cells interacting with B cells through CD40/CD40L interaction, to produce four distinct anti-BMZ antibodies with different specificities. These antibodies bind to their specific target antigen resulting in the production of subepidermal blisters. In addition, the activation of BP180-autoreactive T cells from a cohort of BP patients with *HLA-DQB1*03:01*, was found to be restricted by this BP-associated HLA class II allele (46, 66–70).

1.2.2. Pemphigoid Gestationis

Pemphigoid gestationis (PG) is a rare dermatosis that occurs during pregnancy with a reported incidence rate between 0.5 and 2 per million/year (71–73). It usually affects pregnant women during the third trimenon and, less commonly, during the second trimenon or post-partum period (28, 74, 75). When occurring during the first pregnancy, the disease reoccurs in following pregnancies in 90% of the cases. PG persists and converts to BP in less than 5% of patients. In contrast to BP, blisters are infrequent and usually small in size with predominating urticarial erythema that first affects the periumbilical region. Autoantibodies are mainly directed against *BP180* NC16A and in 10% of the cases against *BP230*. The main IgG subclasses are IgG1 and IgG3 and a strong association with maternal *HLA-DR3* and *HLA-DR4* exists (74, 75).

1.2.3. Epidermolysis Bullosa Acquisita

In epidermolysis bullosa acquisita (EBA), the autoantibodies are directed against type VII collagen, an anchoring fibril at the BMZ. Both skin and mucous membranes can be affected by EBA, albeit the latter to a lesser extent. The EBA incidence rate has been reported to be between 0.2 and 0.5 new cases per million/year (76). Clinically, mechanobullous (classical) EBA and inflammatory EBA can be distinguished. A characterizing feature of the classical variant is fragility of the skin that usually affects the trauma-prone areas, such as the extensor side of joints. The inflammatory subtype can resemble other AIBDs in clinical presentation as well as in serologic and histologic findings. Common to both types is the scarring and formation of milia. The scarring is particularly problematic in mucous membranes as it reduces the tissue function, even after successful suppression of the disorder (73). Inflammatory bowel disease (IBD) has been reported in 20% of the EBA patients. A link between IBD and EBA is strengthened by the presence of type VII collagen in the colon and the finding of its respective autoantibodies in IBD patients (33). EBA has been associated with environmental factors and genetically with the MHC locus *HLA-DR2* notably the *DRB1*15:03* allele in patients of African descent (73).

1.2.4. Anti-p200/Anti-Laminin $\gamma 1$ Pemphigoid

Anti-p200 pemphigoid is a pemphigoid disease with IgG autoantibodies against a 200 kDa protein at the DEJ (77), while IgA reactivity has also been reported (78). In 90% of anti-p200 pemphigoid cases, laminin $\gamma 1$ is the target antigen (34). Therefore, anti-p200 pemphigoid is also known as anti-laminin $\gamma 1$ pemphigoid. However, because reactivity with laminin $\gamma 1$ cannot be demonstrated in all patients with anti-p200 pemphigoid, it is recommended to restrict the term "anti-laminin $\gamma 1$ pemphigoid" to those patients with reactivity against laminin $\gamma 1$ (40). The clinical presentation is highly variable, often resembling BP or the inflammatory variant of EBA, and lesions heal without scarring or milia formation (77). Mucous membranes may be affected (79) and one third of the patients present with psoriasis as a co-morbidity (73). Due to variable clinical representation, histopathology, serological, and direct immunofluorescence microscopy findings, the diagnosis requires specialized assays. Therefore, anti-p200/ anti-laminin $\gamma 1$ pemphigoid might be underdiagnosed (73).

1.2.5. Linear IgA Bullous Dermatosis

Linear IgA bullous dermatosis (LABD) is a pemphigoid disease with an incidence rate of about 0.2–2.3 per million/year. The autoantibodies (mainly IgA) are directed against antigens with various molecular weights, including 97-, 120-, 180-, 200-, 230-, 280-, 285-, and 290-kDa proteins (80–82). In the majority of patients, the autoantibodies target the soluble ectodomain of BP180, LAD-1, and 20% of the sera recognize BP180 NC16A (83). The disorder can affect both children and adults. The age of onset for the adult variant shows two peaks in the teenage years and around 60 years, respectively. The childhood variant has an age onset of 4.5 years (84). A significant association between the HLA locus and LABD has been reported. In particular, the haplotypes B8, DR3 and DQ2 increase the likelihood of an early onset and are thus commonly seen in the chronic bullous disease of childhood (CBDC) variant. In both children and adults alike, the tumor necrosis factor-2 (*TNF-2*) serves as an indicator of the increased duration of the disorder, whereas *TNF-1* indicates a reduced duration and an overall better prognosis (85).

1.2.6. Mucous Membrane Pemphigoid

Mucous membrane pemphigoid (MMP) is a pemphigoid disease which predominantly affects the mucous membranes. It is also known as cicatricial pemphigoid and has an incidence of 0.5–2 new cases per million/year. In contrast to other pemphigoid diseases, a common characteristic of MMP is scarring, which may cause functional limitations of the affected tissue and adds to the severity of the disease. The age of onset varies between 60–65 years of age (71–73). The target antigens are hemidesmosome proteins, such as BP180, BP230, laminin 332, $\alpha 6$, $\beta 4$ integrin, and collagen VII (63, 73).

2. OMICS APPROACHES TO AIBD DIAGNOSIS AND DISEASE ETIOLOGY

Clinical diagnosis of AIBD relies on the combination of clinical representation, i.e., mapping of a patients' symptoms to the aforementioned phenotypic characteristics and detection of tissue-bound auto-antibodies through direct immunofluorescence (DIF) microscopy as the *de facto* standard. Although a robust and successful approach, DIF microscopy requires cryosections of perilesional biopsies and only offers limited information about the target antigen. Circulating autoantibodies can be detected via indirect immunofluorescence

TABLE 2 | Available AIBD microarray or next generation sequencing datasets covering more than the known marker genes.

	Microarray RNA-seq	WES WGS	Microbiome	NGS Amplicon (IgVH Repertoire)	GWAS
	Pemphigus				
PV	–	–	–	(90–93)	(94–97)
PF	(98)	–	–	(91, 92)	(94, 96, 100)
PH	–	–	–	–	–
PNP	–	–	–	–	–
AP	–	–	–	–	–
PE	–	–	–	(101)	–
	Pemphigoid				
BP	–	–	(102)	–	–
PG	–	–	–	–	–
EBA	–	(99)	–	–	–
ALP	–	–	–	–	–
LABD	–	–	–	–	–
MMP	(103)	–	–	–	–

Citations refer to published sets of data. PV, Pemphigus Vulgaris; PF, Pemphigus Foliaceus; PH, Pemphigus Herpetiformis; PNP, Paraneoplastic Pemphigus; AP, IgA Pemphigus; PE, Pemphigus Erythematosus; BP, Bullous Pemphigoid; PG, Pemphigoid Gestationis; EBA, Epidermolysis Bullosa Acquisita; ALP, Anti-Laminin γ1\p200 Pemphigoid; LABD, Linear IgA-Dermatosis; MMP, Mucus Membrane Pemphigoid; WES, Whole Exome Sequencing; WGS, Whole Genome Sequencing; NGS, Next Generation Sequencing; IgVH, Immunoglobulin Variable Region Heavy Chain; GWAS, Genome wide Association Study.

(IIF) microscopy, incubating tissue substrates, e.g., monkey, rabbit or human esophagus with patient serum. Procedures that offer specific information about the autoantigen are, for example, enzyme-linked immunosorbent assays (ELISA), IIF microscopy assays, and immunoblotting/-precipitation (40).

Individual molecules and genetic associations have been unraveled in the context of AIBD pathogenesis. However, AIBDs are complex diseases, with many associations and factors contributing to their etiology (cf. **Table 1**). As such they should be investigated in light of a systems medicine approach on different, feedback-entangled regulatory layers such as the genome, transcriptome, epigenome, proteome, or microbiome (86–88).

However, despite recent developments in next generation sequencing and OMICS technologies, AIBDs are only now becoming the focus of genetic and high-throughput data studies, and are reviewed below.

2.1. OMICS Studies of AIBD

Beyond the directly affected genes and proteins listed in **Table 1**, there are few additional studies addressing unbiased, exploratory approaches to AIBD. We searched for AIBD OMICS datasets using Gene Expression Omnibus (GEO), European Nucleotide Archive (ENA), and the NCBI databases. Additionally, we searched for microbiome studies because of growing evidence on the microbiome-immune system crosstalk (89). All identified datasets are shown in **Table 2**.

Two whole transcriptome studies are currently publicly available. In both studies, microarrays were used to quantify transcriptome differences between patients with AIBD and the controls. Malheiros et al. (98) compared gene expression in isolated CD4+ T cells from 15 PF patients to five controls (Gene Expression Omnibus ID GSE53873). A patient subgroup comparison revealed few (up to 135) differentially regulated genes related to lymphocytes, apoptosis, proliferation and antigen presentation, which may however, be due to the small cohort size and inter-patient heterogeneity. A second, unpublished study quantified gene expression profiles in 12 patients with ocular MMP and 12 controls (Gene Expression Omnibus ID GSE77361).

More recently, the immune repertoire of PV, PF, and PE patients was classified using high-throughput sequencing methods. Two studies investigated four PV patients each (90–93). Additionally, two PF patients were investigated in (91). A third dataset is available that classifies the immune repertoire of two patients with pemphigus, without providing any further details [NCBI Bioproject ID (101)].

During the last decade, genome-wide association studies (GWAS) have become a popular approach to find genetic alterations, and so-called single nucleotide polymorphisms (SNPs) linked to diseases. Such studies compare the genotypes, i.e., a selected set of about 1-2 million SNPs, of large population cohorts in search of point mutations that significantly differ in the trait of interest. So far there are about 6,000 association studies that found more than 70,000 variant-trait associations (104). Further, association studies with gene expression as the trait (eQTL studies) (105) or methylation as the trait (meQTL) have been conducted (106). More recently, GWAS data have also been used for the computation of polygenic risk scores (107). Interestingly, the number of risk loci detected by GWAS studies scales linearly with the cohort size with no sign of saturation (108). Extrapolating on this circumstance, it is most likely that the whole genome of a person contributes to the individual disease risk. In fact, recent perspectives deny the existence of a few core genes that are causing adult-onset of disease. Instead, they argue for polygenicity or an "omnigenic" gene model, in which all mutations contribute with small effect sizes (109, 110). This is due to the robustness of biological systems, which can buffer many deleterious effects such as mutations through multiple back-up mechanisms, redundancy or feedback (111–113).

A number of GWAS for PV and PF were published recently for the Jewish (97) and Han Chinese population (94–96). Besides associations within the HLA locus, all studies found one or multiple significantly associated non-HLA SNPs, however, the associated genes differed between the studies. Another study found long non-coding RNA (lncRNA) polymorphisms associated with PF (100) using SNP data from 229 cases.

Besides the availability of just a small number of datasets for AIBDs, all studies were performed on a rather limited number of cases. Even the number of patients in the GWAS publications is low (between 100 and 365) compared to genome-wide association studies performed in other autoimmune disorders in which tens of thousands of patients were investigated [for review see e.g., (114)]. The small sample sizes lead to a small number of associated variants and genes identified by the use of GWAS.

2.2. Novel Approaches and Technologies in AIBD Research

Recent advances in mass spectrometry technology allows the unbiased quantification of protein abundance in an unprecedented way (115). Alongside proteomics, the field of degradomics has been established, which identifies proteases together with their cleaved substrates, or "degradomes" *in vivo* (116–118). Granzyme serine proteases in particular play important roles in the context of tissue injury and repair (119, 120). Granzyme B (GzmB) is involved in both intracellular and extracellular processes in immune cell-mediated apoptosis and extracellular proteolysis, respectively, which suggests a proteolytic role of GzmB in the pathogenesis of AIBD including BP (121). GzmB accumulated in the DEJ and blister fluid of AIBD, where it cleaved key anchoring proteins in a murine model of EBA. In line with this, GzmB deficiency reduced blistering (121).

A recent field of investigation is concerned with the organisms living in a state of symbiosis on and inside the human body. Only about 43% of cells in the human body are human, while the remaining 57% are comprised of bacterial (microbiome), fungal (mycobiome) and viral (virome) communities (122). Indeed, the total number of genes of the microbiome is ten times larger compared to the roughly 22,000 human genes. Physiological structures have adapted to the interplay between resident communities and the host, e.g., the vagus nerve represents an interface between the gut-microbiome and brain (123). The gut microbiome exists synergistically with its host to shape both metabolism and immunity. Details of this inter-dependency are still largely unknown, and it is unclear whether dysbiosis is an inducing factor leading to the exacerbation of symptoms or an epiphenomenon (124). There is also little understanding of the relationship between the skin microbiome and host defense. The communities populating the stratum corneum contribute to the first defensive line against outside influences. Furthermore, a connection between host genetics and microbial composition has been shown (125).

So far, one study investigated the role of the skin microbiota and BP with a rather limited number of patients and controls [12 per group; (102)], using a variety of skin locations (five different sampling sites). Despite the small sample size and the large heterogeneity of the skin microbiome, a significantly shifted microbiome at perilesional sites was identified.

Apart from detrimental environmental influences or lifestyle choices, e.g., injuries, pathogens and drug use, it is reasonable to assume that the respective diet has an impact. In their work Fedeles et al. (126) summarized research on the influence that dietary factors exert on bullous skin disorders. Both detrimental and advantageous effects of nutritional contents are presented, i.e., associations to exacerbation or even triggering of symptoms are drawn and protective effects are pointed out as well. This linkage is of particular interest with regards to the human microbiome.

A comparable line of investigation is the effect of the mitochondria on cellular processes. As the main source of cellular energy, mitochondria are essential constituents in signaling processes, cellular metabolism as well as inflammatory responses. It has been reported that changes in the mitochondrial genome can lead to pathological conditions and are implicated in various immune diseases. In particular, the mitochondrially encoded *MT-ATP8* gene has been linked to BP susceptibility (127).

Single-cell RNA-sequencing (scRNA-seq) is another recent technology that will have a major impact on elucidating the molecular processes in AIBD. The technology allows the characterization of individual cells, leading to the discovery of new cell types and cellular states that echo the underlying heterogeneity and plasticity of the immune system. scRNA-seq opens up new possibilities to analyze the immune repertoire and its effects on immune cells while in parallel recording both the quantitative gene expression and the repertoire sequence information for both chains (α/β, light/heavy) of the receptor. This additional feature would identify subpopulations of immune cells, that drive the disease to paracrine stimulation or recruitment of further immune cells. Although recent progress in scRNA-sequencing has been achieved, there are currently only a few studies that have investigated the human epidermis. To date, there is still no approach for BP, only for psoriasis, where Cheng et al. (128) analyzed the scRNA-seq profiles of 92,889 human epidermal cells from nine normal and three inflamed skin samples. The analysis of transcriptome levels of keratinocyte subpopulations reflects classical epidermal layers, but also strongly segmented epithelial functions such as cell-cell communication, inflammation, and WNT pathway modulation. The identification of molecular fingerprints of inflammatory skin states, including the enrichment of the CD1C+CD301A+ myeloid dendritic cell population in psoriatic epidermis, provides a critical step toward elucidating epidermal diseases of development, differentiation and inflammation.

2.3. A Computational Approach to AIBD

Since the number of available genetic and/or OMICS datasets is limited and hitherto provides narrow insights into the disease etiology, one can ask whether it is possible to derive phenotype-specific pathways from given gene-sets, i.e., disease specific transcriptome patterns that allow patient stratification and also provide insight about the molecular processes involved. The exploratory approach of choice was a network diffusion in order to determine the impact of each gene-set on its biological neighborhood (129). It was followed by Gene Set Variation Analysis (GSVA) (130), which enables the assignment of sample-wise pathway enrichments on the basis of the calculated diffusion scores.

The inferred pathways do, however, not enable a clear separation of either phenotypes or clinical subclasses. It can be argued that the number of known associated genes is too small for an accurate inference of protein-protein interactions and related pathways, without a significant amount of noise. A closer investigation is warranted merely on account of the heterogeneity of phenotypes and the presumed multifactorial framework of disease genesis.

3. SUMMARY AND OUTLOOK

Autoimmune skin blistering diseases (AIBDs) are complex diseases, mostly with a late onset in life. They are driven by both genetic and environmental factors. So far, most of the research on AIBDs has been conducted on clinical and diagnostic aspects of the diseases. In AIBDs, autoreactive antibodies are generated that target proteins involved in cell-to-cell and cell-to-matrix adhesion in the epidermis/epithelium and at the dermal-epidermal junction. Binding of those autoantibodies leads to inflammation and the loss of function of those proteins. Depending on the autoantigen, AIBDs can be divided into pemphigus and pemphigoid diseases. However, knowledge on detailed disease mechanisms leading to the development of AIBDs is still scarce.

The limited availability of OMICS data-sets in AIBDs (cf. **Table 2**) illustrates the long road ahead in elucidating the causes of AIBDs. Limiting factors include low prevalence and high age of onset. Those factors hinder the acquisition of sufficient suitable test-subjects and also limit perceived importance of this topic, hence lowering the impact of scientific research in this field.

In recent years, significant efforts have been made to remedy the problem of cohort size by establishing programs that advance regional, national, and international cooperation between medical facilities and research institutions. European Reference Networks (ERN) for instance are part of the Directive on Patient Rights in Cross-Border Healthcare of 2011. They are oriented toward the handling of rare disorders through the interconnection of specialists and resources. An example, with regards to AIBDs, is the "Dimethyl fumarate for the treatment of bullous pemphigoid" (DPem) research network that connects study groups from four European countries. This particular initiative is funded by the ERA-Net for Research Programmes on Rare Diseases, an initiative with the expressed purpose of facilitating cooperative research into rare disorders (131, 132). Observance of incidence and distribution of AIBDs is the objective of the Regibul Register (133).

One way to make the best use of the limited patient data is to use theoretical concepts and test the idea of core vs. peripheral genes. Initial genome-wide association studies on bullous pemphigoid have predicted HLA genes as risk factors. These genes are common to autoimmune diseases but not specific to AIBDs and might be considered as core gene candidates. Alternatively, core genes might be those that are strongly linked to the disease phenotype. Therefore, one might expect immune system and cell adhesion related genes to be critical to AIBD. In addition to identifying core genes it will be important to find tissue specific regulatory networks that mediate the effect of the core genes to the phenotype. To study these networks, it might be important to develop further *in vitro* and *in vivo* models, be it active or passive mouse models or organotypic skin models. The latter might be generated from fibroblasts and keratinocytes of AIBD patients or derived from induced pluripotent stem cells, thereby harboring a disease genome. A third approach to better understand disease etiology is the integration of environmental factors through microbiome studies. The effect of microbiome-immune cell interaction is well established but has never been studied in detail in AIBDs. First studies indicate a dysbiosis of the skin microbiome in lesional skin, a mechanistic link to increased immune reaction or decreased barrier function of the skin which still needs to be established.

In summary, an integrated OMICS approach to study skin blistering diseases, comprising genomics, transcriptomics, and proteomics together with the microbiome and novel methods such as single cell RNAseq, is highly warranted. Research in this direction has only recently begun and much work and opportunities still remain. Besides increasing the numbers for further GWAS, we advocate for high-throughput deep phenotyping and whole genome sequencing and investigation of tissue specific gene expression to characterize cellular properties associated with disease-associated genomes. Further, the use of disease models may elucidate the polygenic complexity of the diseases.

AUTHOR CONTRIBUTIONS

All authors reviewed the literature and collected the data, contributed to the manuscript, read, and approved it.

ACKNOWLEDGMENTS

The authors gratefully acknowledge the support and advice by colleagues of the Institute of Dermatology and the Institute for Experimental Dermatology, Lübeck. Furthermore, the authors acknowledge computational support from the OMICS compute cluster at the University of Lübeck. We acknowledge financial support by Land Schleswig-Holstein within the funding programme Open Access Publikationsfonds.

REFERENCES

1. Jordon RE, Beutner EH, Witebsky E, Blumental G, Hale WL, Lever WF. Basement zone antibodies in bullous pemphigoid. *JAMA.* (1967) 200:751–6.
2. Schmidt E, Zillikens D. Pemphigoid diseases. *Lancet.* (2013) 381:320–32.
3. Sequencing Consortium TM. Complete sequence and gene map of a human major histocompatibility complex. *Nature.* (1999) 401:921–23. doi: 10.1038/44853
4. Gough SCL, Simmonds MJ. The HLA region and autoimmune disease: associations and mechanisms of action. *Curr Genom.* (2007) 8:453–65. doi: 10.2174/138920207783591690

5. Whitacre CC. Sex differences in autoimmune disease. *Nat Immunol.* (2001) 2:777 EP. doi: 10.1038/ni0901-777
6. Markle JG, Fish EN. SeXX matters in immunity. *Trends Immunol.* (2014) 35:97–104. doi: 10.1016/j.it.2013.10.006
7. Whitacre CC, Reingold SC, O'Looney PA, Blankenhorn E, Brinley F, Collier E, et al. A gender gap in autoimmunity. *Science.* (1999) 283:1277. doi: 10.1126/science.283.5406.1277
8. Eidinger D, Garrett TJ. Studies of the regulatory effects of the sex hormones on antibody formation and stem cell differentiation. *J Exp Med.* (1972) 136:1098. doi: 10.1084/jem.136.5.1098
9. Weinstein Y, Ran S, Segal S. Sex-associated differences in the regulation of immune responses controlled by the MHC of the mouse. *J Immunol.* (1984) 132:656.
10. Amadori A, Zamarchi R, De Silvestro G, Forza G, Cavatton G, Danieli GA, et al. Genetic control of the CD4/CD8 T-cell ratio in humans. *Nat Med.* (1995) 1:1279–83. doi: 10.1038/nm1295-1279
11. Griffin AC, Whitacre CC. Sex and strain differences in the circadian rhythm fluctuation of endocrine and immune function in the rat: implications for rodent models of autoimmune disease. *J Neuroimmunol.* (1991) 35:53–64. doi: 10.1016/0165-5728(91)90161-Y
12. Schmidt E, Zillikens D. Diagnostik und Therapie bull∧ser Autoimmundermatosen. *Dtsch Arztebl Int.* (2011) 108:399–405.
13. Vodo D, Sarig O, Sprecher E. The genetics of pemphigus vulgaris. *Front Med.* (2018) 5:226. doi: 10.3389/fmed.2018.00226
14. Buonavoglia A, Leone P, Dammacco R, Di Lernia G, Petruzzi M, Bonamonte D, et al. Pemphigus and mucous membrane pemphigoid: an update from diagnosis to therapy. *Autoimmun Rev.* (2019) 18:349–58. doi: 10.1016/j.autrev.2019.02.005
15. Miyagawa S, Amagai M, Iida T, Yamamoto Y, Nishikawa T, Shirai T. Late development of antidesmoglein 1 antibodies in pemphigus vulgaris: correlation with disease progression. *Brit J Dermatol.* (2001) 141:1084–7. doi: 10.1046/j.1365-2133.1999.03209.x
16. Espe S. MalaCards: the human disease database. *J Med Library Assoc.* (2018) 1:106. doi: 10.5195/JMLA.2018.253
17. Borroni G, Biagi F, Ciocca O, Vassallo C, Carugno A, Cananzi R, et al. IgA anti–epidermal transglutaminase autoantibodies: a sensible and sensitive marker for diagnosis of dermatitis herpetiformis in adult patients. *J Eur Acad Dermatol Venereol.* (2012) 27:836–41. doi: 10.1111/j.1468-3083.2012.04586.x
18. Sárdy M, Kárpáti S, Merkl B, Paulsson M, Smyth N. Epidermal transglutaminase (TGase 3) is the autoantigen of dermatitis herpetiformis. *J Exp Med.* (2002) 195:747–57. doi: 10.1084/jem.20011299
19. Mehta V, Balachandran C, Nayak S. Herpetiform pemphigus clinically resembling bullous pemphigoid. *Ind J Dermatol.* (2008) 53:158–9. doi: 10.4103/0019-5154.43218
20. Porro AM, Caetano LV, Maehara LS, Enokihara MM. Non-classical forms of pemphigus: pemphigus herpetiformis, IgA pemphigus, paraneoplastic pemphigus and IgG/IgA pemphigus. *Anais Brasileiros de Dermatologia.* (2014) 89:96–106. doi: 10.1590/abd1806-4841.20142459
21. Wieczorek M, Czernik A. Paraneoplastic pemphigus: a short review. *Clin Cosmet Investigat Dermatol.* (2016) 9:291–5. doi: 10.2147/CCID.S100802
22. Aslanova M, Zito PM. *IgA Pemphigus.* NCBI Bookshelf. (2019). Available online at: https://www.ncbi.nlm.nih.gov/books/NBK519063/
23. Pérez-Pérez ME, Avalos-Dìaz E, Herrera-Esparza R. Autoantibodies in senear-usher syndrome: cross-reactivity or multiple autoimmunity? *Autoimmune Dis.* (2012) 2012:7. doi: 10.1155/2012/296214
24. Liu Y, Li L, Xia Y. BP180 is critical in the autoimmunity of bullous pemphigoid. *Front Immunol.* (2017) 8:1752. doi: 10.3389/fimmu.2017.01752
25. Fang H, Zhang Y, Li L, Wang G, Liu Z. The autoimmune skin disease bullous pemphigoid: the role of mast cells in autoantibody-induced tissue injury. *Front Immunol.* (2018) 9:407. doi: 10.3389/fimmu.2018.00407
26. Iranzo P, López-Lerma I, Teresa Robles M. Bullous pemphigoid associated with mantle cell lymphoma. *Arch Dermatol.* (2005) 140:1496–9. doi: 10.1001/archderm.140.12.1496
27. Baigrie D, Nookala V. *Bullous Pemphigoid* (2018). Available online at: https://www.ncbi.nlm.nih.gov/books/NBK535374/
28. Sävervall C, Thomsen SF. Pemphigoid gestationis: current perspectives. *Clin Cosmet Investigat Dermatol.* (2017) 10:441–9. doi: 10.2147/CCID.S128144
29. Iwata H, Vorobyev A, Koga H, Ludwig RJ, Zillikens D, Prost-Squarcioni C, et al. Meta-analysis of the clinical and immunopathological characteristics and treatment outcomes in epidermolysis bullosa acquisita patients. *Orphanet J Rare Dis.* (2018) 13:153–62. doi: 10.1186/s13023-018-0896-1
30. Shaffer BR. Epidermolysis bullosa acquisita in association with mantle cell lymphoma. *Cutis.* (2018) 101:E13–5.
31. Koga H, Prost-Squacioni C, Iwata H, Jonkman MF, Ludwig RJ, Bieber K. Epidermolysis bullosa acquisita: the 2019 update. *Front Med.* (2019) 5:362. doi: 10.3389/fmed.2018.00362
32. Koga H, Kasprick A, López R, Aulí M, Pont M, Godessart N. Therapeutic effect of a novel phosphatidylinositol-3-kinase δ inhibitor in experimental epidermolysis bullosa acquisita. *Front Immunol.* (2018) 9:1558. doi: 10.3389/fimmu.2018.01558
33. Woodley DT, Chen M, Kim G. *Epidermolysis Bullosa Acquisita.* UpToDate Inc. (2019). Available online at: https://www.uptodate.com/contents/epidermolysis-bullosa-acquisita#H306466519
34. Dainichi T, Kurono S, Zillikens D. Anti-laminin gamma-1 pemphigoid. In: Hakomori S, editor. *Proceedings of the National Academy of Sciences of the United States of America.* Fukuoka: US National Library of Medicine National Institutes of Health (2009). p. 2800–5.
35. Zumelzu C, Alexandre M, Le Roux C, Weber P, Guyot A, Levy A, et al. Mucous membrane pemphigoid, bullous pemphigoid, and anti-programmed death-1/ programmed death-ligand 1: a case report of an elderly woman with mucous membrane pemphigoid developing after pembrolizumab therapy for metastatic melanoma and review of the literature. *Front Med.* (2018) 5:268. doi: 10.3389/fmed.2018.00268
36. Meyer N, Misery L. Geoepidemiologic considerations of auto-immune pemphigus. *Autoimmun Rev.* (2010) 9:A379–A382. doi: 10.1016/j.autrev.2009.10.009
37. Gazit E, Loewenthal R. The immunogenetics of pemphigus vulgaris. *Autoimmun Rev.* (2005) 4:16–20. doi: 10.1016/j.autrev.2004.05.002
38. Aoki V, Millikan RC, Rivitti EA, Hans-Filho G, Eaton DP, Warren SJP, et al. Environmental risk factors in endemic pemphigus foliaceus (fogo selvagem). *J Investigat Dermatol Symp Proc.* (2004) 9:34–40. doi: 10.1111/j.1087-0024.2004.00833.x
39. Shirakata Y, Amagai M, Hanakawa Y, Nishikawa T, Hashimoto K. Lack of mucosal involvement in pemphigus foliaceus may be due to low expression of desmoglein 1. *J Investigat Dermatol.* (1998) 110:76–8. doi: 10.1046/j.1523-1747.1998.00085.x
40. Witte M, Zillikens D. Diagnosis of autoimmune blistering diseases. *Front Med.* (2018) **5**:296. doi: 10.3389/fmed.2018.00296
41. Mimouni D, Bar H, Gdalevich M, Katzenelson V, David M. Pemphigus—analysis of epidemiological factors in 155 patients. *J Eur Acad Dermatol Venereol.* (2008) **22**:1232–5. doi: 10.1111/j.1468-3083.2008.02786.x
42. McPherson T, Venning VV. Management of autoimmune blistering diseases in pregnancy. *Dermatol Clin.* (2011) 29:585–90. doi: 10.1016/j.det.2011.06.008
43. Svecova D, Parnicka Z, Pastyrikova L, Urbancek S, Luha J, Buc M. HLA DRB1* and DQB1* alleles are associated with disease severity in patients with pemphigus vulgaris. *Int J Dermatol.* (2015) 54:168–73. doi: 10.1111/ijd.12418
44. Ahmed AR, Yunis EJ, Khatri K, Wagner R, Notani G, Awdeh Z, et al. Major histocompatibility complex haplotype studies in Ashkenazi Jewish patients with pemphigus vulgaris. *Proc Natl Acad Sci USA.* (1990) 87:7658–62. doi: 10.1073/pnas.87.19.7658
45. Gazit E, Slomov Y, Goldberg I, Brenner S, Loewenthal R. HLA-G is associated with pemphigus vulgaris in jewish patients. *Hum Immunol.* (2004) 65:39–46. doi: 10.1016/j.humimm.2003.09.019
46. Delgado JC, Turbay D, Yunis EJ, Yunis JJ, Morton ED, Bhol K, et al. A common major histocompatibility complex class II allele HLA-DQB1* 0301 is present in clinical variants of pemphigoid. *Proc Natl Acad Sci USA.* (1996) 93:8569–71. doi: 10.1073/pnas.93.16.8569
47. Loiseau P, Lecleach L, Prost C, Lepage V, Busson M, Bastuji-Garin S, et al. HLA class II polymorphism contributes to specify desmoglein derived peptides in pemphigus vulgaris and pemphigus foliaceus. *J Autoimmun.* (2000) 15:67–73. doi: 10.1006/jaut.2000.0388

48. Scharf SJ, Friedmann A, Brautbar C, Szafer F, Steinman L, Horn G, et al. HLA class II allelic variation and susceptibility to pemphigus vulgaris. *Proc Natl Acad Sci USA.* (1988) 85:3504–8. doi: 10.1073/pnas.85.10.3504
49. Cirillo N, Al-Jandan BA. Desmosomal adhesion and pemphigus vulgaris: the first half of the story. *Cell Commun Adhesion.* (2013) 20:1–10. doi: 10.3109/15419061.2013.763799
50. Culton DA, Qian Y, Li N, Rubenstein D, Aoki V, Filhio GH, et al. Advances in pemphigus and its endemic pemphigus foliaceus (Fogo Selvagem) phenotype: a paradigm of human autoimmunity. *J Autoimmun.* (2008) 31:311–24. doi: 10.1016/j.jaut.2008.08.003
51. Bastuji-Garin S, Souissi R, Blum L, Turki H, Nouira R, Jomaa B, et al. Comparative epidemiology of pemphigus in tunisia and France: unusual incidence of pemphigus foliaceus in young tunisian women. *J Investigat Dermatol.* (1995) 104:302–5. doi: 10.1111/1523-1747.ep12612836
52. Kridin K. Pemphigus group: overview, epidemiology, mortality, and comorbidities. *Immunol Res.* (2018) 66:255–70. doi: 10.1007/s12026-018-8986-7
53. Martel P, Gilbert D, Busson M, Loiseau P, Lepage V, Drouot L, et al. Epistasis between DSG1 and HLA class II genes in pemphigus foliaceus. *Genes Immun.* (2002) 3:205–10. doi: 10.1038/sj.gene.6363839
54. Kasperkiewicz M, Kowalewski C, Jabłońska S. Pemphigus herpetiformis: From first description until now. *J Am Acad Dermatol.* (2014) 70:780–7. doi: 10.1016/j.jaad.2013.11.043
55. Kozlowska A, Hashimoto T, Jarzabek-Chorzelska M, Amagai A, Nagata Y, Strasz Z, et al. Pemphigus herpetiformis with IgA and IgG antibodies to desmoglein 1 and IgG antibodies to desmocollin 3. *J Am Acad Dermatol.* (2003) 48:117–22. doi: 10.1067/mjd.2003.23
56. Ishii N, Teye K, Fukuda S, Uehara R, Hachiya T, Koga H, et al. Anti-desmocollin autoantibodies in nonclassical pemphigus. *Brit J Dermatol.* (2015) 173:59–68. doi: 10.1111/bjd.13711
57. Schepens I, Jaunin F, Begre N, Läderach U, Marcus K, Hashimoto T, et al. The protease inhibitor alpha-2-macroglobuline-like-1 is the p170 antigen recognized by paraneoplastic pemphigus autoantibodies in human. *PLoS ONE.* (2010) 5:e12250. doi: 10.1371/journal.pone.0012250
58. Kridin K, Zelber-Sagi S, Comaneshter D, Cohen AD. Coexistent solid malignancies in pemphigus: a population-based study. *JAMA Dermatol.* (2018) 154:435–40. doi: 10.1001/jamadermatol.2017.6334
59. Tajima M, Mitsuhashi Y, Irisawa R, Amagai M, Hashimoto T, Tsuboi R. IgA pemphigus reacting exclusively to desmoglein 3. *Eur J Dermatol.* (2011) 20:626–9. doi: 10.1684/ejd.2010.1021
60. Kárpáti S, Amagai M, Liu WL, Dmochowski M, Hashimoto T, Horváth A. Identification of desmoglein 1 as autoantigen in a patient with intraepidermal neutrophilic IgA dermatosis type of IgA pemphigus. *Exp Dermatol.* (2000) 9:224–8. doi: 10.1034/j.1600-0625.2000.00900 3224.x
61. Sánchez-Pérez J, Garcìa-Dìez A. Pemphigus. *Actas Dermo-Sifiliograficas.* (2005) 96:329–56. doi: 10.1016/S0001-7310(05)73090-8
62. Jordon RE, Beutner EH, Witebsky E, Blumental G, Hale WL, Lever WF. Basement zone antibodies in bullous pemphigoid. *JAMA.* (1967) 200:751–6. doi: 10.1001/jama.200.9.751
63. Di Zenzo G, della Torre R, Zambruno G, Borradori L. Bullous pemphigoid: from the clinic to the bench. *Clin Dermatol.* (2012) 30:3–16. doi: 10.1016/j.clindermatol.2011.03.005
64. Nishie W. Update on the pathogenesis of bullous pemphigoid: an autoantibody-mediated blistering disease targeting collagen XVII. *J Dermatol Sci.* (2014) 73:179–86. doi: 10.1016/j.jdermsci.2013.12.001
65. Horváth B, Niedermeier A, Podstawa E, Müller R, Hunzelmann N, Kárpáti S, et al. IgA autoantibodies in the pemphigoids and linear IgA bullous dermatosis. *Exp Dermatol.* (2010) 19:648–53. doi: 10.1111/j.1600-0625.2010.01080.x
66. Wojnarowska F, Venning VA. Immunobullous diseases. In: *Rook's Textbook of Dermatology*, 7th ed. Blackwell Science. (2004). p. 1–41. Available online at: https://doi.org/10.1002/9780470750520.ch41
67. Zakka LR, Reche P, Ahmed AR. Role of MHC Class II genes in the pathogenesis of pemphigoid. *Autoimmun Rev.* (2011) 11:40–7. doi: 10.1016/j.autrev.2011.07.002
68. Büdinger L, Borradori L, Yee C, Eming R, Ferencik S, Grosse-Wilde H, et al. Identification and characterization of autoreactive T cell responses to bullous pemphigoid antigen 2 in patients and healthy controls. *J Clin Investigat.* (1998) 102:2082–9. doi: 10.1172/JCI3335
69. Büdinger L, Borradori L, Yee C, Eming R, Ferencik S, Grosse-Wilde H, et al. T cell control in autoimmune bullous skin disorders. *J Clin Investigat.* (2006) 116:1159–66. doi: 10.1172/JCI28547
70. Lin M, Diaz LA, Fu C, Giudice GJ, Olague-Marchan M, Lazaro AM, et al. Epitopes targeted by bullous pemphigoid T lymphocytes and autoantibodies map to the same sites on the bullous pemphigoid 180 ectodomain. *J Investigat Dermatol.* (2000) **115**:955–61. doi: 10.1046/j.1523-1747.2000.00153.x
71. Bertram F, Bröcker E, Zillikens D, Schmidt E. Prospective analysis of the incidence of autoimmune bullous disorders in Lower Franconia, Germany. *J Deutschen Dermatologischen Gesellschaft.* (2009) 7:434–9. doi: 10.1111/j.1610-0387.2008.06976.x
72. Joly P, Baricault S, Sparsa A, Bernard P, Bédane C, Duvert-Lehembre S, et al. Incidence and mortality of bullous pemphigoid in France. *J Investigat Dermatol.* (2012) 132:1998–2004. doi: 10.1038/jid.2012.35
73. Schmidt E, Zillikens D. Pemphigoid diseases. *Lancet.* (2013) 381:320–32. doi: 10.1016/S0140-6736(12)61140-4
74. Cobo MF, Santi CG, Maruta CW, Aoki V. Pemphigoid gestationis: clinical and laboratory evaluation. *Clinics (São Paulo, Brazil).* (1999) 64:1043–7. doi: 10.1590/S1807-59322009001100002
75. Jenkins RE, Hern S, Black MM. Clinical features and management of 87 patients with pemphigoid gestationis. *Clin Exp Dermatol.* (2009) 24:255–9. doi: 10.1046/j.1365-2230.1999.00472.x
76. Vorobyev A, Ludwig RJ, Schmidt E. Clinical features and diagnosis of epidermolysis bullosa acquisita. *Exp Rev Clin Immunol.* (2017) 13:157–69. doi: 10.1080/1744666X.2016.1221343
77. Dilling A, Rose C, Hashimoto T, Zillikens D, Shimanovich I. Anti-p200 pemphigoid: a novel autoimmune subepidermal blistering disease. *J Dermatol.* (2007) 34:1–8. doi: 10.1111/j.1346-8138.2007.00208.x
78. Wozniak K, Hashimoto T, Fukuda S, Ohyama B, Ishii N, Koga H, et al. IgA Anti-p200 pemphigoid. *JAMA Dermatol.* (2011) 147:1306–10. doi: 10.1001/archdermatol.2011.303
79. Goletz S, Hashimoto T, Zillikens D, Schmidt E. Anti-p200 pemphigoid. J Am Acad Dermatol. (2014) 71:185–91. doi: 10.1016/j.jaad.2014. 02.036
80. Wojnarowska F, Whitehead P, Leigh IM, Bhogal BS, Black MM. Identification of the target antigen in chronic bullous disease of childhood and linear IgA disease of adults. *Brit J Dermatol.* (1991) 124:157–62. doi: 10.1111/j.1365-2133.1991.tb00425.x
81. Marinkovich MP, Taylor TB, Keene DR, Burgeson RE, Zone JJ. LAD-1, the linear IgA bullous dermatosis autoantigen, is a novel 120-kDa anchoring filament protein synthesized by epidermal cells. *J Investigat Dermatol.* (1996) 106:734–8. doi: 10.1111/1523-1747.ep12345782
82. Zone JJ, Taylor TB, Meyer LJ, Petersen MJ. The 97kDa linear IgA bullous disease antigen is identical to a portion of the extracellular domain of the 180kDa bullous pemphigoid antigen, BPAg2. *J Investigat Dermatol.* (1998) 110:207–10. doi: 10.1046/j.1523-1747.1998.00129.x
83. Zillikens D, Herzele K, Georgi M, Schmidt E, Chimanovitch I, Bröcker E, et al. Autoantibodies in a subgroup of patients with linear IgA disease react with the NC16A domain of BP1801. *J Investigat Dermatol.* (1999) 113:947–53. doi: 10.1046/j.1523-1747.1999.00808.x
84. Chaudhari S, Mobini N. Linear IgA bullous dermatosis: a rare clinicopathologic entity with an unusual presentation. *J Clin Aesthet Dermatol.* (2015) 8:43–6.
85. Collier PM, Wojnarowska F, Welsh K, McGuire W, Black MM. Adult linear IgA disease and chronic bullous disease of childhood: the association with human lymphocyte antigens Cw7, B8, DR3 and tumour necrosis factor influences disease expression. *Brit J Dermatol.* (1999) 141:867–75. doi: 10.1046/j.1365-2133.1999.03110.x
86. Civelek M, Lusis AJ. Systems genetics approaches to understand complex traits. *Nat Rev Genet.* (2014) 15:34–48. doi: 10.1038/nrg3575
87. Yugi K, Kubota H, Hatano A, Kuroda S. Trans-omics: how to reconstruct biochemical networks across multiple 'omic' layers. *Trends Biotechnol.* (2016) 34:276–90. doi: 10.1016/j.tibtech.2015.12.013
88. Durmaz AA, Karaca E, Demkow U, Toruner G, Schoumans J, Cogulu O. Evolution of genetic techniques: past, present, and beyond. *BioMed Res Int.* (2015) 2015:461524–31. doi: 10.1155/2015/461524

89. De Luca F, Shoenfeld Y. The microbiome in autoimmune diseases. *Clin Exp Immunol.* (2019) 195:74–85. doi: 10.1111/cei.13158
90. University of Pennsylvania and University of Maryland Homo sapiens isolate: Human IgG isolate Targeted Locus (Loci). *Data-set: Characterization of Autoantibody Repertoires in Antibody-Mediated Diseases Is Necessary to Understand Pathophysiology and Therapeutic Approaches* (2016). Available online at: https://www.ncbi.nlm.nih.gov/bioproject/309663
91. Chen J, Zheng Q, Hammers CM, Ellebrecht CT, Mukherjee EM, Tang H, et al. Proteomic analysis of pemphigus autoantibodies indicates a larger, more diverse, and more dynamic repertoire than determined by B cell genetics. *Cell Rep.* (2017) 18:237–47. doi: 10.1016/j.celrep.2016.12.013
92. Mukherjee EM, Millar SE, Payne AS, Stanley JR. *Distinct Clonal Relationships Among Autoreactive IgG and IgA B-Cells in Pemphigus Vulgaris. Data-set: Lineage Analysis of Autoreactive B-Cells Can Reveal the Origins of Autoimmunity.* (2018). Available online at: https://www.ncbi.nlm.nih.gov/bioproject/?term=PRJNA437136
93. Ellebrecht CT, Mukherjee EM, Zheng Q, Choi EJ, Reddy SG, Mao X, et al. Autoreactive IgG and IgA B cells evolve through distinct subclass switch pathways in the autoimmune disease pemphigus vulgaris. *Cell Rep.* (2018) 24:2370–80. doi: 10.1016/j.celrep.2018.07.093
94. Sun Y, Liu H, Yang B, Wang C, Foo JN, Bao F, et al. Investigation of the predisposing factor of pemphigus and its clinical subtype through a genome-wide association and next generation sequence analysis. *J Eur Acad Dermatol Venereol.* (2019) 33:410–5. doi: 10.1111/jdv.15227
95. Gao J, Zhu C, Zhang Y, Sheng Y, Yang F, Wang W, et al. Association study and fine-mapping major histocompatibility complex analysis of pemphigus vulgaris in a han chinese population. *J Investigat Dermatol.* (2018) 138:2307–14. doi: 10.1016/j.jid.2018.05.011
96. Zhang SY, Zhou XY, Zhou XL, Zhang Y, Deng Y, Liao F, et al. Subtype-specific inherited predisposition to pemphigus in the Chinese population. *Brit J Dermatol.* (2019) 180:828–35. doi: 10.1111/bjd.17191
97. Sarig O, Bercovici S, Zoller L, Goldberg I, Indelman M, Nahum S, et al. Population-specific association between a polymorphic variant in ST18, encoding a pro-apoptotic molecule, and pemphigus vulgaris. *J Investigat Dermatol.* (2012) 132:1798–805. doi: 10.1038/jid.2012.46
98. Malheiros D, Panepucci RA, Roselino AM, Araújo AG, Zago MA, Petzl-Erler ML. Genome-wide gene expression profiling reveals unsuspected molecular alterations in pemphigus foliaceus. *Immunology.* (2014) 143:381–95. doi: 10.1111/imm.12315
99. Takeichi T, Liu L, Fong K, Ozoemena L, McMillan JR, Salam A, et al. Whole-exome sequencing improves mutation detection in a diagnostic epidermolysis bullosa laboratory. *Brit J Dermatol.* (2015) 172:94–100. doi: 10.1111/bjd.13190
100. Lobo-Alves SC, Augusto DG, Magalhães WCS, Tarazona-Santos E, Lima-Costa MF, Barreto ML, et al. Long non-coding RNA polymorphisms influence susceptibility to endemic pemphigus foliaceus. *Brit J Dermatol.* (2019) 181:324–31. doi: 10.1111/bjd.17640
101. University E. Homo Sapiens Targeted Locus (Loci). *Data-set: Accession: PRJNA260985; ID: 260985* (2014). Available online at: https://www.ncbi.nlm.nih.gov/bioproject/?term=PRJNA260985
102. Miodovnik M, Künstner A, Langan EA, Zillikens D, Gläser R, Sprecher E, et al. A distinct cutaneous microbiota profile in autoimmune bullous disease patients. *Exp Dermatol.* (2017) 11:839–7. doi: 10.1111/exd.13357
103. Ahadome S, Dart J. *Genome Wide Analysis of Gene Expression in Conjunctiva Whole Tissue and Primary Conjunctival Fibroblasts From Patients With Ocular Mucous Membrane Pemphigoid and Control Patients.* (2016). Available online at: https://www.ncbi.nlm.nih.gov/geo/query/acc.cgi?acc=GSE77361
104. Richardson TG, Harrison S, Hemani G, Davey-Smith G. An atlas of polygenic risk score associations to highlight putative causal relationships across the human phenome. *eLife.* (2019) 8:e43657. doi: 10.7554/eLife.43657
105. Gilad Y, Rifkin SA, Pritchard JK. Revealing the architecture of gene regulation: the promise of eQTL studies. *Trends Genet.* (2008) 24:408–15. doi: 10.1016/j.tig.2008.06.001
106. Smith AK, Kilaru V, Kocak M, Almli LM, Mercer KB, Ressler KJ, et al. Methylation quantitative trait loci (meQTLs) are consistently detected across ancestry, developmental stage, and tissue type. *BMC Genom.* (2014) 15:145. doi: 10.1186/1471-2164-15-145
107. Torkamani A, Wineinger NE, Topol EJ. The personal and clinical utility of polygenic risk scores. *Nat Rev Genet.* (2018) 19:581. doi: 10.1038/s41576-018-0018-x
108. Canela-Xandri O, Rawlik K, Tenesa A. An atlas of genetic associations in UK Biobank. *Nat Genet.* (2018) 50:1593–9. doi: 10.1038/s41588-018-0248-z
109. Wray NR, Wijmenga C, Sullivan PF, Yang J, Visscher PM. Common disease is more complex than implied by the core gene omnigenic model. *Cell.* (2018) 173:1573–80. doi: 10.1016/j.cell.2018.05.051
110. Boyle EA, Li YI, Pritchard JK. An expanded view of complex traits: from polygenic to omnigenic. *Cell.* (2017) 169:1177–86. doi: 10.1016/j.cell.2017.05.038
111. Kitano H. Cancer as a robust system: implications for anticancer therapy. *Nat Rev Cancer.* (2004) 4:227–35. doi: 10.1038/nrc1300
112. Masel J, Siegal ML. Robustness: mechanisms and consequences. *Trends Genet.* (2009) 25:395–403. doi: 10.1016/j.tig.2009.07.005
113. Wang X, Goldstein DB. Enhancer redundancy predicts gene pathogenicity and informs complex disease gene discovery. *bioRxiv 459123.* (2018). Available online at: https://www.biorxiv.org/content/10.1101/459123v1
114. Inshaw JRJ, Cutler AJ, Burren OS, Stefana MI, Todd JA. Approaches and advances in the genetic causes of autoimmune disease and their implications. *Nat Immunol.* (2018) 19:674–84. doi: 10.1038/s41590-018-0129-8
115. Aebersold R, Mann M. Mass-spectrometric exploration of proteome structure and function. *Nature.* (2016) 537:347–55. doi: 10.1038/nature19949
116. Savickas S, Auf dem Keller U. Targeted degradomics in protein terminomics and protease substrate discovery. *Biol Chem.* (2017) 399:47–54. doi: 10.1515/hsz-2017-0187
117. Klein T, Eckhard U, Dufour A, Solis N, Overall CM. Proteolytic cleavage-mechanisms, function, and "omic" approaches for a near-ubiquitous posttranslational modification. *Chem Rev.* (2018) 118:1137–68. doi: 10.1021/acs.chemrev.7b00120
118. López-Otín C, Overall CM. Protease degradomics: a new challenge for proteomics. *Nat Rev Mol Cell Biol.* (2002) 3:509–19. doi: 10.1038/nrm858
119. Granville DJ. Granzymes in disease: bench to bedside. *Cell Death Different.* (2010) 17:565–6. doi: 10.1038/cdd.2009.218
120. Turner CT, Lim D, Granville DJ. Granzyme B in skin inflammation and disease. *Matrix Biol.* (2019) 75–76:126–40. doi: 10.1016/j.matbio.2017.12.005
121. Russo V, Klein T, Lim DJ, Solis N, Machado Y, Hiroyasu S, et al. Granzyme B is elevated in autoimmune blistering diseases and cleaves key anchoring proteins of the dermal-epidermal junction. *Sci Rep.* (2018) 8:1–11. doi: 10.1038/s41598-018-28070-0
122. Sender R, Fuchs S, Milo R. Revised estimates for the number of human and bacteria cells in the body. *PLoS Biol.* (2016) 14:e1002533. doi: 10.1371/journal.pbio.1002533
123. Carabotti M, Scirocco A, Maselli MA, Severia C. The gut-brain axis: interactions between enteric microbiota, central and enteric nervous systems. *Ann Gastroenterol.* (2015) 28:203–9.
124. Li B, Selmi C, Tang R, Gershwin ME, Ma X. The microbiome and autoimmunity: a paradigm from the gut-liver axis. *Cell Mol Immunol.* (2018) 15:595–609. doi: 10.1038/cmi.2018.7
125. Ross AA, Müller KM, Weese JS, Neufeld JD. Comprehensive skin microbiome analysis reveals the uniqueness of human skin and evidence for phylosymbiosis within the class Mammalia. *Proc Natl Acad Sci USA.* (2018) 115:E5786–95. doi: 10.1073/pnas.1801302115
126. Fedeles F, Murphy M, Rothe MJ, Grant-Kels JM. Nutrition and bullous skin diseases. *Clin Dermatol.* (2010) 28:627–43. doi: 10.1016/j.clindermatol.2010.03.036
127. Hirose M, Schilf P, Benoit S, Eming R, Gläser R, Homey B, et al. Polymorphisms in the mitochondrially encoded ATP synthase 8 gene are associated with susceptibility to bullous pemphigoid in the German population. *Exp Dermatol.* (2015) 24:715–7. doi: 10.1111/exd.12732
128. Cheng JB, Sedgewick AJ, Finnegan AI, Harirchian P, Lee J, Kwon S, et al. Transcriptional programming of normal and inflamed human epidermis at single-cell resolution. *Cell Rep.* (2018) 25:871–83. doi: 10.1016/j.celrep.2018.09.006
129. Picart-Armada S, Thompson WK, Buil A, Perera-Lluna A. An R package to compute diffusion-based scores on biological networks: diffuStats. *Bioinformatics.* (2017) 34:533–4. doi: 10.1093/bioinformatics/btx632

130. Hänzelmann S, Castelo R, Guinney J. GSVA: gene set variation analysis for microarray and RNA-Seq data. *BMC Bioinformatics.* (2013) 14:7. doi: 10.1186/1471-2105-14-7
131. Ludwig RJ, Martinez A, Bernard P, Savas Y, Kowalewski C. *DPem: Dimethylfumarate for the Treatment of Bullous Pemphigoid.* (2011). Available online at: https://www.orpha.net/consor/cgi-bin/ResearchTrials_Networks.php?lng=EN&data_id=119994&title=DPem---Dimethylfumarate-for-the-treatment-of-bullous-pemphigoid&search=Disease_Search_Simple
132. Julkowska D, Austin CP, Cutillo CM, Gancberg D, Hager C, Halftermeyer J, et al. The importance of international collaboration for rare diseases research: a European perspective. *Nature.* (2017) 24:562–71. doi: 10.1038/gt.2017.29
133. Loget J, Barbe C, Duvert-Lehembre S, Bédane C, Maiziéres M, Joly P, et al. The regibul register: a tool for monitoring the distributionand incidence of autoimmune bullous dermatoses in three french regions, 2010 to 2015. *Acta Dermato Venereol.* (2017) 11:98. doi: 10.2340/00015555-2848

13

Proteases in Pemphigoid Diseases

Sho Hiroyasu [1,2,3]*, Christopher T. Turner* [1,2,3]*, Katlyn C. Richardson* [1,2,3] *and David J. Granville* [1,2,3*]

[1] *International Collaboration On Repair Discoveries (ICORD), Vancouver Coastal Health Research Institute (VCHRI), Vancouver, BC, Canada,* [2] *Department of Pathology and Laboratory Medicine, University of British Columbia (UBC), Vancouver, BC, Canada,* [3] *BC Professional Firefighters' Burn and Wound Healing Group, Vancouver Coastal Health Research Institute (VCHRI), University of British Columbia (UBC), Vancouver, BC, Canada*

Correspondence:
David J. Granville
dgranville@icord.org

Pemphigoid diseases are a subgroup of autoimmune skin diseases characterized by widespread tense blisters. Standard of care typically involves immunosuppressive treatments, which may be insufficient and are often associated with significant adverse events. As such, a deeper understanding of the pathomechanism(s) of pemphigoid diseases is necessary in order to identify improved therapeutic approaches. A major initiator of pemphigoid diseases is the accumulation of autoantibodies against proteins at the dermal-epidermal junction (DEJ), followed by protease activation at the lesion. The contribution of proteases to pemphigoid disease pathogenesis has been investigated using a combination of *in vitro* and *in vivo* models. These studies suggest proteolytic degradation of anchoring proteins proximal to the DEJ is crucial for dermal-epidermal separation and blister formation. In addition, proteases can also augment inflammation, expose autoantigenic cryptic epitopes, and/or provoke autoantigen spreading, which are all important in pemphigoid disease pathology. The present review summarizes and critically evaluates the current understanding with respect to the role of proteases in pemphigoid diseases.

Keywords: pemphigoid diseases, proteases, bullous pemphigoid, epidermolysis bullosa acquisita, mucous membrane pemphigoid, elastase, MMP, granzyme

CHARACTERISTICS OF PEMPHIGOID DISEASES

The term pemphigoid disease is defined as a specific subset of autoimmune subepidermal blistering diseases having autoantibodies against proteins at the dermal epidermal junction (DEJ) (1). This group includes bullous pemphigoid (BP), epidermolysis bullosa acquisita (EBA), pemphigoid gestationis (PG), mucous membrane pemphigoid (MMPh), linear IgA bullous dermatosis also known as linear IgA disease (LABD), anti-laminin $\gamma 1$ pemphigoid, lichen planus pemphigoid (LPP), and other rare diseases. Dermatitis herpetiformis (DH) is not included since its autoantigen (transglutaminase) does not localize at the DEJ (1, 2).

Pemphigoid diseases typically share a similar clinical presentation as either localized or generalized tense blisters and erosion on the skin (1). However, this presentation varies for each disease and there is heterogeneity within the same disease. BP typically presents as generalized blistering eruptions accompanied/preceded by erythema and pruritis (3). Although the presentation of PG is similar to that of BP, it normally develops during the second trimester of pregnancy (4, 5). The clinical features of EBA are also often similar to that of BP (referred to as an inflammatory variant of EBA), however, one third of the patients exhibit less inflammation (classical mechanobullous variant) (6–8). In MMPh, blistering and erosive lesions preferably but not exclusively develop on mucosa, such as the oral cavity and conjunctiva, genitalia, perianal region, pharynx, esophagus, and nasal (9, 10). This may result in critical complications such as blindness and strictures. Unlike other pemphigoid diseases, EBA and MMPh lesions may heal with scarring and/or milia formation (6, 9). LABD presents with generalized tense blisters with eruption characteristically accompanied by pruritus (11).

Histology of blistered skin in pemphigoid diseases normally shows superficial and mid-dermis perivascular inflammation infiltrated by lymphocytes, neutrophils, eosinophils, mast cells, and other immune cells, with the relative abundance and contribution depending on each disease (1, 12). The hallmark of BP lesions is eosinophil infiltration, whilst MMPh and classical variant EBA lesions exhibit minimal inflammation compared to the other pemphigoid diseases (12–14). Direct immunofluorescent microscopy of the patient skin is used diagnostically to visualize the deposition of immunoglobulins and/or complements along the basement membrane zone (1, 9, 11). Further analysis with direct (using patient prelesional skin) and/or indirect (using healthy human skin treated with patient serum) immunofluorescent microscopy of skin treated with 1M NaCl solution (salt-split skin) is sometimes clinically used to test the localization of the immunoglobulins (15, 16). Since this salt-split treatment separates the skin at the level of lamina lucida and the localizations of target autoantigens in each disease are characteristic [detailed in the Pathomechanism(s) of Pemphigoid Diseases section], salt-split skins of BP, PG, LPP, LABD, and most of MMPh show the immunoglobulin deposition in the epidermal side or in both the epidermal and dermal sides. On the other hand, the deposition of immunoglobulins is observed in the dermal side of the salt-split skin in EBA, anti-laminin $\gamma 1$ pemphigoid, and a subset of MMPh (16–18). To more specifically differentiate between the pemphigoid diseases, identification of target antigens for the autoantibodies is required, using enzyme-linked immunosorbent assay (ELISA) and/or western blotting (19–21).

The combined prevalence of pemphigoid diseases was estimated at 380 cases per million people (pmp) (22). BP, the most common disease within this group, was estimated at 259 pmp. The affected population in BP is increasing over time, presumably linked to the increasing risk factors such as aging, pharmacologics, and improved diagnostic techniques (1, 16, 23). In MMPh, prevalence was up to 25 pmp, whilst in EBA it was estimated at about 3 pmp. Other pemphigoid diseases including LABD and anti-laminin $\gamma 1$ pemphigoid were estimated as 5 pmp. PG in expectant mothers was diagnosed in approximately 1 out of 1,700–50,000 pregnancies (4). While BP and MMPh onset occurs typically in the elderly (median age of onset is ~80 and 70 years, respectively), other pemphigoid diseases show different age distributions (22). Onset of EBA is typically in the elderly (20% of patients are over 70 years old), although a second onset peak has been identified in individuals younger than 30 years old (22, 24). LABD onset peaks before the age of 5 and again after 60 years old (25). The mean age of onset in LPP is between 40 and 50 years of age (1), whilst in PG, as the disease develops during pregnancy, the median age of the onset is ~30 years of age (22).

Multiple factors have been reported to trigger pemphigoid disease onset. For BP, several inflammatory skin conditions (such as trauma, burn, ultraviolet irradiation, radiation, surgical wound, ostomy, and skin graft), specific drugs [including aldosterone antagonists, neuroleptics, spironolactone, phenothiazines with aliphatic side chain, loop diuretics, and dipeptidyl peptidase-4 inhibitor (DPP-4i)], vaccination, and viral infection have been indicated to trigger onset (3, 26–34). The association between BP and neurologic diseases such as stroke, epilepsy, Parkinson's disease, multiple sclerosis, dementia, and unipolar or bipolar disorder is well-documented (3, 28, 35). In LABD, skin trauma and exposure to drugs such as vancomycin have been reported as the triggering factors (11, 36, 37). In addition, several case reports have suggested drugs and inflammatory diseases as initiating other pemphigoid diseases (38–41).

Current treatment modalities for pemphigoid diseases mainly non-specifically target the inflammatory response as their main treatment options, corticosteroids, and immunosuppressive drugs target both innate and adaptive immunities (42–44). For BP, systemic corticosteroid administration remains the standard treatment, however, higher doses of prednisolone may cause critical adverse effects such as diabetes, decreased bone density, and increased susceptibility to infection (45, 46). Topical application of high potency corticosteroids is also used in clinical practice (16, 46, 47). Dapsone, a sulfone with antibacterial properties that is responsible for controlling neutrophil-induced inflammation in the skin, may be used in combination with topical/systemic corticosteroids (48). Other treatment options include systemic administration of a combination of nicotinamide and tetracyclines (tetracycline, doxycycline, or minocycline) (49, 50). Adjuvant immunosuppression with either mycophenolate mofetil or azathioprine has been reported (51). Rituximab, intravenous immunoglobulin, omalizumab, and immunoadsorption have been also reported to show positive effect on the disease course (52–55). PG treatment basically follows a similar course to that of BP including topical corticosteroids and/or low dose systemic corticosteroids (4, 47). LABD often responds well with dapsone (47). EBA is normally treated with systemic corticosteroids in combination with other immunosuppressive/modulatory agents (24). While mild cases of MMPh are often treated with dapsone, severe cases with critical mucosal complications are treated with more aggressive immunosuppressive treatments such as pulse intravenous corticosteroids, cyclophosphamide, or rituximab (9). Overall, pemphigoid disease treatment remains non-specific

---

Abbreviations: α1-AT, α1-antitrypsin; ADAM, a disintegrin and metalloprotease; BP, bullous pemphigoid; BPAG, bullous pemphigoid antigen; COPD, chronic obstructive pulmonary disease; DEJ, dermal-epidermal junction; DH, dermatitis herpetiformis; DPP-4i, dipeptidyl peptidase-4 inhibitor; DPPI, dipeptidyl peptidase I; enzyme-linked immunosorbent assay, ELISA; EBA, epidermolysis bullosa acquisita; Gzm, granzyme; human leukocyte antigen, HLA; Kitl, kit ligand; LABD, linear IgA bullous dermatosis; LAD-1, linear IgA disease antigen-1; LABD97, linear IgA bullous disease antigen of 97 kDa; LPP, lichen planus pemphigoid; mMCP-4, Mouse Mast Cell Protease 4; MMP, Matrix metalloproteinase; MMPh, mucous membrane pemphigoid; NE, neutrophil elastase; NK, natural killer; Pas, plasminogen activators; PAR-2, protease-activated receptor 2; PG, pemphigoid gestationis; PI-9, proteinase inhibitor-9; pmp, per million people; ROS, reactive oxygen species; Scf, stem cell factor; TIMP, tissue inhibitor of matrix metalloproteinase.

and often with critical adverse effects. As such, a deeper understanding of the pathology of these diseases is necessary to identify more specific and safer therapeutic approaches.

PATHOMECHANISM(S) OF PEMPHIGOID DISEASES

The hallmark of pemphigoid diseases is the deposition of autoantibodies targeting specific protein(s) at the DEJ (1). The protein or combination of proteins recognized by the autoantibodies vary for each specific pemphigoid disease: collagen XVII [BP180, bullous pemphigoid antigen 2 (BPAG2)] and/or BPAG1e (BP230, dystonin) for BP, PG, and LPP, collagen VII for EBA, collagen XVII, BPAG1e, laminin-332 (laminin-5), laminin-311 (laminin-6), collagen VII, or β4 integrin for MMPh, truncated collagen XVII fragments [linear IgA disease antigen-1 (LAD-1), linear IgA bullous disease antigen of 97 kDa (LABD97)], and/or BPAG1e for LABD, and laminin γ1 for anti-laminin γ1 pemphigoid (56–74). Most of these autoantigens are components or associated proteins of a DEJ anchoring complex, hemidesmosome. Hemidesmosomes are expressed by basal epithelial cells and perform an anchoring function in the skin between the epidermis and dermis (75, 76). In skin, the hemidesmosome consists of transmembrane proteins such as α6β4integrin, collagen XVII, and CD151, and cytoplasmic proteins such as BPAG1e and plectin, to link cytoplasmic keratin with extracellular laminin-332. Laminin-332 binds to collagen VII in the anchoring fibrils. Saliently, genetic mutations of these proteins cause congenital blistering diseases (i.e., epidermolysis bullosa) (77).

It remains unclear as to how immune tolerance is lost in pemphigoid diseases and how/why autoantibodies are formed against hemidesmosome-associated proteins. Several genetical and/or environmental backgrounds, such as human leukocyte antigen (HLA) allele and regulatory T cell dysfunction were suggested to increase autoreactive T and B cells in the pemphigoid diseases (78–85). These autoreactive lymphocytes possibly react with hemidesmosome-associated protein fragments disseminated in the extracellular space by exaggerated proteolytic cleavages at the DEJ during the aforementioned triggering events including skin inflammatory diseases and immunization.

The pathological functions of autoantibodies in blister formation has been studied using passive transfer mouse models. The models involve injections of anti-mouse collagen XVII IgG, anti-mouse collagen VII IgG, anti-laminin-332 IgG, or anti-human LAD-1/LABD97 IgA into healthy wild-type or human skin transplanted mice, resulting in the development of BP, inflammatory variants of EBA, anti-laminin-332 MMPh, or LABD model, respectively (86–91). Most of these animal models demonstrate the deposition of immunoglobulin and complements C3 at the DEJ, infiltration of inflammatory cells, and the presentation of subepidermal blistering. *Ex vivo* skin systems also provide a valuable research tool to reveal pemphigoid disease pathology (92). Cryosections of healthy skin are incubated with patient-derived IgG and leukocytes, leading to the induction of dermal-epidermal separation (93, 94). Based on these studies, it is now recognized that the blisters present in most pemphigoid diseases are triggered by the accumulation of autoantibodies at the DEJ followed by complement recruitment and inflammatory cell infiltration.

Passive-transfer mouse models of MMPh developed by Lazarova et al. and Darling et al. showed subepidermal blisters with IgG and C3 deposition but without obvious inflammation (90, 91). In addition, in one *ex vivo* skin study with anti-laminin-332 MMPh patient IgG, there was a failure to induce leukocyte recruitment and dermal-epidermal separation, suggesting an inflammation-independent mechanism is involved in blister formation in laminin-332 MMPh (19, 95). Conversely, a recent study using the anti-laminin-332 MMPh model developed by Heppe et al. showed complement activation and inflammation are indeed required for blister formation (88). Further studies are therefore needed to further elucidate the mechanisms in anti-laminin-332 MMPh.

Ex vivo skin- and passive transfer murine-models of pemphigoid diseases have demonstrated that neutrophils are especially important amongst the infiltrated inflammatory cells in blister formation (93, 94, 96). The *ex vivo* skin model showed neutrophils to be indispensable for BP and EBA blister formation as the patient IgG induced dermal-epidermal separations were only observed when co-incubated with neutrophils (93, 94). Liu et al. utilized the passive-transfer mouse model to demonstrate the importance of neutrophils in BP pathology, as depletion of circulating neutrophils in the BP mice showed resistance to blistering (96). To fight against pathogens, neutrophils provide reactive oxygen species (ROS), antimicrobial peptides, and proteases (97, 98). Since blister formation should be induced by the loss of epidermis and dermis attachment, it validated subsequent studies focusing on the function of proteases on the cleavage of anchoring proteins at the DEJ, such as hemidesmosomal components.

PROTEASES IN PEMPHIGOID DISEASES

Proteases are classically categorized into six groups based on the catalytic residue; serine, cysteine, aspartic, glutamic, threonine, and metalloproteases (99). Proteases exert both physiological and pathological roles through proteolytic cleavage and degradation of wide variety of substrates such as extracellular matrices, cell surface molecules, transmembrane proteins, growth factors, cytokines, and chemokines. The remainder of this review will summarize the current understanding with respect to the role of proteases in the pathogenesis of pemphigoid diseases.

Neutrophil Elastase

Neutrophil elastase (NE) is a serine protease that exhibits relatively broad cleavage site specificity and has a preference for regions containing several aliphatic amino acids (100). NE is stored in both azurophilic (also called primary) granules and the nuclear envelop of neutrophils as an active-form (101–103). Following bacterial infection and subsequent inflammatory stimulation, neutrophils phagocytose the invading bacteria, with NE contributing to intracellular killing (104, 105). In addition, upon neutrophil activation, NE is also secreted into the extracellular space, acting anti-bacterially to degrade bacterial proteins and various virulence factors such as outer membrane protein, flagellin, and leukotoxin (101, 106–108). NE also cleaves targets within the skin such as chemokines, cytokines, growth factors, cell surface molecules, adhesion proteins, and extracellular matrices (101, 109–113). These proteolytic functions serve to augment inflammation and to repair tissue at early phases of wound healing. However, excessive NE activity may cause unintended pathological consequences. Exaggerated NE-mediated proteolysis has been implicated as a key factor in inflammatory diseases [chronic obstructive pulmonary disease (COPD), cystic fibrosis, acute lung injury, acute respiratory distress syndrome], autoimmune diseases (type 1 diabetes), cancer (squamous cell carcinoma), and inflammatory skin diseases (psoriasis, skin photoaging) (101, 114–120). To defend against excessive NE proteolysis, there are endogenous secretory NE inhibitors such as α1-antitrypsin (α1-AT), serpin B1, proteinase inhibitor-9 (PI-9, serpinB9), chelonianin, and macroglobulin (114). However, an imbalance of local protease-antiprotease activity has been observed, likely due to genetics, environmental factors, or simply an inability to cope with the massive degree of inflammation (101, 120, 121). In this context, the function of NE in pathology and underlying pemphigoid diseases remains a topic of further study.

Abundant NE-positive neutrophils and NE activity have been reported in human BP blister fluid (122–124) (**Table 1**). A direct link between NE and blistering was identified using the passive-transfer BP model with anti-mouse collagen XVII IgG where NE null mutant mice or wild type mice administered NE inhibitors (α1-AT and MeOSuc-AAPV-CH_2Cl) were resistant to blister formation (125, 126). In addition, in the *ex vivo* human skin model, leukocytes and BP patient IgG dependent dermal-epidermal separation was blocked with a NE inhibitor (MeOSuc-AAPV-CK) (95). Using the same model but with IgG from EBA patients, it was confirmed that pathogenic IgG in EBA patients also contributes to NE-dependent blister formation (95). NE-induced blistering in BP and EBA was proposed to be generated by the degradation of hemidesmosomal proteins including collagen XVII (126, 127) (**Figure 1; Table 1**). NE also cleaved laminin-332 *in vitro*, which is another hemidesmosome-associated protein (128).

The degradation of hemidesmosomal proteins might exaggerate the inflammatory response in pemphigoid disease. Mydel et al. and Lin et al. indicated that NE-induced fragments of laminin-332 and collagen XVII are chemotactic for neutrophils (127, 128). Bergh et al. demonstrated that loss of collagen XVII induces IL-8 expression in keratinocytes, which potentially induces further inflammation in BP (129).

Based on its role in pemphigoid diseases, NE has been proposed as a therapeutic target. However, there has been no reported clinical evidence forwarded that supports the use of NE-inhibiting drugs such as sivelestat (ONO-5046) or AZD9668 for pemphigoid diseases (130, 131). One recent paper suggested a possible mechanism which may induce resistance against macromolecular NE inhibitors (132). It was proposed that the closed compartment between neutrophils and immune complexes prohibits the access of inhibitors, which implies NE inhibition as a treatment strategy for pemphigoid diseases may be challenging.

Matrix Metalloproteases (MMPs)

MMPs (also known as matrixins) are a family of calcium-dependent zinc-containing proteases generally consisting of a signaling peptide-, propeptide-, catalytic-, and hemopexin-like-domains (133, 134). To activate these proteolytic functions, the interaction between catalytic domain and propeptide domain needs to be removed normally by other proteases, such as plasmin, trypsin, kallikrein, tryptase, and other MMPs (134–137). Once activated, MMPs are available to cleave a diverse range of substrates such as chemokines, cytokines, growth factors, cell surface molecules, adhesion proteins, extracellular matrices, and other proteases (134, 138). Because of this wide range of substrates, MMPs play a number of roles in physiological processes, including in inflammatory responses, angiogenesis, reproduction, development, wound closure, and tissue remodeling (133, 134, 139–142). To avoid excess host tissue damage and unregulated inflammation, endogenous inhibitors such as α2-macroglobulin and all types of tissue inhibitor of matrix metalloproteinases (TIMPs) block excessive enzymatic activity of MMPs (137, 143). However, and similar to NE, several reasons may create an imbalance between proteases and antiproteases, resulting in multiple diseases. MMPs have been implicated in pathological roles in cancer, inflammatory diseases, autoimmune diseases, neuropsychiatric disorders, central nervous system diseases, cardiovascular diseases, and delayed wound healing (134, 137, 139, 142, 144–146). The pathological functions of MMPs in pemphigoid diseases have been studied, predominantly focusing on MMP-9.

MMP-9, also known as gelatinase B or 92 kDa type IV collagenase, is secreted from several cell types including neutrophils, macrophages, eosinophils, and fibroblasts (147, 148). In neutrophils, MMP-9 is stored in zymogen granules and secreted upon an inflammatory stimulation (149, 150). Conversely, in macrophages, MMP-9 does not accumulate and instead is secreted as a 92-kDa proactive form following synthesis (151). Once activated, the 88-kDa active form of MMP-9 extracellularly cleaves a variety of substrates such as chemokines, cytokines, growth factors, cell surface molecules, transmembrane proteins, extracellular matrices, and proteases (147, 152–154).

While multiple studies report MMP-9 positive keratinocytes, neutrophils, T-cells, mast cells, and eosinophils to be abundant in lesional and perilesional BP skin (**Table 1**), Verraes et al. indicated that blister fluid MMP-9 may present only as proenzyme and therefore not able to degrade collagen XVII (124, 148, 155–159). Moreover, they indicated that TIMP-1 is abundant in the blister fluids, which would likely inhibit activity of MMP-9. On the other hand, Niimi et al. suggested TIMP-1 expression was less compared to MMP-9 at the BP lesion (156). In MMPh, MMP-9 protein levels and the MMP-9/TIMP-1 ratio were increased in patient tears (160, 161) (**Table 1**).

Once activated, and in the absence of inhibition, MMP-9 degrades the extracellular domain of human collagen XVII and the NE inhibitor, α1-AT (124, 125). The role of MMP-9 in BP and

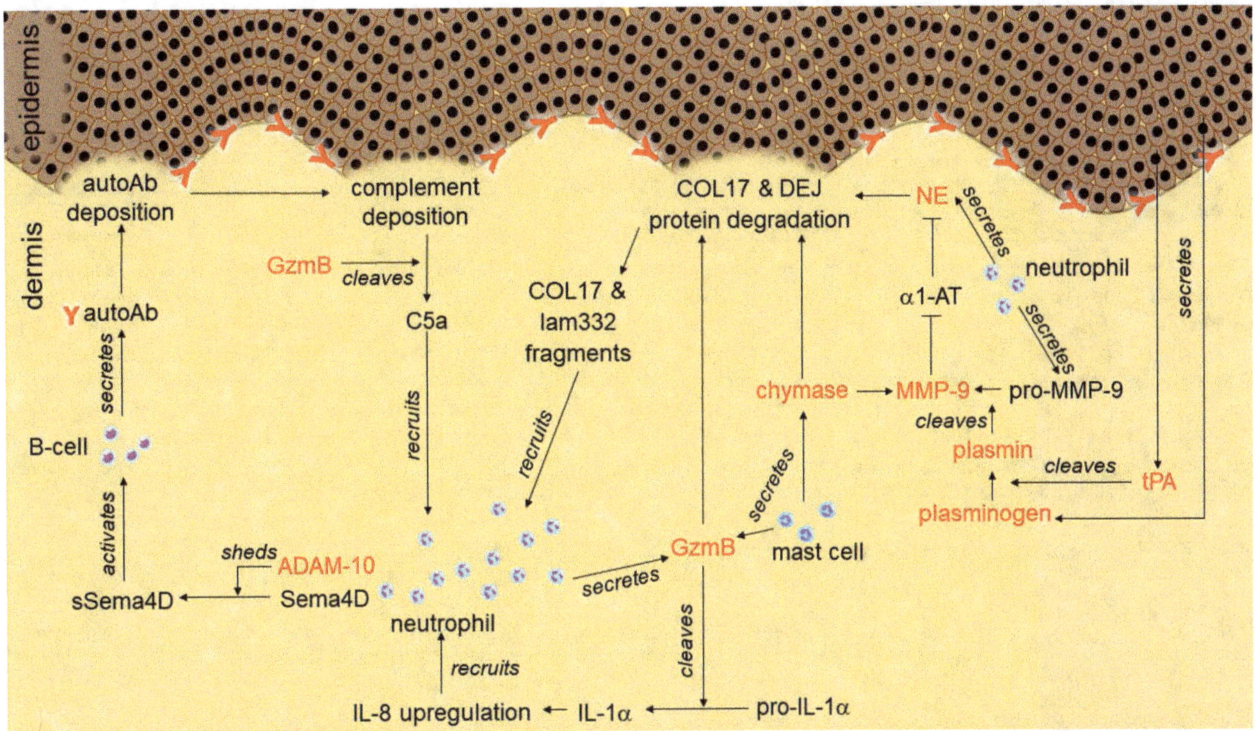

FIGURE 1 | Role of proteases in pemphigoid disease. Tissue-type plasminogen activator (tPA) secreted from keratinocytes activates plasminogen to plasmin. Plasmin activates pro-matrix metalloprotease-9 (pro-MMP-9) to MMP-9. MMP-9 degrades α1-antitrypsin (α1-AT). Without inhibition by α1-AT, neutrophil elastase (NE) cleaves hemidesmosome-associated proteins including collagen XVII (COL17) and laminin-332 (lam332). Granzyme B (GzmB) also cleaves hemidesmosome-associating proteins to induce dermal-epidermal separation. GzmB may induce additional neutrophil infiltration through chemoattractant production such as IL-1α, C5a, and COL17/lam332 fragments. ADAM-10 sheds semaphorin-4D (sema4D) to activate autoantibodies (autoAb) production from B cells.

EBA blistering was confirmed with *ex vivo* human skin models (95). Cryosections of human skin incubated with BP- or EBA-patient IgG and leukocytes created dermal-epidermal separation through an MMP-9-dependent manner as it was blocked by the MMP-9 inhibitor, 3G12scFV. Passive transfer BP mice showed MMP-9 activation at the lesional skin, whilst MMP-9 deficiency induced resistance to blister formation (162, 163). MMP-9 is likely to induce blistering through NE activation by degrading α1-AT, but not through direct-collagen XVII degradation, as direct stimulation with MMP-9 did not induce dermal-epidermal separation in *ex vivo* mouse skin sections (125) (**Figure 1**; **Table 1**). MMP-9 has also been indicated as having a role in complement activation in BP through CD46 shedding (164).

Other than MMP-9, MMP-2, -3, -12, and -13 have been reported to be upregulated in pemphigoid diseases (124, 156, 165–169). MMP-2 (gelatinase A, type IV collagenase) is ubiquitously and constitutively expressed in many cells and tissues including dermal fibroblasts (170). Multiple physiological and pathological roles have been indicated for MMP-2 in angiogenesis, tissue repair, cancer, and inflammation through the cleavage on cytokines, chemokines, cell surface proteins, extracellular matrices, and proMMPs. MMP-2 has been identified in the tears and sera of MMPh patient, blister fluids and lesional skins of BP, and sera of EBA (124, 156, 165, 166) (**Table 1**). MMP-2 is predicted to regulate Hsp-90-dependent blister formation through ROS release in EBA, since MMP-2 is complexed with Hsp-90 to be stabilized by the chaperone in the patient sera (166) (**Table 1**). MMP-2 cleaves some anchoring proteins such as collagen XVII, collagen VII, and laminin-332 *in vitro*, however, the direct function in the pathology remains to be elucidated (171, 172).

MMP-3 (stromelysin-1) exhibits multiple functions in development, inflammation, cancer, wound repair, skin inflammation through proteolyses on cytokines, chemokines, cell surface proteins, extracellular matrices, growth factors, proMMPs, and protease inhibitors (134, 170, 173). Increased MMP-3 has been detected in BP serum and lesional skin (167, 168) (**Table 1**). *In vitro*, MMP-3 can activate MMP-9 (174). However, MMP-3 deficient mice fail to display impaired MMP-9 activation and were still susceptible to experimental BP, suggesting that MMP-3 is dispensable to the pathology of BP (163) (**Table 1**).

MMP-12 (macrophage elastase) is produced in and secreted from mainly macrophages but also detected in other cell types including dermal fibroblast and vascular smooth muscle cells (170, 175). Through the proteolysis of cytokines, chemokines, cell surface proteins, extracellular matrices, proteases, and bacterial cellular membranes, MMP-12 contributes to inflammation, infection, tissue remodeling, and cancer. Increased MMP-12 has been observed in EBA sera and the lesional skin of BP (166, 169) (**Table 1**). In the EBA patient sera, and the same as observed for MMP-2, MMP-12 is complexed with Hsp-90 to regulate Hsp-90-dependent blister formation through ROS release (166) (**Table 1**). The direct function of MMP-12 in pemphigoid diseases remains

TABLE 1 | Major proteases in pemphigoid diseases.

Protease	Class	Location in PD	Functions in PD	References
NE	serine protease	BP—blister fluids	BP, EBA Hemidesmosomal protein degradation (COL17 and laminin-332)	(95, 122–127)
MMP-2 (gelatinase A, 72 kDa type IV collagenase)	Metalloprotease	BP—blister fluids, lesional skin EBA—sera MMPh—tear, sera	EBA Complexed with Hsp-90	(124, 156, 165, 166)
MMP-3 (stromelysin-1)	Metalloprotease	BP—serum, lesional skin	Negative in BP mouse model	(163, 167, 168)
MMP-9 (gelatinase B, 92 kDa type IV collagenase)	Metalloprotease	BP—lesional and perilesional skin, blister fluid MMPh—tear	BP, EBA NE activation through α1-AT degradation CD46 shedding	(96, 124, 125, 148, 155–160, 163, 164)
MMP-12 (macrophage elastase)	Metalloprotease	EBA—sera BP—lesional skin	EBA Complexed with Hsp-90	(166, 169)
MMP-13 (collagenase-3)	Metalloprotease	BP—lesional skin	Unknown	(156)
Plasmin, plasminogen, tPA, and uPA	Serine protease	BP—blister fluid, lesional skin	BP MMP-9 activation COL17 shedding	(163, 201–207)
Chymase/mMCP-4	Serine protease	BP—non lesional skin	BP MMP-9 activation COL17 degradation	(244, 304)
Granzyme B	Serine protease	BP, EBA, DH—lesional skin	DEJ protein degradation (COL7, α6β4 integrins, COL17) IL-1α activation C5a production	(298, 299)
ADAM-8	Metalloprotease	BP—epidermis of lesional skin	Unknown	(159, 258, 259)
ADAM-9	Metalloprotease	BP—epidermis of lesional skin	COL17 shedding	(159, 258, 259)
ADAM-10	Metalloprotease	BP—epidermis of lesional skin	COL17 shedding CD46 shedding Semaphorin 4D shedding	(159, 164, 258, 259)
ADAM-15	Metalloprotease	BP—epidermis of lesional skin	Unknown	(159, 258, 259)
ADAM-17	Metalloprotease	BP—epidermis of lesional skin	(Indirect) COL17 shedding	(159, 258, 259)
Tryptase	Serine protease	BP—blister fluid, sera	Unknown	(302–304)
Cathepsin-G	Serine protease	BP	Negative in BP mouse model	(126, 163, 301)

unknown, however, MMP-12 cleaves laminin-332, suggesting it may directly cause dermal-epidermal separation (128).

MMP-13 (collagenase-3) is distributed in multiple cell types such as in connective tissue, epithelial cells, and neural cells (134, 170). It cleaves cytokines, chemokines, extracellular matrices, proMMPs, and protease inhibitor to exhibit functions in inflammation, cancer, and tissue remodeling. Increased MMP-13 positive cells have been detected in lesional skin of BP (156) (**Table 1**). Although its role in pemphigoid diseases has not been studied, it may contribute to disease through MMP-9 activation, which have been indicated before (176).

As mentioned above, a number of studies implicate MMPs (especially MMP-9) as promising targets for pemphigoid disease treatment. However, it should be noted that therapeutic use of broad spectrum MMP inhibitors have failed in cancer clinical trials with a lack of efficacy and adverse effects possibly caused by inhibiting the essential physiological roles of MMPs (139). Indeed, multiple MMPs appear to exert beneficial functions such as anti-tumorigenesis and/or anti-inflammation and have therefore been proposed as "anti-targets" whereby their inhibitions would cause severe adverse effects (139). For example, since MMP-9 also exhibits aforementioned critical physiological roles, it is not surprising that even the specific MMP-9 inhibitor, andecaliximab showed several adverse effects in the clinical trial, such as nausea, vomiting, fatigue, diarrhea, asthenia, arthralgia, joint stiffness, and dyspnea, which would not be tolerated in treatments for benign diseases such as pemphigoid diseases (177). There are no reports of MMP inhibitors such as andecaliximab being tried as a therapeutic approach to treat pemphigoid diseases. Notably, doxycycline has been reported to regulate MMP-9 activation in other organs (178–181). Although its mechanism in the BP treatment is still unclear, Williams et al. reported 200 mg/day oral doxycycline is as effective as 0.5 mg/kg/day oral prednisolone (50).

Plasmin, Plasminogen, Tissue-Type Plasminogen Activator (tPA), and Urokinase-Type Plasminogen Activator (uPA)

Plasmin is a serine protease well-recognized as functioning in the fibrinolytic cascade (182, 183). Its precursor, plasminogen is created in liver cells and secreted into plasma (184, 185). Subsequently, plasminogen is cleaved by tPA and uPA to generate plasmin. Plasmin preferably cleaves following the arginine or lysine residues (186). As an important factor in the fibrinolytic system, plasmin degrades fibrin clots, thus prevents pathological conditions such as thrombosis (183). In addition to fibrin, plasmin cleaves many other substrates including coagulation factors, complement C3 and C5, hormones, metalloproteases, growth factors, cytokines, chemokines, cell surface molecules, and extracellular matrices (184, 187–194). With this variety of cleavage substrates, plasmin has been linked to multiple physiological processes such as inflammation, wound healing, and tissue remodeling (182, 195, 196). To prevent excessive proteolysis, plasmin activity is regulated by endogenous inhibitor, α2-antiplasmin (184). However, and similar to other proteases, an imbalance between plasmin and its inhibitor trigger pathological conditions, for example in cancer and inflammatory diseases (inflammatory response after the major surgery and trauma, asthma, COPD, and central nervous system inflammation) (182, 197–200).

Elevated levels of active plasmin and tPA are present in blister fluid and the lesional skin of BP patients (201–206) (**Table 1**). Keratinocytes stimulated by BP-patient IgG release tPA (202) (**Figure 1**). The function of the plasminogen/plasmin system in this context was confirmed using the passive-transfer BP model, where the administration of a plasmin inhibitor (α2-antiplasmin) blocked blistering (163). Mice deficient of plasminogen, and both tPA and uPA exhibit delayed and less intense blistering in the passive-transfer BP model. Since all of these deficient mice reconstituted BP with active MMP-9 but not with the proMMP-9, the PA/plasminogen/plasmin cascade is likely to induce blistering through MMP-9 activation (**Figure 1**; **Table 1**).

Intriguingly, Hofmann et al. demonstrated using *in vitro* system that plasmin generates 97-kDa fragments of collagen XVII known as LABD97 (203). Similarly, Nishie et al. showed that BP blister fluid cleaves recombinant collagen XVII into 120-kDa ectodomain in a plasmin-dependent manner (207). They suggested that this plasmin-induced cleavage of NC16a domain in collagen XVII generates neoepitopes possibly involved in the onset of BP and LABD (**Table 1**). As a related topic, Izumi et al. suggested that plasmin inhibition with DPP-4i induced characteristic non-inflammatory BP, possibly through plasmin independent collagen XVII cleavage, and the generation of neoepitopes within different domains by other proteases (208). The physiological role of collagen XVII shedding in re-epithelialization was indicated using a non-shedding collagen XVII mouse model, which exclusively expresses non-sheddable collagen XVII mutant (209).

Anti-plasmin drugs such as ε-aminocaproic acid and tranexamic acid are mostly used to inhibit fibrinolysis (182). Intriguingly, Grando has reported the pemphigoid disease treatment using a combination of oral prednisolone, ε-aminocaproic acid, and aprotinin, which is an inhibitor of serine proteases including plasmin (210). However, the therapeutic effect of this treatment approach compared to the control group (prednisolone alone) has not been reported.

Chymase and Mouse Mast Cell Protease 4 (mMCP-4)

In human tissues, infiltrating and degranulating mast cells were associated with BP (211). The importance of mast cells in the pathology of BP has been suggested, in part through the use of the passive-transfer model with anti-mouse collagen XVII IgG on Kit or Scf [stem cell factor, Kitl (kit ligand)]-mutation dependent mast cell-deficient mice, which failed to develop BP (212). Since intradermal injection of either polymorphonuclear leukocytes or IL-8 (a neutrophil chemoattractant) recovered the lack of phenotypes on Kit- or Scf-mutation mice, they concluded that mast cells play an essential role in neutrophil recruitment in BP. However, as recent studies revealed that Kit- or Scf-mutation affects not only mast cells but also multiple cell types including those of immune- and non-immune origin, this result may be questioned (213, 214). The recently developed Kit- or Scf-mutant independent mast cell deficient mice should be tested for further analysis. It should be also noted that blocking mast cell degranulation with the inhibitor (cromolyn sodium) in BP mice significantly reduced disease phenotype as well, thereby indicating the importance of mast cell granules in BP pathogenesis (212, 215).

Although often believed that the pathological mechanisms operating in BP and inflammatory variant EBA are quite similar, at least in the passive-transfer disease models, mast cells may participate differently in each. Both Kit mutation-dependent and -independent mast cell deficiencies induced consistent blistering phenotypes in passive-transfer mouse model of EBA, even though activated mast cells were abundant in the lesions of the EBA in wild-type mice (216). The results indicate that, in contrast to the BP model, mast cells and secreted proteases appear to be dispensable for the blister formation in EBA.

Human mast cells release proteases including chymase, tryptase, cathepsin G, carboxypeptidase A3, dipeptidtlpeptidase I/cathepsin C, cathepsins L and S, granzyme B, plasminogen activators, and MMPs (217). One of the major granule components of mast cells, chymase, is a serine protease that cleaves peptides after aromatic amino acids, preferably phenylalanine and tyrosine residues (217, 218). It is produced as an inactive form in mast cells and activated by cleavage with dipeptidyl peptidase I (DPPI) within the granules (219). Following stimulation, such as during inflammation or injury, chymase is released into the extracellular space. Chymase is resistant to multiple endogenous inhibitors such as α1-AT, α2-antichymotrypsin, α2-macroglobulin, and eglin C, when bound to heparin proteoglycan (220). While chymase is well-recognized for its ability to convert angiotensin I to its active form, angiotensin II, it also reportedly cleaves cytokines, growth factors, proteases, transmembrane proteins, and extracellular matrices (221–233). Although rodents have multiple isoforms of chymase, mMCP-4 is recognized as the isoform comparable to human chymase because of its biophysical and functional properties and tissue distribution (221). Based on former studies using deficient mice in this functional-equivalent, chymase has been revealed to function in the regulation of inflammatory response and tissue remodeling (221, 234, 235).

Chymase has also been suggested to exert pathological roles in multiple diseases such as cancers, cardiovascular diseases, inflammatory lung diseases (idiopathic pulmonary fibrosis, COPD), renal diseases (diabetic nephropathy, hypertensive nephropathy, rejected kidney allograft), preeclampsia, skin keloid, and atopic dermatitis (220, 221, 236–243).

The critical contribution of mMCP-4 in disease mechanisms is also observed in BP as passive-transfer mouse model with anti-mouse collagen XVII IgG on mMCP-4 deficient mice showed resistant to blistering even neutrophil recruitment was observed (244). Since impaired activation of MMP-9 in the mMCP-4 deficient BP mice and degradation of collagen XVII by mMCP-4 *in vitro* were observed, they indicated that mMCP-4 affects BP pathology by both activating MMP-9 and degrading collagen XVII (**Figure 1**; **Table 1**). On the other hand, cathepsin G/chymase inhibitors (α1-antichymotrypsin or Z-Gly-Leu-Phe-CH_2Cl) did not improve passive-transfer BP model (126).

A few chymase inhibitors were and are being tested in phase II clinical trials for heart failure, diabetic kidney disease, or atopic dermatitis (237). The trial of SUN13834 on atopic dermatitis was discontinued because of adverse side effects. So far, there is no report of chymase inhibitors being tested on pemphigoid disease patients.

A Disintegrin and Metalloproteases (ADAMs)

ADAMs are a family of single-pass transmembrane proteins consisting of an extracellular metalloprotease domain, a disintegrin domain, a cysteine rich domain, a transmembrane domain, and a cytoplasmic tail (245). Although all members of ADAMs contain metalloprotease domains, some of them do not possess functional protease activity. Only ADAMs 8, 9, 10, 12, 15, 17, 19, 20, 21, 28, and 33 are recognized as exhibiting proteolytic activity, requiring removal of the extracellular end prodomain within the cytoplasm (246). These functional ADAM metalloproteases mainly regulate ectodomain shedding on multiple cell surface proteins, which results in regulation of growth factors, cytokines, chemokines, adhesion molecules, and receptors in order to control physiological systems such as inflammation and development (247, 248). These proteolytic activities are controlled by endogenous inhibitors such as TIMPs and by their cellular localizations regulated by endocytosis (249–251). However, as with other proteases, dysregulation is often observed in several diseases. Pathological roles of ADAMs have now been reported in cancers, wound healing, psoriasis, rheumatoid arthritis, inflammatory lung diseases, inflammatory bowel diseases, predominantly functioning through ectodomain shedding of cytokines, chemokines, and chemoattractant (247, 252–257).

In BP, elevated protein levels of ADAMs 8, 9, 10, 15, and 17 in the epidermis of the lesional skins have been indicated (159, 258, 259) (**Table 1**). ADAMs 9, 10, and 17 are regulated by TWEAK/Fn14 pathway and may participate in collagen XVII loss in the skin lesion of BP (159). Upregulated ADAM10 has also been suggested to shed CD46, which results in enhancement of complement activation in BP lesions (164). Moreover, ADAM10 sheds soluble semaphorin 4D from the granulocytes to activate B cells, which results in enhancing autoantibody production in BP (259) (**Figure 1**; **Table 1**).

Intriguingly enough, mainly ADAMs 9 and 10, but also indirectly ADAM17, constitutively shed 120-kDa ectodomain of collagen XVII, LAD-1 (260, 261) (**Table 1**). ADAMs may also play a role in neoepitope production through collagen XVII cleavage, possibly triggering BP and LABD onset (207).

Inhibitors targeting broad spectrum of ADAMs have failed clinical trials primarily due to adverse effects (262). Development of drugs that target specific ADAM is challenging due to structural similarities in ADAMs and MMPs. In addition, many substrates of ADAMs are shared with other ADAMs and MMPs. Therefore, specific ADAM inhibitor may not be sufficient to provide good efficacy. A small molecule inhibitor of ADAMs 10 and 17, INCB7839 has been tested in a breast cancer clinical trial, which was discontinued likely because of increased deep vein thrombosis (263). This drug is now being tested in diffuse large B cell non-Hodgkin lymphoma phase II clinical trial. There is no report of using ADAM inhibitors on pemphigoid diseases.

Granzyme B

Granzymes (Gzms) are a family of serine proteases that includes five members in humans: GzmA, GzmB, GzmH, GzmK, and GzmM (264, 265). Discovered in the granules of cytotoxic T cells and natural killer (NK) cells, granzymes were traditionally considered exclusively as key mediators of granule-induced cell death, targeting cancer or virally infected cells. GzmB initiates apoptosis through caspase-dependent and/or caspase-independent pathways after internalized into target cells (266, 267). For internalization, another granule component, perforin, is required to form pores on the target cell membrane (268, 269). Saliently, not all secreted GzmB is internalized by the target cells as approximately one-third escapes from the immunological synapse and into the extracellular space (270). Moreover, GzmB is secreted by cells not involved in cytotoxicity or perforin release, including immune- (mast cells, neutrophils, macrophages, basophils, dendritic cells, and regulatory T cells) and non-immune (keratinocytes and chondrocytes) cells (271–281). In contrast to other proteases which are tightly regulated in the extracellular spaces, GzmB-mediated proteolysis in the extracellular space is not likely to regulated by the endogenous inhibitors, since the only inhibitor identified thus far in human tissue, PI-9 is located in the cytoplasm and not secreted into the extracellular space (282). Therefore, GzmB is expected to exhibit alternative roles in the extracellular space through its proteolytic activity.

GzmB has cleavage specificity after an aspartic acid or glutamic acid residues (283). Multiple extracellular substrates for GzmB have now been identified *in vitro*, such as cytokines (IL-1α, proIL-18), complements (C3, C5), extracellular proteins (fibronectin, vitronectin, laminin, decorin, biglycan), coagulation/ fibrinolytic factors (von Willebrand factor, plasminogen), and cell surface proteins (VE-cadherin, ZO-1) (284–288). Through these cleavages and degradations in the extracellular spaces, GzmB is expected to regulate inflammation, cell adhesion, cell migration, anoikis, coagulation, fibrinolysis, and cell-cell adhesion. Present at low levels in healthy tissue, GzmB is elevated in numerous pathological conditions such as atherosclerosis, rheumatoid arthritis, transplant rejection, acute graft vs. host disease, discoid lupus, drug eruption, atopic dermatitis, impaired burn wound, and photoaging (279, 289–297). In these diseases, pathological contributions of GzmB are suggested through not only intracellular apoptotic function but also extracellular proteolytic role.

GzmB positive cells localize to blisters in pemphigoid diseases (298, 299) (**Table 1**). However, since GzmB has long been exclusively recognized as a cytotoxic inducer, the proteolytic role of GzmB in the extracellular space had not been tested in pemphigoid diseases until recently (299). GzmB cleaves multiple anchoring proteins such as α6β4 integrins, collagen VII, and collagen XVII *in vitro*. Moreover, GzmB induces dermal-epidermal separation in *ex vivo* human skin. These results suggest that GzmB-induced cleavage of anchoring proteins directly leads to subepidermal blistering in the pemphigoid diseases (**Figure 1**; **Table 1**). Because of its wide variety of substrates in skin and inflammatory conditions, GzmB could exert multiple roles in the pathogenesis of pemphigoid diseases. For example, GzmB proteolytically augments the pro-inflammatory activity of IL-1α, which would be predicted to promote neutrophil accumulation at the lesion through subsequent IL-8 activation (287). In addition, GzmB cleaves C5 to generate a strong chemoattractant, C5a, to cause additional inflammatory cell infiltration (286). Since GzmB directly cleaves collagen XVII, GzmB may also contribute to the neoepitope generation in BP as similar to plasmin and ADAMs. Intriguingly, as GzmB is upregulated with age, it could help to explain its role in age-related autoimmune blistering pathologies such as BP, however further studies are required (3, 300).

Recently, a topical GzmB inhibitor was tested on impaired burn wound murine model, however, there are currently no clinically-approved GzmB inhibitors on the market (289).

Other Proteases

In addition to the above-mentioned proteases, other proteases have been identified as being upregulated in pemphigoid diseases including tryptase and cathepsin G (163, 301–304). Although the functions of these proteases in pemphigoid diseases remain unclear, we enumerate current understanding of these enzymes in the pemphigoid diseases and relating fields.

Tryptase is a serine protease mainly secreted from mast cells (305, 306). It is well-recognized to activate protease-activated receptor 2 (PAR-2) with its proteolytic activity (307). Through PAR-2 dependent and independent mechanisms, tryptase induces the release of cytokines and chemokines from multiple cell types. Other than PAR-2, it cleaves extracellular matrices and coagulant factors and exhibits a role in inflammation, angiogenesis, anticoagulant, tissue remodeling, cancer, allergic inflammatory diseases, and cardiovascular diseases (305, 306). Tryptase has been identified as being elevated in blister fluids and sera from BP patients (302–304) (**Table 1**). Protein levels show at least a partial positive correlation with autoantibody titers, cytokines, and clinical severity, however, its function has not been tested in pemphigoid disease models.

Cathepsin G is a serine protease mainly localized in the azurophilic granules of neutrophils (308, 309). With its proteolytic ability on cytokines, chemokines, cell surface proteins, extracellular matrices, outer membrane of infectant, angiotensin II, and proMMPs, cathepsin G exhibit important roles in inflammation, thrombogenesis, host defense, blood pressure, tumor invasion, and autoimmune diseases. Elevated cathepsin G has been observed in BP samples (163, 301) (**Table 1**). *In vitro* cleavage assays indicated that cathepsin G degrades laminin-332, suggesting it may induce dermal-epidermal separation (128). However, cathepsin G inhibition by α1-antichymotrypsin did not reduce disease severity on passive-transfer mouse model of BP, thus a direct role is yet to be confirmed (126, 163) (**Table 1**).

Together, further studies are required to fully elucidate the contribution of these proteases to pemphigoid disease pathogenicity.

REGULATORS OF PROTEASES IN PEMPHIGOID DISEASES

In addition to the above-described regulatory actions by the endogenous inhibitors, proteases are controlled by other multiple factors such as cytokines and different proteases. Since former studies have characterized that the profiles of cytokines and chemokines in pemphigoid diseases are likely to be unique, these characteristic profiles may be important for protease regulation.

Th2 relating cytokines such as IL-4, IL-5, soluble CD30, CCL5 (RANTES), CCL11 (eotaxin), CCL17 (TARC), CCL18 (PARC), CCL22 (MDC), CCL26 (eotaxin 3), and TSLP are elevated in the sera and/or blister fluids of BP patients (310–326). Elevated Th1 cytokines such as IFN-γ, IL-1β, TNF-α, CXCL9 (MIG), CXCL10 (IP10), and IL-18 have been also identified within the BP patient samples (310, 312, 318, 324, 325, 327). Besides them, IL-6, IL-8, IL-17, IL-21, IL-22, and IL-23 are elevated (310, 320, 324, 328, 329). Intriguingly, serum level of IL-17, IL-23, and CXCL10 in follow-up patients were elevated only in patients who later relapsed (328, 330). Since these cytokines and chemokine regulate MMP-9 secretion from inflammatory cells, it has been suggested that elevated IL-17, IL-23, and CXCL10 could trigger relapse through increased MMP-9 secretion (328, 330). Cytokine and chemokine profiles in other pemphigoid diseases are poorly defined at present, presumably due to the rareness of such diseases. Regarding EBA, serum and skin IL-6 expression are increased, however other cytokines did not show a significant increase due to a high degree of variation (331). In the same study, elevated concentration of IL-4, RANTES, IL-1α, IL-1β, TNF-α, IL-6, IL-10, IL-17, MIP-1α, KC, and GM-CSF are detected in the passive-transfer mouse model of EBA. In MMPh, elevated IL-4, IL-5, IL-13, IL-1α, IL-1β, IL-2, IL-12, TNF-α, IL-6, IL-8, IL-17, and TGF-β1 have been detected in serum and/or lesions of the human patients (161, 332–340).

As indicated above as interaction between NE, MMP-9, chymase, and plasmin, the proteases influence each other directly and indirectly by degrading intermediate proteases or protease inhibitors. Identifying the interaction between the proteases in the diseases is challenging since tissues include many types of proteases and each protease has wide variety of substrates. To conquer this conundrum, the field of degradomics was established (341). Combining genomics, proteomics, and bioinformatics, a whole map of complex protease interactions and networks is beginning to be elucidated not only *in vitro*, but also *in vivo* including in diseases such as COPD and pancreatic tumors (154, 342–344). Resulting from these and other studies, proteases have been recognized as influencing the activities of other proteases and, helping to define the "protease web" (342).

CONCLUSION

Multiple proteases have been identified as being elevated in pemphigoid diseases. Several have been proposed to play key roles in blistering pathology through the cleavage of hemidesmosomal proteins, resulting in dermal-epidermal separation and blister formation. In addition, some proteases have been suggested to contribute to neoepitope generation and dysregulated inflammatory response in the diseases. Despite significant advancements, further research is required to further elucidate the complex role that proteases play in various pemphigoid diseases.

Inhibition of specific proteases in pemphigoid diseases provides a unique, potentially safer therapeutic approach compared to current non-specific immune suppressive treatments that are often plagued with undesirable adverse effects. Thus far, evidence of clinical efficacy is minimal, but this may change as protease function is further defined, more effective inhibitors are developed, and new trials are commenced.

AUTHOR CONTRIBUTIONS

SH, CT, and DG wrote the manuscript. SH and KR prepared the table and figure.

ACKNOWLEDGMENTS

We appreciate Drs. Daisuke Tsuruta and Takashi Hashimoto for their valuable comments. This work was supported by grants-in-aid from the Canadian Institutes for Health Research (CIHR) (DG) and Michael Smith Foundation for Health Research (DG). CT is funded by a CIHR post-doctoral fellowship (F16-05378).

REFERENCES

1. Schmidt E, Zillikens D. Pemphigoid diseases. *Lancet.* (2013) 381:320–32. doi: 10.1016/S0140-6736(12)61140-4
2. Dieterich W, Schuppan D, Laag E, Bruckner-Tuderman L, Reunala T, Kárpáti S, et al. Antibodies to tissue transglutaminase as serologic markers in patients with dermatitis herpetiformis. *J Invest Dermatol.* (1999) 113:133–6. doi: 10.1046/j.1523-1747.1999.00627.x
3. Schmidt E, della Torre R, Borradori L. Clinical features and practical diagnosis of bullous pemphigoid. *Immunol Allergy Clin North Am.* (2012) 32:217–32. doi: 10.1016/j.iac.2012.04.002
4. Ljubojevic S, Bukvić-Mokos Z, Chapsa M, Heyne S, Schneiderat S, Beissert S, et al. Pemphigoid gestationis. *Clin Dermatol.* (2012) 30:51–5. doi: 10.1016/j.clindermatol.2011.03.009
5. Shornick JK, Bangert JL, Freeman RG, Gilliam JN. Herpes gestationis: clinical and histologic features of twenty-eight cases. *J Am Acad Dermatol.* (1983) 8:214–24. doi: 10.1016/S0190-9622(83)70027-7
6. Vorobyev A, Ludwig RJ, Schmidt E. Clinical features and diagnosis of epidermolysis bullosa acquisita. *Expert Rev Clin Immunol.* (2017) 13:157–69. doi: 10.1080/1744666X.2016.1221343
7. Gammon WR, Briggaman RA, Woodley DT, Heald PW, Wheeler CE Jr. Epidermolysis bullosa acquisita—a pemphigoid-like disease. *J Am Acad Dermatol.* (1984) 11:820–32. doi: 10.1016/S0190-9622(84)80459-4
8. Roenigk HH, Ryan JG, Bergfeld WF. Epidermolysis bullosa acquisita. *Arch Dermatol.* (1971) 103:1. doi: 10.1001/archderm.1971.04000130003001
9. Amber KT, Murrell DF, Schmidt E, Joly P, Borradori L. Autoimmune subepidermal bullous diseases of the skin and mucosae: clinical features, diagnosis, and management. *Clin Rev Allergy Immunol.* (2018) 54:26–51. doi: 10.1007/s12016-017-8633-4
10. Thorne JE, Anhalt GJ, Jabs DA. Mucous membrane pemphigoid and pseudopemphigoid. *Ophthalmology.* (2004) 111:45–52. doi: 10.1016/j.ophtha.2003.03.001
11. Venning VA. Linear IgA disease: clinical presentation, diagnosis, and pathogenesis. *Immunol Allergy Clin North Am.* (2012) 32:245–53. doi: 10.1016/j.iac.2012.04.004
12. BinJadeed HF, Alyousef AM, Alsaif FM, Alhumidi AA, Alotaibi HO. Histologic characterization of cellular infiltration in autoimmune subepidermal bullous diseases in a tertiary hospital in Saudi Arabia. *Clin Cosmet Invest Dermatol.* (2018) 11:187–94. doi: 10.2147/CCID.S158388
13. Kasperkiewicz M, Sadik CD, Bieber K, Ibrahim SM, Manz RA, Schmidt E, et al. Epidermolysis bullosa acquisita : from pathophysiology to novel therapeutic options. *J Invest Dermatol.* (2016) 136:24–33. doi: 10.1038/JID.2015.356
14. Kamaguchi M, Iwata H, Nishie W, Toyonaga E, Ujiie H, Natsuga K, et al. The direct binding of collagen XVII and collagen IV is disrupted by pemphigoid autoantibodies. *Lab Invest.* (2018) 99:48–57. doi: 10.1038/s41374-018-0113-9
15. Gammon WR, Kowalewski C, Chorzelski TP, Kumar V, Briggaman RA, Beutner EH. Direct immunofluorescence studies of sodium chloride—separated skin in the differential diagnosis of bullous pemphigoid and epidermolysis bullosa acquisita. *J Am Acad Dermatol.* (1990) 22:664–70. doi: 10.1016/0190-9622(90)70094-X
16. Bernard P, Antonicelli F. Bullous pemphigoid: a review of its diagnosis, associations and treatment. *Am J Clin Dermatol.* (2017) 18:513–28. doi: 10.1007/s40257-017-0264-2
17. Jindal A, Rao R, Bhogal BS. Advanced diagnostic techniques in autoimmune bullous diseases. *Indian J Dermatol.* (2017) 62:268–78. doi: 10.4103/ijd.IJD_196_17
18. Meijer JM, Diercks GFH, Schmidt E, Pas HH, Jonkman MF. Laboratory diagnosis and clinical profile of anti-p200 pemphigoid. *JAMA Dermatol.* (2016) 152:897–904. doi: 10.1001/jamadermatol.2016.1099
19. Kamaguchi M, Iwata H. The diagnosis and blistering mechanisms of mucous membrane pemphigoid. *Front Immunol.* (2019) 10:34. doi: 10.3389/fimmu.2019.00034
20. Antiga E, Caproni M, Fabbri P. Linear immunoglobulin a bullous dermatosis: need for an agreement on diagnostic criteria. *Dermatology.* (2013) 226:329–32. doi: 10.1159/000350818
21. Witte M, Zillikens D, Schmidt E. Diagnosis of autoimmune blistering diseases. *Front Med.* (2018) 5:296. doi: 10.3389/fmed.2018.00296
22. Hübner F, Recke A, Zillikens D, Linder R, Schmidt E. Prevalence and age distribution of pemphigus and pemphigoid diseases in Germany. *J Invest Dermatol.* (2016) 136:2495–8. doi: 10.1016/j.jid.2016.07.013
23. Langan SM, Smeeth L, Hubbard R, Fleming KM, Smith CJP, West J. Bullous pemphigoid and pemphigus vulgaris–incidence and mortality in the UK: population based cohort study. *BMJ.* (2008) 337:a180. doi: 10.1136/bmj.a180

24. Ludwig RJ. Clinical presentation, pathogenesis, diagnosis, and treatment of epidermolysis bullosa acquisita. *ISRN Dermatol.* (2013) 2013:812029. doi: 10.1155/2013/812029
25. Wojnarowska F, Marsden RA, Bhogal B, Black MM. Chronic bullous disease of childhood, childhood cicatricial pemphigoid, and linear IgA disease of adults: a comparative study demonstrating clinical and immunopathologic overlap. *J Am Acad Dermatol.* (1988) 19:792–805. doi: 10.1016/S0190-9622(88)70236-4
26. Bastuji-Garin S, Joly P, Picard-Dahan C, Bernard P, Vaillant L, Pauwels C, et al. Drugs associated with bullous pemphigoid. *Arch Dermatol.* (1996) 132:272–6. doi: 10.1001/archderm.1996.03890270044006
27. Lloyd-Lavery A, Chi C-C, Wojnarowska F, Taghipour K. The associations between bullous pemphigoid and drug use. *JAMA Dermatol.* (2013) 149:58–62. doi: 10.1001/2013.jamadermatol.376
28. Bastuji-Garin S, Joly P, Lemordant P, Sparsa A, Bedane C, Delaporte E, et al. Risk factors for bullous pemphigoid in the elderly: a prospective case–control study. *J Invest Dermatol.* (2011) 131:637–43. doi: 10.1038/jid.2010.301
29. Benzaquen M, Borradori L, Berbis P, Cazzaniga S, Valero R, Richard M-A, et al. Dipeptidyl peptidase IV inhibitors, a risk factor for bullous pemphigoid: retrospective multicenter case-control study from France and Switzerland. *J Am Acad Dermatol.* (2018) 78:1090–6. doi: 10.1016/j.jaad.2017.12.038
30. Kawaguchi Y, Shimauchi R, Nishibori N, Kawashima K, Oshitani S, Fujiya A, et al. Dipeptidyl peptidase-4 inhibitors-associated bullous pemphigoid: a retrospective study of 168 pemphigoid and 9,304 diabetes mellitus patients. *J Diabetes Invest.* (2019) 10:392–8. doi: 10.1111/jdi.12877
31. Mai Y, Nishie W, Sato K, Hotta M, Izumi K, Ito K, et al. Bullous pemphigoid triggered by thermal burn under medication with a dipeptidyl peptidase-IV Inhibitor: a case report and review of the literature. *Front Immunol.* (2018) 9:542. doi: 10.3389/fimmu.2018.00542
32. Stavropoulos PG, Soura E, Antoniou C. Drug-induced pemphigoid: a review of the literature. *J Eur Acad Dermatol Venereol.* (2014) 28:1133–40. doi: 10.1111/jdv.12366
33. Baroero L, Coppo P, Bertolino L, Maccario S, Savino F. Three case reports of post immunization and post viral Bullous Pemphigoid: looking for the right trigger. *BMC Pediatr.* (2017) 17:60. doi: 10.1186/s12887-017-0813-0
34. Blazsek A, Sillo P, Ishii N, Gergely P, Poor G, Preisz K, et al. Searching for foreign antigens as possible triggering factors of autoimmunity: torque Teno virus DNA prevalence is elevated in sera of patients with bullous pemphigoid. *Exp Dermatol.* (2008) 17:446–54. doi: 10.1111/j.1600-0625.2007.00663.x
35. Langan SM, Groves RW, West J. The relationship between neurological disease and bullous pemphigoid: a population-based case-control study. *J Invest Dermatol.* (2011) 131:631–6. doi: 10.1038/jid.2010.357
36. Garel B, Ingen-Housz-Oro S, Afriat D, Prost-Squarcioni C, Tétart F, Bensaid B, et al. Drug-induced linear immunoglobulin A bullous dermatosis: a French retrospective pharmacovigilance study of 69 cases. *Br J Clin Pharmacol.* (2019) 85:570–9. doi: 10.1111/bcp.13827
37. Godfrey K, Wojnarowska F, Leonard J. Linear IgA disease of adults: association with lymphoproliferative malignancy and possible role of other triggering factors. *Br JDermatol.* (1990) 123:447–52. doi: 10.1111/j.1365-2133.1990.tb01448.x
38. Delbaldo C, Chen M, Friedli A, Prins C, Desmeules J, Saurat J-H, et al. Drug-induced epidermolysis bullosa acquisita with antibodies to type VII collagen. *J Am Acad Dermatol.* (2002) 46:S161–4. doi: 10.1067/mjd.2002.107774
39. Marteau J-M, Bercault B, Catros S, Fenelon M, Fricain J-C. Drug-induced oral mucous membrane pemphigoid: a case report. *Méd Buccale Chir Buccale.* (2017) 23:181–3. doi: 10.1051/mbcb/2017005
40. Chen M, Kim GH, Prakash L, Woodley DT. Epidermolysis bullosa acquisita: autoimmunity to anchoring fibril collagen. *Autoimmunity.* (2012) 45:91–101. doi: 10.3109/08916934.2011.606450
41. Xu H-H, Werth VP, Parisi E, Sollecito TP. Mucous membrane pemphigoid. *Dent Clin North Am.* (2013) 57:611–30. doi: 10.1016/j.cden.2013.07.003
42. Bereshchenko O, Bruscoli S, Riccardi C. Glucocorticoids, sex hormones, and immunity. *Front Immunol.* (2018) 9:1332. doi: 10.3389/fimmu.2018.01332
43. Gibson RH, Hotham R, Bojarczuk A, Lewis A, Bielska E, May RC, et al. Mycophenolate mofetil increases susceptibility to opportunistic fungal infection independent of lymphocytes. *biorxiv [Preprint].* (2017). doi: 10.1101/131540
44. Patel AA, Swerlick RA, McCall CO. Azathioprine in dermatology: the past, the present, and the future. *J Am Acad Dermatol.* (2006) 55:369–89. doi: 10.1016/j.jaad.2005.07.059
45. Yamagami J. Recent advances in the understanding and treatment of pemphigus and pemphigoid. *F1000Research.* (2018) 7:1360. doi: 10.12688/f1000research.14474.1
46. Kirtschig G, Middleton P, Bennett C, Murrell DF, Wojnarowska F, Khumalo NP. Interventions for bullous pemphigoid. *Cochrane Database Syst Rev.* (2010) 6:CD002292. doi: 10.1002/14651858.CD002292.pub3
47. Kasperkiewicz M, Zillikens D, Schmidt E. Pemphigoid diseases: pathogenesis, diagnosis, and treatment. *Autoimmunity.* (2012) 45:55–70. doi: 10.3109/08916934.2011.606447
48. Gürcan HM, Ahmed AR. Efficacy of dapsone in the treatment of pemphigus and pemphigoid. *Am J Clin Dermatol.* (2009) 10:383–96. doi: 10.2165/11310740-000000000-00000
49. Fivenson DP, Breneman DL, Rosen GB, Hersh CS, Cardone S, Mutasim D. Nicotinamide and tetracycline therapy of bullous pemphigoid. *Arch Dermatol.* (1994) 130:753–8. doi: 10.1001/archderm.1994.01690060083010
50. Williams HC, Wojnarowska F, Kirtschig G, Mason J, Godec TR, Schmidt E, et al. Doxycycline versus prednisolone as an initial treatment strategy for bullous pemphigoid: a pragmatic, non-inferiority, randomised controlled trial. *Lancet.* (2017) 389:1630–8. doi: 10.1016/S0140-6736(17)30560-3
51. Beissert S, Werfel T, Frieling U, Böhm M, Sticherling M, Stadler R, et al. A comparison of oral methylprednisolone plus azathioprine or mycophenolate mofetil for the treatment of bullous pemphigoid. *Arch Dermatol.* (2007) 143:1536–42. doi: 10.1001/archderm.143.12.1536
52. Kasperkiewicz M, Shimanovich I, Ludwig RJ, Rose C, Zillikens D, Schmidt E. Rituximab for treatment-refractory pemphigus and pemphigoid: a case series of 17 patients. *J Am Acad Dermatol.* (2011) 65:552–8. doi: 10.1016/j.jaad.2010.07.032
53. Ishii N, Hashimoto T, Zillikens D, Ludwig RJ. High-Dose Intravenous Immunoglobulin (IVIG) therapy in autoimmune skin blistering diseases. *Clin Rev Allergy Immunol.* (2010) 38:186–95. doi: 10.1007/s12016-009-8153-y
54. Fairley JA, Baum CL, Brandt DS, Messingham KAN. Pathogenicity of IgE in autoimmunity: successful treatment of bullous pemphigoid with omalizumab. *J Allergy Clin Immunol.* (2009) 123:704–5. doi: 10.1016/j.jaci.2008.11.035
55. Ino N, Kamata N, Matsuura C, Shinkai H, Odaka M. Immunoadsorption for the treatment of bullous pemphigoid. *Ther Apher.* (1997) 1:372–6. doi: 10.1111/j.1744-9987.1997.tb00059.x
56. Giudice GJ, Emery DJ, Diaz LA. Cloning and primary structural analysis of the bullous pemphigoid autoantigen BP180. *J Invest Dermatol.* (1992) 99:243–50. doi: 10.1111/1523-1747.ep12616580
57. Stanley JR, Tanaka T, Mueller S, Klaus-Kovtun V, Roop D. Isolation of complementary DNA for bullous pemphigoid antigen by use of patients' autoantibodies. *J Clin Invest.* (1988) 82:1864–70. doi: 10.1172/JCI113803
58. Domloge-Hultsch N, Gammon WR, Briggaman RA, Gil SG, Carter WG, Yancey KB. Epiligrin, the major human keratinocyte integrin ligand, is a target in both an acquired autoimmune and an inherited subepidermal blistering skin disease. *J Clin Invest.* (1992) 90:1628–33. doi: 10.1172/JCI116033
59. Kirtschig G, Marinkovich MP, Burgeson RE, Yancey KB. Anti-basement membrane autoantibodies in patients with anti-epiligrin cicatricial pemphigoid bind the α subunit of laminin 5. *J Invest Dermatol.* (1995) 105:543–8. doi: 10.1111/1523-1747.ep12323431
60. Tyagi S, Bhol K, Natarajan K, Livir-Rallatos C, Foster CS, Ahmed AR. Ocular cicatricial pemphigoid antigen: partial sequence and biochemical characterization. *Proc Natl Acad Sci USA.* (1996) 93:14714–9. doi: 10.1073/pnas.93.25.14714
61. Bhol KC, Dans MJ, Simmons RK, Foster CS, Giancotti FG, Ahmed AR. The autoantibodies to alpha 6 beta 4 integrin of patients affected by ocular cicatricial pemphigoid recognize predominantly epitopes within the large cytoplasmic domain of human beta 4. *J Immunol.* (2000) 165:2824–9. doi: 10.4049/jimmunol.165.5.2824
62. Rashid KA, Gürcan HM, Razzaque Ahmed A. Antigen specificity in subsets of mucous membrane pemphigoid. *J Invest Dermatol.* (2006) 126:2631–6. doi: 10.1038/sj.jid.5700465

63. Cozzani E, Di Zenzo G, Calabresi V, Carrozzo M, Burlando M, Longanesi L, et al. Autoantibody profile of a cohort of 78 Italian patients with mucous membrane pemphigoid: correlation between reactivity profile and clinical involvement. *Acta Derm Venereol.* (2014) 96:768–73. doi: 10.2340/00015555-2311
64. Peter Marinkovich M, Taylor TB, Keene DR, Burgeson RE, Zone JJ. LAD-1, the linear IgA bullous dermatosis autoantigen, is a novel 120-kDa anchoring filament protein synthesized by epidermal cells. *J Invest Dermatol.* (1996) 106:734–8. doi: 10.1111/1523-1747.ep12345782
65. Zone JJ, Taylor TB, Kadunce DP, Meyer LJ. Identification of the cutaneous basement membrane zone antigen and isolation of antibody in linear immunoglobulin A bullous dermatosis. *J Clin Invest.* (1990) 85:812–20. doi: 10.1172/JCI114508
66. Dainichi T, Kurono S, Ohyama B, Ishii N, Sanzen N, Hayashi M, et al. Anti-laminin gamma-1 pemphigoid. *Proc Natl Acad Sci USA.* (2009) 106:2800–5. doi: 10.1073/pnas.0809230106
67. Giudice GJ, Emery DJ, Zelickson BD, Anhalt GJ, Liu Z, Diaz LA. Bullous pemphigoid and herpes gestationis autoantibodies recognize a common non-collagenous site on the BP180 ectodomain. *J Immunol.* (1993) 151:5742–50. doi: 10.1016/0923-1811(93)90940-Q
68. Morrison LH, Labib RS, Zone JJ, Diaz LA, Anhalt GJ. Herpes gestationis autoantibodies recognize a 180-kD human epidermal antigen. *J Clin Invest.* (1988) 81:2023–6. doi: 10.1172/JCI113554
69. Hsu S, Ghohestani RF, Uitto J. Lichen planus pemphigoides with IgG autoantibodies to the 180 kd bullous pemphigoid antigen (type XVII collagen). *J Am Acad Dermatol.* (2000) 42:136–41. doi: 10.1016/S0190-9622(00)90024-0
70. Skaria M, Salomon D, Jaunin F, Friedli A, Saurat J-H, Borradori L. IgG Autoantibodies from a Lichen planus pemphigoides patient recognize the NC16A domain of the bullous pemphigoid antigen 180. *Dermatology.* (1999) 199:253–5. doi: 10.1159/000018257
71. Chen M, Chan LS, Cai X, O'Toole EA, Sample JC, Woodley DT. Development of an ELISA for rapid detection of anti-type VII collagen autoantibodies in epidermolysis bullosa acquisita. *J Invest Dermatol.* (1997) 108:68–72. doi: 10.1111/1523-1747.ep12285634
72. Oyama N, Setterfield JF, Powell AM, Sakuma-Oyama Y, Albert S, Bhogal BS, et al. Bullous pemphigoid antigen II (BP180) and its soluble extracellular domains are major autoantigens in mucous membrane pemphigoid: the pathogenic relevance to HLA class II alleles and disease severity. *Br J Dermatol.* (2006) 154:90–8. doi: 10.1111/j.1365-2133.2005.06998.x
73. Schmidt E, Skrobek C, Kromminga A, Hashimoto T, Messer G, Brocker E-B, et al. Cicatricial pemphigoid: IgA and IgG autoantibodies target epitopes on both intra- and extracellular domains of bullous pemphigoid antigen 180. *Br J Dermatol.* (2001) 145:778–83. doi: 10.1046/j.1365-2133.2001.04471.x
74. Balding SD, Prost C, Diaz LA, Bernard P, Bedane C, Aberdam D, et al. Cicatricial pemphigoid autoantibodies react with multiple sites on the BP180 extracellular domain. *J Invest Dermatol.* (1996) 106:141–6. doi: 10.1111/1523-1747.ep12329728
75. Walko G, Castañón MJ, Wiche G. Molecular architecture and function of the hemidesmosome. *Cell Tissue Res.* (2015) 360:363–78. doi: 10.1007/s00441-014-2061-z
76. Hopkinson SB, Hamill KJ, Wu Y, Eisenberg JL, Hiroyasu S, Jones JCR. Focal contact and hemidesmosomal proteins in keratinocyte migration and wound repair. *Adv Wound Care.* (2014) 3:247–63. doi: 10.1089/wound.2013.0489
77. Fine JD, Eady RAJ, Bauer EA, Bauer JW, Bruckner-Tuderman L, Heagerty A, et al. The classification of inherited epidermolysis bullosa (EB): Report of the Third International Consensus Meeting on Diagnosis and Classification of EB. *J Am Acad Dermatol.* (2008) 58:931–50. doi: 10.1016/j.jaad.2008.02.004
78. Liu Y, Li L, Xia Y. BP180 is critical in the autoimmunity of bullous pemphigoid. *Front Immunol.* (2017) 8:1752. doi: 10.3389/fimmu.2017.01752
79. Iwata H, Jonkman MF, Koga H, Ludwig RJ, Prost-Squarcioni C, Bieber K. Epidermolysis bullosa acquisita: the 2019 update. *Front Med.* (2019) 5:362. doi: 10.3389/fmed.2018.00362
80. Zakka LR, Reche P, Ahmed AR. Role of MHC class II genes in the pathogenesis of pemphigoid. *Autoimmun Rev.* (2011) 11:40–7. doi: 10.1016/j.autrev.2011.07.002
81. Büdinger L, Borradori L, Yee C, Eming R, Ferencik S, Grosse-Wilde H, et al. Identification and characterization of autoreactive T cell responses to bullous pemphigoid antigen 2 in patients and healthy controls. *J Clin Invest.* (1998) 102:2082–9. doi: 10.1172/JCI3335
82. Gammon WR, Heise ER, Burke WA, Fine J-D, Woodley DT, Briggaman RA. Increased frequency of HLA-DR2 in patients with autoantibodies to epidermolysis bullosa acquisita antigen: evidence that the expression of autoimmunity to type VII collagen is HLA class II allele associated. *J Invest Dermatol.* (1988) 91:228–32. doi: 10.1111/1523-1747.ep12470317
83. Zumelzu C, Le Roux-Villet C, Loiseau P, Busson M, Heller M, Aucouturier F, et al. Black patients of African descent and HLA-DRB1*15:03 frequency overrepresented in epidermolysis bullosa acquisita. *J Invest Dermatol.* (2011) 131:2386–93. doi: 10.1038/jid.2011.231
84. Ujiie H. Regulatory T cells in autoimmune skin diseases. *Exp Dermatol.* (2019) 28:642–6. doi: 10.1111/exd.13535
85. Antiga E, Quaglino P, Volpi W, Pierini I, Del Bianco E, Bianchi B, et al. Regulatory T cells in skin lesions and blood of patients with bullous pemphigoid. *J Eur Acad Dermatol Venereol.* (2014) 28:222–30. doi: 10.1111/jdv.12091
86. Liu Z, Diaz LA, Troy JL, Taylor AF, Emery DJ, Fairley JA, Giudice GJ. A passive transfer model of the organ-specific autoimmune disease, bullous pemphigoid, using antibodies generated against the hemidesmosomal antigen, BP180. *J Clin Invest.* (1993) 92:2480–8. doi: 10.1172/JCI116856
87. Sitaru C, Mihai S, Otto C, Chiriac MT, Hausser I, Dotterweich B, et al. Induction of dermal-epidermal separation in mice by passive transfer of antibodies specific to type VII collagen. *J Clin Invest.* (2005) 115:870–8. doi: 10.1172/JCI200521386
88. Heppe EN, Tofern S, Schulze FS, Ishiko A, Shimizu A, Sina C, et al. Experimental laminin 332 mucous membrane pemphigoid critically involves C5aR1 and reflects clinical and immunopathological characteristics of the human disease. *J Invest Dermatol.* (2017) 137:1709–18. doi: 10.1016/j.jid.2017.03.037
89. Zone JJ, Egan CA, Taylor TB, Meyer LJ. Iga autoimmune disorders: development of a passive transfer mouse model. *J Investig Dermatology Symp Proc.* (2004) 9:47–51. doi: 10.1111/j.1087-0024.2004.00840.x
90. Darling T, Briggaman RA, Yancey KB, Lazarova Z, Yee C. Passive transfer of anti-laminin 5 antibodies induces subepidermal blisters in neonatal mice. *J Clin Invest.* (2008) 98:1509–18. doi: 10.1172/JCI118942
91. Lazarova Z, Hsu R, Yee C, Yancey KB. Human anti-laminin 5 autoantibodies induce subepidermal blisters in an experimental human skin graft model. *J Invest Dermatol.* (2000) 114:178–84. doi: 10.1046/j.1523-1747.2000.00829.x
92. Gammon WR, Merritt CC, Lewis DM, Sams WM, Carlo JR, Wheeler CE. An *in vitro* model of immune complex-mediated basement membrane zone separation caused by pemphigoid antibodies, leukocytes, and complement. *J Invest Dermatol.* (1982) 78:285–90. doi: 10.1111/1523-1747.ep12507222
93. Sitaru C, Schmidt E, Petermann S, Munteanu LS, Brocker EB, Zillikens D. Autoantibodies to bullous pemphigoid antigen 180 induce dermal-epidermal separation in cryosections of human skin. *J Invest Dermatol.* (2002) 118:664–71. doi: 10.1046/j.1523-1747.2002.01720.x
94. Sitaru C, Kromminga A, Hashimoto T, Bro EB. Autoantibodies to type VII collagen mediate Fcg -dependent neutrophil activation and induce dermal-epidermal separation in cryosections of human skin. *Am J Pathol.* (2002) 161:301–11. doi: 10.1016/S0002-9440(10)64182-X
95. Shimanovich I, Mihai S, Oostingh GJ, Ilenchuk TT, Bröcker EB, Opdenakker G, et al. Granulocyte-derived elastase and gelatinase B are required for dermal-epidermal separation induced by autoantibodies from patients with epidermolysis bullosa acquisita and bullous pemphigoid. *J Pathol.* (2004) 204:519–27. doi: 10.1002/path.1674
96. Liu Z, Giudice GJ, Zhou X, Swartz SJ, Troy JL, Fairley JA, et al. A major role for neutrophils in experimental bullous pemphigoid. *J Clin Invest.* (1997) 100:1256–63. doi: 10.1172/JCI119639
97. Teng T-S, Ji A, Ji X-Y, Li Y-Z. Neutrophils and immunity: from bactericidal action to being conquered. *J Immunol Res.* (2017) 2017:1–14. doi: 10.1155/2017/9671604
98. Segal AW. How neutrophils kill microbes. *Annu Rev Immunol.* (2005) 23:197–223. doi: 10.1146/annurev.immunol.23.021704.115653
99. López-Otín C, Bond JS. Proteases: multifunctional enzymes in life and disease. *J Biol Chem.* (2008) 283:30433–7. doi: 10.1074/jbc.R800035200
100. Fu Z, Thorpe M, Akula S, Chahal G, Hellman LT. Extended cleavage specificity of human neutrophil elastase, human proteinase 3, and their

distant ortholog clawed frog PR3 — three elastases with similar primary but different extended specificities and stability. Front Immunol. (2018) 9:2387. doi: 10.3389/fimmu.2018.02387

101. Korkmaz B, Horwitz MS, Jenne DE, Gauthier F. Neutrophil elastase, proteinase 3, and cathepsin G as therapeutic targets in human diseases. *Pharmacol Rev.* (2010) 62:726–59. doi: 10.1124/pr.110.002733
102. Janoff A. Human granulocyte elastase. Further delineation of its role in connective tissue damage. *Am J Pathol.* (1972) 68:579–92.
103. Clark JM, Vaughan DW, Aiken BM, Kagan HM. Elastase-like enzymes in human neutrophils localized by ultrastructural cytochemistry. *J Cell Biol.* (1980) 84:102–19. doi: 10.1083/jcb.84.1.102
104. Kobayashi SD, Voyich JM, Burlak C, DeLeo FR. Neutrophils in the innate immune response. *Arch Immunol Ther Exp.* (2005) 53:505–17. doi: 10.1055/s-2005-870318
105. Belaaouaj A, McCarthy R, Baumann M, Gao Z, Ley TJ, Abraham SN, Shapiro SD. Mice lacking neutrophil elastase reveal impaired host defense against gram negative bacterial sepsis. *Nat Med.* (1998) 4:615–8. doi: 10.1038/nm0598-615
106. López-Boado YS, Espinola M, Bahr S, Belaaouaj A. Neutrophil serine proteinases cleave bacterial flagellin, abrogating its host response-inducing activity. *J Immunol.* (2004) 172:509–15. doi: 10.4049/jimmunol.172.1.509
107. Belaaouaj A, Kim KS, Shapiro SD. Degradation of outer membrane protein A in *Escherichia coli* killing by neutrophil elastase. *Science.* (2000) 289:1185–8. doi: 10.1126/science.289.5482.1185
108. Johansson A, Claesson R, Hänström L, Sandström G, Kalfas S. Polymorphonuclear leukocyte degranulation induced by leukotoxin from *Actinobacillus actinomycetemcomitans. J Periodontal Res.* (2000) 35:85–92. doi: 10.1034/j.1600-0765.2000.035002085.x
109. Benabid R, Wartelle J, Malleret L, Guyot N, Gangloff S, Lebargy F, et al. Neutrophil elastase modulates cytokine expression: contribution to host defense against *Pseudomonas aeruginosa*-induced pneumonia. *J Biol Chem.* (2012) 287:34883–94. doi: 10.1074/jbc.M112.361352
110. Zhu J, Nathan C, Jin W, Sim D, Ashcroft GS, Wahl SM, et al. Conversion of proepithelin to epithelins: roles of SLPI and elastase in host defense and wound repair. *Cell.* (2002) 111:867–78. doi: 10.1016/S0092-8674(02)01141-8
111. Bank U, Ansorge S. More than destructive: neutrophil-derived serine proteases in cytokine bioactivity control. *J Leukoc Biol.* (2001) 69:197–206. doi: 10.1189/JLB.69.2.197
112. Pham CTN. Neutrophil serine proteases : specific regulators of inflammation. *Nat Rev Immunol.* (2006) 6:541–50. doi: 10.1038/nri1841
113. Meyer-Hoffert U. Neutrophil-derived serine proteases modulate innate immune responses. *Front Biosci.* (2009) 14:3462. doi: 10.2741/3462
114. Tsai Y-F, Hwang T-L. Neutrophil elastase inhibitors: a patent review and potential applications for inflammatory lung diseases (2010 – 2014). *Expert Opin Ther Pat.* (2015) 25:1145–58. doi: 10.1517/13543776.2015.1061998
115. Rees DD, Rogers RA, Cooley J, Mandle RJ, Kenney DM, Remold-O'Donnell E. Recombinant human monocyte/neutrophil elastase inhibitor protects rat lungs against injury from cystic fibrosis airway secretions. *Am J Respir Cell Mol Biol.* (1999) 20:69–78. doi: 10.1165/ajrcmb.20.1.3306
116. Churg A, Wang RD, Xie C, Wright JL. α-1-antitrypsin ameliorates cigarette smoke–induced emphysema in the mouse. *Am J Respir Crit Care Med.* (2003) 168:199–207. doi: 10.1164/rccm.200302-203OC
117. Takeuchi H, Gomi T, Shishido M, Watanabe H, Suenobu N. Neutrophil elastase contributes to extracellular matrix damage induced by chronic low-dose UV irradiation in a hairless mouse photoaging model. *J Dermatol Sci.* (2010) 60:151–8. doi: 10.1016/j.jdermsci.2010.09.001
118. Rogalski C, Meyer-Hoffert U, Proksch E, Wiedow O. Human leukocyte elastase induces keratinocyte proliferation *in vitro* and *in vivo*. *J Invest Dermatol.* (2002) 118:49–54. doi: 10.1046/j.0022-202x.2001.01650.x
119. Starcher B, O'Neal P, Granstein RD, Beissert S. Inhibition of neutrophil elastase suppresses the development of skin tumors in hairless mice. *J Invest Dermatol.* (1996) 107:159–63. doi: 10.1111/1523-1747.ep12329559
120. Wang Y, Xiao Y, Zhong L, Ye D, Zhang J, Tu Y, et al. Increased neutrophil elastase and proteinase 3 and augmented NETosis are closely associated with β-cell autoimmunity in patients with type 1 diabetes. *Diabetes.* (2014) 63:4239–48. doi: 10.2337/db14-0480
121. Laurell CB, Eriksson S. The electrophoretic α;1-globulin pattern of serum in α;1-antitrypsin deficiency. *Scand J Clin Lab Invest.* (1963) 15:132–40. doi: 10.1080/00365516309051324
122. Oikarinen AI, Zone JJ, Ahmed AR, Kiistala U, Uitto J. Demonstration of collagenase and elastase activities in the blister fluids from bullous skin diseases. Comparison between dermatitis herpetiformis and bullous pemphigoid. *J Invest Dermatol.* (1983) 81:261–6. doi: 10.1111/1523-1747.ep12518285
123. Oikarinen AI, Reunala T, Zone JJ, Kiistala U, Uitto J. Proteolytic enzymes in blister fluids from patients with dermatitis herpetiformis. *Br J Dermatol.* (1986) 114:295–302. doi: 10.1111/j.1365-2133.1986.tb02820.x
124. Verraes S, Hornebeck W, Polette M, Borradori L, Bernard P. Respective contribution of neutrophil elastase and matrix metalloproteinase 9 in the degradation of BP180 (type XVII collagen) in human bullous pemphigoid. *J Invest Dermatol.* (2001) 117:1091–6. doi: 10.1046/j.0022-202x.2001.01521.x
125. Liu Z, Zhou X, Shapiro SD, Shipley JM, Twining SS, Diaz L, et al. The serpin alpha1-proteinase inhibitor is a critical substrate for gelatinase B/MMP-9 *in vivo*. *Cell.* (2000) 102:647–55. doi: 10.1016/S0092-8674(00)00087-8
126. Liu Z, Fairley JA, Diaz LA, Liu Z, Shapiro SD, Zhou X, et al. A critical role for neutrophil elastase in experimental bullous pemphigoid. *J Clin Invest.* (2000) 105:113–23. doi: 10.1172/JCI3693
127. Lin L, Betsuyaku T, Heimbach L, Li N, Rubenstein D, Shapiro SD, et al. Neutrophil elastase cleaves the murine hemidesmosomal protein BP180/type XVII collagen and generates degradation products that modulate experimental bullous pemphigoid. *Matrix Biol.* (2012) 31:38–44. doi: 10.1016/j.matbio.2011.09.003
128. Mydel P, Shipley JM, Adair-kirk TL, Kelley DG, Broekelmann TJ, Mecham RP, et al. Neutrophil elastase cleaves laminin-332 (laminin-5) generating peptides that are chemotactic for neutrophils. *J Biol Chem.* (2008) 283:9513–22. doi: 10.1074/jbc.M706239200
129. Van den Bergh F, Eliason SL, Burmeister BT, Giudice GJ. Collagen XVII (BP180) modulates keratinocyte expression of the proinflammatory chemokine, IL-8. *Exp Dermatol.* (2012) 21:605–11. doi: 10.1111/j.1600-0625.2012.01529.x
130. Kawabata K, Suzuki M, Sugitani M, Imaki K, Toda M, Miyamoto T. ONO-5046, a novel inhibitor of human neutrophil elastase. *Biochem Biophys Res Commun.* (1991) 177:814–20. doi: 10.1016/0006-291X(91)91862-7
131. Stevens T, Ekholm K, Gränse M, Lindahl M, Kozma V, Jungar C, et al. AZD9668: pharmacological characterization of a novel oral inhibitor of neutrophil elastase. *J Pharmacol Exp Ther.* (2011) 339:313–20. doi: 10.1124/jpet.111.182139
132. Yu X, Akbarzadeh R, Pieper M, Scholzen T, Gehrig S, Schultz C, et al. Neutrophil adhesion is a prerequisite for antibody-mediated proteolytic tissue damage in experimental models of epidermolysis bullosa acquisita. *J Invest Dermatol.* (2018) 138:1990–8. doi: 10.1016/j.jid.2018.03.1499
133. Verma RP, Hansch C. Matrix metalloproteinases (MMPs): chemical-biological functions and (Q)SARs. *Bioorgan Med Chem.* (2007) 15:2223–68. doi: 10.1016/j.bmc.2007.01.011
134. Nissinen L, Kähäri VM. Matrix metalloproteinases in inflammation. *Biochim Biophys Acta.* (2014) 1840:2571–80. doi: 10.1016/j.bbagen.2014.03.007
135. Visse R, Nagase H. Matrix metalloproteinases and tissue inhibitors of metalloproteinases. *Circ Res.* (2003) 92:827–39. doi: 10.1161/01.RES.0000070112.80711.3D
136. Van Wart HE, Birkedal-Hansen H. The cysteine switch: a principle of regulation of metalloproteinase activity with potential applicability to the entire matrix metalloproteinase gene family. *Proc Natl Acad Sci USA.* (1990) 87:5578–82. doi: 10.1073/pnas.87.14.5578
137. Klein T, Bischoff R. Physiology and pathophysiology of matrix metalloproteases. *Amino Acids.* (2011) 41:271–90. doi: 10.1007/s00726-010-0689-x
138. Rodríguez D, Morrison CJ, Overall CM. Matrix metalloproteinases: what do they not do? New substrates and biological roles identified by murine models and proteomics. *Biochim Biophys Acta.* (2010) 1803:39–54. doi: 10.1016/j.bbamcr.2009.09.015
139. Dufour A, Overall CM. Missing the target: matrix metalloproteinase antitargets in inflammation and cancer. *Trends Pharmacol Sci.* (2013) 34:233–42. doi: 10.1016/j.tips.2013.02.004

140. Rundhaug JE. Matrix metalloproteinases and angiogenesis. *J Cell Mol Med.* (2007) 9:267–85. doi: 10.1111/j.1582-4934.2005.tb00355.x
141. Vu TH, Werb Z. Matrix metalloproteinases: effectors of development and normal physiology. *Genes Dev.* (2000) 14:2123–33. doi: 10.1101/gad.815400
142. Caley MP, Martins VLC, O'Toole EA. Metalloproteinases and wound healing. *Adv Wound Care.* (2015) 4:225–34. doi: 10.1089/wound.2014.0581
143. Brew K, Nagase H. The tissue inhibitors of metalloproteinases (TIMPs): An ancient family with structural and functional diversity. *Biochim Biophys Acta.* (2010) 1803:55–71. doi: 10.1016/j.bbamcr.2010.01.003
144. Winer A, Adams S, Mignatti P. Matrix metalloproteinase inhibitors in cancer therapy: turning past failures into future successes. *Mol Cancer Ther.* (2018) 17:1147–55. doi: 10.1158/1535-7163.MCT-17-0646
145. Ram M, Sherer Y, Shoenfeld Y. Matrix metalloproteinase-9 and autoimmune diseases. *J Clin Immunol.* (2006) 26:299–307. doi: 10.1007/s10875-006-9022-6
146. Rybakowski JK. Matrix Metalloproteinase-9 (MMP9)-a mediating enzyme in cardiovascular disease, cancer, and neuropsychiatric disorders. *Cardiovasc Psychiatry Neurol.* (2009) 2009:904836. doi: 10.1155/2009/904836
147. Yabluchanskiy A, Ma Y, Iyer RP, Hall ME, Lindsey ML. Matrix metalloproteinase-9: many shades of function in cardiovascular disease. *Physiology.* (2013) 28:391–403. doi: 10.1152/physiol.00029.2013
148. Ståhle-Bäckdahl M, Inoue M, Giudice GJ, Parks WC. 92-kD gelatinase is produced by eosinophils at the site of blister formation in bullous pemphigoid and cleaves the extracellular domain of recombinant 180-kD bullous pemphigoid autoantigen. *J Clin Invest.* (1994) 93:2022–30. doi: 10.1172/JCI117196
149. Pugin J, Widmer M-C, Kossodo S, Liang C-M, Preas HL, Suffredini AF. Human neutrophils secrete gelatinase B *in vitro* and *in vivo* in response to endotoxin and proinflammatory mediators. *Am J Respir Cell Mol Biol.* (1999) 20:458–464. doi: 10.1165/ajrcmb.20.3.3311
150. Vandooren J, Van Den Steen PE, Opdenakker G. Biochemistry and molecular biology of gelatinase B or matrix metalloproteinase-9 (MMP-9): the next decade. *Crit Rev Biochem Mol Biol.* (2013) 48:222–72. doi: 10.3109/10409238.2013.770819
151. Galis ZS, Sukhova GK, Kranzhöfer R, Clark S, Libby P. Macrophage foam cells from experimental atheroma constitutively produce matrix-degrading proteinases. *Proc Natl Acad Sci USA.* (1995) 92:402–6. doi: 10.1073/pnas.92.2.402
152. Chelladurai P, Seeger W, Pullamsetti SS. Series "matrix metalloproteinases in lung health and disease": matrix metalloproteinases and their inhibitors in pulmonary hypertension. *Eur Respir J.* (2012) 40:766–82. doi: 10.1183/09031936.00209911
153. Xu D, Suenaga N, Edelmann MJ, Fridman R, Muschel RJ, Kessler BM. Novel MMP-9 substrates in cancer cells revealed by a label-free quantitative proteomics approach. *Mol Cell Proteomics.* (2008) 7:2215–28. doi: 10.1074/mcp.M800095-MCP200
154. Prudova A, auf dem Keller U, Butler GS, Overall CM. Multiplex N-terminome analysis of MMP-2 and MMP-9 substrate degradomes by iTRAQ-TAILS quantitative proteomics. *Mol Cell Proteomics.* (2010) 9:894–911. doi: 10.1074/mcp.M000050-MCP201
155. Oikarinen A, Kylmäniemi M, Autio-Harmainen H, Autio P, Salo T. Demonstration of 72-kDa and 92-kDa forms of type IV collagenase in human skin: variable expression in various blistering diseases, induction during re-epithelialization, and decrease by topical glucocorticoids. *J Invest Dermatol.* (1993) 101:205–10. doi: 10.1111/1523-1747.ep12363823
156. Niimi Y, Pawankar R, Kawana S. Increased expression of matrix metalloproteinase-2, matrix metalloproteinase-9 and matrix metalloproteinase-13 in lesional skin of bullous pemphigoid. *Int Arch Allergy Immunol.* (2006) 139:104–13. doi: 10.1159/000090385
157. Zebrowska A, Wagrowska-Danilewicz M, Danilewicz M, Stasikowska-Kanicka O, Kulczycka-Siennicka L, Wozniacka A, et al. Mediators of mast cells in bullous pemphigoid and dermatitis herpetiformis. *Mediators Inflamm.* (2014) 2014:936545. doi: 10.1155/2014/936545
158. Le Jan S, Plée J, Vallerand D, Dupont A, Delanez E, Durlach A, et al. Innate immune cell-produced IL-17 sustains inflammation in bullous pemphigoid. *J Invest Dermatol.* (2014) 134:2908–17. doi: 10.1038/jid.2014.263
159. Liu Y, Peng L, Li L, Liu C, Hu X, Xiao S, et al. TWEAK/Fn14 activation contributes to the pathogenesis of bullous pemphigoid. *J Invest Dermatol.* (2017) 137:1188–9. doi: 10.1016/j.jid.2017.03.019
160. Arafat SN, Suelves AM, Spurr-Michaud S, Chodosh J, Foster CS, Dohlman CH, et al. Neutrophil collagenase, gelatinase, and myeloperoxidase in tears of patients with Stevens-Johnson syndrome and ocular cicatricial pemphigoid. *Ophthalmology.* (2014) 121:79–87. doi: 10.1016/j.ophtha.2013.06.049
161. Chan MF, Sack R, Quigley DA, Sathe S, Vijmasi T, Li S, et al. Membrane array analysis of tear proteins in ocular cicatricial pemphigoid. *Optom Vis Sci.* (2011) 88:1005–9. doi: 10.1097/OPX.0b013e31821ddc6c
162. Liu Z, Shipley JM, Vu TH, Zhou XY, Diaz LA, Werb Z, et al. Gelatinase B-deficient mice are resistant to experimental bullous pemphigoid. *J Exp Med.* (1998) 188:475–82. doi: 10.1084/jem.188.3.475
163. Liu Z, Li N, Diaz LA, Shipley JM, Senior RM, Werb Z. Synergy between a plasminogen cascade and MMP-9 in autoimmune disease. *J Clin Invest.* (2005) 115:879–87. doi: 10.1172/JCI23977
164. Qiao P, Dang E, Cao T, Fang H, Zhang J, Qiao H, et al. Dysregulation of mCD46 and sCD46 contribute to the pathogenesis of bullous pemphigoid. *Sci Rep.* (2017) 7:1–9. doi: 10.1038/s41598-017-00235-3
165. Mair YH, Jhamb T, Visser MB, Aguirre A, Kramer JM. Sera and salivary matrix metalloproteinases are elevated in patients with vesiculoerosive disease: a pilot study. *Oral Surg Oral Med Oral Pathol Oral Radiol.* (2016) 121:520–9. doi: 10.1016/j.oooo.2016.01.002
166. Tukaj S, Hellberg L, Ueck C, Hänsel M, Samavedam U, Zillikens D, et al. Heat shock protein 90 is required for *ex vivo* neutrophil-driven autoantibody-induced tissue damage in experimental epidermolysis bullosa acquisita. *Exp Dermatol.* (2015) 24:471–3. doi: 10.1111/exd.12680
167. Airola K, Vaalamo M, Reunala T, Saarialho-Kere UK. Enhanced expression of interstitial collagenase, stromelysin-1, and urokinase plasminogen activator in lesions of dermatitis herpetiformis. *J Invest Dermatol.* (1995) 105:184–9. doi: 10.1111/1523-1747.ep12317093
168. Airola K, Reunala T, Salo S, Saarialho-Kere UK. Urokinase plasminogen activator is expressed by basal keratinocytes before interstitial collagenase, stromelysin-1, and laminin-5 in experimentally induced dermatitis herpetiformis lesions. *J Invest Dermatol.* (1997) 108:7–11. doi: 10.1111/1523-1747.ep12285610
169. Fujimura T, Kakizaki A, Furudate S, Aiba S. A possible interaction between periostin and CD163+ skin-resident macrophages in pemphigus vulgaris and bullous pemphigoid. *Exp Dermatol.* (2017) 26:1193–8. doi: 10.1111/exd.13157
170. Cui N, Hu M, Khalil RA. Biochemical and biological attributes of matrix metalloproteinases. *Prog Mol Biol Transl Sci.* (2017) 147:1–73. doi: 10.1016/bs.pmbts.2017.02.005
171. Franzke CW, Tasanen K, Schacke H, Zhou Z, Tryggvason K, Mauch C, et al. Transmembrane collagen XVII, an epithelial adhesion protein, is shed from the cell surface by ADAMs. *EMBO J.* (2002) 21:5026–35. doi: 10.1093/emboj/cdf532
172. Li Y, Sun B, Zhao X, Wang X, Zhang D, Gu Q, et al. MMP-2 and MMP-13 affect vasculogenic mimicry formation in large cell lung cancer. *J Cell Mol Med.* (2017) 21:3741–51. doi: 10.1111/jcmm.13283
173. Wang M, Qin X, Mudgett JS, Ferguson TA, Senior RM, Welgus HG. Matrix metalloproteinase deficiencies affect contact hypersensitivity: stromelysin-1 deficiency prevents the response and gelatinase B deficiency prolongs the response. *Proc Natl Acad Sci USA.* (1999) 96:6885–9. doi: 10.1073/pnas.96.12.6885
174. Flores-Pliego A, Espejel-Nuñez A, Castillo-Castrejon M, Meraz-Cruz N, Beltran-Montoya J, Zaga-Clavellina V, et al. Matrix Metalloproteinase-3 (MMP-3) is an endogenous activator of the MMP-9 Secreted by placental leukocytes: implication in human labor. *PLoS ONE.* (2015) 10:e0145366. doi: 10.1371/journal.pone.0145366
175. Tewari A, Grys K, Kollet J, Sarkany R, Young AR. Upregulation of MMP12 and its activity by UVA1 in human skin: potential implications for photoaging. *J Invest Dermatol.* (2014) 134:2598–609. doi: 10.1038/jid.2014.173
176. Knäuper V, Smith B, López-Otin C, Murphy G. Activation of progelatinase B (proMMP-9) by active collagenase-3 (MMP-13). *Eur J Biochem.* (1997) 248:369–73. doi: 10.1111/j.1432-1033.1997.00369.x

177. Shah MA, Starodub A, Sharma S, Berlin J, Patel M, Wainberg ZA, et al. Andecaliximab/GS-5745 alone and combined with mFOLFOX6 in advanced gastric and gastroesophageal junction adenocarcinoma: results from a phase I study. *Clin Cancer Res.* (2018) 24:3829–37. doi: 10.1158/1078-0432.CCR-17-2469
178. Benjamin MM, Khalil RA. Matrix metalloproteinase inhibitors as investigative tools in the pathogenesis and management of vascular disease. *Exp Suppl.* (2013) 103:209–9. doi: 10.1007/978-3-0348-0364-9_7
179. Zhang C, Gong W, Liu H, Guo Z, Ge S. Inhibition of matrix metalloproteinase-9 with low-dose doxycycline reduces acute lung injury induced by cardiopulmonary bypass. *Int J Clin Exp Med.* (2014) 7:4975–82.
180. Sochor M, Richter S, Schmidt A, Hempel S, Hopt UT, Keck T. Inhibition of matrix metalloproteinase-9 with doxycycline reduces pancreatitis-associated lung injury. *Digestion.* (2009) 80:65–73. doi: 10.1159/000212080
181. Lindeman JHN, Abdul-Hussien H, van Bockel JH, Wolterbeek R, Kleemann R. Clinical trial of doxycycline for matrix metalloproteinase-9 inhibition in patients with an abdominal aneurysm. *Circulation.* (2009) 119:2209–16. doi: 10.1161/CIRCULATIONAHA.108.806505
182. Draxler D, Sashindranath M, Medcalf R. Plasmin: a modulator of immune function. *Semin Thromb Hemost.* (2016) 43:143–53. doi: 10.1055/s-0036-1586227
183. Cesarman-Maus G, Hajjar KA. Molecular mechanisms of fibrinolysis. *Br J Haematol.* (2005) 129:307–21. doi: 10.1111/j.1365-2141.2005.05444.x
184. Syrovets T, Lunov O, Simmet T. Plasmin as a proinflammatory cell activator. *J Leukoc Biol.* (2012) 92:509–19. doi: 10.1189/jlb.0212056
185. Raum D, Marcus D, Alper CA, Levey R, Taylor PD, Starzl TE. Synthesis of human plasminogen by the liver. *Science.* (1980) 208:1036–7. doi: 10.1126/science.6990488
186. Weinstein MJ, Doolittle RF. Differential specificities of thrombin, plasmin and trypsin with regard to synthetic and natural substrates and inhibitors. *Biochim Biophys Acta.* (1972) 258:577–90. doi: 10.1016/0005-2744(72)90250-1
187. Amara U, Flierl MA, Rittirsch D, Klos A, Chen H, Acker B, et al. Molecular intercommunication between the complement and coagulation systems. *J Immunol.* (2010) 185:5628–36. doi: 10.4049/jimmunol.0903678
188. Jiang Q, Taupenot L, Mahata SK, Mahata M, O'Connor DT, Miles LA, et al. Proteolytic cleavage of chromogranin A (CgA) by plasmin. Selective liberation of a specific bioactive CgA fragment that regulates catecholamine release. *J Biol Chem.* (2001) 276:25022–9. doi: 10.1074/jbc.M101545200
189. Lijnen HR. Molecular interactions between the plasminogen/plasmin and matrix metalloproteinase systems. *Fibrinolysis Proteolysis.* (2000) 14:175–181. doi: 10.1054/fipr.2000.0065
190. Saksela O, Rifkin DB. Release of basic fibroblast growth factor-heparan sulfate complexes from endothelial cells by plasminogen activator-mediated proteolytic activity. *J Cell Biol.* (1990) 110:767–75. doi: 10.1083/jcb.110.3.767
191. Lyons RM, Keski-Oja J, Moses HL. Proteolytic activation of latent transforming growth factor-beta from fibroblast-conditioned medium. *J Cell Biol.* (1988) 106:1659–65. doi: 10.1083/jcb.106.5.1659
192. Vakili J, Ständker L, Detheux M, Vassart G, Forssmann WG, Parmentier M. Urokinase plasminogen activator and plasmin efficiently convert hemofiltrate CC chemokine 1 into its active. *J Immunol.* (2001) 167:3406–13. doi: 10.4049/jimmunol.167.6.3406
193. Waltz DA, Natkin LR, Fujita RM, Wei Y, Chapman HA. Plasmin and plasminogen activator inhibitor type 1 promote cellular motility by regulating the interaction between the urokinase receptor and vitronectin. *J Clin Invest.* (1997) 100:58–67. doi: 10.1172/JCI119521
194. Deryugina EI, Quigley JP. Cell surface remodeling by plasmin: a new function for an old enzyme. *J Biomed Biotechnol.* (2012) 2012:564259. doi: 10.1155/2012/564259
195. Shen Y, Guo Y, Mikus P, Sulniute R, Wilczynska M, Ny T, et al. Plasminogen is a key proinflammatory regulator that accelerates the healing of acute and diabetic wounds. *Blood.* (2012) 119:5879–87. doi: 10.1182/blood-2012-01-407825
196. Aisina RB, Mukhametova LI. Structure and function of plasminogen/plasmin system. *Russ J Bioorg Chem.* (2014) 40:590–605. doi: 10.1134/S1068162014060028
197. Kwaan HC, McMahon B. *The Role of Plasminogen-Plasmin System in Cancer.* Boston, MA: Springer. 43–66. doi: 10.1007/978-0-387-79962-9_4
198. Kuramoto E, Nishiuma T, Kobayashi K, Yamamoto M, Kono Y, Funada Y, et al. Inhalation of urokinase-type plasminogen activator reduces airway remodeling in a murine asthma model. *Am J Physiol Cell Mol Physiol.* (2009) 296:L337–46. doi: 10.1152/ajplung.90434.2008
199. Schuliga M, Westall G, Xia Y, Stewart AG. The plasminogen activation system: new targets in lung inflammation and remodeling. *Curr Opin Pharmacol.* (2013) 13:386–93. doi: 10.1016/j.coph.2013.05.014
200. Gur-Wahnon D, Mizrachi T, Maaravi-Pinto F-Y, Lourbopoulos A, Grigoriadis N, Higazi A-AR, et al. The plasminogen activator system: involvement in central nervous system inflammation and a potential site for therapeutic intervention. *J Neuroinflammation.* (2013) 10:124. doi: 10.1186/1742-2094-10-124
201. Kramer MD, Reinartz J. The autoimmune blistering skin disease bullous pemphigoid: the presence of plasmin/α2-antiplasmin complexes in skin blister fluid indicates plasmin generation in lesional skin. *J Clin Invest.* (1993) 92:978–83. doi: 10.1172/JCI116674
202. Schmidt E, Wehr B, Tabengwa EM, Reimer S, Bröcker EB, Zillikens D. Elevated expression and release of tissue-type, but not urokinase-type, plasminogen activator after binding of autoantibodies to bullous pemphigoid antigen 180 in cultured human keratinocytes. *Clin Exp Immunol.* (2004) 135:497–504. doi: 10.1111/j.1365-2249.2004.02401.x
203. Hofmann SC, Voith U, Schonau V, Sorokin L, Bruckner-Tuderman L, Franzke CW. Plasmin plays a role in the *in vitro* generation of the linear IgA dermatosis antigen LADB97. *J Invest Dermatol.* (2009) 129:1730–9. doi: 10.1038/jid.2008.424
204. Baird J, Lazarus GS, Belin D, Vassalli JD, Busso N, Gubler P, et al. mRNA for tissue-type plasminogen activator is present in lesional epidermis from patients with psoriasis, pemphigus, or bullous pemphigoid, but is not detected in normal epidermis. *J Invest Dermatol.* (1990) 95:548–52. doi: 10.1111/1523-1747.ep12504901
205. Venning VA, Wojnarowska F, Cederholm-Williams S. An immunohistochemical study of the distribution of plasminogen and plasminogen activators in bullous pemphigoid. *Clin Exp Dermatol.* (1993) 18:119–23. doi: 10.1111/j.1365-2230.1993.tb00990.x
206. Gissler HM, Simon MM, Kramer MD. Enhanced association of plasminogen/plasmin with lesional epidermis of bullous pemphigoid. *Br J Dermatol.* (1992) 127:272–7. doi: 10.1111/j.1365-2133.1992.tb00127.x
207. Nishie W, Schlosser A, Licarete E, Franzke C. Ectodomain shedding generates neoepitopes on collagen XVII, the major autoantigen for bullous pemphigoid. *J Immunol.* (2010) 185:4938–47. doi: 10.4049/jimmunol.1001524
208. Izumi K, Nishie W, Mai Y, Wada M, Natsuga K, Ujiie H, et al. Autoantibody profile differentiates between inflammatory and noninflammatory bullous pemphigoid. *J Invest Dermatol.* (2016) 136:2201–10. doi: 10.1016/j.jid.2016.06.622
209. Jacków J, Schlosser A, Sormunen R, Nyström A, Sitaru C, Tasanen K, et al. Generation of a functional non-shedding collagen XVII mouse model: relevance of collagen XVII shedding in wound healing. *J Invest Dermatol.* (2016) 136:516–25. doi: 10.1016/j.jid.2015.10.060
210. Grando SA. Decompensation in proteinase-inhibitor system and application of proteinase inhibitors in pemphigus and pemphigoid. *J Dermatol Sci.* (1992) 4:95–7. doi: 10.1016/0923-1811(92)90065-J
211. Wintroub BU, Mihm MC, Goetzl EJ, Soter NA, Austen KF. Morphologic and functional evidence for release of mast-cell products in bullous pemphigoid. *N Engl J Med.* (1978) 298:417–21. doi: 10.1056/NEJM197802232980803
212. Chen R, Ning G, Zhao ML, Fleming MG, Diaz LA, Werb Z, et al. Mast cells play a key role in neutrophil recruitment in experimental bullous pemphigoid. *J Clin Invest.* (2001) 108:1151–8. doi: 10.1172/JCI11494
213. Feyerabend TB, Weiser A, Tietz A, Stassen M, Harris N, Kopf M, et al. Cre-mediated cell ablation contests mast cell contribution in models of antibody- and T cell-mediated autoimmunity. *Immunity.* (2011) 35:832–44. doi: 10.1016/j.immuni.2011.09.015
214. Fang H, Zhang Y, Li N, Wang G, Liu Z. The autoimmune skin disease bullous pemphigoid: the role of mast cells in autoantibody-induced tissue injury. *Front Immunol.* (2018) 9:407. doi: 10.3389/fimmu.2018.00407

215. Chen R, Fairley JA, Zhao M-L, Giudice GJ, Zillikens D, Diaz LA, et al. Macrophages, but not T and B lymphocytes, are critical for subepidermal blister formation in experimental bullous pemphigoid: macrophage-mediated neutrophil infiltration depends on mast cell activation. *J Immunol.* (2002) 169:3987–92. doi: 10.4049/jimmunol.169.7.3987
216. Kasprick A, Yu X, Scholten J, Hartmann K, Pas HH, Zillikens D, et al. Conditional depletion of mast cells has no impact on the severity of experimental epidermolysis bullosa acquisita. *Eur J Immunol.* (2015) 45:1462–70. doi: 10.1002/eji.201444769
217. Caughey GH. Mast cell proteases as pharmacological targets. *Eur J Pharmacol.* (2016) 778:44–55. doi: 10.1016/j.ejphar.2015.04.045
218. Caughey GH, Zerweck EH, Vanderslice P. Structure, chromosomal assignment, and deduced amino acid sequence of a human gene for mast cell chymase. *J Biol Chem.* (1991) 266:12956–63.
219. Wolters PJ, Pham CT, Muilenburg DJ, Ley TJ, Caughey GH. Dipeptidyl peptidase I is essential for activation of mast cell chymases, but not tryptases, in mice. *J Biol Chem.* (2001) 276:18551–6. doi: 10.1074/jbc.M100223200
220. Lindstedt L, Lee M, Kovanen PT. Chymase bound to heparin is resistant to its natural inhibitors and capable of proteolyzing high density lipoproteins in aortic intimal fluid. *Atherosclerosis.* (2001) 155:87–97. doi: 10.1016/S0021-9150(00)00544-X
221. Dell'italia LJ, Collawn JF, Ferrario CM. Multifunctional role of chymase in acute and chronic tissue injury and remodeling. *Circ Res.* (2018) 122:319–36. doi: 10.1161/CIRCRESAHA.117.310978
222. Takai S, Jin D. Chymase inhibitor as a novel therapeutic agent for non-alcoholic steatohepatitis. *Front Pharmacol.* (2018) 9:144. doi: 10.3389/fphar.2018.00144
223. Omoto Y, Tokime K, Yamanaka K, Habe K, Morioka T, Kurokawa I, et al. Human mast cell chymase cleaves pro-IL-18 and generates a novel and biologically active IL-18 fragment. *J Immunol.* (2006) 177:8315–9. doi: 10.4049/jimmunol.177.12.8315
224. Fu Z, Thorpe M, Hellman L. rMCP-2, the major rat mucosal mast cell protease, an analysis of its extended cleavage specificity and its potential role in regulating intestinal permeability by the cleavage of cell adhesion and junction proteins. *PLoS ONE.* (2015) 10:e0131720. doi: 10.1371/journal.pone.0131720
225. Tchougounova E, Lundequist A, Fajardo I, Winberg J-O, Abrink M, Pejler G. A key role for mast cell chymase in the activation of pro-matrix metalloprotease-9 and pro-matrix metalloprotease-2. *J Biol Chem.* (2005) 280:9291–6. doi: 10.1074/jbc.M410396200
226. Urata H, Kinoshita A, Misono KS, Bumpus FM, Husain A. Identification of a highly specific chymase as the major angiotensin II-forming enzyme in the human heart. *J Biol Chem.* (1990) 265:22348–57.
227. Vartio T, Seppä H, Vaheri A. Susceptibility of soluble and matrix fibronectins to degradation by tissue proteinases, mast cell chymase and cathepsin G. *J Biol Chem.* (1981) 256:471–7.
228. Tejada T, Tan L, Torres RA, Calvert JW, Lambert JP, Zaidi M, et al. IGF-1 degradation by mouse mast cell protease 4 promotes cell death and adverse cardiac remodeling days after a myocardial infarction. *Proc Natl Acad Sci USA.* (2016) 113:6949–54. doi: 10.1073/pnas.1603127113
229. Urata H. Chymase and matrix metalloproteinase. *Hypertens Res.* (2007) 30:3–4. doi: 10.1291/hypres.30.3
230. Fang KC, Raymond WW, Lazarus SC, Caughey GH. Dog mastocytoma cells secrete a 92-kD gelatinase activated extracellularly by mast cell chymase. *J Clin Invest.* (1996) 97:1589–96. doi: 10.1172/JCI118583
231. Wei C-C, Chen Y, Powell LC, Zheng J, Shi K, Bradley WE, et al. Cardiac kallikrein-kinin system is upregulated in chronic volume overload and mediates an inflammatory induced collagen loss. *PLoS ONE.* (2012) 7:e40110. doi: 10.1371/journal.pone.0040110
232. Lindstedt KA, Wang Y, Shiota N, Saarinen J, Hyytiäinen M, Kokkonen JO, et al. Activation of paracrine TGF-beta1 signaling upon stimulation and degranulation of rat serosal mast cells: a novel function for chymase. *FASEB J.* (2001) 15:1377–88. doi: 10.1096/fj.00-0273com
233. Mizutani H, Schechter N, Lazarus G, Black RA, Kupper TS. Rapid and specific conversion of precursor interleukin 1 beta (IL-1 beta) to an active IL-1 species by human mast cell chymase. *J Exp Med.* (1991) 174:821–5. doi: 10.1084/jem.174.4.821
234. Piliponsky AM, Chen C-C, Rios EJ, Treuting PM, Lahiri A, Abrink M, et al. The chymase mouse mast cell protease 4 degrades TNF, limits inflammation, and promotes survival in a model of sepsis. *Am J Pathol.* (2012) 181:875–86. doi: 10.1016/j.ajpath.2012.05.013
235. Firth JD, Uitto V-J, Putnins EE. Mechanical induction of an epithelial cell chymase associated with wound edge migration. *J Biol Chem.* (2008) 283:34983–93. doi: 10.1074/jbc.M801975200
236. Zheng J, Wei C-C, Hase N, Shi K, Killingsworth CR, Litovsky SH, et al. Chymase mediates injury and mitochondrial damage in cardiomyocytes during acute ischemia/reperfusion in the dog. *PLoS ONE.* (2014) 9:e94732. doi: 10.1371/journal.pone.0094732
237. Ahmad S, Ferrario CM. Chymase inhibitors for the treatment of cardiac diseases: a patent review (2010–2018). *Expert Opin Ther Pat.* (2018) 28:755–64. doi: 10.1080/13543776.2018.1531848
238. Ibaraki T, Muramatsu M, Takai S, Jin D, Maruyama H, Orino T, et al. The relationship of tryptase- and chymase-positive mast cells to angiogenesis in stage I non-small cell lung cancer. *Eur J Cardio-Thoracic Surg.* (2005) 28:617–21. doi: 10.1016/j.ejcts.2005.06.020
239. de Souza Junior DA, Santana AC, da Silva EZM, Oliver C, Jamur MC. The role of mast cell specific chymases and tryptases in tumor angiogenesis. *Biomed Res Int.* (2015) 2015:142359. doi: 10.1155/2015/142359
240. Kosanovic D, Dahal BK, Wygrecka M, Reiss I, Günther A, Ghofrani HA, et al. Mast cell chymase: an indispensable instrument in the pathological symphony of idiopathic pulmonary fibrosis? *Histol Histopathol.* (2013) 28:691–9.
241. Wasse H, Naqvi N, Husain A. Impact of mast cell chymase on renal disease progression. *Curr Hypertens Rev.* (2012) 8:15–23. doi: 10.2174/157340212800505007
242. Wang Y, Alexander JS. Role of chymase in preeclampsia. *Curr Vasc Pharmacol.* (2013) 11:606–15. doi: 10.2174/1570161111311050005
243. Watanabe N, Tomimori Y, Saito K, Miura K, Wada A, Tsudzuki M, et al. Chymase inhibitor improves dermatitis in NC/Nga mice. *Int Arch Allergy Immunol.* (2002) 128:229–34. doi: 10.1159/000064256
244. Lin L, Bankaitis E, Heimbach L, Li N, Abrink M, Pejler G, et al. Dual targets for mouse mast cell protease-4 in mediating tissue damage in experimental bullous pemphigoid. *J Biol Chem.* (2011) 286:37358–67. doi: 10.1074/jbc.M111.272401
245. Seals DF, Courtneidge SA. The ADAMs family of metalloproteases: multidomain proteins with multiple functions. *Genes Dev.* (2003) 17:7–30. doi: 10.1101/gad.1039703
246. Kawaguchi M, Hearing VJ. The roles of ADAMs family proteinases in skin diseases. *Enzyme Res.* (2011) 2011:1–9. doi: 10.4061/2011/482498
247. Dreymueller D, Uhlig S, Ludwig A. ADAM-family metalloproteinases in lung inflammation: potential therapeutic targets. *Am J Physiol Cell Mol Physiol.* (2014) 308:L325–43. doi: 10.1152/ajplung.00294.2014
248. Weber S, Saftig P. Ectodomain shedding and ADAMs in development. *Development.* (2012) 139:3693–709. doi: 10.1242/dev.076398
249. Edwards DR, Handsley MM, Pennington CJ. The ADAM metalloproteinases. *Mol Aspects Med.* (2009) 29:258–89. doi: 10.1016/j.mam.2008.08.001
250. Wisniewska M, Goettig P, Maskos K, Belouski E, Winters D, Hecht R, et al. Structural determinants of the ADAM inhibition by TIMP-3: crystal structure of the TACE-N-TIMP-3 complex. *J Mol Biol.* (2008) 381:1307–19. doi: 10.1016/j.jmb.2008.06.088
251. Lorenzen I, Lokau J, Korpys Y, Oldefest M, Flynn CM, Künzel U, et al. Control of ADAM17 activity by regulation of its cellular localisation. *Sci Rep.* (2016) 6:35067 doi: 10.1038/srep35067
252. Moriyama H, Tsukida T, Inoue Y, Yokota K, Yoshino K, Kondo H, et al. Azasugar-based MMP/ADAM inhibitors as antipsoriatic agents. *J Med Chem.* (2004) 47:1930–8. doi: 10.1021/jm0304313
253. Dreymueller D, Ludwig A. Considerations on inhibition approaches for proinflammatory functions of ADAM proteases. *Platelets.* (2017) 28:354–61. doi: 10.1080/09537104.2016.1203396
254. Kataoka H. EGFR ligands and their signaling scissors, ADAMs, as new molecular targets for anticancer treatments. *J Dermatol Sci.* (2009) 56:148–53. doi: 10.1016/j.jdermsci.2009.10.002

255. Mauch C, Zamek J, Abety AN, Grimberg G, Fox JW, Zigrino P. Accelerated wound repair in ADAM-9 knockout animals. *J Invest Dermatol.* (2010) 130:2120–30. doi: 10.1038/jid.2010.60
256. Oh ST, Schramme A, Stark A, Tilgen W, Gutwein P, Reichrath J. Overexpression of ADAM 10 and ADAM 12 in lesional psoriatic skin. *Br J Dermatol.* (2008) 158:1371–3. doi: 10.1111/j.1365-2133.2008.08513.x
257. Charbonneau M, Harper K, Grondin F, Pelmus M, McDonald PP, Dubois CM. Hypoxia-inducible factor mediates hypoxic and tumor necrosis factor alpha-induced increases in tumor necrosis factor-alpha converting enzyme/ADAM17 expression by synovial cells. *J Biol Chem.* (2007) 282:33714–24. doi: 10.1074/jbc.M704041200
258. Zebrowska A, Wagrowska-Danilewicz M, Danilewicz M, Wodz K, Sokolowska M, Erkiert-Polguj A, et al. Expression of selected ADAMs in bullous pemphigoid and dermatitis herpetiformis. *J Dermatol Sci.* (2009) 56:58–61. doi: 10.1016/j.jdermsci.2009.06.018
259. Shen S, Zhang J, Fang H, Ke Y, Zhang T, Wang G, et al. Semaphorin 4D from CD15+ granulocytes via ADAM10-induced cleavage contributes to antibody production in bullous pemphigoid. *J Invest Dermatol.* (2017) 138:588–97. doi: 10.1016/j.jid.2017.09.037
260. Franzke CW, Tasanen K, Borradori L, Huotari V, Bruckner-Tuderman L. Shedding of collagen XVII/BP180. Structural motifs influence cleavage from cell surface. *J Biol Chem.* (2004) 279:24521–9. doi: 10.1074/jbc.M308835200
261. Franzke CW, Bruckner-Tuderman L, Blobel CP. Shedding of collagen XVII/BP180 in skin depends on both ADAM10 and ADAM9. *J Biol Chem.* (2009) 284:23386–96. doi: 10.1074/jbc.M109.034090
262. Ieguchi K, Maru Y. Savior or not: ADAM17 inhibitors overcome radiotherapy-resistance in non-small cell lung cancer. *J Thorac Dis.* (2016) 8:E813–5. doi: 10.21037/jtd.2016.07.56
263. Moss ML, Minond D. Recent advances in ADAM17 research: a promising target for cancer and inflammation. *Mediators Inflamm.* (2017) 2017:9673537. doi: 10.1155/2017/9673537
264. Masson D, Nabholz M, Estrade C, Tschopp J. Granules of cytolytic T-lymphocytes contain two serine esterases. *EMBO J.* (1986) 5:1595–600. doi: 10.1002/j.1460-2075.1986.tb04401.x
265. Bots M, Medema JP. Granzymes at a glance. *J Cell Sci.* (2006) 119:5011–4. doi: 10.1242/jcs.03239
266. Li P, Nijhawan D, Budihardjo I, Srinivasula SM, Ahmad M, Alnemri ES, et al. Cytochrome c and dATP-dependent formation of Apaf-1/Caspase-9 complex initiates an apoptotic protease cascade. *Cell.* (1997) 91:479–89. doi: 10.1016/S0092-8674(00)80434-1
267. Darmon AJ, Nicholson DW, Bleackley RC. Activation of the apoptotic protease CPP32 by cytotoxic T-cell-derived granzyme B. *Nature.* (1995) 377:446–8. doi: 10.1038/377446a0
268. Kägi D, Ledermann B, Bürki K, Seiler P, Odermatt B, Olsen KJ, et al. Cytotoxicity mediated by T cells and natural killer cells is greatly impaired in perforin-deficient mice. *Nature.* (1994) 369:31–7. doi: 10.1038/369031a0
269. Kägi D, Vignaux F, Ledermann B, Bürki K, Depraetere V, Nagata S, et al. Fas and perforin pathways as major mechanisms of T cell-mediated cytotoxicity. *Science.* (1994) 265:528–30. doi: 10.1126/science.7518614
270. Isaaz S, Baetz K, Olsen K, Podack E, Griffiths GM. Serial killing by cytotoxic T lymphocytes: T cell receptor triggers degranulation, re-filling of the lytic granules and secretion of lytic proteins via a non-granule pathway. *Eur J Immunol.* (1995) 25:1071–9. doi: 10.1002/eji.1830250432
271. Horiuchi K, Saito S, Sasaki R, Tomatsu T, Toyama Y. Expression of granzyme B in human articular chondrocytes. *J Rheumatol.* (2003) 30:1799–810.
272. Hernandez-Pigeon H, Jean C, Charruyer A, Haure MJ, Titeux M, Tonasso L, et al. Human keratinocytes acquire cellular cytotoxicity under UV-B irradiation: implication of granzyme B and perforin. *J Biol Chem.* (2006) 281:13525–32. doi: 10.1074/jbc.M512694200
273. Grossman WJ, Verbsky JW, Tollefsen BL, Kemper C, Atkinson JP, Ley TJ. Differential expression of granzymes A and B in human cytotoxic lymphocyte subsets and T regulatory cells. *Blood.* (2004) 104:2840–8. doi: 10.1182/blood-2004-03-0859
274. Vernooy JHJ, Möller GM, van Suylen RJ, van Spijk MP, Cloots RHE, Hoet PH, et al. Increased granzyme A expression in type II pneumocytes of patients with severe chronic obstructive pulmonary disease. *Am J Respir Crit Care Med.* (2007) 175:464–72. doi: 10.1164/rccm.200602-169OC
275. Hirst CE, Buzza MS, Sutton VR, Trapani JA, Loveland KL, Bird PI. Perforin-independent expression of granzyme B and proteinase inhibitor 9 in human testis and placenta suggests a role for granzyme B-mediated proteolysis in reproduction. *Mol Hum Reprod.* (2001) 7:1133–42. doi: 10.1093/molehr/7.12.1133
276. Jeng MY, Hull PA, Fei M, Kwon H-S, Tsou C-L, Kasler H, et al. Metabolic reprogramming of human CD8+ memory T cells through loss of SIRT1. *J Exp Med.* (2018) 215:51–62. doi: 10.1084/jem.20161066
277. Namekawa T, Wagner UG, Goronzy JJ, Weyand CM. Functional subsets of CD4 T cells in rheumatoid synovitis. *Arthritis Rheum.* (1998) 41:2108–16. doi: 10.1002/1529-0131(199812)41:12<2108::AID-ART5>3.0.CO;2-Q
278. Pardo J, Wallich R, Ebnet K, Iden S, Zentgraf H, Martin P, et al. Granzyme B is expressed in mouse mast cells *in vivo* and *in vitro* and causes delayed cell death independent of perforin. *Cell Death Differ.* (2007) 14:1768–79. doi: 10.1038/sj.cdd.4402183
279. Choy JC, McDonald PC, Suarez AC, Hung VHY, Wilson JE, McManus BM, et al. Granzyme B in atherosclerosis and transplant vascular disease: association with cell death and atherosclerotic disease severity. *Mod Pathol.* (2003) 16:460–70. doi: 10.1097/01.MP.0000067424.12280.BC
280. Wagner C, Iking-Konert C, Denefleh B, Stegmaier S, Hug F, Hänsch GM. Granzyme B and perforin: constitutive expression in human polymorphonuclear neutrophils. *Blood.* (2003) 103:1099–104. doi: 10.1182/blood-2003-04-1069
281. Rissoan M-C, Duhen T, Bridon J-M, Bendriss-Vermare N, Péronne C, de Saint Vis B, et al. Subtractive hybridization reveals the expression of immunoglobulin-like transcript 7, Eph-B1, granzyme B, and 3 novel transcripts in human plasmacytoid dendritic cells. *Blood.* (2002) 100:3295–303. doi: 10.1182/blood-2002-02-0638
282. Kaiserman D, Bird PI. Control of granzymes by serpins. *Cell Death Differ.* (2010) 17:586–95. doi: 10.1038/cdd.2009.169
283. Sun J, Whisstock JC, Harriott P, Walker B, Novak A, Thompson PE, et al. Importance of the P4' residue in human granzyme B inhibitors and substrates revealed by scanning mutagenesis of the proteinase inhibitor 9 reactive center loop. *J Biol Chem.* (2001) 276:15177–84. doi: 10.1074/jbc.M006645200
284. Turner CT, Lim D, Granville DJ. Granzyme B in skin inflammation and disease. *Matrix Biol.* (2019) 75–76:126–40. doi: 10.1016/j.matbio.2017.12.005
285. Akeda T, Yamanaka K, Tsuda K, Omoto Y, Gabazza EC, Mizutani H. CD8+ T cell granzyme B activates keratinocyte endogenous IL-18. *Arch Dermatol Res.* (2014) 306:125–30. doi: 10.1007/s00403-013-1382-1
286. Perl M, Denk S, Kalbitz M, Huber-Lang M. Granzyme B: a new crossroad of complement and apoptosis. *Adv Exp Med Biol.* (2012). 946:135–46. doi: 10.1007/978-1-4614-0106-3_8
287. Afonina IS, Tynan GA, Logue SE, Cullen SP, Bots M, Lüthi AU, et al. Granzyme B-dependent proteolysis acts as a switch to enhance the proinflammatory activity of IL-1α. *Mol Cell.* (2011) 44:265–78. doi: 10.1016/j.molcel.2011.07.037
288. Buzza MS, Zamurs L, Sun J, Bird CHCH, Smith AI, Trapani JA, Froelich CJ, Nice EC, Bird PI. Extracellular matrix remodeling by human granzyme B via cleavage of vitronectin, fibronectin, and laminin. *J Biol Chem.* (2005) 280:23549–58. doi: 10.1074/jbc.M412001200
289. Shen Y, Zeglinski MR, Turner CT, Raithatha SA, Wu Z, Russo V, et al. Topical small molecule granzyme B inhibitor improves remodeling in a murine model of impaired burn wound healing. *Exp Mol Med.* (2018) 50:68. doi: 10.1038/s12276-018-0095-0
290. Saito A, Okiyama N, Kubota N, Nakamura Y, Fujisawa Y, Watanabe R, et al. Blockade of granzyme B remarkably improves mucocutaneous diseases with keratinocyte death in interface dermatitis. *J Invest Dermatol.* (2018) 138:2079–83. doi: 10.1016/j.jid.2018.03.1507
291. Mac QD, Mathews DV, Kahla JA, Stoffers CM, Delmas OM, Holt BA, et al. Non-invasive early detection of acute transplant rejection via nanosensors of granzyme B activity. *Nat Biomed Eng.* (2019) 3:281–91. doi: 10.1038/s41551-019-0358-7
292. Kim W-J, Kim H, Suk K, Lee W-H. Macrophages express granzyme B in the lesion areas of atherosclerosis and rheumatoid arthritis. *Immunol Lett.* (2007) 111:57–65. doi: 10.1016/j.imlet.2007.05.004

293. Goldbach-Mansky R, Suson S, Wesley R, Hack CE, El-Gabalawy HS, Tak PP. Raised granzyme B levels are associated with erosions in patients with early rheumatoid factor positive rheumatoid arthritis. *Ann Rheum Dis.* (2005) 64:715–21. doi: 10.1136/ard.2003.007039
294. Parkinson LG, Toro A, Zhao H, Brown K, Tebbutt SJ, Granville DJ. Granzyme B mediates both direct and indirect cleavage of extracellular matrix in skin after chronic low-dose ultraviolet light irradiation. *Aging Cell.* (2015) 14:67–77. doi: 10.1111/acel.12298
295. Kamata Y, Kimura U, Matsuda H, Tengara S, Kamo A, Umehara Y, et al. Relationships among plasma granzyme B level, pruritus and dermatitis in patients with atopic dermatitis. *J Dermatol Sci.* (2016) 84:266–71. doi: 10.1016/j.jdermsci.2016.09.009
296. Abdou AG, Shoeib M, Bakry OA, El-Bality H. Immunohistochemical expression of granzyme B and perforin in discoid lupus erythematosus. *Ultrastruct Pathol.* (2013) 37:408–16. doi: 10.3109/01913123.2013.816400
297. Posadas SJ, Padial A, Torres MJ, Mayorga C, Leyva L, Sanchez E, et al. Delayed reactions to drugs show levels of perforin, granzyme B, and Fas-L to be related to disease severity. *J Allergy Clin Immunol.* (2002) 109:155–61. doi: 10.1067/mai.2002.120563
298. Hussein MR, Ali FMN, Omar A-EMM. Immunohistological analysis of immune cells in blistering skin lesions. *J Clin Pathol.* (2007) 60:62–71. doi: 10.1136/jcp.2006.037010
299. Russo V, Klein T, Lim DJ, Solis N, Machado Y, Hiroyasu S, et al. Granzyme B is elevated in autoimmune blistering diseases and cleaves key anchoring proteins of the dermal-epidermal junction. *Sci Rep.* (2018) 8:1–11. doi: 10.1038/s41598-018-28070-0
300. Belal KM, Yousef AA, Almahdy MA, Alsalahy MM, Essawy TS. Study of serum Granzyme B in heavy cigarette smokers with and without chronic obstructive pulmonary disease. *Egypt J Chest Dis Tuberc.* (2014) 63:815–9. doi: 10.1016/j.ejcdt.2014.07.009
301. Antonicelli F, Le Jan S, Plée J, Bernard P. Inflammation in bullous pemphigoid, a skin autoimmune disease. *Immun Inflamm Heal Dis.* (2018)213–22. doi: 10.1016/B978-0-12-805417-8.00017-2
302. D'Auria L, Pietravalle M, Cordiali-Fei P, Ameglio F. Increased tryptase and myeloperoxidase levels in blister fluids of patients with bullous pemphigoid: correlations with cytokines, adhesion molecules and anti-basement membrane zone antibodies. *Exp Dermatol.* (2000) 9:131–7. doi: 10.1034/j.1600-0625.2000.009002131.x
303. Bieber K, Ernst AL, Tukaj S, Holtsche MM, Schmidt E, Zillikens D, et al. Analysis of serum markers of cellular immune activation in patients with bullous pemphigoid. *Exp Dermatol.* (2017) 26:1248–52. doi: 10.1111/exd.13382
304. Kaminska R, Naukkarinen A, Glinski W, Horsmanheimo M, Harvima IT. Mast cells in developing subepidermal bullous diseases: Emphasis on tryptase, chymase and protease inhibitors. *Acta Derm Venereol.* (1999) 79:351–5. doi: 10.1080/000155599750010247
305. Payne V, Kam PCA. Mast cell tryptase: a review of its physiology and clinical significance. *Anaesthesia.* (2004) 59:695–703. doi: 10.1111/j.1365-2044.2004.03757.x
306. Ni W-W, Cao M-D, Huang W, Meng L, Wei J-F. Tryptase inhibitors: a patent review. *Expert Opin Ther Pat.* (2017) 27:919–28. doi: 10.1080/13543776.2017.1322064
307. Lan RS, Stewart GA, Henry PJ. Role of protease-activated receptors in airway function: a target for therapeutic intervention? *Pharmacol Ther.* (2002) 95:239–57. doi: 10.1016/S0163-7258(02) 00237-1
308. Gao S, Zhu H, Zuo X, Luo H. Cathepsin G and its role in inflammation and autoimmune diseases. *Arch Rheumatol.* (2018) 33:498–504. doi: 10.5606/ArchRheumatol.2018.6595
309. Kosikowska P, Lesner A. Inhibitors of cathepsin G: a patent review (2005 to present). *Expert Opin Ther Pat.* (2013) 23:1611–24. doi: 10.1517/13543776.2013.835397
310. Giusti D, Jan S Le, Pham BN, Antonicelli F, Gatouillat G, Bernard P, et al. Biomarkers related to bullous pemphigoid activity and outcome. *Exp Dermatol.* (2017) 26:1240–7. doi: 10.1111/exd.13459
311. Zhang Y, Hwang B-J, Liu ZZ, Li N, Lough K, Williams SE, et al. BP180 dysfunction triggers spontaneous skin inflammation in mice. *Proc Natl Acad Sci USA.* (2018) 115:6434–9. doi: 10.1073/pnas.1721805115
312. Nakashima H, Fujimoto M, Asashima N, Watanabe R, Kuwano Y, Yazawa N, et al. Serum chemokine profile in patients with bullous pemphigoid. *Br J Dermatol.* (2007) 156:454–9. doi: 10.1111/j.1365-2133.2006.07601.x
313. Saeki H, Tamaki K. Thymus and activation regulated chemokine (TARC)/CCL17 and skin diseases. *J Dermatol Sci.* (2006) 43:75–84. doi: 10.1016/j.jdermsci.2006.06.002
314. Nin-Asai R, Muro Y, Sekiya A, Sugiura K, Akiyama M. Serum thymus and activation-regulated chemokine (TARC/CCL17) levels reflect the disease activity in a patient with bullous pemphigoid. *J Eur Acad Dermatol Venereol.* (2016) 30:327–8. doi: 10.1111/jdv.12719
315. Günther C, Carballido-Perrig N, Kopp T, Carballido JM, Pfeiffer C. CCL18 is expressed in patients with bullous pemphigoid and parallels disease course. *Br J Dermatol.* (2009) 160:747–55. doi: 10.1111/j.1365-2133.2008.08979.x
316. Günther C, Wozel G, Meurer M, Pfeiffer C. Up-regulation of CCL11 and CCL26 is associated with activated eosinophils in bullous pemphigoid. *Clin Exp Immunol.* (2011) 166:145–53. doi: 10.1111/j.1365-2249.2011.04464.x
317. Wakugawa M, Nakamura K, Hino H, Toyama K, Hattori N, Okochi H, et al. Elevated levels of eotaxin and interleukin-5 in blister fluid of bullous pemphigoid: correlation with tissue eosinophilia. *Br J Dermatol.* (2000) 143:112–6. doi: 10.1046/j.1365-2133.2000.03599.x
318. D'Auria L, Cordiali Fei P, Ameglio F. Cytokines and bullous pemphigoid. *Eur Cytokine Netw.* (1999) 10:123–34.
319. De Pitá O, Frezzolini A, Cianchini G, Ruffelli M, Teofoli P, Puddu P. T-helper 2 involvement in the pathogenesis of bullous pemphigoid: role of soluble CD30 (sCD30). *Arch Dermatol Res.* (1997) 289:667–70. doi: 10.1007/s004030050259
320. Inaoki M, Takehara K. Increased serum levels of interleukin (IL)-5, IL-6 and IL-8 in bullous pemphigoid. *J Dermatol Sci.* (1998) 16:152–7. doi: 10.1016/S0923-1811(97)00044-3
321. Engineer L, Bhol K, Kumari S, Razzaque Ahmed A. Bullous pemphigoid: Interaction of interleukin 5, anti-basement membrane zone antibodies and eosinophils. A preliminary observation. *Cytokine.* (2001) 13:32–8. doi: 10.1006/cyto.2000.0791
322. Endo H, Iwamoto I, Fujita M, Okamoto S, Yoshida S. Increased immunoreactive interleukin-5 levels in blister fluids of bullous pemphigoid. *Arch Dermatol Res.* (1992) 284:312–4. doi: 10.1007/BF00372588
323. Shrikhande T, Hunziker LR, Braa M, Hunziker T, Braathen LR, Pichler WJ, et al. Increased coexpression of eotaxin and interleukin 5 in bullous pemphigoid. *Acta Derm Venereol.* (2000) 80:277–80. doi: 10.1080/000155500750012162
324. Ameglio F, D'Auria L, Bonifati C, Ferraro C, Mastroianni A, Giacalone B. Cytokine pattern in blister fluid and serum of patients with bullous pemphigoid: relationships with disease intensity. *Br J Dermatol.* (1998) 138:611–4. doi: 10.1046/j.1365-2133.1998.02169.x
325. Giacalone B, D'Auria L, Bonifati C, Ferraro C, Riccardi E, Mussi A, et al. Decreased interleukin-7 and transforming growth factor-betal levels in blister fluids as compared to the respective 'serum levels in patients with bullous pemphigoid. Opposite behavior of TNF-alpha, interleukin-4 and interleukin-10. *Exp Dermatol.* (1998) 7:157–61. doi: 10.1111/j.1600-0625.1998.tb00317.x
326. D'Auria L, Pietravalle M, Mastroianni A, Ferraro C, Mussi A, Bonifati C, et al. IL-5 levels in the serum and blister fluid of patients with bullous pemphigoid: correlations with eosinophil cationic protein, RANTES, IgE and disease severity. *Arch Dermatol Res.* (1998) 290:25–7. doi: 10.1007/s004030050272
327. Fang H, Shao S, Cao T, Lei J, Dang E, Zhang J, et al. Increased expression of NLRP3 inflammasome components and interleukin-18 in patients with bullous pemphigoid. *J Dermatol Sci.* (2016) 83:116–23. doi: 10.1016/j.jdermsci.2016.04.009
328. Plée J, Le Jan S, Giustiniani J, Barbe C, Joly P, Bedane C, et al. Integrating longitudinal serum IL-17 and IL-23 follow-up, along with autoantibodies variation, contributes to predict bullous pemphigoid outcome. *Sci Rep.* (2015) 5:18001. doi: 10.1038/srep18001
329. Li Q, Liu Z, Dang E, Jin L, He Z, Yang L, et al. Follicular Helper T Cells (Tfh) and IL-21 involvement in the pathogenesis of bullous pemphigoid. *PLoS ONE.* (2013) 8:e68145. doi: 10.1371/journal.pone.0068145
330. Riani M, Le Jan S, Plée J, Durlach A, Le Naour R, Haegeman G, et al. Bullous pemphigoid outcome is associated with CXCL10-induced matrix metalloproteinase 9 secretion from monocytes and neutrophils

but not lymphocytes. *J Allergy Clin Immunol.* (2016) 139:863–72.e3. doi: 10.1016/j.jaci.2016.08.012
331. Samavedam UKSRL, Kalies K, Scheller J, Sadeghi H, Gupta Y, Jonkman MF, et al. Recombinant IL-6 treatment protects mice from organ specific autoimmune disease by IL-6 classical signalling-dependent IL-1ra induction. *J Autoimmun.* (2013) 40:74–85. doi: 10.1016/j.jaut.2012.08.002
332. Lee SJ, Li Z, Sherman B, Foster CS. Serum levels of tumor necrosis factor-alpha and interleukin-6 in ocular cicatricial pemphigoid. *Invest Ophthalmol Vis Sci.* (1993) 34:3522–5.
333. Saw VPJ, Offiah I, Dart RJ, Galatowicz G, Dart JKG, Daniels JT, et al. Conjunctival interleukin-13 expression in mucous membrane pemphigoid and functional effects of interleukin-13 on conjunctival fibroblasts *in vitro*. *Am J Pathol.* (2009) 175:2406–15. doi: 10.2353/ajpath.2009.090579
334. Suelves AM, Zhao TZ, Siddique SS, Foster CS. Profile of local interleukin expression in a cohort of ocular cicatricial pemphigoid patients. *Invest Opthalmol Vis Sci.* (2012) 53:8112. doi: 10.1167/iovs.11-9322
335. Saw VPJ, Dart RJC, Galatowicz G, Daniels JT, Dart JKG, Calder VL. Tumor necrosis factor-α in ocular mucous membrane pemphigoid and its effect on conjunctival fibroblasts. *Invest Opthalmol Vis Sci.* (2009) 50:5310. doi: 10.1167/iovs.08-3345
336. Caproni M, Calzolari A, Salvatore E, Giomi B, Volpi W, D'Agata A, et al. Cytokine profile and supposed contribution to scarring in cicatricial pemphigoid. *J Oral Pathol Med.* (2003) 32:34–40. doi: 10.1034/j.1600-0714.2003.00028.x
337. Kumari S, Bhol KC, Rehman F, Foster CS, Ahmed AR. Interleukin 1 components in cicatricial pemphigoid. Role in intravenous immunoglobulin therapy. *Cytokine.* (2001) 14:218–24. doi: 10.1006/cyto.2001.0877
338. Razzaque MS, Ahmed BS, Foster CS, Ahmed AR. Effects of IL-4 on conjunctival fibroblasts: possible role in ocular cicatricial pemphigoid. *Invest Ophthalmol Vis Sci.* (2003) 44:3417–23. doi: 10.1167/iovs.02-1084
339. Letko E, Bhol K, Colon J, Foster SC, Ahmed RA. Biology of interleukin-5 in ocular cicatricial pemphigoid. *Graefe's Arch Clin Exp Ophthalmol.* (2002) 240:565–9. doi: 10.1007/s00417-002-0497-4
340. Bernauer W, Wright P, Dart JK, Leonard JN, Lightman S. Cytokines in the conjunctiva of acute and chronic mucous membrane pemphigoid: an immunohistochemical analysis. *Graefe's Arch Clin Exp Ophthalmol.* (1993) 231:563–70. doi: 10.1007/BF00936519
341. López-Otín C, Overall CM. Protease degradomics: a new challenge for proteomics. *Nat Rev Mol Cell Biol.* (2002) 3:509–19. doi: 10.1038/nrm858
342. Fortelny N, Cox JH, Kappelhoff R, Starr AE, Lange PF, Pavlidis P, et al. Network analyses reveal pervasive functional regulation between proteases in the human protease web. *PLoS Biol.* (2014) 12:e1001869. doi: 10.1371/journal.pbio.1001869
343. Mallia-Milanes B, Dufour A, Philp C, Solis N, Klein T, Fischer M, et al. TAILS proteomics reveals dynamic changes in airway proteolysis controlling protease activity and innate immunity during COPD exacerbations. *Am J Physiol Cell Mol Physiol.* (2018) 315:L1003–14. doi: 10.1152/ajplung.00175.2018
344. Prudova A, Gocheva V, auf dem Keller U, Eckhard U, Olson OC, Akkari L, et al. TAILS N-terminomics and proteomics show protein degradation dominates over proteolytic processing by cathepsins in pancreatic tumors. *Cell Rep.* (2016) 16:1762–73. doi: 10.1016/j.celrep.2016.06.086

14

Complement Receptor 1 (CR1, CD35) Polymorphisms and Soluble CR1: A Proposed Anti-Inflammatory Role to Quench the Fire of "Fogo Selvagem" Pemphigus Foliaceus

Luana Caroline Oliveira[1], *Gabriela Canalli Kretzschmar*[1], *Andressa Cristina Moraes dos Santos*[1], *Carolina Maciel Camargo*[1], *Renato Mitsunori Nisihara*[2], *Ticiana Della Justina Farias*[1], *Andre Franke*[3], *Michael Wittig*[3], *Enno Schmidt*[4,5], *Hauke Busch*[4], *Maria Luiza Petzl-Erler*[1] and *Angelica Beate Winter Boldt*[1*]

[1] Laboratory of Human Molecular Genetics, Department of Genetics, Federal University of Paraná, Curitiba, Brazil, [2] Laboratory of Molecular Immunopathology, Department of Clinical Pathology, Clinical Hospital, Federal University of Paraná, Curitiba, Brazil, [3] Institute of Clinical Molecular Biology, Christian-Albrechts-University of Kiel, Kiel, Germany, [4] Lübeck Institute of Experimental Dermatology, University of Lübeck, Lübeck, Germany, [5] Department of Dermatology, University of Lübeck, Lübeck, Germany

***Correspondence:**
Angelica Beate Winter Boldt
angelicaboldt@gmail.com

Pemphigus foliaceus is an autoimmune disease that is sporadic around the world but endemic in Brazil, where it is known as fogo selvagem (FS). Characterized by autoantibodies against the desmosomal cadherin desmoglein 1, FS causes painful erosions, and crusts that may be widespread. The recognition of antigens, including exposed sugar moieties, activates the complement system. Complement receptor 1 (CR1, CD35), which is responsible for the Knops blood group on erythrocytes (York and McCoy antigens), is also expressed by antigen-presenting cells. This regulates the complement system by removing opsonized antigens, blocking the final steps of the complement cascade. Membrane-bound CR1 also fosters antigen presentation to B cells, whereas soluble CR1 has anti-inflammatory properties. *CR1* gene polymorphisms have been associated with susceptibility to complex diseases. In order to investigate the association of *CR1* polymorphisms with FS susceptibility, we developed a multiplex sequence-specific assay to haplotype eleven polymorphisms in up to 367 FS patients and 242 controls from an endemic area and 289 from a non-endemic area. We also measured soluble CR1 (sCR1) in the serum of 53 FS patients and 27 controls and mRNA levels in the peripheral blood mononuclear cells of 63 genotyped controls. The haplotypes *CR1*3B2B* (with the York antigen–encoded by p.1408Met) and *CR1*3A2A* (with p.1208Arg) were associated with protection against FS (OR = 0.57, $P = 0.027$, and OR = 0.46, $P = 0.014$, respectively). In contrast, the *CR1*1* haplotype (with the McCoy antigen – encoded by p.1590Glu) was associated with FS susceptibility (OR = 4.97, $P < 0.001$). Heterozygote *rs12034383*A/G* individuals presented higher mRNA expression than homozygotes with the *G* allele ($P = 0.04$). The lowest sCR1 levels occurred in patients with active disease before treatment ($P = 0.036$). Patients in remission had higher levels of sCR1 than did healthy controls ($P = 0.013$). Among those under treatment, patients with localized lesions also presented higher sCR1 levels than those with generalized lesions ($P = 0.0073$). In conclusion, the Knops blood group seems to modulate susceptibility to the disease. Furthermore, corticosteroid treatment might increase sCR1 serum levels, and higher levels may play an anti-inflammatory role in patients with FS, limiting the distribution of lesions. Based on these results, we suggest CR1 as a potential new therapeutic target for the treatment of FS.

Keywords: pemphigus foliaceus, complement receptor 1, CR1, CD35, polymorphism, York blood antigen, McCoy blood antigen, fogo selvagem

INTRODUCTION

Pemphigus foliaceus (PF) is an autoimmune blistering skin disease presenting with erosions and crusts that may be widespread and painful (1). Around the world, PF occurs sporadically, with an incidence of 0.75–5 cases/million per year (2, 3). In Brazil, it reaches up to 3% prevalence and is also known as *fogo selvagem* (FS, meaning "wild fire" in Portuguese) (2–6). While major immunopathological and histological characteristics are similar in both endemic and sporadic forms, the clinical presentation may differ (3, 7). The etiology of FS is little understood, but environmental factors are being considered. The bites of black mosquitoes (*Simuliidae*) and sand flies (*Phlebotominae*) are associated with an almost five times increased susceptibility to FS. Elements delivered in the saliva of these hematophagous insects are thought to trigger a cross-reaction against keratinocyte surface epitopes in genetically susceptible individuals living in endemic regions (8–10).

The intraepidermal blisters of PF are due to keratinocyte detachment, a process known as acantholysis (11). FS patients generate pathogenic IgG4 autoantibodies against desmoglein 1 (Dsg1) and occasionally and to a much lesser extent, against Dsg3, which are important structural components of desmosomes (1, 12). Altered cell-associated molecular patterns activate the complement system, and this is responsible for the recurrent observation of C3 component deposits along the basement membrane zone and in intercellular spaces of the perilesional and lesional epidermis of FS patients (13–16). Deposits of complement membrane attack complexes, in contrast, were only found in injured skin, whereas pathogenic IgG4 anti-desmoglein 1 autoantibodies—which cannot activate complement—were also abundant in apparently healthy tissue in FS patients (14, 17).

Although not required to initiate blister formation (18, 19), complement activation enhances acantholysis in cell culture (20, 21). Furthermore, FS patients with active disease present enhanced expression of the *C1QA* gene (an initiator molecule of the classical pathway) and increased serum levels of C3 and C-reactive protein (opsonins), of the cleaved factors resulting from the activation of the alternative pathway (Ba factor), or of the classical/lectin complement pathways (C4d factor), as well as a trend to decreased mannose-binding lectin serine protease 2 levels, reflecting activation of the lectin pathway (14, 22–24).

Complement receptor 1 (CR1, CD35) is a glycoprotein with ~200 kDa encoded by the *CR1* gene (on chromosome region 1q32). The extracellular domain of the most common form of CR1 is composed of a series of 30 repeating units named short consensus repeats (SCRs). The SCRs are distributed in four long homologous repeats (LHRs A, B, C, and D), arising from duplication of a seven-SCR unit (**Figure 1**) (26–28). CR1 is primarily expressed in erythrocytes, B and T cells, neutrophils, monocytes, and dendritic cells, as well as in neurons, microglia, and the choroid plexus of the brain, in the membrane or in soluble form (29). The soluble CR1 (sCR1) form results from proteolytic cleavage in terminal secretory vesicles or in the cell membrane (30, 31). Both CR1 forms act to regulate complement activity by binding cleaved C3b and C4b components as well as the complement cascade initiation molecules mannose-binding lectin (MBL-2), ficolins (FCN1, FCN2, and FCN3), and C1q deposited in altered cell components or pathogens. CR1 competes with serine proteases (MASPs) for the same binding sites on the collagenous tails of MBL and FCNs, inhibiting the initiation of the lectin pathway of complement (32). Upon binding, the membrane-bound form of CR1 internalizes the opsonized elements or presents them to other immune cells, preventing the formation of the C5 convertase. This blocks the formation of the membrane attack complex (MAC). CR1 might also prevent excessive complement activation, acting as a cofactor for the Factor I-mediated cleavage of soluble/bound C3b and C4b (33). On the other hand, binding of opsonized elements fosters antigen presentation to lymphocytes, increasing antibody production, and the humoral response (29, 34). In the presence of excess interleukin 2, CR1 expressed on activated T lymphocytes generates regulatory T cells in secondary lymphoid organs, where they may interact with B cells (35). In fact, CR1 ligation inhibits B cell receptor-mediated activation and differentiation to plasma cells (36).

In a recent study by our group that encompassed polymorphisms of all genes encoding complement components, we found evidence for an association with gene variants of almost all complement elements previously detected in the epidermis or with altered serum levels in FS patients. In addition, we identified the association of four opsonin-binding complement receptors (CR1-4, encoded by *CR1*, *CR2*, *ITGAM*, and *ITGAX*) (37). Among them, we found that a *CR1* haplotype with the major *rs6656401**G* allele was associated with increased susceptibility to FS (37). This prompted us to thoroughly investigate the *CR1*

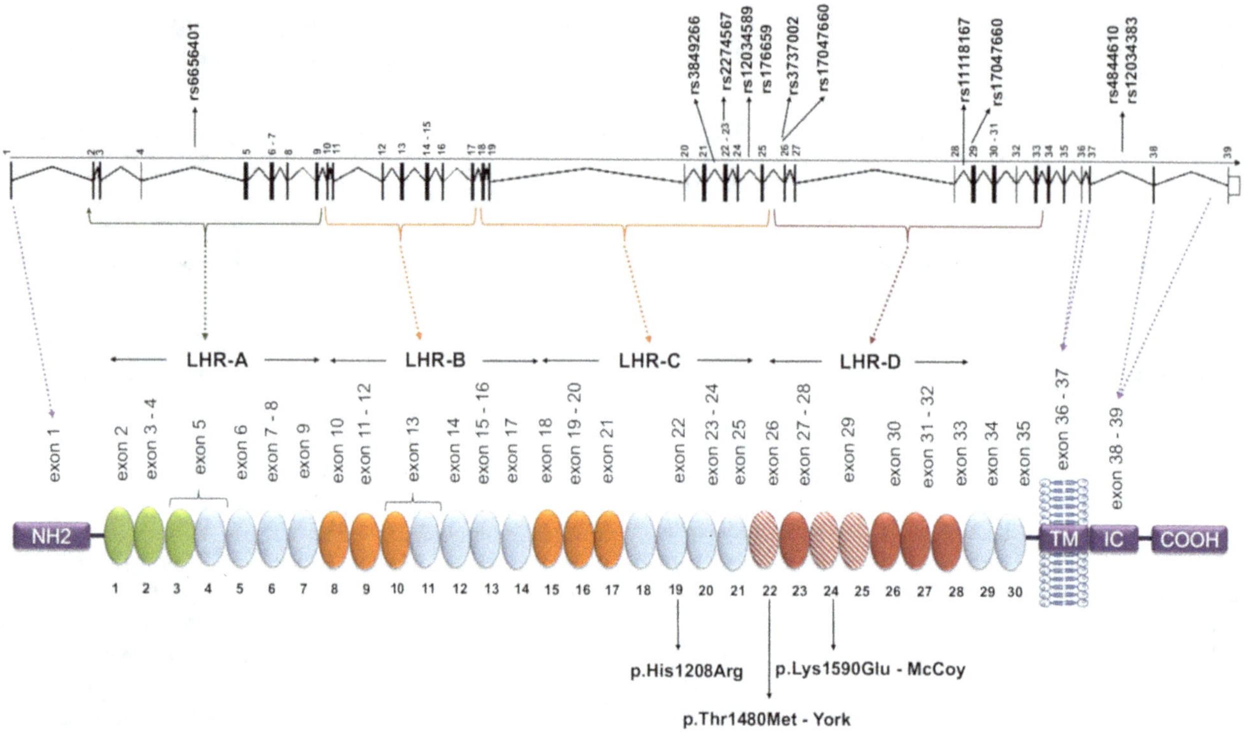

FIGURE 1 | *CR1* gene and protein structure and localization of the investigated SNPs. Each circular block represents a SCR (short consensus repeat, numbered 1–30), encoded by the exons 2–35, listed immediately above. There are three C4b binding sites (SCR 1-3, 8-10, and 15-17, in green and orange) and two C3b binding sites (SCR 8-10 and 15-17, both in orange). SCRs 22-28 bind C1q, MBL, and ficolins, and SCRs 22, 24, and 25 (red dashed blocks) carry Knops blood group antigens. The SNPs analyzed in this study are indicated in the gene, and the amino acid substitutions resulting from polymorphisms located in exons are indicated on the protein. The dashed lines indicate coding exons of the main parts: the aminoterminal region (NH2, exon 1), transmembrane domain (TM, exons 36-37), the intracytoplasmic carboxi-terminal domain (IC COOH, exons 38-39), and the four long homologous repeats (LHR), responsible for complement decay-accelerating, and cofactor activities (exons 1-7, 8-14, 15-21, 22-28). The functional sites in 8-10 and 15-17 are nearly identical. Repeats in green are required for C4b binding and decay-accelerating activity, while those in orange are required for C3b and C4b binding and cofactor activity [adapted of (25)].

gene for other polymorphisms, including those encoding blood group antigens that may affect the binding of C1q, MBL, and FCNs, as well as to measure the expression of this gene at the mRNA and soluble protein levels.

MATERIALS AND METHODS

Ethics Statement

This transversal case-control study was approved by the National Committee for Ethics in Research (CONEP 02727412.4.0000.0096, protocol 505.988). All study participants were informed about the research and signed a term of informed consent.

Research Participants

For the association study, a total of 367 FS patients and 242 controls from an endemic area and 289 individuals from a non-endemic area (among accompanying persons, health workers, and other volunteers) were analyzed. The participants were recruited from four centers: Hospital Adventista do Pênfigo (Campo Grande-MS, Central Western Brazil), Lar da Caridade (Uberaba-MG, Southwestern Brazil), Hospital das Clínicas da Faculdade de Medicina de Ribeirão Preto (Ribeirão Preto-SP, Southwestern Brazil), and Hospital das Clínicas da Universidade Federal do Paraná (UFPR) (Curitiba-PR, South Brazil). Data for both patients and controls were collected through interviews and medical records. Inclusion criteria were: written informed consent, being a resident in the endemic region, and for the patients, FS diagnosis based on clinical evidence and positive anti-Dsg1 serology. Exclusion criteria were: consanguinity with a control or a patient and a familial history of autoimmune diseases. All subjects were classified according to ancestral origin, based on physical characteristics and self-reported ancestry, as previously described (38, 39). The demographic characteristics of the participants in this study are listed in **Table 1**.

For the analysis of sCR1 levels in serum, we selected 53 FS patients and 27 healthy controls, matched for sex, age, and previously genotyped for *CR1* polymorphisms. Eighteen of the patients were in complete remission, nine were without treatment and nine were under immunosuppressive treatment; 35 patients presented with active fogo selvagem, six of whom were still untreated and 29 of whom were already being treated. Among all treated patients with known information regarding the distribution of lesions, five had localized lesions, and 21 had generalized lesions.

In order to evaluate a possible correlation between *CR1* polymorphisms and mRNA levels from peripheral blood mononuclear cells (PBMC), we also genotyped 158 healthy unrelated Euro-Brazilian volunteers, resident in Curitiba, Brazil, and surrounding areas. We selected 63 individuals from this group with the following inclusion criteria: no previous history of an autoimmune disease, an obvious skin disease, and presenting *CR1* alleles and haplotypes associated with the disease (to quantify mRNA levels).

TABLE 1 | Demographic data on endemic pemphigus foliaceus patients and controls.

	Controls		FS patients		
	Endemic $n = 204$	Non-endemic $n = 256$	Patients $n = 265$	Localized lesions $n = 44$	Generalized lesions $n = 80$
Epidemiologic data					
Male (%)	99 (48.5)	106 (41.4)	121 (45.7)	18 (40.9)	32 (40.0)
Average age (min-max)	44.75 (13–86)	33.64 (17–66)	37.42 (12–88)	28.5 (16–73)	38.55 (14–85)
Demographic data					
Central-Western (%)	177 (86.8)	0	206 (77.7)	31 (70.5)	57 (71.3)
Southwestern (%)	5 (2.5)	0	56 (21.1)	12 (27.3)	21 (26.3)
South (%)	22 (10.8)	256 (100)	3 (1.1)	1 (2.3)	2 (2.5)

N, number of individuals; Central-Western, Campo Grande-MS; Southwestern, Ribeirão Preto-SP. South, Curitiba-PR.
The total number of patients with localized or generalized lesions did not sum 265 due to lack of proper diagnostic classification of some individuals.

CR1 Genotyping

Blood was collected with anticoagulant EDTA, and DNA was extracted from PBMC as previously described, using phenol-chloroform-isoamyl alcohol (40).

We selected 11 single nucleotide polymorphisms (SNPs) based on [1] being previously associated with a disease, [2] being a tag SNP with $r^2 \geq 0.8$ in the European (Utah—USA), Mexican, Colombian, or Yoruba populations of the 1000 Genomes Project (41); and/or [3] by presenting a minor allele frequency higher than 0.05. The *CR1* SNPs evaluated were: *rs6656401*a>G* (intron 4); *rs3849266*c>T* (intron 21); *rs2274567*a>G* (exon 22, p.His1208Arg); *rs12034598*a>G* (intron 24), *rs1746659*t>A* (intron 24), *rs3737002*c>T* (exon 26, p.Thr1408Met, responsible for the York blood group antigen); *rs11118131*c>T* (intron 26); *rs11118167*t>C* (intron 28); *rs17047660*a>G* (exon 29, p.Lys1590Glu, responsible for the McCoy blood group antigen); *rs4844610*a>C* (intron 37); *rs12034383*g>A* (intron 37).

We developed two multiplex Polymerase Chain Reaction-Sequence Specific Primer (PCR-SSP) reactions for simultaneous identification of four SNPs and two simple PCR-SSPs for one SNP each. All PCRs co-amplified a Human Growth Hormone (*HGH*) or Human Leukocyte E antigen (*HLA-E*) fragment as internal control. The sequences of specific and control primers are shown in **Table 2**. All reactions were carried out in a final volume of 8 μl, containing 20 ng of genomic DNA, 0.2 mM each of dNTP and 1x Coral Buffer (Invitrogen Life Technologies, Carlsbad, USA)

TABLE 2 | Primers for *CR1* sequence-specific amplification.

	Forward Primers			Reverse primers			
	SNP	Localization	5′→3′ Sequence	SNP	Localization	5′→3′ Sequence	Fragment
Simple PCR 1	**rs6656401**	Intron 4	CTCTGTCTCCATCTTCTC**A** CTCTGTCTCCATCTTCTC**G**	**Generic Primer**	Intron 4	CATAGTTGTAGTTGGGGATT**G**	257 bp
Multi 1	**rs3849266**	Intron 21	CTGATGGCTTGGGGTA**T** CTGATGGCTTGGGGTA**C**	**rs2274567**	Exon 22	CTCAATCTGCATTGATCCA**C** CTCAATCTGCATTGATCCA**T**	667 bp
Simple PCR 1	**rs12034598**	Intron 24	GCCTGGCATCATCAAGAAA**A** GCCTGGCATCATCAAGAAA**G**	**rs1746659**	Intron 24	GGTTAGTGTTCAGAGGCAG**A** GGTTAGTGTTCAGAGGCAG**T**	1068 bp
Multi 2	**rs3737002**	Exon 26	CCATTTGCCAGTCCTA**C** CCATTTGCCAGTCCTA**T**	**rs11118131**	Intron 26	CAAGAAGAAGGGGTGAT**G** CAAGAAGAAGGGGTGAT**A**	457 bp
Multi 2	**rs11118167**	Intron 28	GCCAATATGTGAATATTATTATCTTA**T** GCCAATATGTGAATATTATTATCTTA**C**	**rs17047660**	Exon 29	TTCTGGAGCTGTGCATT**T** TTCTGGAGCTGTGCATT**C**	746 bp
Multi 1	**rs4844610**	Intron 37	CTACACAAAACAGCCTTGT**A** CTACACAAAACAGCCTTGT**C**	**rs12034383**	Intron 37	AGATGTCCATGCCTTAA**C** AGATGTCCATGCCTTAA**T**	1080 bp
	Control primers						
Simple PCR 1, 2 and muli 1	*HGHf*		TGCCTTCCCAACCATTCCCTTA		*HGHr*	CCACTCACGGATTTCTGTTGTGTTTC	431 bp
Multi 2	*HLA-Ef*		CGGGACTGACTAAGGGGCGG		*HLA-Er*	GTAGCCCTGTGGACCCTCTTAC	324 bp

In bold: variant nucleotide. SNP, single nucleotide polymorphism; bp, base pairs; HGH, human growth hormone; HLA-E, Human leukocyte E antigen; f, forward; r, reverse; Multi, multiplex PCR-SSP.

TABLE 3 | Primers for the *CR1* Sequenom massARRAY iPLEX Platform.

SNP	Localization	5′→3′ Forward Primer Sequence	5′→3′ Reverse Primer Sequence	5′→3′ Extended Primer Sequence
rs6656401	Intron 4	ACGTTGGATGGCATCATTTCCTTCTCTGTC	ACGTTGGATGGACAGAAGAGCAAAGGACAC	GTTTTTTCTCTGTCTCCATCTTCTC
rs3849266	Intron 21	ACGTTGGATGATAACTCGCCCCTCAATCTG	ACGTTGGATGGCAGGCAACTGTGTTTATAC	ACCTCAATCTGCATTGATCCA
rs3737002	Exon 26	ACGTTGGATGTCCAGGTCACTGTAAAACCC	ACGTTGGATGAAGATGTCCCGACTGGAAAC	CTATCAGTTTCCATTTGCCAGTCCTA
rs11118131	Intron 26	ACGTTGGATGGATGTCTATATTTGCCCAAG	ACGTTGGATGGCATCTAGTCAAGGTTCAGG	GGTATAAAGGAAAGGATGGTCTTGTA
rs11118167	Intron 28	ACGTTGGATGATGTGTGTAGTCACTTAGCC	ACGTTGGATGATAATGGCAGATTTAAGGGC	GCCAATATGTGAATATTATTATCTTA
rs17047660	Exon 29	ACGTTGGATGCAAGTTGGTGTTTGGAGCAG	ACGTTGGATGGCATTTTCAACTTCTGGAGC	TCACCTTCTGGAGCTGTGCATT

SNP, single nucleotide polymorphism.

(**Supplementary Table 1**). Thermal cycling began with 95°C for 5 min, followed by 33 (PCR-SSP-1) or 30 (PCR-SSP-2, 3 and 4) cycles, for which each cycle began with 94°C for 20 s and ended with 72°C (extension step) for 40 s (**Supplementary Table 1**). We submitted the amplified fragments to an electrophoretic run on 1% agarose gel, stained with Sybersafe (Invitrogen Life Technologies, Carlsbad, USA).

Genotyping of the rs6656401, rs3849266, rs3737002, rs11118131, rs11118167, rs17047660, and rs12034383 polymorphisms was performed with the iPLEX platform of the MassARRAY system (Agena Bioscience, San Diego, USA) at the Insitut für Klinische Molekularbiologie (IKMB), Christian-Albrechts-Universität, Kiel, Germany (42), in order to technically validate the results obtained by PCR-SSP. Genotypes were called using the software MassARRAY Typer (v4.0) (Agena Bioscience, San Diego, USA) with standard settings. The sequences of specific and control primers are shown in **Table 3**.

sCR1 Quantification

We measured sCR1 levels in the serum (collected without anticoagulant) by using a SEB123Hu ELISA kit (USCN Life Science Inc., Wuhan, China) according to the manufacturer's instructions. Anti-Dsg1 and anti-Dsg3 levels were previously measured using commercial ELISA kits (RG-M7593-D and RG-7680-EC-D, respectively) (MBL, Woburn, USA) (43).

mRNA Quantification

Total RNA was isolated from PBMC lysed in TRIzol (Ambion, Austin, USA) and reverse-transcribed with a High Capacity cDNA Reverse Transcription Kit (Applied Biosystems, Foster City, USA). Gene expression levels were quantified by qPCR using TaqMan (Applied Biosystems, Foster City, USA) chemistry for the *CR1* (Hs00559348_m1, the most common CR1 transcript) and the housekeeping Glucuronidase Beta (*GUSB*) gene (4333767F). All assays were performed in triplicate, and the relative mRNA levels were normalized for mRNA expression of the *GUSB* gene. Cq values (threshold cycle) were calculated using the Viia 7 Software v1.2 Kit (Applied Biosystems, Foster City, USA), and gene expression was calculated via the comparative Cq method 2-ΔΔCq (44).

Statistical and Bioinformatics Analysis

We obtained allele, genotype and two-SNP haplotype frequencies by direct counting, and the hypothesis of Hardy-Weinberg equilibrium was calculated with the exact test of Guo & Thompson. We also compared haplotype distribution between the investigated groups, using the exact test of population differentiation of Raymond and Rousset. All tests were performed in Arlequin v.5.1, a population genetics software package (45).

We reconstructed extended haplotypes based on linkage disequilibrium (LD) and phase information about the two-SNP haplotypes obtained by PCR-SSP amplification, compared the results with the haplotypes estimated using the EM algorithm (Expectation-Maximization) implemented in PLINK software (46), and found 2.9% of haplotypes with discrepant results in accordance with the literature (47). We also used PLINK for analysis of possible SNP interactions and evaluated LD with Haploview 4.2 (48). We used Mega Software v.6 to name the haplotypes according to the phylogenetic nomenclature suggested by the literature (49) and adapted them for recombinant haplotypes (**Figure 2**). We further compared the distribution of polymorphisms and haplotypes in patients and controls adjusted for the proportion of ancestry groups using the Fisher exact test in the online software VassarStats (VassarStats: Website for Statistical Computation; available at: http://vassarstats.net). We adjusted all associations for the possible effects of confounding factors (age, sex, ancestry group) by logistic regression in total patient and control groups using the software STATA v.9.2 (Statacorps, Lakeway Drive, USA). To check for false discovery rate, we used the correction of Benjamini and Hochberg (50) on all significant results ("q" values lower than 0.05 were considered significant).

Normality tests (D'Agostino & Pearson and Shapiro-Wilk), correlation tests (Spearman), and non-parametric comparisons of *CR1* mRNA and sCR1 levels (Mann-Whitney and Kruskal-Wallis tests) were carried out using GraphPad Prism v.5.01 (GraphPad Software). The use of different dosages of corticosteroids was evaluated in the group of patients undergoing treatment in order to verify whether there were differences between them.

To predict the functional effects of associated SNPs, we explored data from the ENCODE project contained in the Regulome-DB (51) and Haploreg (52) databases. To evaluate the effect of non-synonymous SNPs, we used Polyphen-2 (53) and SNiPA (54).

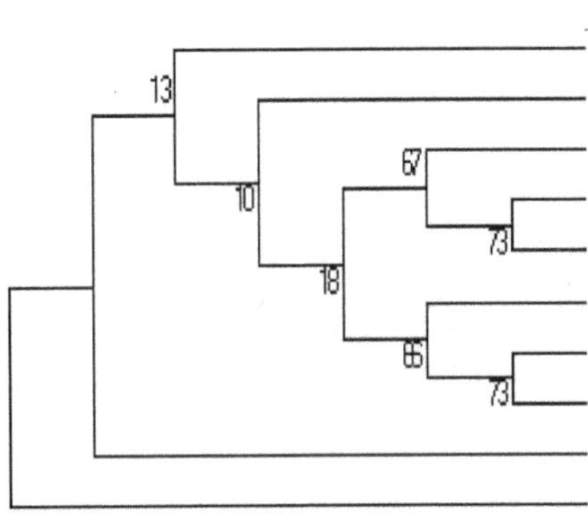

Phylogenetic Nomenclature	rs6656401	rs3849266	rs2274567	rs3737002	rs11118131	rs11118167	rs17047660	rs4844610	rs12034383
*1	G	C	H	T	C	T	K	C	G
*2							E		
*3A1			R						
*3A2A			R		T				
*3A2B			R		T				
*3B1									A
*3B2A		T							A
*3B2B		T		M					A
*4	A							A	
PAN									
*1.3A2B.3B2B						C		C	A
*2.3B2B							E		A
*1.3B2B	G			M					A
*3B2B.3A2B	G	T		M		C			A

FIGURE 2 | Maximum parsimony tree of *CR1* haplotypes with nucleotide changes and phylogenetic nomenclature. Underlined: amino acid substitutions.

RESULTS

CR1 Polymorphisms and Susceptibility to Fogo Selvagem

None of the groups had genotype distributions that deviated from those predicted under Hardy-Weinberg equilibrium. The allele frequencies for each SNP did not differ between controls and the Iberian population from the 1,000 Genomes Project. In contrast, *CR1* haplotype distributions differed between the endemic and non-endemic controls, even within each ancestry group ($P < 0.0001$). This led us to compare the patient group with endemic and non-endemic control groups separately. We found differences between the allelic distributions of isolated SNPs of non-endemic controls and patients.

Comparing these two groups (**Table 4, Supplementary Table 2**), we found evidence for a disease association with the minor allele of *rs17047660*G* in exon 29. This variant encodes p.1590Glu, which is responsible for positive McCoy blood group antigen. Its allelic frequency was higher among FS patients [OR = 3.77 (95%CI = 1.52–9.35), q = 0.005]. *rs17047660*A/G* heterozygote individuals were more frequent among those with generalized lesions [OR = 3.06 (95%CI = 1.09–8.56), q = 0.025]. The rs3849266 within intron 21 occurs in a region with enhancer histone H3K4me1 marks, binding at least 23 different regulatory proteins, according to the ENCODE Database. *rs3849266*C/T* presented an association with increased susceptibility to the disease [OR = 1.54 (95%CI = 1.03–2.31), q = 0.030]. We also found an additive effect of carrying the "wild type" haplotype with *rs3737002*C* in exon 26 (p.1408Thr, York negative) and *rs11118131*C* in intron 26 [OR = 1.5 (95%CI = 1.00–2.26), q = 0.049] with susceptibility to severe FS. The minor allele *rs2274567*G*, encoding p.1208Arg, occurred more frequently among non-endemic controls than among patients [OR = 0.58 (95%CI = 0.38–0.87), q = 0.035].

There was strong pairwise LD between the SNPs in intron 21 (rs3849266), exon 22 (rs2274567), exon 26 (rs3737002), and intron 37 (rs12034383) (**Supplementary Figure 1**). Based on LD and phase information, we haplotyped all SNPs in a subset of 146 FS patients and 126 controls from an endemic area and 156 from a non-endemic area and identified 21 haplotypes (**Figure 2**). In fact, we obtained the most conspicuous association results with *CR1* haplotypes (**Table 5**), revealing synergistic, additive/epistatic effects between variants located on the same DNA string. The carrier status of the **3B2B* haplotype (*GTHMCTKCA*), the most common haplotype encoding the York blood group antigen (rs3737002, p.1408Met), protects against FS [OR = 0.57 (95%CI = 0.35–0.93), q = 0.042] as well as against the localized form of the disease [OR = 0.25 (95%CI = 0.089–0.72), q = 0.01]. In contrast with all other results, this association agreed for comparisons with both endemic and non-endemic controls. A similar protective effect was observed from carrying the **3A2A* (*GCRTTTKCG*) haplotype, presenting p.1208Arg and p.1408Thr [OR = 0.46 (95%CI = 0.25–0.85), q = 0.033]. This protective effect agreed with the aforementioned association results of rs2274567 (p.His1208Arg). In contrast, the frequency of the **1* haplotype (*GCHTCTKCG*) was higher among FS patients with both localized and generalized distributions of cutaneous lesions than in controls (OR = 5.50 [95%CI = 1.84–16.45], q = 0.016 and OR = 4.33 [95%CI = 1.74–10.77], q = 0.002, respectively).

TABLE 4 | Association of *CR1* variants with endemic pemphigus foliaceus.

		Controls		FS patients				
***CR1* genetic variants**	**Iberian *n* = 214 (%)**	**Endemic control *n* (%)**	**Non-endemic control *n* (%)**	**Patient *n* (%)**	**Localized lesion *n* (%)**	**Generalized lesion *n* (%)**	**Patient vs. Non-endemic control**	
rs6656401 A>G		*n* = 203	*n* = 234	*n* = 265	*N* = 44	*N* = 81	**OR [95% CI]**	**P (q) value**
A	27 (12.60)	46 (11.33)	63 (13.46)	59 (11.13)	8 (9.09)	20 (12.35)		
AA	2 (1.90)	2 (0.99)	1 (0.43)	2 (0.75)	1 (2.27)	0		
AG	23 (21.50)	42 (20.69)	61 (26.07)	55 (20.75)	6 (13.64)	20 (24.69)		
GG	82 (76.60)	159 (78.33)	172 (73.50)	208 (78.49)	37 (84.09)	61 (75.31)		
A+		44 (21.67)	62 (26.50)	57 (21.51)	7 (15.91)	20 (24.69)		
rs3849266 C>T		*n* = 182	*n* = 238	*n* = 233	*n* = 41	*n* = 76		
T	68 (31.80)	103 (28.30)	122 (25.63)	125 (26.82)	19 (23.17)	38 (25.00)		
CC	50 (46.70)	90 (49.45)	134 (56.30)	120 (51.50)	24 (58.54)	41 (53.95)		
CT	46 (43.00)	81 (44.51)	86 (36.13)	101 (43.35)	15 (36.59)	32 (42.11)	1.54 [1.03–2.31]	0.036 (0.030)
TT	11 (10.30)	11 (6.04)	18 (7.56)	12 (5.15)	2 (4.88)	3 (3.95)		
T+		92 (50.55)	104 (43.70)	113 (48.50)	17 (41.46)	35 (46.05)		
***rs2274567 A>G* (p.His1208Arg)**		*n* = 148	*n* = 232	*n* = 158	*n* = 28	*n* = 54		
G	36 (16.80)	65 (21.96)	138 (29.74)	73 (23.10)	15 (26.79)	22 (20.37)	0.70 [0.51–0.98]	0.048 (0.035)
AA	73 (68.20)	94 (63.51)	110 (47.41)	93 (58.86)	14 (50.00)	32 (59.26)		
AG	32 (29.90)	43 (29.05)	106 (45.69)	57 (36.08)	13 (46.43)	22 (40.74)		
GG	2 (1.90)	11 (7.43)	16 (6.90)	8 (5.06)	1 (3.57)	0		
G+		54 (36.49)	122 (52.59)	65 (41.14)	14 (50.00)	22 (40.74)		
***rs3737002 C>T* (p.Thr1408Met)**		n= 192	n= 246	n= 253	n= 43	n= 79		
T	68 (31.80)	109 (28.39)	134 (27.24)	127 (25.10)	18 (20.93)	36 (22.78)		
CC	50 (46.70)	103 (53.65)	133 (54.07)	144 (56.92)	27 (62.79)	47 (59.49)		
CT	46 (43.00)	69 (35.94)	92 (37.40)	91 (35.97)	14 (32.56)	28 (35.44)		
TT	11 (10.30)	20 (10.42)	21 (8.54)	18 (7.11)	2 (4.65)	4 (5.06)		
T+		89 (46.35)	113 (45.93)	109 (43.08)	16 (37.21)	32 (40.51)		
rs11118131 C>T		*n* = 177	*n* = 208	*n* = 225	*n* = 49	*n* = 71		
T	35 (16.40)	75 (21.19)	103 (24.76)	89 (19.78)	15 (19.23)	26 (18.31)	0.74 [0.54–1.03]	0.08
CC	74 (69.20)	114 (64.41)	120 (57.69)	147 (65.33)	25 (64.10)	45 (63.38)		
CT	31 (29.00)	51 (28.81)	73 (35.10)	67 (29.78)	13 (33.33)	26 (36.62)		
TT	2 (1.90)	12 (6.78)	15 (7.21)	11 (4.89)	1 (2.56)	0		
T+		63 (35.59)	88 (42.31)	78 (34.67)	14 (35.90)	26 (36.62)		
rs11118167 T>C		*n* = 179	*n* = 232	*n* = 234	*n* = 41	*n* = 77		
C	35 (16.40)	65 (18.16)	91 (19.61)	82 (17.52)	18 (21.95)	28 (18.18)		
CC	2 (1.90)	4 (2.23)	5 (2.16)	7 (2.99)	2 (4.88)	2 (2.60)		
CT	31 (29.00)	57 (31.84)	81 (34.91)	68 (29.06)	14 (34.15)	24 (31.17)		
TT	74 (69.20)	118 (65.92)	146 (62.93)	159 (67.95)	25 (60.98)	51 (66.23)		
C+		61 (34.08)	86 (37.07)	75 (32.05)	16 (39.02)	26 (33.77)		
***rs17047660 A>G* (p.Lys1590Glu)**		*n* = 185	*n* = 235	*n* = 247	*n* = 42	*n* = 77		
G	3 (1.40)	10 (2.70)	6 (1.28)	23 (4.66)	4 (4.76)	9 (5.84)	3.77 [1.52–9.35]	0.002 (0.005)
AA	104 (97.20)	175 (94.59)	229 (97.45)	224 (90.69)	38 (90.48)	68 (88.31)		
AG	3 (2.80)	10 (5.41)	6 (2.55)	23 (9.31)	4 (9.52)	9 (11.69)	3.56 [1.37–9.27]	0.009 (0.015)
GG	0	0	0	0	0	0	2.38 [1.01–5.62]	0.048 (0.035)
G+		10 (5.41)	6 (2.55)	23 (9.31)	4 (9.52)	9 (11.69)	2.93 [1.18–7.24]	0.020 (0.020)

(Continued)

TABLE 4 | Continued

		Controls		FS patients				
***CR1* genetic variants**	**Iberian $n = 214$ (%)**	**Endemic control *n* (%)**	**Non-endemic control *n* (%)**	**Patient *n* (%)**	**Localized lesion *n* (%)**	**Generalized lesion *n* (%)**	**Patient vs. Non-endemic control**	
rs4844610 A>C		$n = 203$	$n = 234$	$n = 265$	$n = 44$	$n = 81$		
A	23 (10.70)	47 (11.58)	63 (13.46)	59 (11.13)	8 (9.09)	20 (12.35)		
AA	1 (0.90)	2 (0.99)	1 (0.43)	2 (0.75)	1 (2.27)	0		
AC	21 (19.60)	43 (21.18)	61 (26.07)	55 (20.75)	6 (13.64)	20 (24.69)		
CC	85 (79.40)	158 (77.83)	172 (73.50)	208 (78.49)	37 (84.09)	61 (75.31)		
A+		45 (22.17)	62 (26.50)	57 (21.51)	7 (15.91)	20 (24.69)		
rs12034383 G>A		$n = 191$	$n = 242$	$n = 252$	$n = 43$	$n = 78$		
G	71 (33.20)	188 (49.21)	231 (47.73)	249 (49.40)	46 (53.49)	82 (52.56)	3.95 [1.08–14.34]	0.029
AA	44 (41.10)	50 (26.18)	70 (28.93)	69 (27.38)	10 (23.26)	17 (21.79)		
AG	55 (51.40)	94 (49.21)	113 (46.69)	117 (46.43)	20 (46.51)	40 (51.28)		
GG	8 (7.50)	47 (24.61)	59 (24.38)	66 (26.19)	13 (30.23)	21 (26.92)		
G+		141 (73.82)	172 (71.07)	183 (72.62)	33 (76.74)	61 (78.21)		

All genotype distributions were in Hardy–Weinberg equilibrium. Associations were corrected for age, sex, and, if independent, for ancestry group distribution. P values were checked for false discovery rate using the correction of Benjamini and Hochberg ("q" statistical significance level remained 0.05). n, number of individuals; OR, odds ratio in binary logistic regression; CI, confidence interval; q, Benjamini-Hochberg corrected p-value.

sCR1 Levels and Susceptibility to Fogo Selvagem

sCR1 levels differed according to treatment and disease manifestations but not according to the genotypes of the investigated SNPs and haplotypes (**Figure 3**). Patients in complete remission on treatment had higher sCR1 levels (median 1.82 ng/mL) than did controls and patients that had not yet initiated therapy (medians 1.23 and 0.61 ng/mL, $P = 0.013$ and 0.036, respectively). On the other hand, there was no difference between sCR1 levels in controls and patients with active fogo selvagem on treatment (medians 1.2 ng/mL vs. 1.39 ng/mL, respectively, $P = 0.188$). However, those with localized lesions revealed higher sCR1 levels than did patients with generalized lesions (medians 2.39 ng/mL vs. 1.24 ng/mL, respectively, $P = 0.0073$). The sCR1 levels of patients with localized lesions on immunosuppressive treatment were also significantly higher than in controls ($P = 0.0112$). Of note, no difference in sCR1 levels was found between patients treated with low and high corticosteroid doses ($P = 0.1897$, data not shown).

CR1 mRNA Expression Levels

One out of eleven *CR1* SNPs analyzed (rs12034383) was associated with differential mRNA expression levels. Controls with the *rs12034383*A/G* genotype had higher mRNA levels than controls with the *rs12034383*G/G* genotype (median fold changes 0.96 vs. 0.62, respectively, $P = 0.04$) (**Figure 4**). Carriers of the protective *GTHMCTKCA* haplotype, which includes the *rs12034383*A* allele, presented instead lower mRNA expression ($P = 0.03$) (**Figure 5**).

DISCUSSION

CR1 plays a major role in inhibiting the complement system, removing immune complexes, and activating B cells, important events that are deregulated in autoimmune diseases (35, 55, 56). Polymorphisms that alter *CR1* gene expression or protein activity are also common worldwide (57–60) and have been associated with different infectious, autoimmune, and neurological/neurodegenerative diseases (61–67). Those in exon 29 encode antigens of the Knops blood group system, the 22nd system recognized by the International Society of Blood Transfusion (68): e.g., rs3737002 (p.Thr1408Met) defines the York blood antigen and rs17047660 (p.Lys1590Glu), the McCoy blood antigen (69, 70). These polymorphisms may modulate the success of *Plasmodium falciparum* and *Leishmania major*, as well as mycobacteria that invade erythrocytes and macrophages, respectively (71–75). Most of the time, however, disease associations are related to complement subversion/deregulation and consequent alterations in phagocytosis and cytokine release, even in infectious diseases (29, 76–78). For example, in HIV infection, CR1 molecules expressed on erythrocytes bind C3b-opsonized HIV particles. They act as cofactors for factor I conversion of C3b to inactivated iC3b. This allows the virus to survive anti-retroviral therapy and spread as iC3b-opsonized particles, captured by CR2 on B cells, and presented to other lymphocytes (79). In systemic lupus erythematosus, a low CR1 density on neutrophils and other phagocytes causes excessive C3 activation, the release of proinflammatory cytokines, and immune-complex overload (80–82). The risk for Alzheimer's disease increases with the preferential, low expression of a long CR1 isoform, which is ineffective in the removal of beta-amyloid plaques (83–86). Furthermore, *CR1* polymorphisms also modulate the response to eculizumab therapy, which targets complement protein C5 (87).

Here, the York blood group, encoded by the *CR1*3B2B* haplotype, was associated with higher protection against FS. The p.1408Met amino acid substitution (*rs3737002*T*) is responsible for this antigen and is considered as "probably damaging"

TABLE 5 | Association of *CR1* haplotypes with endemic pemphigus foliaceus.

Phylogenetic Haplotype	Nucleotide sequence	Patient groups n/n total (%)	Control groups n/n total (%)	OR	95% CI	P (q)	Model
*3B2B	GTHMCTKCA	Patient 57/292 (19.5)	Endemic 66/252 (26.2)	0.57	0.35–0.93	0.027 (0.042)	Dominant
		Localized lesion 5/25 (20)	Endemic 66/252 (26.2)	0.25	0.089–0.72	0.010 (0.025)	Dominant
		Localized lesion 5/25 (20)	Endemic 66/252 (26.2)	0.26	0.093–0.72	0.010 (0.029)	Additive
		Localized lesion 5/25 (20)	Non-endemic 71/312 (22.8)	0.35	0.12–1.00	0.052 (0.050)	Dominant
		Localized lesion 5/25 (20)	Non-endemic 71/312 (22.8)	0.35	0.12–0.99	0.049 (0.045)	Additive
*1	GCHTCTKCG	Patient 36/292 (12.3)	Non-endemic 32/252 (12.7)	4.97	2.13–11.59	$<10^3$ (0.004)	Dominant
		Patient 36/292 (12.3)	Non-endemic 32/252 (12.7)	4.76	2.08–10.87	$<10^3$ (0.008)	Additive
		Generalized lesion 9/52 (17.3)	Non-endemic 32/252 (12.7)	4.33	1.74–10.77	0.002 (0.012)	Dominant and additive
		Localized lesion 3/25 (12)	Non-endemic 32/252 (12.7)	5.50	1.84–16.45	0.002 (0.016)	Dominant
		Localized lesion 3/25 (12)	Non-endemic 32/252 (12.7)	5.32	1.85–15.24	0.002 (0.021)	Additive
*3A2A	GCRTTTKCG	Patient 25/292 (8.6)	Non-endemic 43/252 (12.8)	0.46	0.25–0.85	0.014 (0.033)	Dominant
		Patient 25/292 (8.6)	Non-endemic 43/252 (12.8)	0.49	0.27–0.89	0.020 (0.037)	Additive

Haplotypes represented nine investigated CR1 SNPs (rs6656401, rs3849266, rs2274567, rs3737002, rs11118131, rs11118167, rs17047660, rs4844610, and rs12034383). One-letter, underlined amino acid symbols are given instead of nucleotide substitutions, where appropriate. n, number of chromosomes; OR, odds ratio, corrected for age, ancestry group, and sex distribution; CI, confidence interval.

**Fisher's exact test. Dominant model: individuals with the haplotype were more frequent in one of the groups, regardless of whether homozygous or heterozygous. Additive model: homozygote individuals were overrepresented in one of the groups, followed by heterozygotes, meaning that the haplotype presents an additive effect for increasing resistance/protection against the disease.*

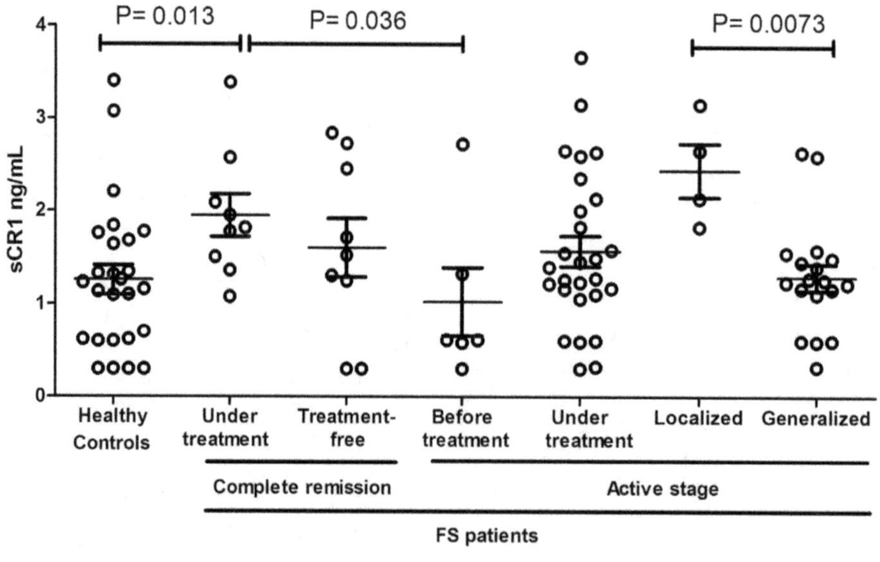

FIGURE 3 | sCR1 serum levels in endemic controls and FS patients. *P*-values were obtained with the Mann-Whitney test. Interquartile median and range are indicated. We excluded two outliers with very high levels (one with 7.14 ng/mL in controls and another with 10.2 ng/mL in FS patients with active disease, but under treatment).

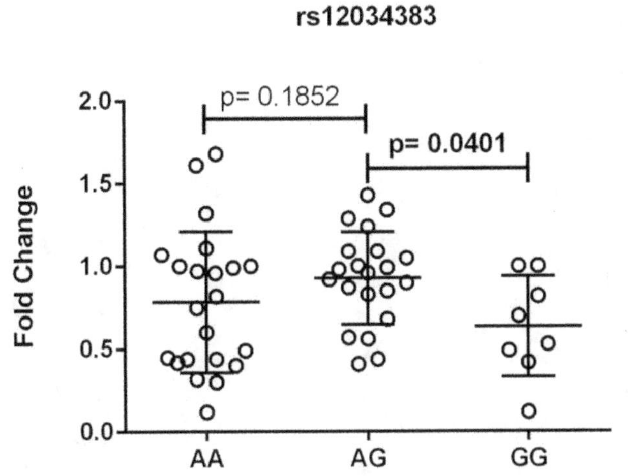

FIGURE 4 | Association between the expression of *CR1* mRNA and *CR1* rs12034383 polymorphism. Fold-change values were calculated through the 2–ΔΔCt method. The horizontal bars in the clusters indicate the median. *P*-values indicate a statistical significance at the 0.05 level and were calculated by Mann–Whitney's test. Scatter plots were constructed from the raw non-normalized, fold change data using GraphPad 6.0 software (La Jolla, California, USA).

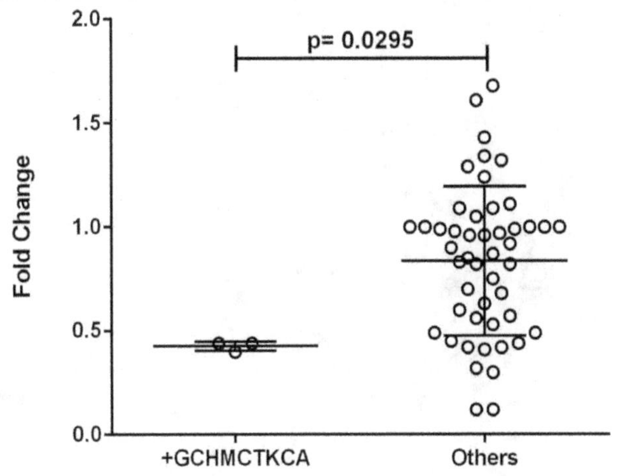

FIGURE 5 | Association between the expression of CR1 mRNA and the **1.3B2B– GCHMCTKCA* haplotype. *+GCHMCTKCA*: homozygote or heterozygote individuals. Fold-change values were calculated through the 2–ΔΔCt method. The horizontal bars in the clusters indicate the median. *P*-values indicate a statistical significance at the 0.05 level and were calculated by Mann–Whitney's test. Scatter plots were constructed from the raw non-normalized, fold change data using GraphPad 6.0 software (La Jolla, California, USA).

(a Polyphen-2 score of 0.9 or higher and a CADD score of 19.52). This substitution modifies the first SCR in the LHR-D module (SCR 22), responsible for the recognition of the initiation molecules of the classical (C1q) and lectin (MBL and FCNs) pathways, and may reduce the recognition of IgG1-bound C1q as well as of MBL/FCNs (32) bound to exposed glycosilated/acetylated residues on desmosomes and epithelial cells, decreasing internalization of neoantigens by antigen-presenting cells (**Figure 6**).

As expected, the most ancestral **1* haplotype, encoding p.1408Thr, seems to increase susceptibility to FS. Interestingly, although this association was found by comparing patients with non-endemic controls, a *CR1* haplotype with p.1408Thr was found to increase FS susceptibility 1.4x within the endemic population in our previous study (37). Furthermore, the same haplotype has recently been associated with increased susceptibility to the more severe multibacillary clinical forms of leprosy (25).

On the other hand, the p.1408Met amino acid substitution was also recently associated with susceptibility to idiopathic pulmonary fibrosis (88). Affected patients present an increase of serum proteins of the complement cascade and higher complement activation in the lung (89). The same allele was also reported to increase the susceptibility to late-onset Alzheimer's disease in Han Chinese (90). Compared to the York antigen, the opposite is expected to occur with the amino acid substitution that creates the McCoy "b" antigen in SCR25, namely p.Lys1590Glu (*rs17047660*G*). This SNP is also deemed to be damaging (although with a low Polyphen score: 0.597) or deleterious, according to SIFT (score of 0.02). It increases the amount of glutamic acid residues in a sequence of only 10 residues, strengthening the negative charge already provided by Glu at the 1595 and 1597 positions and thus most probably increasing the affinity of this LHR-D domain for C1q/MBL/FCNs (91). This could explain the association found with increased susceptibility to FS, since it could potentially increase the capture of complement-opsonized elements, their internalization, and consequent B cell activation (**Figure 6**). The association found with the McCoy antigen (p.1590Glu), however, did not resist correction for demographic factors, which may stem from its higher frequency in African-derived populations and the small sample size of this study. Interestingly, homozygosity for p.1590Glu was also associated with higher susceptibility to repetitive malaria-associated seizures in patients with cerebral malaria (66). The susceptibility associations found for the intronic polymorphisms *rs6656401*G* and *rs3849266*T* are in accordance with our previous results (37), but the latter may also result from strong linkage disequilibrium with rs3737002.

Last, but not least, we found a protective association with the **3A2A* haplotype, containing the p.1208Arg (*rs2274567*G*) amino acid substitution. Among the investigated SNPs, this allele was, as expected, also associated with FS resistance. However, both associations only occurred when comparing patients with non-endemic controls. Thus, we recommend caution in interpreting these results until they are replicated in an independent sample.

In accordance with the proposed anti-inflammatory role of the York antigen in disease resistance, we found an association of higher levels of sCR1, a molecule known for its anti-inflammatory properties (92), with less severe clinical presentation of FS, disease remission, and corticoid therapy. This leads us to suggest that sCR1 plays a protective role in the evolution of the disease. The soluble CR1 molecule shares all LHR domains with exosomal-bound CR1 and cell

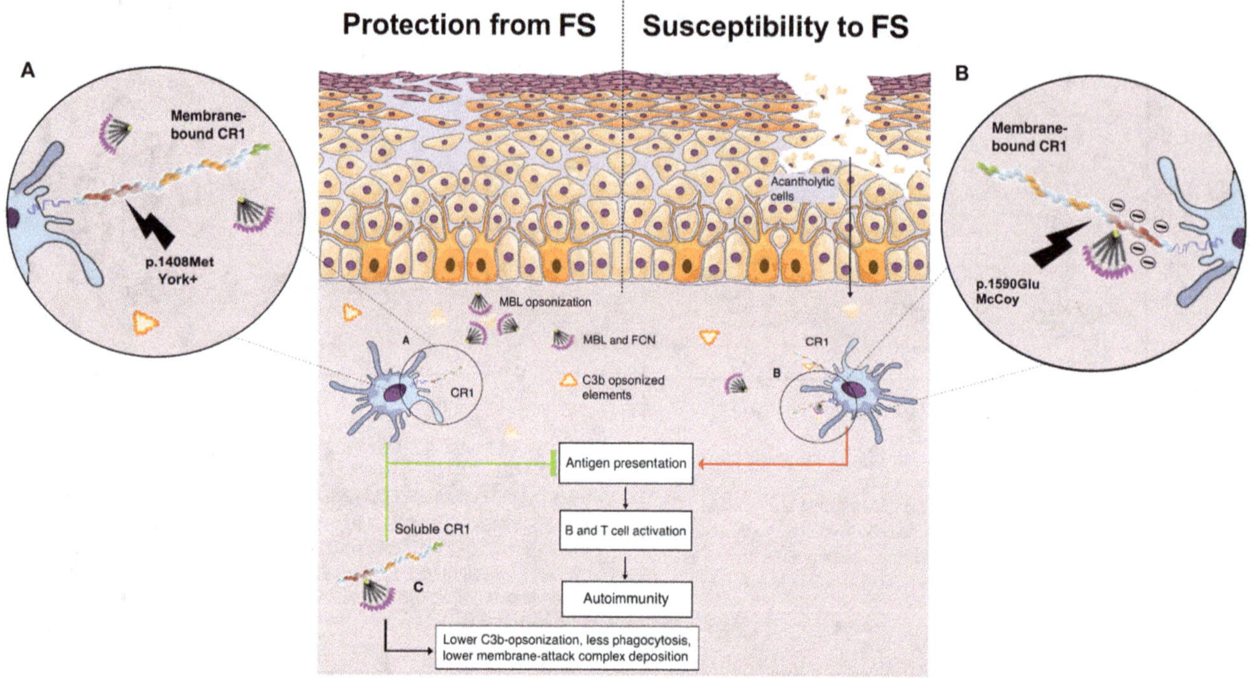

FIGURE 6 | Proposed role of *CR1* polymorphisms of the Knop blood group and soluble CR1 in susceptibility to endemic pemphigus foliaceus. **(A)** The p.1408Met amino acid substitution (York antigen) in the SCR22 module of the protein is proposed to reduce the affinity of CR1 molecules for C1q/collectin/ficolin to IgG1-bound C1q as well to exposed glycosilated/acetylated residues on desmosomes and epithelial cells, decreasing internalization of neoantigens by antigen-presenting cells. **(B)** In contrast, CR1 molecules with p.1590Glu (McCoy antigen) are proposed to have enhanced affinity for C1q/collectin/ficolins due to a negative charge already provided by Glu at the 1595 and 1597 positions, increasing the internalization of cell debris and other opsonized complexes, fostering the autoimmune reaction by renewing the presentation of self-peptides, and consequent B and T cell activation. **(C)** The soluble CR1 molecule has anti-inflammatory properties. As cell membrane-bound CR1, sCR1 acts as a cofactor for the Factor I-mediated cleavage of soluble/bound C3b and C4b, reducing opsonization and phagocytosis. Furthermore, sCR1 and exosomal-bound CR1 are unable to mediate the LHR-D-mediated internalization of opsonized complexes by phagocytes, inhibiting both complement activation, and complement-driven phagocytosis (by the author).

membrane-bound CR1, as well as all functions mediated by LHRs A-C, including the ability to cleave C4b, accelerating the decay of C3 and C5 convertases, and to cleave C3b, reducing opsonization and phagocytosis (27, 93). Nevertheless, sCR1 and exosomal-bound CR1 are unable to mediate the LHR-D-mediated internalization of opsonized complexes by phagocytes, thus acting as a "sink" for initiation molecules of the complement cascade and inhibiting both complement activation and complement-driven phagocytosis (92). Taking into account that human sCR1 has been demonstrated to reduce acute inflammation and autoimmunity, even preventing disease progression in a rat arthritis model (94, 95), and as the potential application of sCR1 in therapeutic settings has been shown (96), its role in susceptibility to pemphigus and its clinical evolution might be highly relevant. A longitudinal follow-up study would be necessary to find out whether patients with localized lesions that have progressed to the generalized form also present a decline in sCR1 concentration. In the present study, *CR1* genotypes were not correlated with sCR1 serum levels, which might rely on the fact that the sCR1 form does not result from alternative splicing of the gene but from proteolytic cleavage (31).

CR1 gene expression was higher in healthy individuals with the genotype *A/G* (rs12034383) than in *G/G* homozygotes. This latter genotype is also associated with impaired removal of amyloid Aß in the cerebrospinal fluid of Alzheimer patients compared with *A/A* homozygotes (83). Interestingly, the recombinant **1.3B2B* (*GCHMCTKCA*) haplotype, containing the proposed protective York antigen (p.1408Met), was associated with lower gene expression, lending support to the hypothesis that low CR1 levels would protect against the production of autoantibodies, as previously discussed.

In conclusion, our data lead us to suggest that *CR1* polymorphisms of the Knops blood group modulate susceptibility to FS. Furthermore, higher sCR1 levels may limit FS lesions and promote/accelerate disease remission. CR1 may thus be regarded as a candidate for new therapeutic interventions in the disease.

ETHICS STATEMENT

The studies involving human participants were reviewed and approved by The National Committee for Ethics in Research (CONEP 02727412.4.0000.0096, protocol 505.988). Written informed consent to participate in this study was provided by the participants' legal guardian/next of kin.

AUTHOR CONTRIBUTIONS

AB administered the project and supervised this work. AB and LO contributed to the conception of the work and curated and analyzed the data. LO, GK, AS, RN, TF, AF, and MW performed the investigation. CC obtained and prepared samples. LO and GK further provided methodological input by developing the multiplex PCR-SSP method used in this study. MP-E provided the samples, and ES and HB provided resources for analysis. AB, MP-E, ES, and HB acquired the funding. LO drafted the manuscript, which was further edited by AB. All authors revised the work critically for intellectual content and approved the final version of the work.

ACKNOWLEDGMENTS

We thank the patients and healthy controls for volunteering for this study, and the staff of the Hospital Adventista do Pênfigo, Lar da Caridade (Uberaba, MG), Hospital das Clínicas at the Faculdade de Medicina de Ribeirão Preto, and Hospital de Clínicas at the Federal University of Paraná for their support. Deep thanks also to the staff of the Laboratório de Genética Molecular Humana/UFPR and to Mariana Basso Spadoni, Gabriel Adelman Cipolla, Liana Alves de Oliveira, and Danillo Gardenal Augusto for technical assistance and helpful discussions.

SUPPLEMENTARY MATERIAL

Supplementary Figure 1 | Pairwise linkage disequilibrium plot based on investigated *CR1* SNPs. Colors are indicative of D'/logarithm of odds (LOD), and values correspond to r^2. Bright red represents LOD score for LD $\geq$ 2 and D = 1, shades of pink/red represent LOD $\geq$ 2 and D < 1, blue represents D = 1 but LOD < 2, and white squares represent LOD< 2 and D < 1. **(A)** Euro-Brazilian patients. **(B)** Euro-Brazilian controls. **(C)** Afro-Brazilian patients. **(D)** Afro-Brazilian controls. The SNPs rs12034598 and rs1746659 are not represented in the plot because they were not genotyped for all individuals.

Supplementary Table 1 | PCR conditions. *HGH* was used as an internal amplification control for simple PCR 1, 2 and multiplex 1; *HLA-E* was used as an internal amplification control for multiplex PCR 2; Simple PCR 1: *CR1* forward primer-1 pair detects rs6656401 alleles; Simple PCR 2: *CR1* forward primer-1 pair detects rs12034598 alleles and *CR1* reverse primer-1 pair detects rs1746659 alleles; Multiplex PCR 1: *CR1* forward primer-1 pair detects rs3849266 alleles and *CR1* reverse primer-1 pair detects rs2274567 alleles; and *CR1* forward primer-2 pair detects rs4844610 alleles and *CR1* reverse primer-2 pair detects rs12034383 alleles; Multiplex PCR 2: CR1 forward primer-1 pair detects rs3737002 alleles and *CR1* reverse primer-1 pair detects rs11118131 alleles; and *CR1* forward primer-2 pair detects rs11118167 alleles and *CR1* reverse primer-2 pair detects rs17047660 alleles; C, Celsius; min: minute; sec: seconds.

Supplementary Table 2 | Allele and genotype distributions of *CR1* polymorphisms investigated in this study.

REFERENCES

1. Schmidt E, Kasperkiewicz M, Joly P. Pemphigus. *Lancet*. (2019) 394:882–94. doi: 10.1016/S0140-6736(19)31778-7
2. Meyer N, Misery L. Geoepidemiologic considerations of auto-immune pemphigus. *Autoimmun Rev*. (2010) 9:A379–82. doi: 10.1016/j.autrev.2009.10.009
3. Alpsoy E, Akman-Karakas A, Uzun S. Geographic variations in epidemiology of two autoimmune bullous diseases: pemphigus and bullous pemphigoid. *Arch Dermatol Res*. (2015) 307:291. doi: 10.1007/s00403-014-1531-1
4. Castro R, Roscoe J, Sampaio S. Brazilian pemphigus foliaceus. *Clin Dermatol*. (1983) 1:22–41. doi: 10.1016/0738-081X(83)90021-4
5. Bastuji-Garin S, Souissi R, Blum L, Turki H, Nouira R, Jomaa B, et al. Comparative epidemiology of pemphigus in Tunisia and France: unusual incidence of pemphigus foliaceus in young Tunisian women. *J Invest Dermatol*. (1995) 104:302–5. doi: 10.1111/1523-1747.ep12612836
6. Diaz L, Sampaio SA, Rivitti E, Martins C, Cunha P, Lombardi C, et al. Endemic pemphigus foliaceus. (Fogo Selvagem) II. Current and historic epidemiologic studies. *J Invest Dermatol*. (1989) 92:4–12. doi: 10.1111/1523-1747.ep13070394
7. Baum S, Sakka N, Artsi O, Trau H, Barzilai A. Diagnosis and classification of autoimmune blistering diseases. *Autoimmun Rev*. (2014) 13:482–9. doi: 10.1016/j.autrev.2014.01.047
8. Lombardi C, Borges PC, Chaul A, Sampaio SA, Rivitti E, Friedman H, et al. Environmental risk factors in the endemic pemphigus foliaceus. (fogo selvagem). *J Invest Dermatol*. (1992) 98:847–5. doi: 10.1111/1523-1747.ep12456932
9. Vernal S, Pepinelli M, Casanova C, Goulart TM, Kim O, Paula NA De, et al. Insights into the epidemiological link between biting flies and pemphigus foliaceus in southeastern Brazil. *Acta Tropica*. (2017) 176:455–62. doi: 10.1016/j.actatropica.2017.09.015
10. Qian Y, Culton DA, Jeong JS, Trupiano N, Valenzuela JG, Diaz LA. Non-infectious environmental antigens as a trigger for the initiation of an autoimmune skin disease. *Autoimmun Rev*. (2016) 15:923–30. doi: 10.1016/j.autrev.2016.07.005
11. Amagai M, Stanley JR. Desmoglein as a target in skin disease and beyond. *J Invest Dermatol*. (2012) 132:776–84. doi: 10.1038/jid.2011.390
12. Culton DA, Qian Y, Li N, Rubenstein D, Aoki V, Filhio GH, et al. Advances in pemphigus and its endemic pemphigus foliaceus. (Fogo Selvagem) phenotype: a paradigm of human autoimmunity. *J Autoimmun*. (2008) 31:311–24. doi: 10.1016/j.jaut.2008.08.003
13. Messias IT, von Kuster LC, Santamaria J, Kajdacsy-Balla A. Complement and antibody deposition in Brazilian pemphigus foliaceus and correlation of disease activity with circulating antibodies. *Arch Dermatol*. (1988) 124:1664–8. doi: 10.1001/archderm.124.11.1664
14. Pegas JRP, dos Reis VMS. Direct immunofluorescence on uninvolved, lesional and perilesional skin in patients with endemic pemphigus foliaceus. (fogo selvagem). *Med Sci Monitor*. (2004) 10:CR657–61.
15. Odo M, Rodrigues R, Miyauchi L. Direct immunofluorescence in skin biopsy of Brazilian pemphigus foliaceus. *An Bras Dermatol*. (1981) 56:1–5.
16. Hernandez C, Amagai M, Chan L. Pemphigus foliaceus : preferential binding of IgGl and C3 at the upper epidermis. *Br J Dermatol*. (1997) 136:249–52. doi: 10.1046/j.1365-2133.1997.d01-1180.x
17. Abreu-Velez AM, Upegui-Zapata YA, Valencia-Yepes CA, Upegui-Quiceno E, Mesa-Herrera N-R, Jiménez-Echavarria AM, et al. Membrane attack complex. (C5b-9 complex or Mac), is strongly present in lesional skin from patients with endemic pemphigus foliaceus in El Bagre, Colombia. *J Cuton Pathol*. (2019) 1–5. doi: 10.1111/cup.13565

18. Rock B, Labib RS, Diaz LA. Monovalent Fab′ immunoglobulin fragments from endemic pemphigus foliaceus autoantibodies reproduce the human disease in neonatal Balb/c mice. *J Clin Invest.* (1990) 85:296–9. doi: 10.1172/JCI114426
19. España A, Diaz LA, Mascaró JM, Giudice GJ, Fairley JA, Till GO, et al. Mechanisms of acantholysis in pemphigus foliaceus. *Clin Immunol Immunopathol.* (1997) 85:83–9. doi: 10.1006/clin.1997.4407
20. Xia P, Jordon RE, Geoghegan WD. Complement fixation by pemphigus Antibodt. *Science.* (1988) 82:1939–47. doi: 10.1172/JCI113813
21. Hashimoto K, Shafran K, Webber P, Lazarus G, Singer K. Anti-cell surface pemphigus autoantibody stimulates plasminogen activator activity of human epidermal cells – a mechanism for the loss of epidermal cohesion and blister formation. *J Exp Med.* (1983) 157:259–72. doi: 10.1084/jem.157.1.259
22. Ablin R. Levels of C'3 in the serum of patients with pemphigus. *J Invest Dermatol.* (1971) 56:450–3. doi: 10.1111/1523-1747.ep12261375
23. Franquini J, Adad S, Murta A, de Morais C, Teixeira Vde P, Júnior V. Tests of inflammatory activity in endemic pemphigus foliaceus. *Rev Soc Bras.* (1994) 27:25–9. doi: 10.1590/S0037-86821994000100006
24. Messias-Reason I, Bosco DG, Nisihara RM, Jakobsen LH, Petzl-Erler ML, Jensenius JC. Circulating levels of mannan-binding lectin. (MBL) and MBL-associated serine protease 2 in endemic pemphigus foliaceus. *Clin Exp Dermatol.* (2008) 33:495–7. doi: 10.1111/j.1365-2230.2008.02743.x
25. Kretzschmar GC, Oliveira LC, Nisihara RM, Velavan TP, Stinghen ST, Stahlke ERS, et al. Complement receptor 1 (CR1, CD35) association with susceptibility to leprosy. *PLoS Neglected Trop Dis.* (2018) 12:1–16. doi: 10.1371/journal.pntd.0006705
26. Klickstein BYLB, Wong WW, Smith JA, Weis JH, Wilson JG, Fearon DT. HUMAN C3b/C4b RECEPTOR. (CR1) - demonstration of long homologous repeating domains that are composed of the short consensus repeats characteristic of C3/C4 binding proteins. *J Exp.* (1987) 165:1095–112. doi: 10.1084/jem.165.4.1095
27. Wong WW, Cahill JM, Rosen MD, Kennedy CA, Bonaccio ET, Morris MJ, et al. Structure of the human CR1 gene. Molecular basis of the structural and quantitative polymorphisms and identification of a new CR1-like allele. *J Exp Med.* (1989) 169:847–63. doi: 10.1084/jem.169.3.847
28. Moulds JM, Zimmerman PA, Doumbo OK, Kassambara L, Sagara I, Diallo DA, et al. Molecular identification of Knops blood group polymorphisms found in long homologous region D of complement receptor 1. *Blood.* (2001) 97:2879–85. doi: 10.1182/blood.V97.9.2879
29. Khera R, Das N. Complement Receptor 1: disease associations and therapeutic implications. *Mol Immunol.* (2009) 46:761–72. doi: 10.1016/j.molimm.2008.09.026
30. Danielsson C, Pascual M, French L, Steiger G, Schifferli JA. Soluble complement receptor type 1. (CD35) is released from leukocytes by surface cleavage. *Eur J Immunol.* (1994) 24:2725–31. doi: 10.1002/eji.1830241123
31. Hamer I, Paccaud J, Belin D, Maeder C, Carpentier J. Soluble form of complement C3b/C4b receptor. (CR1) results from a proteolytic cleavage in the C-terminal region of CR1 transmembrane domain. *Biochem J.* (1998) 190:183–90. doi: 10.1042/bj3290183
32. Furtado PB, Huang CY, Ihyembe D, Hammond R, Marsh HC, Perkins SJ. The partly folded back solution structure arrangement of the 30 SCR domains in human complement receptor type 1. (CR1) permits access to its C3b and C4b ligands. *J Mol Biol.* (2008) 375:102–18. doi: 10.1016/j.jmb.2007.09.085
33. Liu D, Niu Z-X. The structure, genetic polymorphisms, expression and biological functions of complement receptor type 1. (CR1/CD35). *Immunopharmacol Immunotoxicol.* (2009) 31:524–35. doi: 10.3109/08923970902845768
34. Anna S, Heyman B. Specific IgM and regulation of antibody responses. *Curr Top Microbiol Immunol.* (2017) 408:67–87. doi: 10.1007/82_2017_24
35. Török K, Dezso B, Bencsik A, Uzonyi B, Erdei A. Complement receptor type 1 (CR1/CD35) expressed on activated human CD4+ T cells contributes to generation of regulatory T cells. *Immunol Lett.* (2015) 164:117–24. doi: 10.1016/j.imlet.2015.02.009
36. Jozsi M, Prechl J, Bajtay Z, Erdei a. Complement receptor type 1 (CD35) mediates inhibitory signals in human B lymphocytes. *J Immunol.* (2002) 168:2782–8. doi: 10.4049/jimmunol.168.6.2782
37. Bumiller-Bini V, Cipolla GA, Almeida RC De, Ludwig RJ, Beate A, Boldt W. Sparking fire under the skin? Answers from the association of complement genes with pemphigus foliaceus. *Front Immunol.* (2018) 9:1–9. doi: 10.3389/fimmu.2018.00695
38. Probst CM, Bompeixe EP, Pereira NF. HLA polymorphism and evaluation of European, African, and Amerindian contribution to the white and mulatto populations from Paraná, Brazil. *Hum Biol.* (2000) 72:597–617. doi: 10.1590/S0001-37652000000400010
39. Braun-Prado K, Vieira Mion AL, Farah Pereira N, Culpi L, Petzl-Erler ML. HLA class I polymorphism, as characterised by PCR-SSOP, in a Brazilian exogamic population. *Tissue Antigens.* (2000) 56:417–27. doi: 10.1034/j.1399-0039.2000.560504.x
40. Sambrook JR. *Molecular Cloning: A Laboratory Manual* Cold Spring, NY: CSHL Press (2001).
41. Durbin RM, Abecasis GR, Altshuler DL, Bentley DR, Chakravarti A, Clark AG, et al. A map of human genome variation from population-scale sequencing. *Nature.* (2010) 467:1061–73. doi: 10.1038/nature09534
42. Gabriel S, Ziaugra L, Tabbaa D. SNP genotyping using the sequenom massARRAY iPLEX Platform. *Curr Protocols Hum Genet.* (2009) Chapter 2:Unit 2.12. doi: 10.1002/0471142905.hg0212s60
43. Oliveira LA, Marquart-filho A, Trevilato G, Timóteo RP, Mukai M, Roselino AMF, et al. Anti-desmoglein 1 and 3 autoantibody levels in endemic pemphigus foliaceus and pemphigus vulgaris from Brazil. *Clin Lab.* (2016) 62:1209–16. doi: 10.7754/Clin.Lab.2015.150628
44. Livak KJ, Schmittgen TD. Analysis of relative gene expression data using real-time quantitative PCR and 2CT Method. *Methods.* (2001) 25:402–8. doi: 10.1006/meth.2001.1262
45. Excoffier L, Lischer HE. Arlequin suite ver 3.5: a new series of programs to perform population genetics analyses under Linux and Windows. *Mol Ecol Resour.* (2010) 10:564–7. doi: 10.1111/j.1755-0998.2010.02847.x
46. Purcell S, Neale B, Todd-Brown K, Thomas L, Ferreira MAR, Bender D, et al. PLINK: a tool set for whole-genome association and population-based linkage analyses. *Am J Hum Genet.* (2007) 81:559–75. doi: 10.1086/519795
47. Boldt ABW, Messias-Reason IJ, Meyer D, Schrago CG, Lang F, Lell B, et al. Phylogenetic nomenclature and evolution of mannose-binding lectin (MBL2) haplotypes. *BMC Genet.* (2010) 11:38. doi: 10.1186/1471-2156-11-38
48. Barrett JC, Fry B, Maller J, Daly MJ. Haploview: analysis and visualization of LD and haplotype maps. *Bioinformatics.* (2005) 21:263–5. doi: 10.1093/bioinformatics/bth457
49. Nebert DW. Proposal for an allele nomenclature system based on the evolutionary divergence of haplotypes. *Hum Mutat.* (2002) 20:463–72. doi: 10.1002/humu.10143
50. Benjamini Y, Hochberg Y. Controlling the false discovery rate : a practical and powerful approach to multiple testing. *JR Statist Soc.* (1995) 57:289–300. doi: 10.1111/j.2517-6161.1995.tb02031.x
51. Boyle AP, Hong EL, Hariharan M, Cheng Y, Schaub MA, Kasowski M, et al. Annotation of functional variation in personal genomes using RegulomeDB. *Genome Res.* (2012) 22:1790–1797. doi: 10.1101/gr.137323.112
52. Ward LD, Kellis M. HaploReg: a resource for exploring chromatin states, conservation, and regulatory motif alterations within sets of genetically linked variants. *Nucl Acids Res.* (2012) 40:930–4. doi: 10.1093/nar/gkr917
53. Adzhubei IA, Schimidt S, Peshkin L, Ramensky VE, Gerasimova A, et al. A method and server for predicting damaging missense mutations. *Nat Methods.* (2010) 7:248–9. doi: 10.1038/nmeth0410-248
54. Arnold M, Raffler J, Pfeufer A, Suhre K, Kastenmüller G. SNiPA: an interactive, genetic variant-centered annotation browser. *Bioinformatics.* (2015) 31:1334–6. doi: 10.1093/bioinformatics/btu779
55. Arora V, Grover R, Kumar A, Anand D, Das N. Relationship of leukocyte CR1 transcript and protein with the pathophysiology and prognosis of systemic lupus erythematosus: a follow-up study. *Lupus.* (2011) 20:1010–8. doi: 10.1177/0961203311400112
56. Donius LR, Handy JM, Weis JJ, Weis JH. Optimal germinal center B cell activation and T-dependent antibody responses require the expression of the mouse complement receptor Cr1. *J Immunol.* (2013) 191:434–47. doi: 10.4049/jimmunol.1203176
57. Birmingham DJ, Irshaid F, Gavit KF, Nagaraja HN, Yu CY, Rovin BH, et al. A polymorphism in the type one complement receptor (CR1) involves an additional cysteine within the C3b/C4b binding domain that inhibits ligand

binding. *Mol Immunol.* (2007) 44:3510–6. doi: 10.1016/j.molimm.2007.03.007

58. Duru KC, Noble JA, Guindo A, Yi L, Imumorin IG, Diallo DA, et al. Extensive genomic variability of Knops blood group polymorphisms is associated with sickle cell disease in Africa. *Evol Bioinform.* (2015) 11:25–34. doi: 10.4137/EBO.S23132
59. Yoon JH, Oh S, Shin S, Park JS, Roh EY, Song EY, et al. The polymorphism of Knops blood group system in Korean population and their relationship with HLA system. *Hum Immunol.* (2013) 74:196–8. doi: 10.1016/j.humimm.2012.10.024
60. Xiang L, Rundles JR, Hamilton DR, Wilson JG. Quantitative alleles of CR1: coding sequence analysis and comparison of haplotypes in two ethnic groups. *J Immunol.* (1999) 1:4939–45.
61. Luo J, Li S, Qin X, Song L, Peng Q, Chen S, et al. Meta-analysis of the association between CR1 polymorphisms and risk of late-onset Alzheimer's disease. *Neurosci Lett.* (2014) 578:165–70. doi: 10.1016/j.neulet.2014.06.055
62. Fontes AM, Kashima S, Bonfim-Silva R, Azevedo R, Abraham KJ, Roberto S, et al. Association between Knops blood group polymorphisms and susceptibility to malaria in an endemic area of the Brazilian Amazon. *Genet Mol Biol.* (2011) 34:539–45. doi: 10.1590/S1415-47572011005000051
63. Sweet RA, Seltman H, Emanuel JE, Lopez OL, Becker JT, Bis JC, et al. Effect of Alzheimer' s disease risk genes on trajectories of cognitive function in the cardiovascular health study. *Am J Psychiatr.* (2012) 169:954–62. doi: 10.1176/appi.ajp.2012.11121815
64. Keenan BT, Shulman JM, Chibnik LB, Raj T, Tran D, Sabuncu MR, et al. A coding variant in CR1 interacts with APOE-ε4 to influence cognitive decline. *Hum Mol Genet.* (2012) 21:2377–88. doi: 10.1093/hmg/dds054
65. Arakelyan A, Zakharyan R, Khoyetsyan A, Poghosyan D, Aroutiounian R, Mrazek F, et al. Functional characterization of the complement receptor type 1 and its circulating ligands in patients with schizophrenia. *BMC Clin Pathol* (2011) 11:1–7. doi: 10.1186/1472-6890-11-10
66. Kariuki SM, Rockett K, Clark TG, Reyburn H, Agbenyega T, Taylor TE, et al. The genetic risk of acute seizures in African children with falciparum malaria. *Epilepsia.* (2013) 54:990–1001. doi: 10.1111/epi.12173
67. Shen N, Chen B, Jiang Y, Feng R, Liao M, Zhang L, et al. An updated analysis with 85,939 samples confirms the association between CR1 rs6656401 polymorphism and Alzheimer's disease. *Mol Neurobiol.* (2014) 1–7. doi: 10.1007/s12035-014-8761-2
68. Daniels GL, Fletcher A, Garratty G, Henry S, Jørgensen J, Judd WJ, et al. Blood group terminology 2004 : from the International Society of Blood Transfusion committee on terminology for red cell surface antigens. *Vox Sanguinis.* (2004) 87:304–16. doi: 10.1111/j.1423-0410.2004.00564.x
69. Moulds JM, Thomas BJ, Doumbo O, Diallo DA, Lyke KE, Plowe CV, et al. Identification of the Kna / Knb polymorphism and a method for Knops genotyping. *Transfusion.* (2010) 44:164–9. doi: 10.1111/j.1537-2995.2004.00615.x
70. Veldhuisen B, Ligthart PC, Vidarsson G, Roels I, Folman CC, van der Schoot CE, et al. Molecular analysis of the York antigen of the Knops blood group system. *Transfusion.* (2011) 51:1389–96. doi: 10.1111/j.1537-2995.2010.02999.x
71. Awandare GA, Spadafora C, Moch JK, Dutta S, Haynes JD, Stoute JA. *Plasmodium falciparum* field isolates use complement receptor 1 (CR1) as a receptor for invasion of erythrocytes. *Mol Biochem Parasitol.* (2011) 177:57–60. doi: 10.1016/j.molbiopara.2011.01.005
72. Schlesinger LS, Horwitz MA. Phagocytosis of leprosy bacilli is mediated by complement receptors CR1 and CR3 on human monocytes and complement component C3 in serum. *J Clin Invest.* (1990) 85:1304–14. doi: 10.1172/JCI114568
73. Bermudez LE, Young LS, Enkel H. Interaction of *Mycobacterium avium* complex with human macrophages : roles of membrane receptors and serum proteins. *Infect Immun.* (1991) 59:1697–702.
74. Noumsi GT, Tounkara A, Diallo H, Billingsley K, Moulds JJ. Knops blood group polymorphism and susceptibility to Mycobacterium tuberculosis infection. *Transfusion.* (2011) 51:2462–9. doi: 10.1111/j.1537-2995.2011.03161.x
75. Rosenthal LA, Sutterwala FS, Kehrli ME, Mosser DM. Leishmania major - Human Macrophage Interactions: cooperation between Mac-1 (CD11b/CD18) and Complement Receptor Type 1 (CD35) in Promastigote Adhesion. *Infect Immun.* (1996) 64:2206–15.
76. Fernandez-Arias C, Lopez JP, Hernandez-Perez JN, Bautista-Ojeda MD, Branch O, Rodriguez A. Malaria inhibits surface expression of complement receptor-1 in monocyte/macrophages causing decreased immunecomplex internalization. *J Immunol.* (2014) 190:3363–72. doi: 10.4049/jimmunol.1103812
77. Teeranaipong P, Ohashi J, Patarapotikul J, Kimura R, Nuchnoi P, Hananantachai H, et al. A functional single-nucleotide polymorphism in the CR1 promoter region contributes to protection against cerebral malaria. *J Infect Dis.* (2008) 198:1880–91. doi: 10.1086/593338
78. Gomes JAS, Campi-Azevedo AC, Teixeira-Carvalho A, Silveira-Lemos D, Vitelli-Avelar D, Sathler-Avelar R, et al. Impaired phagocytic capacity driven by downregulation of major phagocytosis-related cell surface molecules elicits an overall modulatory cytokine profile in neutrophils and monocytes from the indeterminate clinical form of Chagas disease. *Immunobiology.* (2012) 217:1005–16. doi: 10.1016/j.imbio.2012.01.014
79. Bánki Z, Wilflingseder D, Ammann CG, Pruenster M, Müllauer B, Holländer K, et al. Factor I-mediated processing of complement fragments on HIV immune complexes targets HIV to CR2-expressing B cells and facilitates B cell-mediated transmission of opsonized HIV to T cells. *J Immunol.* (2006) 177:3469–76. doi: 10.4049/jimmunol.177.5.3469
80. Arora V, Verma J, Dutta R, Marwah V, Kumar A, Das N. Reduced complement receptor 1 (CR1, CD35) transcription in systemic lupus erythematosus. *Mol Immunol.* (2004) 41:449–56. doi: 10.1016/j.molimm.2004.03.004
81. Arora V, Matin A, Grover R, Kumar A, Chattopadhyay P, Das N. Modulation of CR1 transcript in systemic lupus erythematosus (SLE) by IFN- γ and immune complex. *Mol Immunol.* (2007) 44:1722–8. doi: 10.1016/j.molimm.2006.07.300
82. Kavai M. Immune complex clearance by complement receptor type 1 in SLE. *Autoimmun Rev.* (2008) 8:160–4. doi: 10.1016/j.autrev.2008.06.002
83. Brouwers N, Van Cauwenberghe C, Engelborghs S, Lambert J-C, Bettens K, Le Bastard N, et al. Alzheimer risk associated with a copy number variation in the complement receptor 1 increasing C3b/C4b binding sites. *Mol Psychiatr.* (2012) 17:223–33. doi: 10.1038/mp.2011.24
84. Hazrati L-N, Van Cauwenberghe C, Brooks PL, Brouwers N, Ghani M, Sato C, et al. Genetic association of CR1 with Alzheimer's disease: a tentative disease mechanism. *Neurobiol Aging.* (2012) 33:2949.e5–e12. doi: 10.1016/j.neurobiolaging.2012.07.001
85. Mahmoudi R, Kisserli A, Novella J-L, Donvito B, Dramé M, Réveil B, et al. Alzheimer's disease is associated with low density of the long CR1 isoform. *Neurobiol Aging.* (2015) 36:1766.e5–12. doi: 10.1016/j.neurobiolaging.2015.01.006
86. Mahmoudi R, Feldman S, Kisserli A, Tabary T, Bertholon L, Badr S, et al. Inherited and Acquired Decrease in Complement Receptor 1 (CR1) density on red blood cells associated with high levels of soluble CR1 in alzheimer's disease. *Int J Mol Sci.* (2018) 19:1–18. doi: 10.3390/ijms19082175
87. Rondelli T, Risitano AM, Latour RP De, Sica M, Peruzzi B, Barcellini W, et al. Polymorphism of the complement receptor 1 gene correlates with the hematologic response to eculizumab in patients with paroxysmal nocturnal hemoglobinuria. *Hematologica.* (2014) 9:262–6. doi: 10.3324/haematol.2013.090001
88. Deng Y, Li Z, Liu J, Wang Z, Cao Y, Mou Y, et al. Targeted resequencing reveals genetic risks in patients with sporadic idiopathic pulmonary fibrosis. *Hum Mutat.* (2018) 39:1238–45. doi: 10.1002/humu.23566
89. Gu H, Mickler EA, Cummings OW, Sandusky GE, Weber DJ, Gracon A, et al. Crosstalk between TGF-β1 and complement activation augments epithelial injury in pulmonary fibrosis. *FASEB J.* (2014) 28:4223–34. doi: 10.1096/fj.13-247650
90. Ma XY, Yu JT, Tan MS, Sun FR, Miao D, Tan L. Missense variants in CR1 are associated with increased risk of Alzheimer' disease in Han Chinese. *Neurobiol Aging.* (2014) 35:443:e17–21. doi: 10.1016/j.neurobiolaging.2013.08.009
91. Jacquet M, Lacroix M, Ancelet S, Gout E, Gaboriaud C, Thielens NM, et al. Deciphering complement receptor type 1 interactions with recognition proteins of the lectin complement pathway. *J Immunol.* (2013) 190:3721–31. doi: 10.4049/jimmunol.1202451
92. Hess C, Sadallah S, Hefti A, Landmann R, Schifferli JA. Ectosomes Released by human neutrophils are specialized functional units. *J Immunol.* (1999) 163:4564–73.
93. Krych-goldberg M, Atkinson JP. Structure-function relationships

of complement receptor type 1. *Immunol Rev.* (2001) 180:112–22. doi: 10.1034/j.1600-065X.2001.1800110.x

94. Goodfellow RM, Williams AS, Levin JL, Williams BD, Morgan BP. Local therapy with soluble complement receptor 1 (sCR1) suppresses inflammation in rat mono-articular arthritis. *Clin Exp Immunol.* (1997) 110:45–52. doi: 10.1046/j.1365-2249.1997.5111408.x
95. Dreja H, Annenkov A, Chernajovsky Y. Soluble complement receptor 1 (CD35) delivered by retrovirally infected syngeneic cells or by naked DNA injection prevents the progression of collagen-induced arthritis. *Arthr Rheumat.* (2000) 43:1698–709. doi: 10.1002/1529-0131(200008)43:8<1698::AID-ANR5>3.0.CO;2-8
96. Keshavjee S, Davis RD, Zamora MR, de Perrot M, Patterson GA. A randomized, placebo-controlled trial of complement inhibition in ischemia-reperfusion injury after lung transplantation in human beings. *J Thor Cardiovascul Surg.* (2005) 129:423–8. doi: 10.1016/j.jtcvs.2004.06.048

15

Learning from Success and Failure: Biologics for Non-Approved Skin Diseases

Reinhart Speeckaert*, Jo Lambert and Nanja van Geel

Department of Dermatology, Ghent University Hospital, Ghent, Belgium

Correspondence:
Reinhart Speeckaert
reinhart.speeckaert@ugent.be

The impressive potential of biologics has been demonstrated in psoriasis, hidradenitis suppurativa, and urticaria. Numerous biologicals are entering the field for a restricted number of skin disorders. Off-label use of biologics in other recalcitrant skin diseases has increased. Mounting data point to the potential of already existing biologics acting on the IL-17/IL-23 pathway in skin disorders with epidermal hyperkeratosis (e.g., pityriasis rubra pilaris), acneiform inflammation (e.g., hidradenitis suppurativa), and loss of mucosal integrity (e.g., aphthosis). TNF-α blockers are also effective in the latter conditions but seem of particular value in granulomatous (e.g., granuloma annulare) and neutrophilic disorders (e.g., pyoderma gangrenosum). Failure of IL-17 blockade in skin diseases resulting from immune-mediated cell destruction (e.g., alopecia areata and vitiligo) illustrates its limited involvement in Th1-dependent skin immunology. Overall, disappointing results of TNF-α blockers in alopecia areata and vitiligo point to the same conclusion although promising results in toxic epidermal necrolysis suggest TNF-α exerts at least some *in vivo* Th1-related activities. Acting on both the Th1 and Th17 pathway, ustekinumab has a rather broad potential with interesting results in lupus and alopecia areata. The efficacy of omalizumab in bullous pemphigoid has revealed an IgE-mediated recruitment of eosinophils leading to bullae formation. Reconsidering reimbursement criteria for less common but severe diseases seems appropriate if substantial evidence is available (e.g., pityriasis rubra pilaris). For other disorders, investigator- and industry-initiated randomized clinical trials should be stimulated. They are likely to improve patient outcome and advance our understanding of challenging skin disorders.

Keywords: biologics, off-label, TNF-α, IL-1, IL-12, IL-23, IgE, CD20

INTRODUCTION

A large number of dermatological disorders is mediated by a deregulated skin immune response. In the last 2 decades, biologics have revolutionized the traditional approach by achieving unprecedented results with limited adverse events. Unfortunately, their use is restricted to a very small number of diseases (psoriasis, urticaria, and hidradenitis suppurativa). The promise of a targeted approach triggers clinicians to test these drugs in recalcitrant disorders despite their off-label status. More than 100 articles have been published on the off-label use of biologics. This is in obvious contrast with the limited number of prospective randomized trials that have been carried out. In this review we summarize the evidence of the currently available biologics targeting IL-1, IL-12/IL-23, IL-17, IL-23, TNF-α, CD20, and IgE in different "off-label" skin conditions (**Supplementary Table S1**).

DISORDERS BASED ON TARGETED IMMUNE-BASED CELL DESTRUCTION: ALOPECIA AREATA AND VITILIGO

Given the role of TNF-α in the Th1 response, it made sense to test TNF-α inhibitors in alopecia areata and vitiligo. Nonetheless, adalimumab fails to induce hair regrowth in most alopecia areata patients (1). Several cases have been published mentioning *de novo* development of alopecia areata due to TNF-α blockers (2, 3). However, some successful cases have also been reported (4). The risk of vitiligo is significantly increased in patients receiving this class of biologics [hazard ratio: 1.99 (95% confidence interval: 1.06–3.75)] (5). Overall, repigmentation using TNF-α blockers is limited in vitiligo and this approach was considered to be ineffective (6). Nonetheless, TNF-α inhibitors can be useful to halt disease progression in active vitiligo (7). No data on the combination of TNF-α inhibitors and phototherapy are available.

Increased IL-17 levels and Th17 lymphocytes have been observed in the skin and blood of patients with alopecia areata and vitiligo (8, 9). Unfortunately, most alopecia areata patients did not show any response to secukinumab, an anti-IL17 monoclonal antibody (10). The same result was observed in our trial using secukinumab in progressive vitiligo which showed that 7/8 patients developed new skin depigmentations leading to an early halt of further recruitment. In subsequent experiments, we showed that Th17.1 cells rather than Th17 cells are increased in active vitiligo (11). Th17.1 lymphocytes are a subgroup of Th17 cells gradually differentiating into non-classical Th1 cells. IL-12 and IL-23 (in combination with low TGF-β) are the main cytokines driving Th17 > Th1 polarization. In that regard, ustekinumab, a combined anti-IL12/23 monoclonal antibody, might represent an attractive treatment option. Despite some reports mentioning new onset vitiligo and alopecia areata during ustekinumab, cases showing repigmentation have been published (12). In alopecia areata, some impressive cases of hair regrowth following the initiation of ustekinumab illustrate the interesting potential of this biologic (13, 14). Increased serum levels of IL-23 have been found in vitiligo although no clinical data are available for IL-23 blockers (15).

ACNEIFORM DISORDERS WITH NEUTROPHILS: HIDRADENITIS SUPPURATIVA AND ACNE CONGLOBATA

The introduction of TNF-α blockers in the therapeutic arsenal of hidradenitis suppurativa has increased the scientific interest for this disorder. The improvement of abscesses and pustules with beneficial effects on the quality of life are clear although treatment failure is more common compared to psoriasis (16).

IL-17 is considered to be an important factor in the detrimental inflammatory responses in HS. Case reports and a small pilot trial mention clear improvement in HS patients receiving secukinumab (17, 18). In contrast, an *ex vivo* study on lesional skin samples showed a more pronounced decrease in pro-inflammatory cytokine production and antimicrobial peptides with TNF-α inhibitors compared to IL-17 inhibition (19). Treatment with ustekinumab leads to moderate-marked responses in 82% of HS patients (20). In a retrospective analysis, guselkumab showed improvement in 8/11 (73%) of HS patients (21, 22).

In a small randomized controlled trial (RCT) (10:10), anakinra—a recombinant IL-1 receptor antagonist—displayed promising results with a 67% decreased activity score compared to 20% in the placebo arm (23). Nonetheless, some HS patients fail to improve with both anakinra and canakinumab (= monoclonal antibody against IL-1β) (24, 25). Up till now, large RCTs are missing.

Acne conglobata can be a disfiguring disease with limited treatment options in case of failure of systemic retinoids. Sand and Thomsen reported benefit from TNF-α inhibitors in 64% (7/11) of patients with severe refractory acne conglobata (26). Propionibacterium acnes stimulates keratinocytes to produce IL-1α and TNF-α. Additionally, peripheral blood mononuclear cells (PBMCs) of acne patients stimulated with P. acnes produce increased amounts of TNF-α and IL-8 pointing to the central role of TNF-α in this condition (27). P. acnes also promotes Th17 and Th17.1 responses (28) although no data have been published on the efficacy of IL-17 blockers or ustekinumab.

SYSTEMIC DISORDERS: LUPUS AND DERMATOMYOSITIS

A phase II RCT of patients with active systemic lupus erythematosus (SLE) demonstrated that the addition of ustekinumab to standard care resulted in an improved efficacy (29). After 6 months, a Systemic Lupus Erythematosus Responder Index (SRI)-4 response was achieved in 62% of ustekinumab treated patients compared to 33% in the placebo group. Although some patients have been reported to exhibit lupus-like cutaneous disorders following ustekinumab, several successfully treated cases of subacute and discoid cutaneous lupus can be found in literature with ustekinumab (30–32). Regarding TNF-α blockers, lupus is a well-known adverse event which can display diverse presentation patterns (33).

Rituximab showed promising results in open-label studies but failed to reach the primary endpoints in 2 RCTs (34, 35). However, some confounding factors such as concomitant immunosuppressive medication and problems in study design (e.g., outcome measures with limited sensitivity) might have played a role. Nonetheless, cutaneous lesions of SLE showed beneficial results in a retrospective study. At 6 months, 76% of patients ($n = 50$) showed improvement in mucocutaneous lesions with 40% complete responses. The response to rituximab in subacute cutaneous lupus erythematosus and chronic cutaneous lupus erythematosus seems more variable (36).

Omalizumab was tested in a small RCT ($n = 15$) which enrolled SLE patients with increased levels of IgE anti-dsDNA, anti-Sm or anti-SSA autoantibodies. A significant improvement in Systemic Lupus Erythematosus Disease Activity Index 2000 (SLEDAI-2k) scores was found at 16 weeks although the difference was lower than the clinically minimal important change (37).

A similar pattern emerges with anti-TNF-α antibodies in dermatomyositis which can develop during therapy. Nonetheless, an RCT demonstrated that infliximab can be of value in a subset of patients despite failure to reach the endpoints after 16 weeks (38).

In a retrospective series of patients with refractory idiopathic inflammatory myopathies (including antisynthetase syndrome, dermatomyositis and polymyositis) rituximab resulted in a significantly decreased dependency on glucocorticoids and favorable clinical responses (39).

Abnormal IL-1 receptor antagonist production has been observed in dermatomyositis and polymyositis. 4/15 (36.4%) patients with dermatomyositis or polymyositis improved with anakinra (40).

APHTHOSIS (AND BEHCET'S SYNDROME)

Anti-TNF-α inhibitors were useful in resistant cases of recurrent aphthous stomatitis. Adalimumab, etanercept and infliximab have all shown good efficacy. Complete responses have been documented in approximately two-thirds of patients treated with adalimumab (41). Adalimumab is also effective to reduce other manifestations of Behcet's syndrome including the resolution of venous thrombosis (42).

Secukinumab showed benefit in five patients with Behcet's syndrome (and concomitant ankylosing spondylitis or psoriatic arthritis) refractory to conventional treatment and anti-TNF-α therapy. Improvement of active mucocutaneous manifestations was evident. Especially the rapid resolution of oral ulcerations was remarkable (43). Different studies have confirmed the involvement of IL-17 in the pathogenesis. Ustekinumab was also effective in a small prospective study of 14 patients. After 12 weeks, complete response was seen in 64%, partial response in 21% with 14% non-responders (44).

IL-1 antagonism (Anakinra) is mainly tested on uveitis in Behcet's syndrome although a small pilot study has investigated the effect on the mucocutaneous complaints. In five of six patients the severity and number of ulcers improved with two cases of complete response (45).

NEUTROPHILIC DISORDERS: PYODERMA GANGRENOSUM (PG)

Infliximab is the only biologic with an RCT for classic PG showing improvement in 20/29 patients (46). Etanercept and adalimumab have variable efficacy in small studies. Paradoxical new onset PG has also been linked to TNF-α inhibitors. Beneficial results have been ascribed to ustekinumab in case reports (47). This is in line with the role of the IL-17/23 pathway in neutrophil migration (48). A retrospective study found complete responses for infliximab in 63.6% (n = 33), for adalimumab in 57.1% (n = 28), for etanercept in 71.4% (n = 7) and for ustekinumab in 66.6% (n = 9) of patients. These results were all superior to corticosteroids (48.8%; n = 78) (49). Anakinra and canakinumab lead to variable outcomes (50, 51).

Occurrence of Sweet syndrome is possible during anti-TNF-α treatment although it can also be effective in pre-existing Sweet syndrome (52, 53). Some isolated cases responded to IL-1 inhibition (anakinra) (54, 55). Neutrophilic dermatoses associated with auto-inflammatory disorders (e.g., Schnitzler syndrome, Muckle-Wells syndrome) respond well to IL-1 inhibitors (56).

BULLOUS DISORDERS: BULLOUS PEMPHIGOID (BP) AND OTHER BULLOUS DISEASES

Remarkable improvements have been seen for omalizumab in BP. A systematic review found 22 reported cases with 84% complete responses. Anti-BP180 IgE antibodies correlate with disease activity in BP supporting their pathogenic relevance (57). IgE autoantibodies against BP180 and BP230 were found in, respectively 21/36 (58.3%) and 18/36 (50%) BP sera (58). The favorable safety profile of omalizumab makes it an attractive treatment option for BP (59).

Rituximab (anti-CD20) also led to 85% complete responses in BP (in 62 patients). Rituximab was associated with lower recurrence rates and a longer disease-free period compared to omalizumab (60). Patients that first did not respond to omalizumab but improved using rituximab (61), but also cases with improvement on omalizumab after failure to rituximab have been published.

Development of BP using anti-TNF-α treatment can occur sporadically although this link remains controversial. Both for ustekinumab and secukinumab cases of successful treatment of BP and new onset BP during treatment have been described (62–65). IL-17 production by innate immune cells, especially neutrophils, is characteristic in lesional BP skin. IL-17 upregulates matrix-metalloproteinase-9 and neutrophil elastase expression which are involved in blister formation (66). Elevated serum concentrations of IL-23 were confirmed in BP patients and rising levels were associated with disease relapse. This pathway could therefore be potentially interesting in BP (66).

Besides pemphigus, rituximab has been administered successfully in other autoimmune bullous diseases. In a retrospective cohort, mucous membrane pemphigoid (n= 14) exhibited disease control in 85.7% (partial response: 64.3%, complete response: 28.6%) (67). Similarly, some encouraging data have been obtained in ocular cicatricial pemphigoid (68). A meta-analysis showed that rituximab is also a promising option in epidermolysis bullosa acquisita (69).

PSORIASIFORM DISORDERS: PITYRIASIS RUBRA PILARIS

Off-label use of biologics has been extensively performed in PRP given its high clinical and pathogenic similarity with psoriasis. Anti-TNF-α, anti-IL-17 and anti-IL-12/23 treatments are all effective with marked to complete responses ranging around 50–78%. Partial responses were seen in 11–25% of patients and lack of response in 11–25% (70). Infliximab exhibited superior results compared to adalimumab while ustekinumab is currently most widely used for this disorder. Recent case series on IL-17 inhibition (secukinumab and ixekizumab) show a fast clearance and limited risk of recurrence after therapy withdrawal (71, 72). Nonetheless, treatment response is difficult to predict due to the heterogeneity of the disease (73). Both cases with progression using IL-17 inhibition that subsequently improved using ustekinumab (74) as a patient with limited response to ustekinumab who benefited from secukinumab, have been published (73).

GRANULOMATOUS DISORDERS: GRANULOMA ANNULARE

The role of TNF-α producing macrophages in granuloma formation points to a key role of this cytokine in granuloma annulare. A summary of published cases showed that 20/26 patients with granuloma annulare responded to anti-TNF-α treatment (75). Overall, these data support a high efficacy of TNF-α inhibitors in granuloma annulare although well-designed RCTs are missing. Nonetheless, granuloma annulare has also been reported as a side effect of biologics including adalimumab, infliximab and etanercept but also during treatment with secukinumab (76–78).

MASTOCYTOSIS

Given its excellent efficacy in urticaria, the use of omalizumab in other mast cell mediated diseases such as mastocytosis looks promising. Most published cases report excellent efficacy on systemic symptoms (e.g., gastrointestinal problems, pruritus). Some interesting patients with resolution of cutaneous lesions have been observed (79, 80). A multicenter RCT with 7 patients receiving omalizumab and 9 placebo was conducted. After 6 months, improvement in French Association for the Initiatives of Research on Mastocyte and Mastocytosis (AFIRMM) score was higher in the omalizumab group (52–26 vs. 104–102) although significance was not reached (81).

TOXIC EPIDERMAL NECROLYSIS

Being one of the most life-threatening skin disorders, treatment of toxic epidermal necrolysis is extremely important. TNF-α has been identified in the blister fluid and serum of TEN patients (82). Most evidence is gathered from case series and case reports. Nonetheless, the majority of cases show excellent responses with improved outcomes compared to the expected mortality (83). An interesting case series of 10 patients with excellent outcome using etanercept was published (84). Adequate screening for infections is necessary given the high prevalence of soft tissue infections (*S. aureus, P. aeruginosa, K. pneumoniae*) (83). An RCT comparing etanercept ($n = 48$) with corticosteroids ($n = 43$) showed a lower mortality rate after etanercept (8.3%) compared to predicted outcome (17.7%). The difference with the corticosteroid group (16.3%) was not significant although the time for complete skin healing was lower (85). Nonetheless, more than 50 cases have been described developing TEN despite concurrent treatment with TNF-α blockers.

LICHEN PLANUS

Lichenoid drug eruptions are a well-known side effect of TNF-α blockade (86). Cutaneous and oral lichen planus, lichen planopilaris and lichen striatus have all developed in patients receiving anti-TNF- α treatment. Nonetheless, in some cases of extensive lichen planus adalimumab showed improvement and isolated cases of oral lichen planus and nail lichen planus improved using etanercept (87–89). Despite some promising reports, rituximab failed to show efficacy in a small trial with five consecutive patients with erosive lichen planus (90). Data on other biologics are very limited.

DISCUSSION

Several promising results have been obtained by the off-label use of biologics and by pilot trials (**Table 1**, **Figure 1**) although disappointing results can be equally important to clarify the underlying pathogenic pathways. Failure of both TNF-α inhibitors and IL-17A-blockers in alopecia areata and vitiligo limits the involvement of these cytokines in the immune-mediated destruction of skin cells (10, 11). However, the apparent efficacy of TNF-α inhibitors in toxic epidermal necrolysis and occasional cases of alopecia areata and vitiligo suggest that the role of TNF-α is more complex (4, 7, 91). Alopecia areata and vitiligo remain biologic orphan diseases although some exciting cases have been published showing hair regrowth after initiation of ustekinumab (13, 14).

Promising early data concerning the blockage of the IL-23/IL17 pathway in HS confirm that this pathway is an important initiator of a suppurative neutrophilic inflammation (19, 20, 22, 92). The benefit of blocking IL-17 in aphthosis is in agreement with its defensive capacities against mucosal invasion of pathogens and its protective actions to maintain epithelial barrier integrity.

The results of the phase II trial of ustekinumab in lupus could be a major breakthrough although phase III trials have to be awaited. Increased IL-12 and IL-23 levels have been reported in SLE patients and genetic research links the IL-12 pathway with an increased susceptibility for SLE (29). In general, interferon is considered the main driving factor in lupus. In contrast, the efficacy of ustekinumab was independent of interferon levels (29, 31, 32).

One of the most remarkable findings was undoubtedly the impressive resolution of bullae in BP following the administration of anti-IgE antibodies (59, 59, 60, 93, 94). This confirms the pathogenic role of anti-IgE antibodies which seem actively involved in the development of bullae. Mice injected with IgE autoantibodies from BP patients in grafted human skin developed erythema and infiltration of eosinophils in the skin and ultimately histological dermal-epidermal separation (95). Further studies on omalizumab in bullous pemphigoid seem of particular value given its efficacy and improved safety profile compared to the alternative options.

While current biologics cover mainly the Th17 pathway, strong inhibition of important Th1 cytokines such as IFN-γ is not (yet) available leading to disappointing results in vitiligo

TABLE 1 | Biologics and their efficacy in off-label skin diseases.

	Anti-TNF-α		Anti-IL12/23		Anti-IL17		Anti-IL23		Anti-IL1		Anti-IgE		Anti-CD20	
	Efficacy	**Evidence**	**Efficacy**	**Evidence**	**Efficacy**	**Evidence**	**Efficacy**	**Evidence**	**Efficacy**	**Evidence**	**Efficacy**	**Evidence**	**Efficacy**	**Evidence**
Alopecia areata	–	CR	+	CR	–	PT								
	AE	CR												
Vitiligo	–/(+)	PT			–	PT								
	AE	RCS												
Hidradenitis suppurativa	+	RCT	+	PT	+	CR			+	RCT				
Acne conglobata	+	CR												
Lupus	AE	CR	+	RCT					+/–	PT, CR	+/–	RCT	+	CR, PT
													–	RCT
Dermatomyositis	+/–	RCT							+/–	CR			+	CR
Aphthosis/behcet	+	RCT	+	PT	+	CR			+	CR				
Pyoderma gangrenosum	+	RCT	+	CR					+	CR				
	AE	CR												
Bullous pemphigoid	AE	CR	AE	CR	AE	CR					+	CR	+	CR
			+	CR	+	CR								
Pityriasis rubra pilaris	+	PT	+	PT	+	CR								
Granuloma annulare	+	PT, CR												
Toxic epidermal necrolysis	+	RCT											AE	CR
Lichen planus	+	CR											–	PT
	AE	CR											+	CR

Evidence: CR (white), case reports (at least 2 case reports); PT (gray), pilot trials; RCT (black), randomized controlled trials; RCS, retrospective cohort study; + (green), positive evidence; +/– (orange), unclear/conflicting results; – (red), no clear benefit; AE (blue), reported as adverse event.

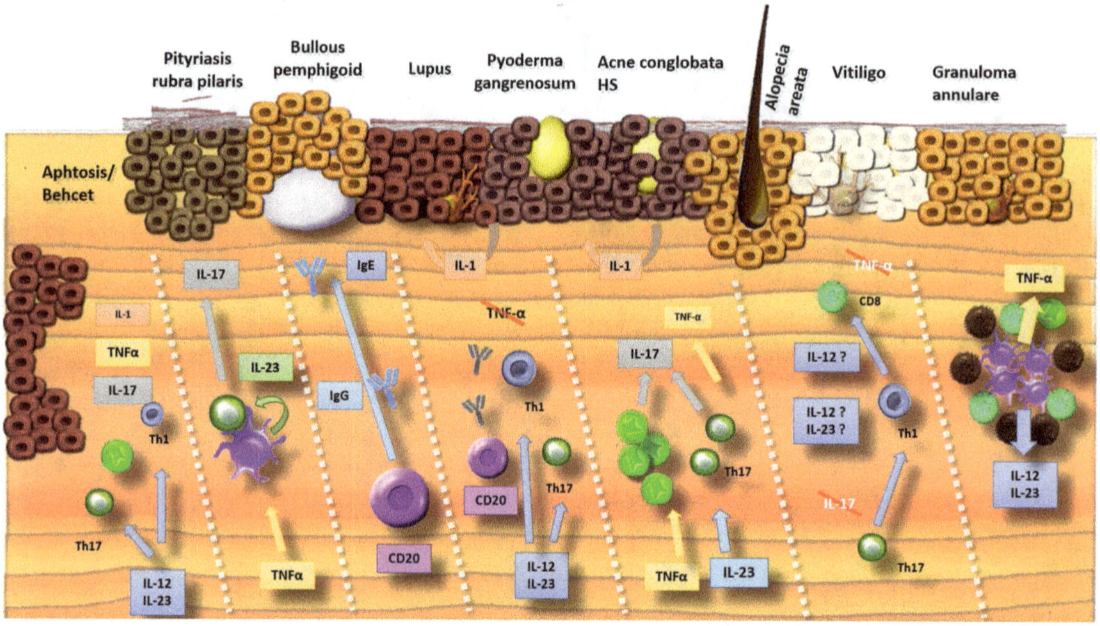

FIGURE 1 | Summary of the involved cytokines in cutaneous disorders (Crossed interleukins: trials were conducted but failed). Mucosal ulceration involves a wide range of cytokines and therefore biologics inhibiting different pathways (IL-1, TNF-α, and IL-17/23) result in improvement. Pityriasis rubra pilaris has a psoriasis-like pathophysiology with a TNF-α stimulated production of IL-23 by dendritic cells. This results in the release of IL-17. Bullous pemphigoid is an antibody-mediated disorder where both inhibition of B lymphocytes (e.g., rituximab) as binding of IgE-antibodies with omalizumab is efficacious. The pathophysiology of lupus is complex with a possible driving role for IL-12 and IL-23. Mixed results for inhibition of B-lymphocytes with rituximab were obtained. TNF-α inhibitors are associated with drug-induced lupus. In neutrophilic pustular disorders (pyoderma gangrenosum, acne, hidradenitis), the IL-17 pathway seems crucial with beneficial results if cytokines of this pathway are targeted (IL-17, IL-23, and TNF-α). In alopecia areata and vitiligo, antibodies against TNF-α and IL-17 were disappointing. Some evidence exists for a role of ustekinumab (IL-12/23) in alopecia areata. TNF-α and IL-12/23 can be targeted in granuloma annulare.

and alopecia areata. Dupilumab, a monoclonal antibody directed against IL-4 and IL-13, developed for atopic dermatitis interferes with key cytokines in the Th2 pathway and offers new possibilities for off-label use. Case reports of good response to different types of chronic itch including prurigo nodularis, uremic pruritus and genital pruritus illustrate the interesting potential of dupilumab (96–99). New development of alopecia areata has been observed during treatment with dupilumab (100–102). Nonetheless, patients with both atopic dermatitis and alopecia areata treated with dupilumab have repeatedly demonstrated hair regrowth (103–105). Furthermore, some isolated cases were published with beneficial results in bullous pemphigoid (106), eosinophilic annular erythema (107), and papuloerythroderma of Ofuji (108).

Biologics have been linked to the occasional development of alopecia areata, vitiligo, lupus, dermatomyositis and bullous diseases. However, as we have learned from TNF-α antagonists in psoriasis, this finding does not exclude their efficacy. Increased serum or lesional levels of specific interleukins do not ensure the efficacy of the corresponding biologic. As seen in alopecia areata and vitiligo, numerous studies documented increased TNF-α and IL-17 levels while the inhibition of both cytokines failed in these disorders (10, 11). Unfortunately, the lack of convincing mouse models for most dermatologic disorders limits the evidence that can be obtained before conducting a clinical trial.

Getting biologics approved and reimbursed for these new indications is another challenge. Weighing economic implications vs. health improvement will remain a difficult balance in the next decades. The rise of biosimilars may improve access to off-label use in disorders which are unlikely to be of economic interest due to their rare incidence or limited patients with severe disease requiring biologics (109). An increased appreciation and funding of investigator-initiated clinical trials seem of particular relevance to explore the full capacity of biologics.

AUTHOR CONTRIBUTIONS

RS reviewed the literature, drafted the manuscript, and made the figures. JL and NvG critically revised the manuscript.

REFERENCES

1. Bolduc C, Bissonnette R. Safety and efficacy of adalimumab for the treatment of severe alopecia areata: case series of three patients. *J Cutan Med Surg.* (2012) 16:257–60. doi: 10.1177/120347541201600407
2. Melé-Ninot G, Expósito-Serrano V, Quintana Codina M, Iglesias Sancho M, Sánchez-Regaña M, Umbert Millet P, et al. Adalimumab-related alopecia in a patient affected by psoriasis. *Dermatol Online J.* (2017) 23.
3. Ostojic P, Pavlov-Dolijanovic S. Alopecia universalis in a patient with rheumatoid arthritis developed during treatment with adalimumab. *Z Rheumatol.* (2018) 77:412–5. doi: 10.1007/s00393-018-0464-z
4. Gorcey L, Gordon Spratt EA, Leger MC. Alopecia universalis successfully treated with adalimumab. *JAMA Dermatol.* (2014) 150:1341–4. doi: 10.1001/jamadermatol.2014.1544
5. Bae JM, Kim M, Lee HH, Kim K-J, Shin H, Ju HJ, et al. Increased risk of vitiligo following anti-tumor necrosis factor therapy: a 10-year population-based cohort study. *J Invest Dermatol.* (2018) 138:768–74. doi: 10.1016/j.jid.2017.11.012
6. Alghamdi KM, Khurrum H, Taieb A, Ezzedine K. Treatment of generalized vitiligo with anti-TNF-α Agents. *J Drugs Dermatol.* (2012) 11:534–9.
7. Webb KC, Tung R, Winterfield LS, Gottlieb AB, Eby JM, Henning SW, et al. Tumour necrosis factor-α inhibition can stabilize disease in progressive vitiligo. *Br J Dermatol.* (2015) 173:641–50. doi: 10.1111/bjd.14016
8. Bassiouny DA, Shaker O. Role of interleukin-17 in the pathogenesis of vitiligo. *Clin Exp Dermatol.* (2011) 36:292–7. doi: 10.1111/j.1365-2230.2010.03972.x
9. Atwa MA, Youssef N, Bayoumy NM. T-helper 17 cytokines (interleukins 17, 21, 22, and 6, and tumor necrosis factor-α) in patients with alopecia areata: association with clinical type and severity. *Int J Dermatol.* (2016) 55:666–72. doi: 10.1111/ijd.12808
10. Guttman-Yassky E, Nia JK, Hashim PW, Mansouri Y, Alia E, Taliercio M, et al. Efficacy and safety of secukinumab treatment in adults with extensive alopecia areata. *Arch Dermatol Res.* (2018) 310:607–14. doi: 10.1007/s00403-018-1853-5
11. Speeckaert R, Mylle S, van Geel N. IL-17A is not a treatment target in progressive vitiligo. *Pigm Cell Mel Res.* (2019). doi: 10.1111/pcmr.12789. [Epub ahead of print].
12. Elkady A, Bonomo L, Amir Y, Vekaria AS, Guttman-Yassky E. Effective use of ustekinumab in a patient with concomitant psoriasis, vitiligo, and alopecia areata. *JAAD Case Rep.* (2017) 3:477–9. doi: 10.1016/j.jdcr.2017.07.009
13. Guttman-Yassky E, Ungar B, Noda S, Suprun M, Shroff A, Dutt R, et al. Extensive alopecia areata is reversed by IL-12/IL-23p40 cytokine antagonism. *J Allergy Clin Immunol.* (2016) 137:301–4. doi: 10.1016/j.jaci.2015.11.001
14. Aleisa A, Lim Y, Gordon S, Her MJ, Zancanaro P, Abudu M, et al. Response to ustekinumab in three pediatric patients with alopecia areata. *Pediatr Dermatol.* (2018) 36:e44–5. doi: 10.1111/pde.13699
15. Vaccaro M, Cannavò SP, Imbesi S, Cristani M, Barbuzza O, Tigano V, et al. Increased serum levels of interleukin-23 circulating in patients with non-segmental generalized vitiligo. *Int J Dermatol.* (2015) 54:672–4. doi: 10.1111/ijd.12392
16. Kyriakou A, Trigoni A, Galanis N, Sotiriadis D, Patsatsi A. Efficacy of adalimumab in moderate to severe hidradenitis suppurativa: real life data. *Dermatol Rep.* (2018) 10:7859. doi: 10.4081/dr.2018.7859
17. Prussick L, Rothstein B, Joshipura D, Saraiya A, Turkowski Y, Abdat R, et al. Open-label, investigator-initiated, single-site exploratory trial evaluating secukinumab, an anti-interleukin-17A monoclonal antibody, for patients with moderate-to-severe hidradenitis suppurativa. *Br J Dermatol.* (2019). doi: 10.1111/bjd.17822. [Epub ahead of print].
18. Schuch A, Fischer T, Boehner A, Biedermann T, Volz T. Successful treatment of severe recalcitrant hidradenitis suppurativa with the interleukin-17A antibody secukinumab. *Acta Derm Venereol.* (2018) 98:151–2. doi: 10.2340/00015555-2794
19. Vossen ARJV, Ardon CB, van der Zee HH, Lubberts E, Prens EP. The anti-inflammatory potency of biologics targeting TNF-α, IL-17A, IL-12/23 and CD20 in hidradenitis suppurativa: an *ex vivo* study. *Br J Dermatol.* (2019) 181. doi: 10.1111/bjd.17641
20. Blok JL, Li K, Brodmerkel C, Horvátovich P, Jonkman MF, Horváth B. Ustekinumab in hidradenitis suppurativa: clinical results and a search for potential biomarkers in serum. *Br J Dermatol.* (2016) 174:839–46. doi: 10.1111/bjd.14338
21. Casseres RG, Kahn JS, Her MJ, Rosmarin D. Guselkumab in the treatment of hidradenitis suppurativa: a retrospective chart review. *J Am Acad Dermatol.* (2018) 81:265–7. doi: 10.1016/j.jaad.2018.12.017
22. Kovacs M, Podda M. Guselkumab in the treatment of severe Hidradenitis suppurativa. *J Eur Acad Dermatol Venereol.* (2018) 33:e140–1. doi: 10.1111/jdv.15368
23. Tzanetakou V, Kanni T, Giatrakou S, Katoulis A, Papadavid E, Netea MG, et al. Safety and efficacy of anakinra in severe hidradenitis suppurativa: a randomized clinical trial. *JAMA Dermatol.* (2016) 152:52–9. doi: 10.1001/jamadermatol.2015.3903
24. Russo V, Alikhan A. Failure of anakinra in a case of severe hidradenitis suppurativa. *J Drugs Dermatol.* (2016) 15:772–4.
25. Tekin B, Salman A, Ergun T. Hidradenitis suppurativa unresponsive to canakinumab treatment: a case report. *Indian J Dermatol Venereol Leprol.* (2017) 83:615–7. doi: 10.4103/ijdvl.IJDVL_147_16
26. Sand FL, Thomsen SF. Off-label use of TNF-alpha inhibitors in a dermatological university department: retrospective evaluation of 118 patients. *Dermatol Ther.* (2015) 28:158–65. doi: 10.1111/dth.12222
27. Yiu ZZN, Madan V, Griffiths CEM. Acne conglobata and adalimumab: use of tumour necrosis factor-α antagonists in treatment-resistant acne conglobata, and review of the literature. *Clin Exp Dermatol.* (2015) 40:383–6. doi: 10.1111/ced.12540
28. Kistowska M, Meier B, Proust T, Feldmeyer L, Cozzio A, Kuendig T, et al. Propionibacterium acnes promotes Th17 and Th17/Th1 responses in acne patients. *J Invest Dermatol.* (2015) 135:110–8. doi: 10.1038/jid.2014.290
29. van Vollenhoven RF, Hahn BH, Tsokos GC, Wagner CL, Lipsky P, Touma Z, et al. Efficacy and safety of ustekinumab, an IL-12 and IL-23 inhibitor, in patients with active systemic lupus erythematosus: results of a multicentre, double-blind, phase 2, randomised, controlled study. *Lancet.* (2018) 392:1330–9. doi: 10.1016/S0140-6736(18)32167-6
30. Winchester D, Duffin KC, Hansen C. Response to ustekinumab in a patient with both severe psoriasis and hypertrophic cutaneous lupus. *Lupus.* (2012) 21:1007–10. doi: 10.1177/0961203312441982
31. De Souza A, Ali-Shaw T, Strober BE, Franks AG. Successful treatment of subacute lupus erythematosus with ustekinumab. *Arch Dermatol.* (2011) 147:896–8. doi: 10.1001/archdermatol.2011.185
32. Dahl C, Johansen C, Kragballe K, Olesen AB. Ustekinumab in the treatment of refractory chronic cutaneous lupus erythematosus: a case report. *Acta Derm Venereol.* (2013) 93:368–9. doi: 10.2340/00015555-1467
33. Shovman O, Tamar S, Amital H, Watad A, Shoenfeld Y. Diverse patterns of anti-TNF-α-induced lupus: case series and review of the literature. *Clin Rheumatol.* (2018) 37:563–8. doi: 10.1007/s10067-017-3884-2
34. Scherlinger M, Carcaud C, Truchetet M-E, Barnetche T, Duffau P, Couzi L, et al. Rituximab in moderate to severe non-renal systemic lupus erythematosus: a reanalysis of the EXPLORER study. *Ann Rheum Dis.* (2019) 78:1007–10. doi: 10.1136/annrheumdis-2018-214833
35. Merrill JT, Neuwelt CM, Wallace DJ, Shanahan JC, Latinis KM, Oates JC, et al. Efficacy and safety of rituximab in moderately-to-severely active systemic lupus erythematosus: the randomized, double-blind, phase II/III systemic lupus erythematosus evaluation of rituximab trial. *Arthritis Rheum.* (2010) 62:222–33. doi: 10.1002/art.27233
36. Quelhas da Costa R, Aguirre-Alastuey ME, Isenberg DA, Saracino AM. Assessment of response to B-cell depletion using rituximab in cutaneous lupus erythematosus. *JAMA Dermatol.* (2018) 154:1432–40. doi: 10.1001/jamadermatol.2018.3793
37. Hasni S, Gupta S, Davis M, Poncio E, Temesgen-Oyelakin Y, Joyal E, et al. Safety and tolerability of omalizumab, a randomized clinical trial of humanized anti-IgE monoclonal antibody in systemic lupus erythematosus? *Arthritis Rheumatol.* (2019) 71: 1135–40. doi: 10.1002/art.40828
38. Schiffenbauer A, Garg M, Castro C, Pokrovnichka A, Joe G, Shrader J, et al. A randomized, double-blind, placebo-controlled trial of infliximab in refractory polymyositis and dermatomyositis. *Semin Arthritis Rheum.* (2018) 47:858–64. doi: 10.1016/j.semarthrit.2017.10.010
39. de Souza FHC, Miossi R, de Moraes JCB, Bonfá E, Shinjo SK. Favorable rituximab response in patients with refractory idiopathic inflammatory myopathies. *Adv Rheumatol.* (2018) 58:31. doi: 10.1186/s42358-018-0030-z

40. Svensson J, Tjärnlund A, Askling J, Dastmalchi M, Hanna B, Bucher SM, et al. FRI0197 use of BIOLOGICS in PM and DM in Sweden - a national register study. *Ann Rheum Dis.* (2014) 73:453–4. doi: 10.1136/annrheumdis-2014-eular.4966
41. Ranganath SP, Pai A. Is optimal management of recurrent aphthous stomatitis possible? A reality check. *J Clin Diagn Res.* (2016) 10:ZE08–13. doi: 10.7860/JCDR/2016/19519.8643
42. Emmi G, Bettiol A. Adalimumab-based treatment versus disease-modifying antirheumatic drugs for venous thrombosis in Behçet's syndrome: a retrospective study of seventy patients with vascular involvement. *Arthritis Rheumatol.* (2018) 70:1500–7. doi: 10.1002/art.40531
43. Di Scala G, Bettiol A, Cojan RD, Finocchi M, Silvestri E, Emmi G. Efficacy of the anti-IL 17 secukinumab in refractory Behçet's syndrome: a preliminary study. *J Autoimmun.* (2019) 97:108–13. doi: 10.1016/j.jaut.2018.09.002
44. Mirouse A, Barete S, Monfort J-B, Resche-Rigon M, Bouyer A-S, Comarmond C, et al. Ustekinumab for Behçet's disease. *J Autoimmun.* (2017) 82:41–6. doi: 10.1016/j.jaut.2017.05.002
45. Grayson PC, Yazici Y, Merideth M, Sen HN, Davis M, Novakovich E, et al. Treatment of mucocutaneous manifestations in Behçet's disease with anakinra: a pilot open-label study. *Arthritis Res Ther.* (2017) 19:69. doi: 10.1186/s13075-017-1222-3
46. Brooklyn TN, Dunnill MGS, Shetty A, Bowden JJ, Williams JDL, Griffiths CEM, et al. Infliximab for the treatment of pyoderma gangrenosum: a randomised, double blind, placebo controlled trial. *Gut.* (2006) 55:505–9. doi: 10.1136/gut.2005.074815
47. de Risi-Pugliese T, Seksik P, Bouaziz J-D, Chasset F, Moguelet P, Gornet J-M, et al. Ustekinumab treatment for neutrophilic dermatoses associated with Crohn's disease: a multicenter retrospective study. *J Am Acad Dermatol.* (2019) 80:781–4. doi: 10.1016/j.jaad.2018.06.065
48. Ahn C, Negus D, Huang W. Pyoderma gangrenosum: a review of pathogenesis and treatment. *Expert Rev Clin Immunol.* (2018) 14:225–33. doi: 10.1080/1744666X.2018.1438269
49. Herberger K, Dissemond J, Brüggestrat S, Sorbe C, Augustin M. Biologics and immunoglobulins in the treatment of pyoderma gangrenosum - analysis of 52 patients. *J Dtsch Dermatol Ges.* (2019) 17:32–41. doi: 10.1111/ddg.13741
50. Sun NZ, Ro T, Jolly P, Sayed CJ. Non-response to Interleukin-1 Antagonist canakinumab in two patients with refractory pyoderma gangrenosum and hidradenitis suppurativa. *J Clin Aesthet Dermatol.* (2017) 10:36–8.
51. Beynon C, Chin MF, Hunasehally P, Bhagwandas K, Bevan M, Taylor M, et al. Successful treatment of autoimmune disease-associated pyoderma gangrenosum with the IL-1 receptor antagonist anakinra: a case series of 3 patients. *J Clin Rheumatol.* (2017) 23:181–3. doi: 10.1097/RHU.0000000000000511
52. Banse C, Sobocinski V, Savoye G, Avenel G, Vittecoq O. Occurrence of sweet syndrome under anti-TNF. *Clin Rheumatol.* (2015) 34:1993–4. doi: 10.1007/s10067-015-3054-3
53. Agarwal A, Barrow W, Selim MA, Nicholas MW. Refractory subcutaneous sweet syndrome treated with adalimumab. *JAMA Dermatol.* (2016) 152:842–4. doi: 10.1001/jamadermatol.2016.0503
54. Kluger N, Gil-Bistes D, Guillot B, Bessis D. Efficacy of anti-interleukin-1 receptor antagonist anakinra (Kineret®) in a case of refractory Sweet's syndrome. *Dermatology (Basel).* (2011) 222:123–7. doi: 10.1159/000326112
55. Delluc A, Limal N, Puéchal X, Francès C, Piette JC, Cacoub P. Efficacy of anakinra, an IL1 receptor antagonist, in refractory Sweet syndrome. *Ann Rheum Dis.* (2008) 67:278–9. doi: 10.1136/ard.2006.068254
56. Lipsker D, Lenormand C. Indications and modes of use for interleukin (IL)-1 antagonists in inflammatory dermatosis: a new therapeutic approach to immune-mediated inflammatory diseases. *Ann Dermatol Venereol.* (2012) 139:459–67. doi: 10.1016/j.annder.2012.03.012
57. van Beek N, Lüttmann N, Huebner F, Recke A, Karl I, Schulze FS, et al. Correlation of serum levels of IgE autoantibodies against BP180 with bullous pemphigoid disease activity. *JAMA Dermatol.* (2017) 153:30–8. doi: 10.1001/jamadermatol.2016.3357
58. Hashimoto T, Ohzono A, Teye K, Numata S, Hiroyasu S, Tsuruta D, et al. Detection of IgE autoantibodies to BP180 and BP230 and their relationship to clinical features in bullous pemphigoid. *Br J Dermatol.* (2017) 177:141–51. doi: 10.1111/bjd.15114
59. James T, Salman S, Stevenson B, Bundell C, Kelly G, Nolan D, et al. IgE blockade in autoimmunity: omalizumab induced remission of bullous pemphigoid. *Clin Immunol.* (2018) 198:54–6. doi: 10.1016/j.clim.2018.12.015
60. Kremer N, Snast I, Cohen ES, Hodak E, Mimouni D, Lapidoth M, et al. Rituximab and omalizumab for the treatment of bullous pemphigoid: a systematic review of the literature. *Am J Clin Dermatol.* (2018) 20:209–16. doi: 10.1007/s40257-018-0401-6
61. Bilgiç Temel A, Bassorgun CI, Akman-Karakaş A, Alpsoy E, Uzun S. Successful treatment of a bullous pemphigoid patient with rituximab who was refractory to corticosteroid and omalizumab treatments. *Case Rep Dermatol.* (2017) 9:38–44. doi: 10.1159/000452828
62. Loget J, Plée J, Antonicelli F, Bernard P. A successful treatment with ustekinumab in a case of relapsing bullous pemphigoid associated with psoriasis. *J Eur Acad Dermatol Venereol.* (2017) 31:e228–30. doi: 10.1111/jdv.14002
63. Le Guern A, Alkeraye S, Vermersch-Langlin A, Coupe P, Vonarx M. Bullous pemphigoid during ustekinumab therapy. *JAAD Case Rep.* (2015) 1:359–60. doi: 10.1016/j.jdcr.2015.07.014
64. Kamata M, Asano Y, Shida R, Maeda N, Yoshizaki A, Miyagaki T, et al. Secukinumab decreased circulating anti-BP180-NC16a autoantibodies in a patient with coexisting psoriasis vulgaris and bullous pemphigoid. *J Dermatol.* (2019) 46:e216–7. doi: 10.1111/1346-8138.14760
65. Ho P-H, Tsai T-F. Development of bullous pemphigoid during secukinumab treatment for psoriasis. *J Dermatol.* (2017) 44:e2201. doi: 10.1111/1346-8138.13909
66. Le Jan S, Plée J, Vallerand D, Dupont A, Delanez E, Durlach A, et al. Innate immune cell-produced IL-17 sustains inflammation in bullous pemphigoid. *J Invest Dermatol.* (2014) 134:2908–17. doi: 10.1038/jid.2014.263
67. Lamberts A, Euverman HI, Terra JB, Jonkman MF, Horváth B. Effectiveness and safety of rituximab in recalcitrant pemphigoid diseases. *Front Immunol.* (2018) 9:248. doi: 10.3389/fimmu.2018.00248
68. You C, Lamba N, Lasave AF, Ma L, Diaz MH, Foster CS. Rituximab in the treatment of ocular cicatricial pemphigoid: a retrospective cohort study. *Graefes Arch Clin Exp Ophthalmol.* (2017) 255:1221–8. doi: 10.1007/s00417-017-3603-3
69. Iwata H, Vorobyev A, Koga H, Recke A, Zillikens D, Prost-Squarcioni C, et al. Meta-analysis of the clinical and immunopathological characteristics and treatment outcomes in epidermolysis bullosa acquisita patients. *Orphanet J Rare Dis.* (2018) 13:153. doi: 10.1186/s13023-018-0896-1
70. Napolitano M, Abeni D, Didona B. Biologics for pityriasis rubra pilaris treatment: a review of the literature. *J Am Acad Dermatol.* (2018) 79:353–9 e11. doi: 10.1016/j.jaad.2018.03.036
71. Bonomo L, Levitt JO. Secukinumab emerges as a rapidly effective therapy for pityriasis rubra pilaris. *Cutis.* (2018) 101:367–9.
72. Heibel MD, Heibel HD. Successful treatment of type I pityriasis rubra pilaris with ixekizumab. *JAAD Case Rep.* (2018) 4:774–6. doi: 10.1016/j.jdcr.2018.05.006
73. Wain T, Choy B, Satchell AC, Woods JA, Frew JW. Secukinumab in pityriasis rubra pilaris: a case series demonstrating variable response and the need for minimal clinical datasets. *JAAD Case Rep.* (2018) 4:500–5. doi: 10.1016/j.jdcr.2018.02.007
74. Matsuda T, Yamazaki F, Ueda-Hayakawa I, Kambe N, Okamoto H. Case of pityriasis rubra pilaris progressed to generalized erythroderma following blockade of interleukin-17A, but improved after blockade of interleukin-12/23 p40. *J Dermatol.* (2019) 46:70–2. doi: 10.1111/1346-8138.14709
75. Chen A, Truong AK, Worswick S. The role of biologics in the treatment of chronic granuloma annulare. *Int J Dermatol.* (2019) 58:622–6. doi: 10.1111/ijd.14350
76. Ratnarathorn M, Raychaudhuri SP, Naguwa S. Disseminated granuloma annulare: a cutaneous adverse effect of anti-tnf agents. *Indian J Dermatol.* (2011) 56:752–4. doi: 10.4103/0019-5154.91847
77. Voulgari PV, Markatseli TE, Exarchou SA, Zioga A, Drosos AA. Granuloma annulare induced by anti-tumour necrosis factor therapy. *Ann Rheum Dis.* (2008) 67:567–70. doi: 10.1136/ard.2007.075663
78. Bonomo L, Ghoneim S, Levitt J. A case of granuloma annulare associated with secukinumab use. *Case Rep Dermatol Med.* (2017) 2017:5918708. doi: 10.1155/2017/5918708

79. Lieberoth S, Thomsen SF. Cutaneous and gastrointestinal symptoms in two patients with systemic mastocytosis successfully treated with omalizumab. *Case Rep Med.* (2015) 2015:903541. doi: 10.1155/2015/903541
80. Hinojosa T, Lewis DJ, Vangipuram R, Laraib Safeer BA, Mui UN, Haley C, et al. The efficacy of omalizumab in cutaneous mastocytosis: a case series. *Dermatol Ther.* (2019) 32:e12848. doi: 10.1111/dth.12848
81. Distler M, Maul T, Steiner U, Jandus P, Murer C, Graf N, et al. The effect of omalizumab in mastocytosis patients. Prospective double-blind, placebo-controlled multicentre study. *J Allergy Clin Immunol.* (2019) 143:Supplement (AB134). doi: 10.1016/j.jaci.2018.12.407
82. Wang F, Ye Y, Luo Z-Y, Gao Q, Luo D-Q, Zhang X. Diverse expression of TNF-α and CCL27 in serum and blister of Stevens–Johnson syndrome/toxic epidermal necrolysis. *Clin Transl Allergy.* (2018) 8:12. doi: 10.1186/s13601-018-0199-6
83. Woolridge KF, Boler PL, Lee BD. Tumor necrosis factor alpha inhibitors in the treatment of toxic epidermal necrolysis. *Cutis.* (2018) 101:E15–21.
84. Paradisi A, Abeni D, Bergamo F, Ricci F, Didona D, Didona B. Etanercept therapy for toxic epidermal necrolysis. *J Am Acad Dermatol.* (2014) 71:278–83. doi: 10.1016/j.jaad.2014.04.044
85. Wang C-W, Yang L-Y, Chen C-B, Ho H-C, Hung S-I, Yang C-H, et al. Randomized, controlled trial of TNF-α antagonist in CTL-mediated severe cutaneous adverse reactions. *J Clin Invest.* (2018) 128:985–96. doi: 10.1172/JCI93349
86. Garcovich S, De Simone C, Genovese G, Berti E, Cugno M, Marzano AV. Paradoxical skin reactions to biologics in patients with rheumatologic disorders. *Front Pharmacol.* (2019) 10:282. doi: 10.3389/fphar.2019.00282
87. Holló P, Szakonyi J, Kiss D, Jokai H, Horváth A, Kárpáti S. Successful treatment of lichen planus with adalimumab. *Acta Derm Venereol.* (2012) 92:385–6. doi: 10.2340/00015555-1249
88. Yarom N. Etanercept for the management of oral lichen planus. *Am J Clin Dermatol.* (2007) 8:121. doi: 10.2165/00128071-200708020-00010
89. Chao TJ. Adalimumab in the management of cutaneous and oral lichen planus. *Cutis.* (2009) 84:325–8.
90. Tétu P, Monfort J-B, Barbaud A, Francès C, Chasset F. Failure of rituximab in refractory erosive lichen planus. *Br J Dermatol.* (2018) 179:980–1. doi: 10.1111/bjd.16704
91. Woolridge KF, Boler PL, Lee BD. Tumor necrosis factor alpha inhibitors in the treatment of toxic epidermal necrolysis. *Cutis.* (2018) 101:E15–21.
92. Thorlacius L, Theut Riis P, Jemec GBE. Severe hidradenitis suppurativa responding to treatment with secukinumab: a case report. *Br J Dermatol.* (2018) 179:182–5. doi: 10.1111/bjd.15769
93. Balakirski G, Alkhateeb A, Merk HF, Leverkus M, Megahed M. Successful treatment of bullous pemphigoid with omalizumab as corticosteroid-sparing agent: report of two cases and review of literature. *J Eur Acad Dermatol Venereol.* (2016) 30:1778–82. doi: 10.1111/jdv.13758
94. Menzinger S, Kaya G, Schmidt E, Fontao L, Laffitte E. Biological and clinical response to omalizumab in a patient with bullous pemphigoid. *Acta Derm Venereol.* (2018) 98:284–6. doi: 10.2340/00015555-2845
95. Fairley JA, Burnett CT, Fu C-L, Larson DL, Fleming MG, Giudice GJ. A pathogenic role for IgE in autoimmunity: bullous pemphigoid IgE reproduces the early phase of lesion development in human skin grafted to nu/nu mice. *J Invest Dermatol.* (2007) 127:2605–11. doi: 10.1038/sj.jid.5700958
96. Rambhia PH, Levitt JO. Recalcitrant prurigo nodularis treated successfully with dupilumab. *JAAD Case Rep.* (2019) 5:471–3. doi: 10.1016/j.jdcr.2019.03.016
97. Silverberg JI, Brieva J. A successful case of dupilumab treatment for severe uremic pruritus. *JAAD Case Rep.* (2019) 5:339–41. doi: 10.1016/j.jdcr.2019.01.024
98. Yang EJ, Murase JE. Recalcitrant anal and genital pruritus treated with dupilumab. *Int J Womens Dermatol.* (2018) 4:223–6. doi: 10.1016/j.ijwd.2018.08.010
99. Mollanazar NK, Elgash M, Weaver L, Valdes-Rodriguez R, Hsu S. Reduced itch associated with dupilumab treatment in 4 patients with prurigo nodularis. *JAMA Dermatol.* (2019) 155:121–2. doi: 10.1001/jamadermatol.2018.3906
100. Kanda N, Koto M, Hoashi T, Saeki H. Case of alopecia areata during dupilumab treatment for atopic dermatitis. *J Dermatol.* (2019). doi: 10.1111/1346-8138.14880. [Epub ahead of print].
101. Maloney NJ, Worswick S, Cheng K. Development of alopecia in patients treated with dupilumab. *Dermatol Ther.* (2019) 32:e12869. doi: 10.1111/dth.12869
102. Yazdanyar S, Jemec GBE. Alopecia areata after treatment with dupilumab. *Dermatitis.* (2019) 30:175–6. doi: 10.1097/DER.0000000000000458
103. Darrigade A-S, Legrand A, Andreu N, Jacquemin C, Boniface K, Taïeb A, et al. Dual efficacy of dupilumab in a patient with concomitant atopic dermatitis and alopecia areata. *Br J Dermatol.* (2018) 179:534–6. doi: 10.1111/bjd.16711
104. Dobkin H, Mullen R, Zirwas M. Alopecia universalis and atopic dermatitis improvement with dupilumab: demonstration of a shared pathophysiology and clinical efficacy. *Skinmed.* (2019) 17:139–40.
105. Ludriksone L, Elsner P, Schliemann S. Zwei patienten mit abheilung einer alopecia areata unter dupilumab. *J Dtsch Dermatol Ges.* (2019) 17(Suppl. 2):1–3. doi: 10.1111/ddg.13778
106. Kaye A, Gordon SC, Deverapalli SC, Her MJ, Rosmarin D. Dupilumab for the treatment of recalcitrant bullous pemphigoid. *JAMA Dermatol.* (2018) 154:1225–6. doi: 10.1001/jamadermatol.2018.2526
107. Gordon SC, Robinson SN, Abudu M, Her M, Deverapalli S, Levin A, et al. Eosinophilic annular erythema treated with dupilumab. *Pediatr Dermatol.* (2018) 35:e255–6. doi: 10.1111/pde.13533
108. Teraki Y, Taguchi R, Takamura S, Fukuda T. Use of dupilumab in the treatment of papuloerythroderma of ofuji. *JAMA Dermatol.* (2019). doi: 10.1001/jamadermatol.2019.0946
109. Zhao S, Nair JR, Moots RJ. Biosimilars: from extrapolation into off label use. *Curr Pharm Des.* (2017) 23:6746–51. doi: 10.2174/1381612824666171129193258

16

MALT1-Deficient Mice Develop Atopic-Like Dermatitis Upon Aging

Annelies Demeyer[1,2], *Elien Van Nuffel*[1,2], *Griet Baudelet*[1,2], *Yasmine Driege*[1,2], *Marja Kreike*[1,2], *David Muyllaert*[1,2], *Jens Staal*[1,2*†] *and Rudi Beyaert*[1,2*†]

[1] VIB Center for Inflammation Research, Ghent, Belgium, [2] Department of Biomedical Molecular Biology, Ghent University, Ghent, Belgium

***Correspondence:**
Jens Staal
jens.staal@irc.vib-ugent.be
Rudi Beyaert
rudi.beyaert@irc.vib-ugent.be

† These authors share last authorship

MALT1 plays an important role in innate and adaptive immune signaling by acting as a scaffold protein that mediates NF-κB signaling. In addition, MALT1 is a cysteine protease that further fine tunes proinflammatory signaling by cleaving specific substrates. Deregulated MALT1 activity has been associated with immunodeficiency, autoimmunity, and cancer in mice and humans. Genetically engineered mice expressing catalytically inactive MALT1, still exerting its scaffold function, were previously shown to spontaneously develop autoimmunity due to a decrease in Tregs associated with increased effector T cell activation. In contrast, complete absence of MALT1 does not lead to autoimmunity, which has been explained by the impaired effector T cell activation due to the absence of MALT1-mediated signaling. However, here we report that MALT1-deficient mice develop atopic-like dermatitis upon aging, which is preceded by Th2 skewing, an increase in serum IgE, and a decrease in Treg frequency and surface expression of the Treg functionality marker CTLA-4.

Keywords: atopic dermatitis, skin inflammation, MALT1, lymphocytes, Tregs, Th2, aging

INTRODUCTION

MALT1 (Mucosa-associated lymphoid tissue lymphoma translocation protein 1) is an intracellular signaling protein that plays an important role in several cell types, including lymphoid and myeloid cells as well as non-hematopoietic cells (1). MALT1 is best known for its role as a scaffold protein in T cell receptor (TCR)- and B cell receptor (BCR)-induced nuclear factor-κB (NF-κB) signaling, leading to the activation and proliferation of T and B cells, respectively (2, 3). Moreover, MALT1-mediated NF-κB signaling plays a key role in the proliferation of certain B cell lymphomas, such as MALT1 lymphoma and activated B cell-like diffuse large B cell lymphoma (ABC-DLBCL) (4–13). TCR or BCR stimulation, as well as oncogenic mutations in specific signaling proteins, leads to the formation of a so-called CBM signaling complex, consisting of CARD11 (also known as CARMA1), BCL10 and MALT1 (8, 14–18). In this complex, MALT1 acts as an adaptor to recruit the E3 ubiquitin ligase TRAF6, whose activity facilitates the recruitment and activation of downstream NF-κB signaling proteins (19–21). The importance of the CBM complex is illustrated by the impaired TCR-induced NF-κB activation in T cells isolated from *Card11*-, *Bcl10*-, and *Malt1*-knock-out (KO) mice, respectively (2, 3, 22, 23).

In addition to its scaffold function, MALT1 also acts as a cysteine protease. TCR stimulation leads to the MALT1-mediated cleavage of several substrates including BCL10, the deubiquitinases A20 and CYLD, the NF-κB family member RelB, the RNA-binding and RNA-destabilizing proteins Roquin-1/2, Regnase-1, and N4BP1, the E3 ubiquitin ligase HOIL1, and MALT1 itself (24–34).

Although the specific biological role of cleavage of each of these substrates is still largely unclear, MALT1 proteolytic activity contributes to the fine-tuning of TCR-induced gene expression, lymphocyte activation and proliferation, and regulatory T cell (Treg) development and function. Consequently, inhibition of MALT1 proteolytic activity has been proposed as an interesting therapeutic approach for autoimmune diseases and certain cancers, which is further supported by promising results with MALT1 protease inhibitors in preclinical mouse models (12, 13, 35–37). Of note, MALT1 mutation in humans, causing the absence or very low expression of MALT1, leads to combined immunodeficiency (CID), which is characterized by several bacterial, fungal, and viral infections, indicating that targeting MALT1 activity may not be without risk (38–43). Moreover, it was recently shown that *Malt1* protease-dead (PD) knock-in mice expressing a catalytically inactive MALT1 mutant spontaneously develop multi-organ inflammation due to defects in T cell homeostasis (44–49). This was rather unexpected since inflammation was never described for mice that are completely deficient in MALT1. However, in the present paper we show that *Malt1*-KO mice develop atopic-like dermatitis upon aging.

RESULTS

Malt1-KO Mice Spontaneously Develop Skin Lesions, Accompanied by Elevated Serum Cytokine Levels

Malt1-KO mice were housed under SPF conditions and monitored for macroscopic clinical signs on a regular basis. Interestingly, the mice were found to develop skin lesions upon aging, with an average disease onset of 161 days (**Figures 1A,B**). The *Malt1*-KO mice suffer from erosive lesions in the neck and face region, with the epidermis showing acanthosis, hyperkeratosis, and parakeratotic scaling, as well as $CD3^+$ T cell infiltration (**Figure 1C**). Similar lesions were observed in another independent *Malt1*-KO LacZ reporter mouse line (**Figure 1A**), indicating that the observed phenotype is strain-independent. Next to full body *Malt1*-KO mice, also T cell-specific ($Malt1^{FL/FL}CD4\text{-}Cre^{Tg/+}$) and keratinocyte-specific ($Malt1^{FL/FL}K5\text{-}Cre^{Tg/+}$) *Malt1-KO* mice were monitored for skin lesions over time, but these mice did not develop any skin lesions (**Figure 1B**), indicating that absence of MALT1 in T cells or keratinocytes, as such, is not sufficient to induce skin inflammation. *Malt1*-KO mice that develop skin inflammation were found to have increased serum levels of the pro-inflammatory cytokines IL-2, IL-4, IL-6, IL-17, IFN-γ, and TNF (**Figure 1D**). To assess if increased serum cytokine levels reflect a more general inflammation in MALT1-deficient mice, we analyzed H&E stained sections of lung, liver, stomach, colon, small intestine, lacrimal glands and salivary glands. However, no differences were observed between *Malt1*-KO and WT mice for all these tissues (**Figure 2A**). In addition, we checked blood glucose levels in young (±20 weeks) and older mice (7–8 months) to determine possible pancreatic inflammation, but also here MALT1 deficiency had no effect (**Figure 2B**). Together, our data demonstrate that MALT1 deficiency in mice specifically results in an inflammatory skin phenotype upon aging.

MALT1 Deficiency Results in Defective Treg Development and CTLA-4 Expression via a T Cell Intrinsic Mechanism in Both Young and old Mice

Malt1-KO mice are known to have a defect in Treg development (44, 46, 50, 51), which could be responsible for the skin inflammation in aging MALT1-deficient mice. However, it has been reported by Brüstle et al. that whereas young *Malt1*-KO mice have severely reduced numbers of Tregs in blood and thymus, 1 year old *Malt1*-KO mice have normal Treg numbers in blood, which was suggested to reflect the generation of inducible Tregs (iTregs) in aging mice (51). Of note, this study did not mention the development of skin lesions in aged mice. We therefore analyzed the number of Tregs ($Foxp3^+CD25^+CD4^+$ T cells) in young and aged (±7 months old) *Malt1*-KO mice. In agreement with the above mentioned previous studies, Treg numbers were reduced in thymus, lymph nodes (LN), and spleen of lesion-free young mice. However, in contrast to the study by Brüstle et al., we found that the number of Tregs were equally reduced in thymus, LN and spleen of aged *Malt1*-KO mice that developed skin lesions (**Figures 3A,B** and gating strategy in **Supplementary Figures 1**, **2**). The reason for this discrepancy is still unclear, but different findings may reflect specific differences in mouse housing conditions. Similar to the full *Malt1*-KO mice, also T cell specific *Malt1*-KO mice had a reduced Treg frequency in their thymus, spleen, and LN (**Figure 3C**), indicating a T cell intrinsic role of MALT1 in Treg development. We next investigated whether the remaining MALT1-deficient Tregs are functional. CTLA-4 expression on Tregs is known to compete with CD28 on T cells for binding to CD80 and CD86, as well as to reduce the surface expression of CD80 and CD86 on antigen presenting cells, resulting in reduced T cell proliferation and cytokine production (52, 53). We therefore assessed CTLA-4 surface expression on splenocytes from WT and *Malt1*-KO mice that were stimulated *in vitro* for 4 h with phorbol myristic acid/Ionomycine (PMA/IO). As shown in **Figure 3D**, a reduced frequency of Tregs that express surface CTLA-4 could be observed in *Malt1*-KO mice compared to WT mice, suggesting that the remaining MALT1-deficient Tregs are functionally impaired (gating strategy in **Supplementary Figure 2**).

Activation and CTLA-4 Surface Expression of $CD4^+$ T Cells Is Altered in *Malt1*-KO Mice

Since we observed increased $CD3^+$ T cell infiltration in the diseased skin of *Malt1*-KO mice, we further investigated whether the proliferation and activation of $CD4^+$ T cells is affected in MALT1-deficient mice. For this purpose, we purified $CD4^+$ T cells and labeled them with CFSE to measure their proliferation after 72 h stimulation with anti-CD3 and anti-CD28. This showed that MALT1-deficient $CD4^+$ T cells can proliferate, albeit to a lesser extent than WT $CD4^+$ T cells (**Figure 4A**), which is similar to what has previously been described (45). To assess

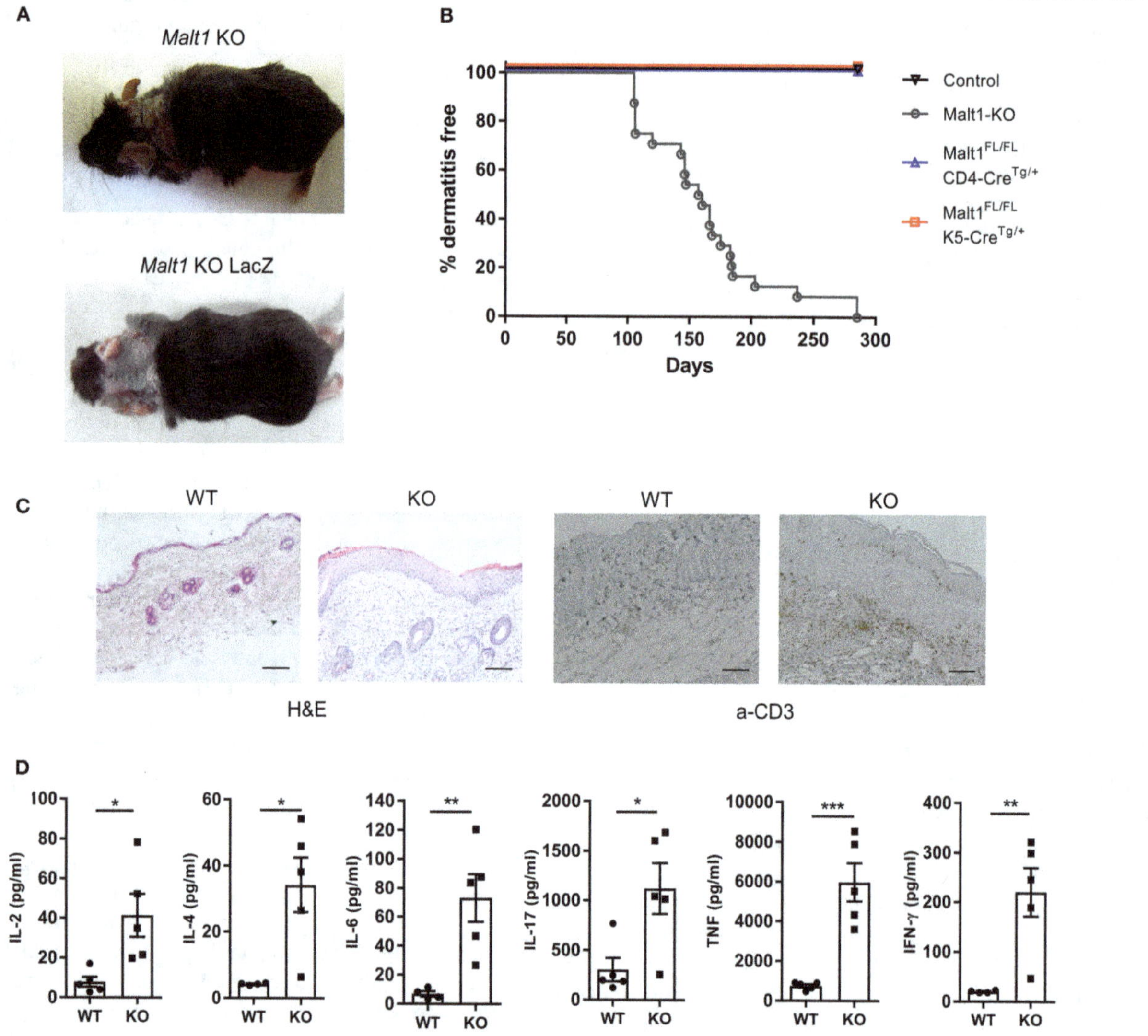

FIGURE 1 | *Malt1*-KO mice develop skin lesions at late age accompanied by elevated serum cytokine levels. **(A)** Skin lesion in the neck of a *Malt1*-KO and *Malt1*-KO LacZ mouse. **(B)** Incidence of dermatitis in *Malt1*-KO mice ($n = 8$ for controls, $n = 24$ for *Malt1-KO*, $n = 6$ for *Malt1*$^{FL/FL}$ *CD4-Cre*$^{Tg/+}$, and $n = 6$ for *Malt1*$^{FL/FL}$ *K5-Cre*$^{Tg/+}$). **(C)** H&E staining on WT and *Malt1*-KO skin (scale bar 100 μm), showing epidermal thickening and parakeratosis in *Malt1*-KO skin and α-CD3 staining on WT and *Malt1*-KO skin (scale bar 100 μm), showing increased CD3 staining in *Malt1*-KO skin. **(D)** Elevated serum levels of IL-2, IL-4, IL-6, IL-17, IFN-γ, and TNF in *Malt1*-KO mice compared to WT mice (both $n = 5$ and >30 weeks, and *Malt1*-KO mice have AD). Open circles (WT) and black squares (KO) represent individual mice. The mean ± SEM is indicated on the graphs. The statistical significance between groups was calculated with an unpaired 2-tailed Student's *t*-test: $^{*}P < 0.05$, $^{**}P < 0.01$, and $^{***}P < 0.001$.

the activation of CD4$^+$ MALT1-deficient T cells, we stimulated splenocytes for 4 h with PMA/IO and determined the frequency of CD44$^+$CD4$^+$ T cells, so-called effector CD4$^+$ T cells. Notably, *Malt1*-KO mice had a reduced frequency of effector CD4$^+$ T cells (**Figure 4B**), which is consistent with previous findings (2).

Since not only Tregs but also effector CD4$^+$ T cells can use surface CTLA-4 to suppress proliferation of effector CD4$^+$ T cells (54–56), we assessed the expression of CTLA-4 on the surface of effector CD4$^+$ T cells from *Malt1*-KO and WT mice. In contrast to WT mice, *Malt1*-KO mice showed a strong reduction in the frequency of effector CD4$^+$ T cells that express surface CTLA-4 (**Figure 4C** and gating strategy in **Supplementary Figure 2**). In addition, the expression of CTLA-4 on the remaining MALT1-deficient surface CTLA-4$^+$ effector CD4$^+$ T cells was also reduced, as determined by the surface CTLA-4 mean fluorescent intensity (**Figure 4D**). These data clearly show that besides being important for CTLA-4 expression on the surface of Tregs, MALT1 is similarly important for the expression of CTLA-4 on the surface of effector CD4$^+$ T cells. Together, these data show that although MALT1 deficiency leads to reduced activation and proliferation of stimulated CD4$^+$ T cells, it also lowers the immune suppressive functions of both Tregs and effector CD4$^+$ T cells, which could contribute to disease development.

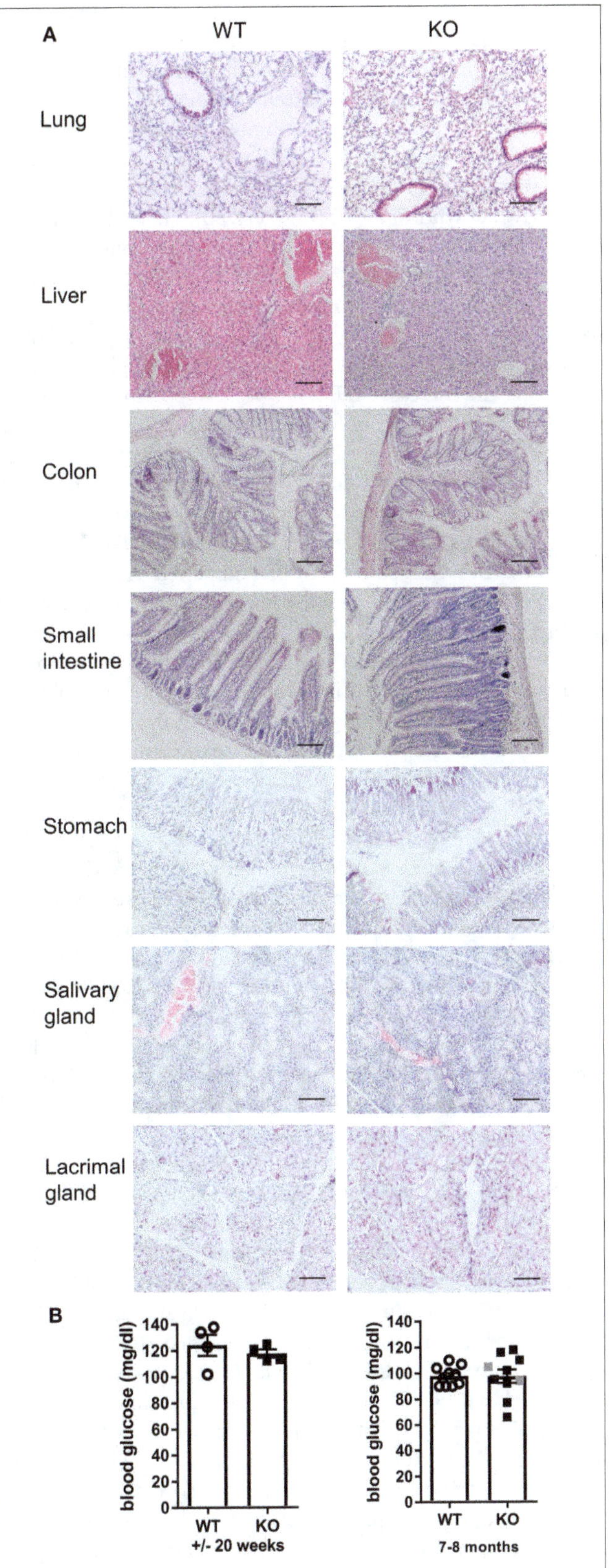

FIGURE 2 | *Malt1*-KO mice do not develop multi-organ inflammation. **(A)** H&E staining (scale bar 100 μm) of several organs from WT and *Malt1*-KO mice *(Continued)*

FIGURE 2 | (*Malt1*-KO mice had skin lesions and the WT and KO mice were between 30 and 40 weeks old). **(B)** Blood glucose levels in mice of ±20 weeks (left, WT: $n = 5$ and KO: $n = 4$) and mice of 7–8 months (right, WT: $n = 10$ and KO: $n = 8$). Open circles (WT), gray squares (KO), and black squares (KO + AD = KO mice with atopic dermatitis) represent individual mice. The mean ± SEM is indicated on the graphs. The statistical significance between groups was calculated with an unpaired 2-tailed Student's *t*-test: no significant difference was found.

MALT1 Deficiency Causes Th2 Skewing Accompanied by Increased Serum IgE Levels

We next investigated whether the impaired Treg development in *Malt1*-KO mice has an impact on the T-helper (Th) cell populations. To this end, we stimulated splenocytes with PMA, IO, and Brefeldin A for 4 h, and determined the percentage of Th2 (IL-4 producing $CD44^+CD4^+$ T cells) (**Figure 5A**) and Th1 cells (IFN-γ producing $CD44^+CD4^+$ T cells) (**Figure 5B**), respectively (gating strategy in **Supplementary Figure 3**). MALT1-deficient mice (±20 weeks, skin lesion free) repeatedly showed largely similar levels of IFN-γ-producing Th1 cells, while the IL-4 producing Th2 cells were significantly increased. Since IL-4, secreted by Th2 cells, is known to induce B cell Ig isotype switching from IgM to IgE (57), we determined the serum IgE levels from *Malt1*-KO and WT mice of several ages. In agreement with the increased Th2 frequency, IgE levels were clearly elevated in *Malt1*-KO mice at any time point tested and preceded lesion onset (**Figure 5C**). Furthermore, in the ear skin of *Malt1*-KO mice with lesions, we found elevated mRNA levels of *Tslp* and *Il22* (**Figure 5D**), which are both known to promote Th2 responses (58, 59). Collectively, these data indicate that MALT1 deficiency leads to Th2 skewing and IgE production, which might contribute to skin lesion development.

DISCUSSION

We report that aging *Malt1*-KO mice suffer from atopic-like dermatitis accompanied by elevated serum cytokine levels and preceded by Th2 skewing and elevated serum IgE levels. No inflammation could be observed at other sites of the body. In contrast to *Malt1*-KO mice, skin lesions were never reported in mice fully deficient in one of the other components of the CBM complex, BCL10 and CARD11, or in the upstream activator PKCθ, even though BCL10 and PKCθ deficient mice were followed up until 6 months of age (22, 60). Notably, despite being part of the same signaling pathway, MALT1, BCL10, and PKC-θ deficiency have also been reported to differentially affect TCR-induced proliferation, IL-2 production, and NF-κB activation in T cells, with MALT1-deficient T cells showing a milder impairment than BCL10- and PKCθ-deficient T cells, suggesting they may have divergent functions and act in additional signaling pathways (61).

We further report that atopic-like dermatitis in aging *Malt1*-KO mice is associated with a decrease in the number and function of Tregs in the thymus and periphery. We propose that the

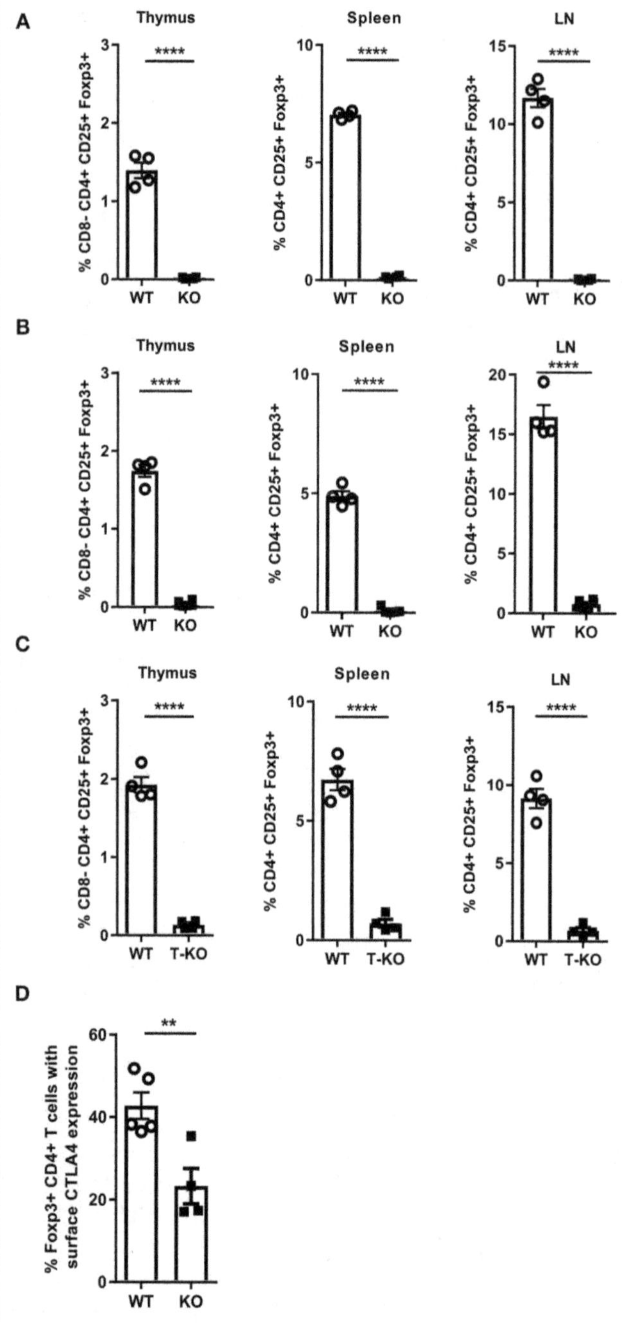

FIGURE 3 | MALT1 plays a T cell-intrinsic role in Treg development. **(A)** Percentage of Tregs (Foxp3$^+$CD25$^+$CD4$^+$ T cells) in the thymus, spleen and lymph nodes of *Malt1*-WT and *Malt1*-KO mice without skin lesions (WT: $n = 4$ and KO: $n = 4$, age 10–12 weeks). **(B)** Percentage of Tregs (Foxp3$^+$CD25$^+$ CD4$^+$ T cells) in the thymus, spleen and lymph nodes of older WT and *Malt1*-KO mice with skin lesions (WT: $n = 4$ and KO: $n = 6$, age 6.5–8.5 months). **(C)** Percentage of Tregs (Foxp3$^+$CD25$^+$CD4$^+$ T cells) in the thymus, spleen and lymph nodes of WT (*Malt1$^{FL/FL}$CD4-Cre$^{+/+}$*, $n = 4$), and T-KO (*Malt1$^{FL/FL}$CD4-Cre$^{Tg/+}$*, $n = 4$) mice. **(D)** Percentage of splenic Tregs (Foxp3$^+$CD4$^+$ T cells) expressing CTLA-4 on their surface after stimulation for 4 h with PMA and IO in WT ($n = 5$) and *Malt1*-KO ($n = 5$) mice. The mean ± SEM is indicated on the graphs. The statistical significance between groups was calculated with an unpaired 2-tailed Student's *t*-test: $^{**}P < 0.01$ and $^{****}P < 0.0001$.

reduction in immune suppressive Tregs leads to a disruption of normal immune homeostasis and contributes to the activation of effector T cells and allergic skin inflammation. In this context, we could measure more Th2 cells producing IL-4, which is known to play multiple roles in promoting atopic-like dermatitis (62). A severe Treg reduction is also seen in patients suffering from immunodysregulation polyendocrinopathy enteropathy X-linked (IPEX) syndrome (OMIM #304790), caused by mutations in the *FOXP3* gene (63) as well as mice with a mutation in the *Foxp3* gene, so called scurfy mice (64). The scurfy mice and the IPEX patients illustrate variable autoimmune disorders. IPEX patients can suffer from type 1 diabetes mellitus and thyroid disease, increased IgE levels, asthma and food allergies, while dermatitis and increased IgE levels are also present in the scurfy mice (63, 65–67). A lack of functional Tregs is a common feature in *Malt1*-KO mice, scurfy mice and IPEX patients (44, 46, 50, 51, 68–70). Moreover, a scurfy-like phenotype was described for mice (*Malt1$^{FL/FL}$Foxp3-cre$^{Tg/+}$*) with a specific deletion of *Malt1* in Tregs (36, 49). However, while *Malt1*-KO mice as well as MALT1 CID patients display impaired T cell activation (3, 22, 38–47), this is not the case for IPEX patients, scurfy mice and mice only lacking *Malt1* in Tregs, where there is a failure to control T cell activation due to the absence of Tregs or the reduced functionality of Tregs leading to lymphoproliferation and autoimmunity, resulting in death (36, 49, 63, 65–67, 71).

CTLA-4 is a known functionality marker on Tregs and is required for their inhibitory function (52, 53). We show that the remaining Tregs in *Malt1*-KO mice are also functionally impaired as demonstrated by a reduced CTLA-4 expression. The reduced Treg frequency and functionality we observed in *Malt1*-KO mice is associated with an increased Th2 frequency. Th2 cells were previously shown to expand disproportionally upon depletion of Tregs, which tightly control the Th2 population via induction of apoptosis of Th2, but not Th1 cells (72). Moreover, Tian et al. showed that addition of recombinant CTLA-4-Ig to Treg depleted mice induces Th2 apoptosis and thus reduces the Th2 expansion, illustrating the tight control by Tregs on the Th2 population (72). In addition to Tregs, also effector CD4$^+$ T cells make use of surface CTLA-4 to inhibit effector CD4$^+$ T cells, albeit with much lower efficiency than Tregs (54–56). Notably, we show that CTLA-4 expression is also reduced on effector CD4$^+$ T cells in *Malt1*-KO mice, which may also contribute to disease pathogenesis. Interestingly, CTLA-4 mRNA is post-transcriptionally regulated by the endonuclease Regnase-1 and the RNA-binding proteins Roquin-1 and-2, which were shown to be inactivated by MALT1-mediated cleavage, leading to stabilization of CTLA-4 and many other mRNA molecules (28, 29). Most likely, reduced CTLA4 expression in MALT1-deficient Tregs and effector CD4$^+$ T cells reflects the absence of Regnase-1 and Roquin cleavage, leading to CTLA-4 mRNA degradation and reduced CTLA-4 protein expression.

Mice that are completely deficient in MALT1 as well as mice expressing a catalytically inactive (protease-dead) mutant MALT1 have a reduced number of Tregs, but only *Malt1*-PD mice develop severe autoimmune symptoms (44–51). Impaired TCR-mediated effector T cell activation, normally mediated by the MALT1 scaffold function, has been proposed to prevent

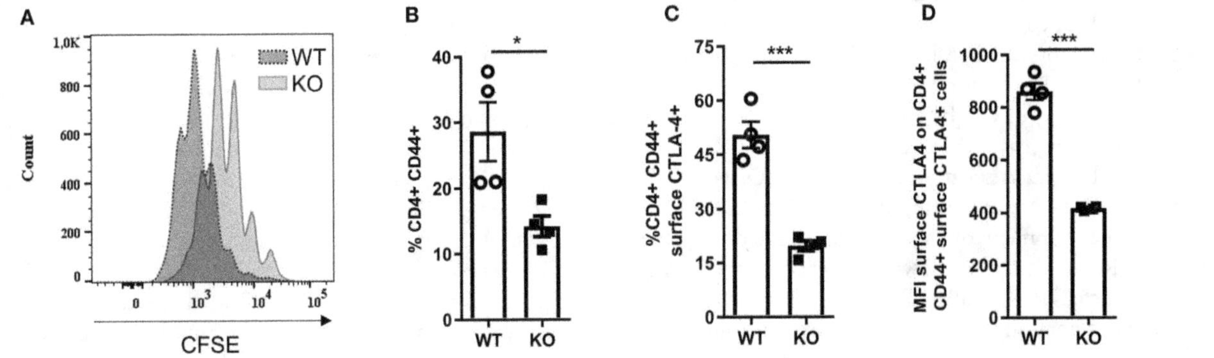

FIGURE 4 | Activation of *Malt1*-KO CD4$^+$ T is altered. **(A)** CFSE labeled CD4$^+$ T cells stimulated for 72 h with plate bound α-CD3 and soluble α-CD28. The CFSE overlaid histograms displaying the proliferation of WT or *Malt1*-KO CD4$^+$ T cells (age mice: 10 weeks lesion-free). **(B)** Splenocytes were stimulated for 4 h with PMA and IO (same for C and D) in order to determine the percentage of CD44$^+$ CD4$^+$ T cells. **(C)** Percentage of CD44$^+$CD4$^+$ T cells that express CTLA-4 on their surface. **(D)** Mean fluorescence intensity (MFI) of CTLA-4 on CD44$^+$CD4$^+$ T cells that express CTLA-4 on their surface. For **(B–D)** open circles (WT: $n = 4$) and black squares (KO: $n = 4$) represent individual mice. The mean ± SEM is indicated on the graphs. The statistical significance between groups was calculated with an unpaired 2-tailed Student's *t*-test: $^{*}P < 0.05$ and $^{***}P < 0.001$.

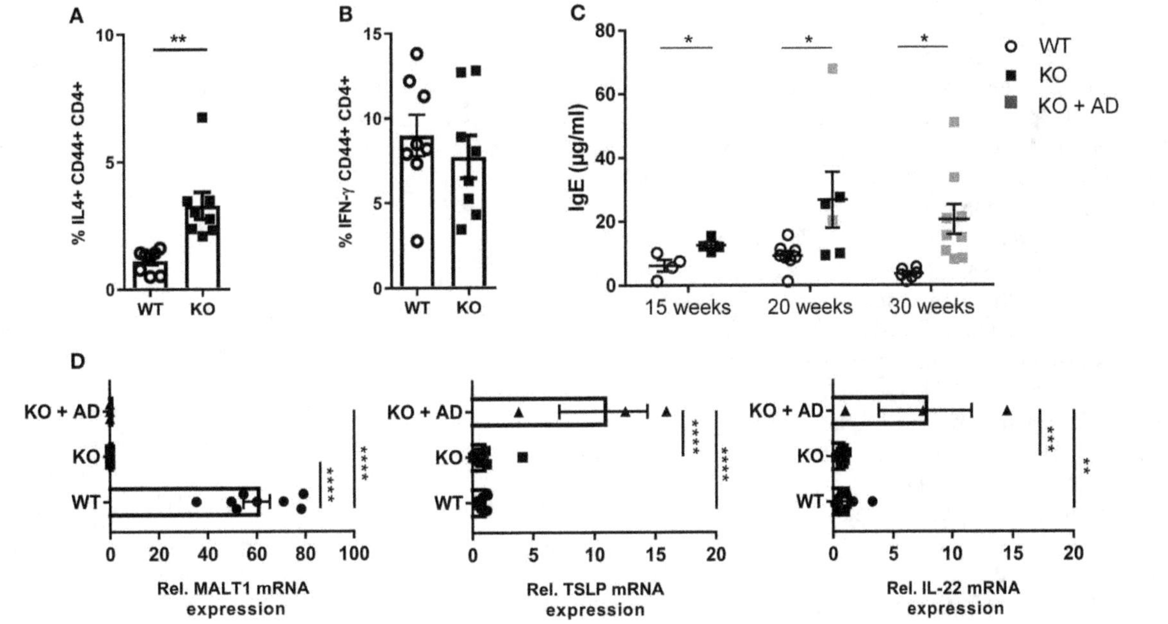

FIGURE 5 | Th2 skewing and elevated IgE levels in *Malt1*-KO mice. **(A)** Splenocytes of 20 weeks old mice without skin lesions were stimulated for 4 h with PMA and IO (same for B), in order to determine the percentage of CD44$^+$CD4$^+$ T cells expressing IL-4 (WT and KO: $n = 8$). **(B)** Percentage of CD44$^+$ CD4$^+$ T cells expressing IFN-γ (WT and KO: $n = 8$). **(C)** IgE levels in serum collected from WT and *Malt1*-KO mice of ±15, ±20, and >30 weeks (15 weeks WT and KO: $n = 4$, at 20 weeks WT: $n = 8$ and KO: $n = 6$ and at 30 weeks WT: $n = 6$ and KO: $n = 9$). Open circles (WT), black squares (KO), and gray squares (KO + AD) represent individual mice. **(D)** mRNA expression levels of *Malt1*, *Tslp*, and *IL22* (relative to reference genes *Hprt1* and *Ubc*) in ears of *Malt1*-WT mice ($n = 7$), *Malt1*-KO mice ($n = 11$), and *Malt1*-KO + AD mice ($n = 3$) suffering from dermatitis. The mean ± SEM is indicated on the graphs. For **(A–C)** all results were obtained by flow cytometry the statistical significance between groups was calculated with an unpaired 2-tailed Student's *t*-test. For **(D)** the statistical significance between groups was calculated with a one-way ANOVA with a Tukey's multiple comparison test. $^{*}P < 0.05$, $^{**}P < 0.01$, $^{***}P < 0.001$, and $^{****}P < 0.0001$.

spontaneous inflammation in full *Malt1*-KO mice (1). Our present finding that *Malt1*-KO mice spontaneously develop skin inflammation upon aging, implicates a role for MALT1-independent antigen or cytokine receptor signaling leading to low or intermediate T cell activation. The reduced frequency of functional Tregs in combination with a lowered effector T cell activation causes a gradual and selective expansion of Th2 cells, culminating in allergic skin inflammation without autoimmunity or generalized inflammation.

Skin inflammation in atopic dermatitis is assumed to arise due to a misdirected immune response against harmless antigens on the one hand, and to skin barrier defects on the other hand

(73). We propose that scratching may cause local skin barrier defects, which in combination with the Treg deficiency and the Th2 skewing favors the specific development of skin lesions in *Malt1*-KO mice. This is further supported by a report showing that tape stripping in combination with Treg depletion results in skin thickening, increased IL-4 and IL-13 mRNA levels in the skin, and elevated serum IgE levels (74). Of note, whereas an increase in IL-4 was already detectable in *Malt*1-KO mice before the development of skin lesions, elevated levels of *Tslp* and *Il22* mRNA, which are known to promote expression of Th2 cytokines, such as IL-4, could only be detected in lesional ear skin. A possible explanation might be that increased *Tslp* and *Il22* levels only occur upon skin barrier disruption in skin lesions, which is in agreement with an observed increase in TSLP expression upon tape stripping (75, 76).

Persistent severe dermatitis (7/9) and increased serum IgE levels (4/8) have been described in patients with loss of function mutations in MALT1 (38, 40–43). Similarly, dermatitis has been reported in genome-wide association studies for *CARD11* (77) and is also one of the clinical features found in most patients with loss of function mutations in *CARD11* (78–80). Also mice that have hypomorphic mutations in *Card11* display dermatitis, reduced Tregs, and increased IgE and Th2 levels (81–83). The proposed mechanism for disease development is the tight relationship between Tregs and Th2 cell levels (72, 82). However, our T cell-specific *Malt1*-KO mice did not develop skin lesions, suggesting that absence of MALT1 in T cells only is not sufficient to drive skin inflammation in aging mice. CARD11 is a member of the CARD-CC protein family, which also contains CARD9, CARD10 (also known as CARMA3), and CARD14 (also known as CARMA2) (84), which can all form distinct CBM complexes in a cell-type specific manner. Recently, Peled at al. reported that two loss-of-function mutations in *CARD14* are associated with atopic dermatitis (85). CARD14 is mainly expressed in keratinocytes and activates MALT1 signaling in keratinocytes (86, 87), which led us hypothesize that MALT1 deficiency in keratinocytes was driving atopic-like dermatitis. However, we also did not observe any skin lesions in keratinocyte-specific *Malt1*-KO mice. Possibly, combined deficiency in T cells and keratinocytes is needed to induce the atopic skin phenotype in aged mice. Alternatively, we cannot exclude a role for other cell types as well.

In general, the here established relationship between impaired MALT1-dependent TCR signaling, partial Treg deficiency, and dysregulated accumulation of Th2 cells, may provide a mechanistic basis to explain the allergic responses in patients carrying *MALT1* and *CARD11* mutations, and invites future studies investigating associations between atopy and genetic variations in other components of the TCR-MALT1 signaling pathway.

MATERIALS AND METHODS

Mice

Malt1-KO mice (backcrossed for more than 10 generations into C57BL/6 background) were a kind gift from Dr. T. Mak (Toronto, Canada). Another *Malt1* allele from EUCOMM ($Malt1^{tm1a(EUCOMM)Hmgu/+}$) was derived from ES cells and subsequently back-crossed to germline-expressing *Flpe*-deleter mice (88) to generate a conditional *Malt1*-deficient allele ($Malt1^{FL/+}$). The ES cells were also backcrossed to a germline-expressing *Cre*-deleter mouse (89) to obtain an alternative full deficient allele with a LacZ reporter ($Malt1^{IRES-LacZ/+}$). To generate a T-cell specific knock-out, $Malt1^{FL/+}$ was further crossed to $CD4\text{-}Cre^{Tg/+}$ mice (90) and $K5\text{-}Cre^{Tg/+}$ (91) and offspring was inter-crossed to select for Flpe-deleter-negative T cell-specific ($Malt1^{FL/FL}CD4\text{-}Cre^{Tg/+}$) and skin-specific ($Malt1^{FL/FL}$ $K5\text{-}Cre^{Tg/+}$) MALT1-deficient mice. *CD4-Cre* is always kept heterozygote by selecting one parent $CD4\text{-}Cre^{Tg/+}$ and the other parent as *Cre*-negative. The specificity of *CD4-Cre* was confirmed via western blot (**Supplementary Figure 4**) using rabbit monoclonal anti-MALT1 (SC-28246, Santa Cruz) and anti-Cre (6905-3, Merck Millipore). The *K5-Cre* is always kept heterozygote by selecting a male $K5\text{-}Cre^{Tg/+}$ and a female as *Cre*-negative, to avoid female germline transmission (91). Mice were housed in individually ventilated cages in a specific pathogen-free (SPF) facility. Mice were supplied with water and food *ad libitum* and experiments were performed in compliance with the guidelines of the University of Ghent Ethics Committee for the use of laboratory animals (EC2011-024 and 2013-066). Mice were monitored regularly for signs of dermatitis, consisting of hair loss in the facial, ear and neck region, together with redness, skin thickening, and scratching.

Genotyping

For *Malt1*-KO-mice we used the primers MALT1-F (GTGCTC TTGTAA TTTTCTGTGCTC), MALT1 WT-R (GGGTACATC ATGGCCTGAACAGTTG), and MALT1 KO-R (GGGTGGGAT TAGATAAATGCCTGCTC), resulting in 172 bp (WT) and 272 bp (KO) PCR products. The genotypings were made using GoTaq Green Hot Start (Promega) master mix, with a typical PCR program: 5 min 94°C denaturation, 35–40 cycles [45 s 94°C|30 s 60°C|45 s 72°C] and 10 min 72°C final elongation.

For the $Malt1^{tm1a(EUCOMM)Hmgu/+}$ derived mice we monitored the *Malt1* Flox-allele or KO allele with the primers MALTcKO-F (GTTTCTCAGGTCTTTAGTTCATGTC), CoMLT-3-R (TAT ACTCTACATCTCCATGGT), MALTcKO-R (TTGTTTTGC AGATCTCTGCC), and MLT-LacZ-F (TCGCTACCATTACCA GTTGGT) resulting in 280 bp (WT), 400 bp (FL), 345 (KO), or 514 bp (KO-LacZ) PCR products. *Flp* was detected with the primers Flp-F (TTAGTTCAGCAGCACATGATG) and Flp-R (GGAGGATTTGATATTCACCTG), resulting in a 370 bp PCR fragment. K5-Cre was detected with the primers Cre-F (TGC CACGACCAAGTGACAGCAATG) and Cre-R (AGAGAC GGAAATCCATCGCTCG) producing a 374 bp PCR fragment. CD4-Cre was detected with primers CD4-Cre-R (TCAAGG CCAGACTAGGCTGCCTAT) and CD4-Cre-F2 (TCTCTGTGG CTGGCAGTTTCTCCA) producing a 300 bp PCR fragment. The genotypings were made using the GoTaq Green Hot Start (Promega) master mix, with a typical PCR program: 5 min 95°C denaturation, 35–40 cycles [30 s 95°C|30 s 55–60°C|60 s 72°C] and 10 min 72°C final elongation.

Histology and Immunohistochemistry

Skin, lung, liver, colon, small intestine, stomach, lacrimal gland, and salivary gland samples were fixed with 4% paraformaldehyde and imbedded in paraffin. Sections (5 µm) were stained with hematoxylin and eosin. Skin sections were also stained with anti-CD3 (clone CD3-12; Serotec). Images were acquired with a BX51 discussion microscope (Olympus) with PixeLink camera under 100× magnification.

RNA Extraction, cDNA Synthesis, and Quantitative Real-Time PCR

After sacrifice, ears were collected and incubated overnight in RNA later at 4°C before long term storage at −70°C. For RNA extraction, the ears were transferred to TRIzol reagent (Invitrogen) and homogenized using the Precellys 24 (Bertin technologies with CK26 beads). After phenol/chloroform phase separation, RNA was isolated using the Aurum total RNA mini kit (Bio-Rad). cDNA was synthesized using the SensiFAST™ cDNA synthesis kit (Bioline), according to manufacturer's instructions. Quantitative PCR was done with a LightCycler 480 (Roche) using sensiFAST™ SYBR No-ROX kit (Bioline) with a total of 10 ng cDNA and 300 nM of specific primers in a 10 µl reaction. Real-time reactions were done in triplicates. The following specific primers were used (5′-3′): *Hprt1* Fwd AGTGTTGGATACAGGCCA GAC and *Hprt* Rev CGTGATTCAAATCCCTGAAGT; *Ubc* Fwd AGGTCAAACAGGAAGACAGACGTA and *Ubc* Rev TCA CACCCAAGAACAAGCACA; *Malt1* Fwd GGACAAAGTCGC CCTTTTGAT and Rev TCCACAGCGTTACACATCTCA; *Il22* Fwd AGACAGGTTCCAGCCCTACAT and *Il22* Rev TCT TCTGGATGTTCTGGTCGT; *Tslp* Fwd TCTCAGGAGCCT CTTCATCCT and *Tslp* Rev CTCACAGTCCTCGATTTGCT. Analysis was done with qBase software (Biogazelle). Values were normalized to two reference genes, as determined by Genorm analysis.

Blood Glucose Levels

A drop of blood from the tail was applied to a test strip and the glucose level was measured with a Freestyle lite glucose meter (Abbot).

Flow Cytometry

Detection of Tregs

Single cell suspensions of thymus, spleen, and lymph nodes were surfaced stained with Aqua Live/dead fixable stain (Life Technologies) or Fixable Viability Dye eFluor 506 (eBioscience), anti-CD16/CD32 Fc block (clone 2.4G2; BD Biosciences), anti-CD3-V450 (clone 17A2; BD Biosciences) or anti-CD3 eFluor450 (clone 17A2; eBioscience), anti-CD4-FITC (clone GK1.5; BD Biosciences or eBioscience), anti-CD25-PercPcy5.5 (clone PC61; BD Biosciences) for 20 min. Next, cells were permeabilized for 30 min, followed by 30 min of intracellular staining for anti-Foxp3-PE (clone FJK-16s; eBioscience). For the intracellular staining, the Foxp3 buffer set (eBioscience) was used and all incubation steps were done on ice.

CTLA-4 Expression of Tregs and CD44$^+$CD4$^+$ Effector T Cells

Splenocytes cultured in complete medium (RPMI 1640 medium supplemented with 10% FCS, Sodium Pyruvate, L-glutamine, antibiotics, and 2-Mercaptoethanol) were stimulated with PMA (50 ng/ml) and ionomycin (IO) (1 µg/ml) for 4 h at 37°C. The cells were stained as mentioned above, but anti-CD44-APC-efluor780 (clone IM7; eBioscience) and anti-CTLA-4 PE-eFluor610 (clone UC10-4B9; eBioscience) were also included in the surface staining.

Analysis of Cytokines by Intracellular Cytokine Staining

Splenocytes were cultured in complete medium and stimulated with PMA (50 ng/ml), IO (500 ng/ml) and Brefeldin A (1 µg/ml) for 4–5 h at 37°C. Stimulated cells were washed, surface stained with anti-CD16/CD32, Aqua Live/dead fixable stain or Fixable Viability Dye eFluor 506, anti-CD3-v450 or anti-CD3 eFluor450, anti-CD4-FITC, APC-anti-CD44-APC eFluor780, for 20 min. Next, cells were fixed and permeabilized for 30 min. using the Foxp3 buffer set, followed by intracellular staining with anti-IL4-APC (clone 11B11; eBioscience) and anti-IFNγ-PE-Cy7 (clone XMG1.2; BD Pharmingen) for 30 min.

Proliferation of CD4$^+$ T Cells

CD4$^+$ T cells isolated with the MACS CD4$^+$ T cell isolation kit II were labeled with 2.5 µM CellTrace™ CFSE (Life Technologies) according to the manufacturer's protocol. The cells were cultured in complete medium for 72 h with 5 µg/ml plate bound anti-CD3 (145-2C11; BD Pharmingen) and 1 µg/ml soluble anti-CD28 (37.51; BD Pharmingen) and 50 IU/ml recombinant mIL-2 (PSF, VIB). Cells were surface stained with Aqua Live/dead fixable stain, anti-CD4-FITC and fixed as mentioned above.

All data were obtained with a LSRII flow cytometer (BD Biosciences) and FlowJo Software (Treestar, Inc, Ashland, Ore) was used for data analysis.

Analysis of IgE and Cytokines in Serum

Peripheral blood samples were collected for serum preparation. The level of IgE in serum was determined using the mouse IgE ELISA Ready-SET-Go kit (eBioscience) and the concentration of IgE was calculated using GraphPad Prism 6 (GraphPad Software, Inc). The levels of IL-2 (171-G5003M), IL-4 (171-G5005M), IL-6 (171-G5007M), IL-17 (171-G5013M), IFN-γ (171-G5017M), and TNF (171-G5023M) was determined by Bio-Plex (Biorad) according to the manufacturer's conditions.

Statistical Analysis

Statistical analysis (indicated in the figure legends) was performed with GraphPad Prism 7.

ETHICS STATEMENT

The animal study was reviewed and approved by University of Ghent Ethics Committee for the use of laboratory animals (EC2011-024 and 2013-066).

AUTHOR CONTRIBUTIONS

AD, DM, JS, and RB designed the experiments. AD performed all the experiments, except for **Figure 1C** (done by DM). EV and GB provided the technical assistance for **Figure 5D** and YD provided the technical assistance for **Figure 3B**. YD and MK assisted with the genotyping of mice. AD, JS, and RB contributed to the scientific discussion and wrote the manuscript.

Foundation Against Cancer; Ghent University Concerted Research Actions (GOA), the VIB Grand Challenges Program (VIB-GC01-C01). AD was supported by a pre-doctoral fellowship from the Agency for Innovation by Science and Technology (IWT). JS and DM were supported by a post-doctoral fellowship from the FWO.

ACKNOWLEDGMENTS

We would like to thank the VIB Flow Core and VIB Bioimaging Core for training, support, and access to the instrument park.

REFERENCES

1. Demeyer A, Staal J, Beyaert R. Targeting MALT1 proteolytic activity in immunity, inflammation and disease: good or bad? *Trends Mol Med.* (2016) 22:135–50. doi: 10.1016/j.molmed.2015.12.004
2. Ruland J, Duncan GS, Wakeham A, Mak TW. Differential requirement for Malt1 in T and B cell antigen receptor signaling. *Immunity.* (2003) 19:749–58. doi: 10.1016/S1074-7613(03)00293-0
3. Ruefli-Brasse AA, French DM, Dixit VM. Regulation of NF-kappaB-dependent lymphocyte activation and development by paracaspase. *Science* (2003) 302:1581–4. doi: 10.1126/science.1090769
4. Akagi T, Motegi M, Tamura A, Suzuki R, Hosokawa Y, Suzuki H, et al. A novel gene, MALT1 at 18q21, is involved in t(11;18)(q21;q21) found in low-grade B-cell lymphoma of mucosa-associated lymphoid tissue. *Oncogene.* (1999) 18:5785–94. doi: 10.1038/sj.onc.1203018
5. Dierlamm J, Baens M, Wlodarska I, Stefanova-Ouzounova M, Hernandez JM, Hossfeld DK, et al. The apoptosis inhibitor gene API2 and a novel 18q gene, MLT, are recurrently rearranged in the t(11;18)(q21;q21) associated with mucosa-associated lymphoid tissue lymphomas. *Blood.* (1999) 93:3601–9.
6. Morgan JA, Yin Y, Borowsky AD, Kuo F, Nourmand N, Koontz JI, et al. Breakpoints of the t(11;18)(q21;q21) in mucosa-associated lymphoid tissue (MALT) lymphoma lie within or near the previously undescribed gene MALT1 in chromosome 18. *Cancer Res.* (1999) 59:6205–13.
7. Streubel B, Lamprecht A, Dierlamm J, Cerroni L, Stolte M, Ott G, et al. T(14;18)(q32;q21) involving IGH and MALT1 is a frequent chromosomal aberration in MALT lymphoma. *Blood.* (2003) 101:2335–9. doi: 10.1182/blood-2002-09-2963
8. Lucas PC, Yonezumi M, Inohara N, McAllister-Lucas LM, Abazeed ME, Chen FF, et al. Bcl10 and MALT1, independent targets of chromosomal translocation in malt lymphoma, cooperate in a novel NF-kappa B signaling pathway. *J Biol Chem.* (2001) 276:19012–9. doi: 10.1074/jbc.M009984200
9. Ferch U, Kloo B, Gewies A, Pfander V, Duwel M, Peschel C, et al. Inhibition of MALT1 protease activity is selectively toxic for activated B cell-like diffuse large B cell lymphoma cells. *J Exp Med.* (2009) 206:2313–20. doi: 10.1084/jem.20091167102109c
10. Hailfinger S, Lenz G, Ngo V, Posvitz-Fejfar A, Rebeaud F, Guzzardi M, et al. Essential role of MALT1 protease activity in activated B cell-like diffuse large B-cell lymphoma. *Proc Natl Acad Sci USA.* (2009) 106:19946–51. doi: 10.1073/pnas.0907511106
11. Hu S, Du MQ, Park SM, Alcivar A, Qu L, Gupta S, et al. cIAP2 is a ubiquitin protein ligase for BCL10 and is dysregulated in mucosa-associated lymphoid tissue lymphomas. *J Clin Invest.* (2006) 116:174–81. doi: 10.1172/JCI25641
12. Fontan L, Yang C, Kabaleeswaran V, Volpon L, Osborne MJ, Beltran E, et al. MALT1 small molecule inhibitors specifically suppress ABC-DLBCL *in vitro* and *in vivo*. *Cancer Cell.* (2012) 22:812–24. doi: 10.1016/j.ccr.2012.11.003
13. Nagel D, Spranger S, Vincendeau M, Grau M, Raffegerst S, Kloo B, et al. Pharmacologic inhibition of MALT1 protease by phenothiazines as a therapeutic approach for the treatment of aggressive ABC-DLBCL. *Cancer Cell.* (2012) 22:825–37. doi: 10.1016/j.ccr.2012.11.002
14. Langel FD, Jain NA, Rossman JS, Kingeter LM, Kashyap AK, Schaefer BC. Multiple protein domains mediate interaction between Bcl10 and MALT1. *J Biol Chem.* (2008) 283:32419–31. doi: 10.1074/jbc.M800670200
15. Sommer K, Guo B, Pomerantz JL, Bandaranayake AD, Moreno-Garcia ME, Ovechkina YL, et al. Phosphorylation of the CARMA1 linker controls NF-kappaB activation. *Immunity.* (2005) 23:561–74. doi: 10.1016/j.immuni.2005.09.014
16. Matsumoto R, Wang D, Blonska M, Li H, Kobayashi M, Pappu B, et al. Phosphorylation of CARMA1 plays a critical role in T Cell receptor-mediated NF-kappaB activation. *Immunity.* (2005) 23:575–85. doi: 10.1016/j.immuni.2005.10.007
17. Li S, Yang X, Shao J, Shen Y. Structural insights into the assembly of CARMA1 and BCL10. *PLoS ONE.* (2012) 7:e42775. doi: 10.1371/journal.pone.0042775
18. Knies N, Alankus B, Weilemann A, Tzankov A, Brunner K, Ruff T, et al. Lymphomagenic CARD11/BCL10/MALT1 signaling drives malignant B-cell proliferation via cooperative NF-kappaB and JNK activation. *Proc Natl Acad Sci USA.* (2015) 112:E7230–8. doi: 10.1073/pnas.1507459112
19. Sun L, Deng L, Ea CK, Xia ZP, Chen ZJ. The TRAF6 ubiquitin ligase and TAK1 kinase mediate IKK activation by BCL10 and MALT1 in T lymphocytes. *Mol Cell.* (2004) 14:289–301. doi: 10.1016/S1097-2765(04)00236-9
20. Oeckinghaus A, Wegener E, Welteke V, Ferch U, Arslan SC, Ruland J, et al. Malt1 ubiquitination triggers NF-kappaB signaling upon T-cell activation. *EMBO J.* (2007) 26:4634–45. doi: 10.1038/sj.emboj.7601897
21. Wu CJ, Ashwell JD. NEMO recognition of ubiquitinated Bcl10 is required for T cell receptor-mediated NF-kappaB activation. *Proc Natl Acad Sci USA.* (2008) 105:3023–8. doi: 10.1073/pnas.0712313105
22. Ruland J, Duncan GS, Elia A, del Barco Barrantes I, Nguyen L, Plyte S, et al. Bcl10 is a positive regulator of antigen receptor-induced activation of NF-kappaB and neural tube closure. *Cell.* (2001) 104:33–42. doi: 10.1016/S0092-8674(01)00189-1
23. Egawa T, Albrecht B, Favier B, Sunshine MJ, Mirchandani K, O'Brien W, et al. Requirement for CARMA1 in antigen receptor-induced NF-kappa B activation and lymphocyte proliferation. *Curr Biol.* (2003) 13:1252–8. doi: 10.1016/S0960-9822(03)00491-3
24. Rebeaud F, Hailfinger S, Posevitz-Fejfar A, Tapernoux M, Moser R, Rueda D, et al. The proteolytic activity of the paracaspase MALT1 is key in T cell activation. *Nat Immunol.* (2008) 9:272–81. doi: 10.1038/ni1568
25. Coornaert B, Baens M, Heyninck K, Bekaert T, Haegman M, Staal J, et al. T cell antigen receptor stimulation induces MALT1 paracaspase-mediated cleavage of the NF-kappaB inhibitor A20. *Nat Immunol.* (2008) 9:263–71. doi: 10.1038/ni1561
26. Staal J, Driege Y, Bekaert T, Demeyer A, Muyllaert D, Van Damme P, et al. T-cell receptor-induced JNK activation requires proteolytic inactivation of CYLD by MALT1. *EMBO J.* (2011) 30:1742–52. doi: 10.1038/emboj.2011.85
27. Hailfinger S, Nogai H, Pelzer C, Jaworski M, Cabalzar K, Charton JE, et al.

Malt1-dependent RelB cleavage promotes canonical NF-kappaB activation in lymphocytes and lymphoma cell lines. *Proc Natl Acad Sci USA.* (2011) 108:14596–601. doi: 10.1073/pnas.1105020108
28. Jeltsch KM, Hu D, Brenner S, Zoller J, Heinz GA, Nagel D, et al. Cleavage of roquin and regnase-1 by the paracaspase MALT1 releases their cooperatively repressed targets to promote T(H)17 differentiation. *Nat Immunol.* (2014) 15:1079–89. doi: 10.1038/ni.3008
29. Uehata T, Iwasaki H, Vandenbon A, Matsushita K, Hernandez-Cuellar E, Kuniyoshi K, et al. Malt1-induced cleavage of regnase-1 in CD4(+) helper T cells regulates immune activation. *Cell.* (2013) 153:1036–49. doi: 10.1016/j.cell.2013.04.034
30. Klein T, Fung SY, Renner F, Blank MA, Dufour A, Kang S, et al. The paracaspase MALT1 cleaves HOIL1 reducing linear ubiquitination by LUBAC to dampen lymphocyte NF-kappaB signalling. *Nat Commun.* (2015) 6:8777. doi: 10.1038/ncomms9777
31. Elton L, Carpentier I, Staal J, Driege Y, Haegman M, Beyaert R. MALT1 cleaves the E3 ubiquitin ligase HOIL-1 in activated T cells, generating a dominant negative inhibitor of LUBAC-induced NF-kappaB signaling. *FEBS J.* (2016) 283:403–12. doi: 10.1111/febs.13597
32. Douanne T, Gavard J, Bidere N. The paracaspase MALT1 cleaves the LUBAC subunit HOIL1 during antigen receptor signaling. *J Cell Sci.* (2016) 129:1775–80. doi: 10.1242/jcs.185025
33. Baens M, Bonsignore L, Somers R, Vanderheydt C, Weeks SD, Gunnarsson J, et al. MALT1 auto-proteolysis is essential for NF-kappaB-dependent gene transcription in activated lymphocytes. *PLoS ONE.* (2014) 9:e103774. doi: 10.1371/journal.pone.0103774
34. Yamasoba D, Sato K, Ichinose T, Imamura T, Koepke L, Joas S, et al. N4BP1 restricts HIV-1 and its inactivation by MALT1 promotes viral reactivation. *Nat Microbiol.* (2019) 4:1532–44. doi: 10.1038/s41564-019-0460-3
35. Mc Guire C, Elton L, Wieghofer P, Staal J, Voet S, Demeyer A, et al. Pharmacological inhibition of MALT1 protease activity protects mice in a mouse model of multiple sclerosis. *J Neuroinflammation.* (2014) 11:124. doi: 10.1186/1742-2094-11-124
36. Rosenbaum M, Gewies A, Pechloff K, Heuser C, Engleitner T, Gehring T, et al. Bcl10-controlled Malt1 paracaspase activity is key for the immune suppressive function of regulatory T cells. *Nat Commun.* (2019) 10:2352. doi: 10.1038/s41467-019-10203-2
37. Di Pilato M, Kim EY, Cadilha BL, Prussmann JN, Nasrallah MN, Seruggia D, et al. Targeting the CBM complex causes Treg cells to prime tumours for immune checkpoint therapy. *Nature.* (2019) 570:112–6. doi: 10.1038/s41586-019-1215-2
38. McKinnon ML, Rozmus J, Fung SY, Hirschfeld AF, Del Bel KL, Thomas L, et al. Combined immunodeficiency associated with homozygous MALT1 mutations. *J Allergy Clin Immunol.* (2013) 133:1458–62, 1462.e1–7. doi: 10.1016/j.jaci.2013.10.045
39. Jabara HH, Ohsumi T, Chou J, Massaad MJ, Benson H, Megarbane A, et al. A homozygous mucosa-associated lymphoid tissue 1 (MALT1) mutation in a family with combined immunodeficiency. *J Allergy Clin Immunol.* (2013) 132:151–8. doi: 10.1016/j.jaci.2013.04.047
40. Punwani D, Wang H, Chan AY, Cowan MJ, Mallott J, Sunderam U, et al. Combined immunodeficiency due to MALT1 mutations, treated by hematopoietic cell transplantation. *J Clin Immunol.* (2015) 35:135–46. doi: 10.1007/s10875-014-0125-1
41. Charbit-Henrion F, Jeverica AK, Begue B, Markelj G, Parlato M, Avcin SL, et al. Deficiency in mucosa-associated lymphoid tissue lymphoma translocation 1: a novel cause of IPEX-like syndrome. *J Pediatr Gastroenterol Nutr.* (2017) 64:378–84. doi: 10.1097/MPG.0000000000001262
42. Wiegmann H, Reunert J, Metze D, Marquardt T, Engel T, Kunde V, et al. Refining the dermatological spectrum in primary immunodeficiency: MALT1 deficiency mimicking Netherton- and Omenn syndrome. *Br J Dermatol.* (2019). doi: 10.1111/bjd.18091. [Epub ahead of print].
43. Frizinsky S, Rechavi E, Barel O, Najeeb RH, Greenberger S, Lee YN, et al. Novel MALT1 mutation linked to immunodeficiency, immune dysregulation, and an abnormal T cell receptor repertoire. *J Clin Immunol.* (2019) 39:401–13. doi: 10.1007/s10875-019-00629-0
44. Jaworski M, Marsland BJ, Gehrig J, Held W, Favre S, Luther SA, et al. Malt1 protease inactivation efficiently dampens immune responses but causes spontaneous autoimmunity. *EMBO J.* (2014) 33:2765–81. doi: 10.15252/embj.201488987
45. Yu JW, Hoffman S, Beal AM, Dykon A, Ringenberg MA, Hughes AC, et al. MALT1 protease activity is required for innate and adaptive immune responses. *PLoS ONE.* (2015) 10:e0127083. doi: 10.1371/journal.pone.0127083
46. Bornancin F, Renner F, Touil R, Sic H, Kolb Y, Touil-Allaoui I, et al. Deficiency of MALT1 paracaspase activity results in unbalanced regulatory and effector T and B cell responses leading to multiorgan inflammation. *J Immunol.* (2015) 194:3723–34. doi: 10.4049/jimmunol.1402254
47. Gewies A, Gorka O, Bergmann H, Pechloff K, Petermann F, Jeltsch KM, et al. Uncoupling Malt1 threshold function from paracaspase activity results in destructive autoimmune inflammation. *Cell Rep.* (2014) 9:1292–305. doi: 10.1016/j.celrep.2014.10.044
48. Demeyer A, Skordos I, Driege Y, Kreike M, Hochepied T, Baens M, et al. MALT1 proteolytic activity suppresses autoimmunity in a T cell intrinsic manner. *Front Immunol.* (2019) 10:1898. doi: 10.3389/fimmu.2019.01898
49. Cheng L, Deng N, Yang N, Zhao X, Lin X. Malt1 protease is critical in maintaining function of regulatory T cells and may be a therapeutic target for antitumor immunity. *J Immunol.* (2019) 202:3008–19. doi: 10.4049/jimmunol.1801614
50. Mc Guire C, Wieghofer P, Elton L, Muylaert D, Prinz M, Beyaert R, et al. Paracaspase MALT1 deficiency protects mice from autoimmune-mediated demyelination. *J Immunol.* (2013) 190:2896–903. doi: 10.4049/jimmunol.1201351
51. Brüstle A, Brenner D, Knobbe-Thomsen CB, Cox M, Lang PA, Lang KS, et al. MALT1 is an intrinsic regulator of regulatory T cells. *Cell Death Differ.* (2017) 24:1214–23. doi: 10.1038/cdd.2015.104
52. Walker LS, Sansom DM. The emerging role of CTLA4 as a cell-extrinsic regulator of T cell responses. *Nat Rev Immunol.* (2011) 11:852–63. doi: 10.1038/nri3108
53. Walker LS, Sansom DM. Confusing signals: recent progress in CTLA-4 biology. *Trends Immunol.* (2015) 36:63–70. doi: 10.1016/j.it.2014.12.001
54. Wang CJ, Kenefeck R, Wardzinski L, Attridge K, Manzotti C, Schmidt EM, et al. Cutting edge: cell-extrinsic immune regulation by CTLA-4 expressed on conventional T cells. *J Immunol.* (2012) 189:1118–22. doi: 10.4049/jimmunol.1200972
55. Tai X, Van Laethem F, Pobezinsky L, Guinter T, Sharrow SO, Adams A, et al. Basis of CTLA-4 function in regulatory and conventional CD4(+) T cells. *Blood.* (2012) 119:5155–63. doi: 10.1182/blood-2011-11-388918
56. Corse E, Allison JP. Cutting edge: CTLA-4 on effector T cells inhibits in trans. *J Immunol.* (2012) 189:1123–7. doi: 10.4049/jimmunol.1200695
57. Geha RS, Jabara HH, Brodeur SR. The regulation of immunoglobulin E class-switch recombination. *Nat Rev Immunol.* (2003) 3:721–32. doi: 10.1038/nri1181
58. Lou H, Lu J, Choi EB, Oh MH, Jeong M, Barmettler S, et al. Expression of IL-22 in the skin causes Th2-biased immunity, epidermal barrier dysfunction, and pruritus via stimulating epithelial Th2 cytokines and the GRP pathway. *J Immunol.* (2017) 198:2543–55. doi: 10.4049/jimmunol.1600126
59. Cianferoni A, Spergel J. The importance of TSLP in allergic disease and its role as a potential therapeutic target. *Expert Rev Clin Immunol.* (2014) 10:1463–74. doi: 10.1586/1744666X.2014.967684
60. Van Beek M, Oravecz-Wilson KI, Delekta PC, Gu S, Li X, Jin X, et al. Bcl10 links saturated fat overnutrition with hepatocellular NF-kB activation and insulin resistance. *Cell Rep.* (2012) 1:444–52. doi: 10.1016/j.celrep.2012.04.006
61. Kingeter LM, Schaefer BC. Loss of protein kinase C theta, Bcl10, or Malt1 selectively impairs proliferation and NF-kappa B activation in the CD4+ T cell subset. *J Immunol.* (2008) 181:6244–54. doi: 10.4049/jimmunol.181.9.6244
62. Sehra S, Yao Y, Howell MD, Nguyen ET, Kansas GS, Leung DY, et al. IL-4 regulates skin homeostasis and the predisposition toward allergic skin inflammation. *J Immunol.* (2010) 184:3186–90. doi: 10.4049/jimmunol.0901860
63. d'Hennezel E, Bin Dhuban K, Torgerson T, Piccirillo CA. The immunogenetics of immune dysregulation, polyendocrinopathy, enteropathy, X linked (IPEX) syndrome. *J Med Genet.* (2012) 49:291–302. doi: 10.1136/jmedgenet-2012-100759
64. Ramsdell F, Ziegler SF. FOXP3 and scurfy: how it all began. *Nat Rev Immunol.* (2014) 14:343–9. doi: 10.1038/nri3650
65. Wildin RS, Smyk-Pearson S, Filipovich AH. Clinical and molecular features of the immunodysregulation, polyendocrinopathy, enteropathy, X linked (IPEX) syndrome. *J Med Genet.* (2002) 39:537–45. doi: 10.1136/jmg.39.8.537

66. Godfrey VL, Wilkinson JE, Russell LB. X-linked lymphoreticular disease in the scurfy (sf) mutant mouse. *Am J Pathol.* (1991) 138:1379–87.
67. Ju ST, Sharma R, Gaskin F, Kung JT, Fu SM. The biology of autoimmune response in the scurfy mice that lack the CD4+Foxp3+ regulatory T-cells. *Biology.* (2012) 1:18–42. doi: 10.3390/biology1010018
68. Lahl K, Mayer CT, Bopp T, Huehn J, Loddenkemper C, Eberl G, et al. Nonfunctional regulatory T cells and defective control of Th2 cytokine production in natural scurfy mutant mice. *J Immunol.* (2009) 183:5662–72. doi: 10.4049/jimmunol.0803762
69. Fontenot JD, Gavin MA, Rudensky AY. Foxp3 programs the development and function of CD4+CD25+ regulatory T cells. *Nat Immunol.* (2003) 4:330–6. doi: 10.1038/ni904
70. Bacchetta R, Barzaghi F, Roncarolo MG. From IPEX syndrome to FOXP3 mutation: a lesson on immune dysregulation. *Ann N Y Acad Sci.* (2016) 1417:5–22. doi: 10.1111/nyas.13011
71. Brunkow ME, Jeffery EW, Hjerrild KA, Paeper B, Clark LB, Yasayko SA, et al. Disruption of a new forkhead/winged-helix protein, scurfin, results in the fatal lymphoproliferative disorder of the scurfy mouse. *Nat Genet.* (2001) 27:68–73. doi: 10.1038/83784
72. Tian L, Altin JA, Makaroff LE, Franckaert D, Cook MC, Goodnow CC, et al. Foxp3(+) regulatory T cells exert asymmetric control over murine helper responses by inducing Th2 cell apoptosis. *Blood.* (2011) 118:1845–53. doi: 10.1182/blood-2011-04-346056
73. Roesner LM, Werfel T, Heratizadeh A. The adaptive immune system in atopic dermatitis and implications on therapy. *Expert Rev Clin Immunol.* (2016) 12:787–96. doi: 10.1586/1744666X.2016.1165093
74. Fyhrquist N, Lehtimaki S, Lahl K, Savinko T, Lappetelainen AM, Sparwasser T, et al. Foxp3+ cells control Th2 responses in a murine model of atopic dermatitis. *J Invest Dermatol.* (2012) 132:1672–80. doi: 10.1038/jid.2012.40
75. Oyoshi MK, Larson RP, Ziegler SF, Geha RS. Mechanical injury polarizes skin dendritic cells to elicit a T(H)2 response by inducing cutaneous thymic stromal lymphopoietin expression. *J Allergy Clin Immunol.* (2010) 126:976–84, 84.e1–5. doi: 10.1016/j.jaci.2010.08.041
76. Leyva-Castillo JM, Hener P, Jiang H, Li M. TSLP produced by keratinocytes promotes allergen sensitization through skin and thereby triggers atopic march in mice. *J Invest Dermatol.* (2013) 133:154–63. doi: 10.1038/jid.2012.239
77. Hirota T, Takahashi A, Kubo M, Tsunoda T, Tomita K, Sakashita M, et al. Genome-wide association study identifies eight new susceptibility loci for atopic dermatitis in the Japanese population. *Nat Genet.* (2012) 44:1222–6. doi: 10.1038/ng.2438
78. Ma CA, Stinson JR, Zhang Y, Abbott JK, Weinreich MA, Hauk PJ, et al. Germline hypomorphic CARD11 mutations in severe atopic disease. *Nat Genet.* (2017) 49:1192–201. doi: 10.1038/ng.3898
79. Dadi H, Jones TA, Merico D, Sharfe N, Ovadia A, Schejter Y, et al. Combined immunodeficiency and atopy caused by a dominant negative mutation in caspase activation and recruitment domain family member 11 (CARD11). *J Allergy Clin Immunol.* (2017) 141:1818–30.e2. doi: 10.1016/j.jaci.2017.06.047
80. Dorjbal B, Stinson JR, Ma CA, Weinreich MA, Miraghazadeh B, Hartberger JM, et al. Hypomorphic caspase activation and recruitment domain 11 (CARD11) mutations associated with diverse immunologic phenotypes with or without atopic disease. *Jo Allergy Clin Immunol.* (2019) 143:1482–95. doi: 10.1016/j.jaci.2018.08.013
81. Barnes MJ, Krebs P, Harris N, Eidenschenk C, Gonzalez-Quintial R, Arnold CN, et al. Commitment to the regulatory T cell lineage requires CARMA1 in the thymus but not in the periphery. *PLoS Biol.* (2009) 7:e51. doi: 10.1371/journal.pbio.1000051
82. Altin JA, Tian L, Liston A, Bertram EM, Goodnow CC, Cook MC. Decreased T-cell receptor signaling through CARD11 differentially compromises forkhead box protein 3-positive regulatory versus T(H)2 effector cells to cause allergy. *J Allergy Clin Immunol.* (2011) 127:1277–85.e5. doi: 10.1016/j.jaci.2010.12.1081
83. Policheni A, Horikawa K, Milla L, Kofler J, Bouillet P, Belz GT, et al. CARD11 is dispensable for homeostatic responses and suppressive activity of peripherally-induced FOXP3+ regulatory T cells. *Immunol Cell Biol.* (2019) 97:740–52. doi: 10.1111/imcb.12268
84. Staal J, Driege Y, Haegman M, Borghi A, Hulpiau P, Lievens L, et al. Ancient origin of the CARD-coiled coil/Bcl10/MALT1-like paracaspase signaling complex indicates unknown critical functions. *Front Immunol.* (2018) 9:1136. doi: 10.3389/fimmu.2018.01136
85. Peled A, Sarig O, Sun G, Samuelov L, Ma CA, Zhang Y, et al. Loss-of-function mutations in caspase recruitment domain-containing protein 14 (CARD14) are associated with a severe variant of atopic dermatitis. *J Allergy Clin Immunol.* (2019) 143:173–81.e10. doi: 10.1016/j.jaci.2018.09.002
86. Afonina IS, Van Nuffel E, Baudelet G, Driege Y, Kreike M, Staal J, et al. The paracaspase MALT1 mediates CARD14-induced signaling in keratinocytes. *EMBO Rep.* (2016) 17:914–27. doi: 10.15252/embr.201642109
87. Van Nuffel E, Schmitt A, Afonina IS, Schulze-Osthoff K, Beyaert R, Hailfinger S. CARD14-mediated activation of paracaspase MALT1 in keratinocytes: implications for psoriasis. *J Invest Dermatol.* (2017) 137:569–75. doi: 10.1016/j.jid.2016.09.031
88. Rodriguez CI, Buchholz F, Galloway J, Sequerra R, Kasper J, Ayala R, et al. High-efficiency deleter mice show that FLPe is an alternative to Cre-loxP. *Nat Genet.* (2000) 25:139–40. doi: 10.1038/75973
89. Betz UA, Vosshenrich CA, Rajewsky K, Muller W. Bypass of lethality with mosaic mice generated by Cre-loxP-mediated recombination. *Curr Biol.* (1996) 6:1307–16. doi: 10.1016/S0960-9822(02)70717-3
90. Wolfer A, Bakker T, Wilson A, Nicolas M, Ioannidis V, Littman DR, et al. Inactivation of Notch 1 in immature thymocytes does not perturb CD4 or CD8T cell development. *Nat Immunol.* (2001) 2:235–41. doi: 10.1038/85294
91. Ramirez A, Page A, Gandarillas A, Zanet J, Pibre S, Vidal M, et al. A keratin K5Cre transgenic line appropriate for tissue-specific or generalized Cre-mediated recombination. *Genesis.* (2004) 39:52–7. doi: 10.1002/gene.20025

17

In silico Analyses of Skin and Peripheral Blood Transcriptional Data in Cutaneous Lupus Reveals CCR2-A Novel Potential Therapeutic Target

Rama Dey-Rao and Animesh A. Sinha**

Department of Dermatology, Jacobs School of Medicine and Biomedical Sciences, University at Buffalo, Buffalo, NY, United States

***Correspondence:**
Rama Dey-Rao
dey@buffalo.edu
Animesh A. Sinha
aasinha@buffalo.edu

Cutaneous lesions feature prominently in lupus erythematosus (LE). Yet lupus and its cutaneous manifestations exhibit extraordinary clinical heterogeneity, making it imperative to stratify patients with varying organ involvement based on molecular criteria that may be of clinical value. We conducted several *in silico* bioinformatics-based analyses integrating chronic cutaneous lupus erythematosus (CCLE)-skin and blood expression profiles to provide novel insights into disease mechanisms and potential future therapy. In addition to substantiating well-known prominent apoptosis and interferon related response in both tissue environments, the overrepresentation of GO categories in the datasets, in the context of existing literature, led us to model a "disease road-map" demonstrating a coordinated orchestration of the autoimmune response in CCLE reflected in three phases: (1) initiation, (2) amplification, and (3) target damage in skin. Within this framework, we undertook *in silico* interactome analyses to identify significantly "over-connected" genes that are potential key functional players in the metabolic reprogramming associated with skin pathology in CCLE. Furthermore, overlapping and distinct transcriptional "hot spots" within CCLE skin and blood expression profiles mapping to specified chromosomal locations offer selected targets for identifying disease-risk genes. Lastly, we used a novel *in silico* approach to prioritize the receptor protein CCR2, whose expression level in CCLE tissues was validated by qPCR analysis, and suggest it as a drug target for use in future potential CCLE therapy.

Keywords: CCLE, cutaneous lupus, skin, autoimmune, therapeutic, bioinformatics, expression profiles

INTRODUCTION

Lupus erythematosus (LE) is a complex (1) autoimmune disease that spans a tremendous variety of forms, degrees, and phenotype expressions ranging from relatively well-defined cutaneous manifestations to a rapidly progressive, lethal, multi-organ involvement in the systemic disease (SLE) (2, 3). Cutaneous features represent a major and medically significant component of LE and are evidenced as a wide range of clinical manifestations, some of which are disfiguring and debilitating. CCLE, which encompasses discoid lupus erythematosus (DLE), represents the most common category of cutaneous lupus erythematosus (CLE). While it is clear that CLE pathogenesis is multifactorial, with distinct roles for genetic, environmental, immunologic as well as epigenetic factors, large gaps in knowledge remain regarding the exact causes, mechanisms and biological interactions leading to the development of autoimmune attack on the skin. A number of trigger factors have been reported to influence the course and prognosis of cutaneous lupus including, UV light, medication, and smoking. Additional factors such as race, sex, age of onset and genetic predisposition, among others also impact disease manifestation (4–9). Although susceptibility to CCLE has been linked to genes within the HLA (HLA-DQ and/or DR), as well as outside the HLA region (*HSP70-1, TNF-α/β, C4* null, *C2, IL-1,* and *IL10*) (10–19) the molecular and genetic basis of disease initiation, progression, and response to treatment is poorly understood.

In large part due to the gap in knowledge regarding disease susceptibility and pathomechanisms, the current therapeutic armamentum in cutaneous LE does not include any approved systemic drugs (20) and needs to be empirically determined for individual patients. Thus, an enhanced understanding of the molecular and genetic basis of disease is a requisite to advance the search for novel therapeutic targets, particularly those that are more targeted and even personalized.

In the present study, gene enrichment analyses of the CCLE skin and blood transcriptional datasets were conducted to illuminate shared, over-represented, disease-related pathways and processes across both tissue environments. Our findings corroborate the involvement of a generalized immune dysregulation and altered apoptosis as central drivers of the cutaneous lupus phenotypes (21, 22). Through our integrative analytical approach we propose a detailed "disease road-map" tethered upon functional enrichments that illuminate a potential orchestration from initiation, amplification to tissue targeting in skin as linked steps in the autoimmune response of CCLE. This framework allowed us to assign existing and emerging therapies within the "disease road-map" based on mechanism of action of specific medications. *In silico* based interactome analysis identified 3 "over-connected" genes as potential key functional players in the metabolic reprogramming associated with skin pathology in CCLE. Subsequently, drug target analyses allowed us to narrow the search and prioritize *CCR2* as the druggable target receptor that needs further research to test viability in potential future disease therapy.

MATERIALS AND METHODS

Recruitment of CCLE/CLE (more specifically the most common subtype, discoid LE DLE), age- and sex-matched patients, and healthy control individuals, tissue procurement and handling has been described in detail along with IRB approval number, consent, demographic data and raw data in our earlier reports (21–24). None of the patients were positive for ANA or met any criteria for SLE. No systemic or topical medications had been used by any of the patients for 2 months prior to sampling. The procedures for blood and tissue handling, peripheral blood mononuclear cell extractions, total RNA preparation, cDNA synthesis and microarray processing have also been described previously (21, 22, 25, 26). The transcriptional data analyzed was from skin of 6 lesional and 4 non-lesional biopsies from patients with CCLE and blood from 3 CCLE patients and 3 healthy controls. There was an overlap of 2 patients (1008 and 1009) between blood and skin analysis. The range of sample size reflects the limited human samples that were available for the rare autoimmune disorder CCLE/DLE.

Differentially Expressed Genes (DEGs)

For the present study, we re-analyzed the CCLE-blood expression dataset to define a new DEGs list based on statistical criteria identical to our previously published CCLE-skin (21) thus allowing a more direct comparison. Briefly, we controlled the *p*-value at ≤ 0.05 and fold change (FC) $\geq \pm 1.1$ and identified 783 non-redundant CCLE- peripheral blood DEGs (337 UP and 446 DOWN), that distinguished patients from healthy controls. The low FC cut off was chosen for this study because: (1) minimal expression differences may be biologically significant (27) and (2) it allowed us to start with a larger pool of significant genes from both transcriptional profiles with which to perform downstream statistical analyses with high stringencies, in order to streamline our search to only "over-connected" DEGs.

Bioinformatics tools in DAVID (28), (https://david.ncifcrf.gov/) and MetaCore^{TM} v6.21 (Thomson Reuters, St Joseph, MI) were used (http://www.genego.com) to analyze and compare the two gene expression profiles (29). Unique gene symbols from the DEGs lists were mapped to "network objects" and used to probe the MetaCore database (metabase) (30). Using the disease terms "lupus" or "cutaneous lupus" we were able to generate and analyze several disease-associated canonical pathway maps followed by similar investigations in the Gene Ontology (GO) and KEGG databases. This allowed us to dissect each known overlapping disease-related biological pathway/process between the two tissue environments.

We compiled lists of interferon (IFN) inducible genes and those linked to apoptosis related pathways as described earlier (22). We also consolidated one hundred and five *potential* SLE susceptibility loci from genome-wide association studies (GWAS) recorded (31–44) in the National Human Genome Research Institute (NHGRI-EBI) catalog (http://www.ebi.ac.uk/gwas/search?query=lupus) and the SLEGEN study as well as susceptibility loci for CLE in a recent GWAS study (16) for comparison.

The DEG lists were analyzed for their chromosomal enrichment by leveraging the gene expression data to detect regions of the chromosomes with a statistically significant proportion of DEGs (called transcriptional "hot spots") (45–49). We used DNA-Chip Analyzer (dCHIP) (www.dchip.org) for the purpose of gene mapping using the "genome" tool with masked duplicate probe sets. *P-value* ≤ 0.001 was calculated for all stretches of chromosomes ("hot spots") that contained ≥ 5 DEGs (CCLE-blood DEGs used for this analysis) (50). We overlaid a similar map generated from our previous site-matched lesional

Abbreviations: C/C/LE, chronic/cutaneous/lupus erythematosus; SLE, systemic lupus erythematosus; DLE, Discoid lupus erythematosus; HLA, human leukocyte antigen; DEGs, differentially expressed genes; DAVID, Database for Annotation, Visualization and Integrated Discovery; MHC, major histocompatibility complex; DC, dendritic cells; IFN, interferon; CTL, cytotoxic T-lymphocytes; IC, immune complex, GO, gene ontology; FC, fold change, NF-kB, nuclear factor kappa-light-chain-enhancer of activated B cells; qPCR/RT-qPCR, quantitative polymerase chain reaction/ real-time quantitative polymerase chain reaction.

vs. non-lesional skin analysis (from CCLE patients) (21) on the CCLE -blood chromosomal map. We explored the overlapping and unique genes that were significantly associated or not with systemic or cutaneous disease in previous gene expression and GWAS studies.

Quantifying Gene Expression Using RT-qPCR

Total RNA was isolated as described previously (22, 26) using TRIzol reagent (Invitrogen, San Diego, CA, USA) per manufacturer's protocol and treated with DNase, purified and quantified by Nanodrop ND-1000. We used reverse transcription quantitative real-time PCR (RT-qPCR) to quantify gene expression from peripheral blood of an entirely different set of 5 CCLE patients (LE 1013, 1014, 1016, 1017, and 1018) and 5 healthy controls (CR, 221, 220, 231, 1042, and 1032). cDNA was synthesized from 400 ng total RNA using Promega Kit (Promega Corp., Madison, WI, USA) and quantitative real-time PCR was subsequently carried out using the FastStart Universal SYBR Green Master (ROX) from Roche (Roche Diagnostics,Mannheim, Germany) according to carefully standardized protocols. Intron-spanning primers were designed using Primer3 v. 4.0.0 (http://bioinfo.ut.ee/primer3/) for the following selected DEGs: *CCR2, IFI30, OAS1, OAS2, STAT1 TNFAIP3, ERBB3,* and *FGFR2,* based on published human gene sequences in the Ensemble Genome Browser (http://useast.ensembl.org/index.html). Primers were checked with a BLAT search (http://genome.ucsc.edu/cgi-bin/hgBlat). Amplicons were designed to be <150 bp in most cases (**Table 1**). Duplicate experiments were run for the 5 biological replicates in each of the patient and control group. The resulting qPCR cycle times (C_t) were normalized against the β-actin (*ACTB*) housekeeping gene to obtain ΔC_t. Fold changes in expression were calculated using the $2^{-\Delta\Delta Ct}$ method (51) relative to one control sample taken as unity (**Figure 6**). The fold changes in gene expression obtained by qPCR were compared to those observed by microarray analysis.

Interactome and Drug Target Analysis

We started out with the broadest pool of statistically significant genes, and subsequently employ downstream bioinformatics-based statistical tools with high stringency to assign disease relevance. To go beyond simply cataloging disease-related molecules we subjected our DEGs from CCLE skin and blood to an interactome analysis by protein function" (52). The relative connectivity of a gene (encoded protein) mirrors its functional significance to the disease under investigation (53) and is calculated by the number of interactions between the experimental gene with the genes on the experimental list normalized to the number of interactions it has with all genes in the human database (in MetaCore). The ranking of importance is related to the "knowledge based" analysis that takes into consideration experimental DEGs in the context of their known interactions in complex gene/protein and molecular networks. The localization of receptors in membranes that allows the extracellular domains to be targeted by specific ligands and drugs was key to narrowing the search to the "over-connected" 3 receptors that were shared between the skin and blood transcriptional profiles. Finally, we were able to prioritize one DEG *CCR2* based on several analytical criteria discussed above. Network generating algorithms in MetaCore were based on auto-expand by one interaction including both up- and downstream reactions. We further categorized the genes by their association with SLE-genes (either expressed or as susceptibility loci). A "drug target analysis" was performed via MetaCore along with a literature search on all three receptor proteins, to discover novel drug/target combinations that offer the best potential to be used in the treatment of CLE.

RESULTS

Differentially Expressed Genes (DEGs) and Ontology Enrichment Analysis

We generated a blood gene expression profile of 783 non-redundant DEGs (**Supplementary Table 1**) for comparison with the skin profile (776 DEGs) described previously (21). Both

A

Milieu	Total DEGs #	up	down
Skin	776	457	319
Blood	783	337	446

B

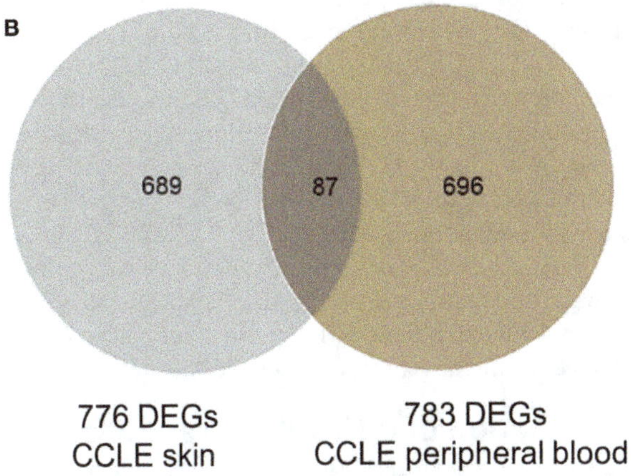

FIGURE 1 | Gene expression analysis in CCLE blood and lesional skin. **(A)** Differentially expressed genes (DEGs) were generated from blood (CCLE vs. healthy control) and skin (lesional vs. non-lesional) of CCLE patients and healthy controls that were able to distinguish between compared phenotypes via hierarchical clustering. **(B)** An overlap of 11% (87 DEGs) between the two lists is shown by the Venn diagram. The majority of genes in both lists are distinct to the respective environment (skin and blood) from which they are generated.

lists were generated using the same fold change and *p*-value cut off (**Figure 1A**). Of the 87 DEGs (**Figure 1B**) common between the blood and skin transcriptional profiles, 65 were dysregulated in the same direction in both tissues (upregulated = UP or down-regulated = DOWN) and 22 were in the opposite direction (**Supplementary Table 2**).

Pathways and Processes Based Enrichment Analyses

Ontology enrichment analysis was processed through two different analytical platforms (DAVID and MetaCore) to identify enriched disease-related biological functions, pathways and processes. We uncovered prominent apoptotic and type I interferon (IFN) signatures in both tissue environments. The overall number of DEGs in the activated immune response related pathways and processes are consistently higher in lesional skin than in peripheral blood. However, processes associated with lysome/proteasome related breakdown were more pronounced in peripheral blood than in skin. The differences and similarities in the two tissue environments forms the basis of our present analysis aimed at elucidating specific local and systemic disturbances linked to pathomechanisms related to CCLE (**Figure 2**).

Integration and synthesis of CCLE blood and skin transcriptional data in the context of existing literature regarding SLE/CCLE-related processes suggests a coordinated orchestration of the autoimmune response leading to organ-specific tissue damage in the skin that can be viewed in 3 phases: (1) initiation, (2) amplification of immune response, and (3) target damage in skin (**Figure 3**).

Identification of Risk Loci

We leveraged the blood transcriptional profile to locate genomic regions in which the 783 CCLE-DEGs cluster more frequently than would be expected by chance.(47, 49) 16 transcriptional "hot spots" were identified on chromosomes 1, 3, 5, 6, 11 (2), 12 (2), 14, 15, 16, 19, 20, 21, 22, and X, harboring 177 CCLE-blood DEGs. We had previously described 13 CCLE-skin specific "hot spots" on chromosomes (21). Seven transcriptionally active regions (chromosome 1, 3, 6, 11, 19, 22, and X) overlapped between skin and blood profiles (**Figure 4A**). Twelve dysregulated genes including *AIM2, ANP32E, CD48, EFNA1, CCR2, CAP2, PSMB8, FEN1, ECH1, LGALS2, TST,* and *APOBEC3G* were common to skin and blood within the overlapping "hot spots" (**Figure 4B**). See **Supplementary Table 3** for details on the 177 DEGs contained within the sixteen CCLE-blood "hot spots."

Identification of a Novel Therapeutic Target

Using our transcriptional datasets, CCLE-specific gene regulation was evaluated through enrichment by "protein function" revealing a significantly high number of ligands, proteases, receptors and other protein classes (**Supplementary Table 4**). Overall interaction topology reveals a high level of incoming and outgoing connections within the CCLE-experimental dataset as well as to and from the CCLE-datasets to the metabase (**Supplementary Table 5**).

We leveraged our expression dataset to search for key drivers of mechanisms underlying CCLE pathogenesis. We reveal 44 DEGs shared between blood and skin that are statistically "over-connected" to objects within the two CCLE datasets as well as the larger human database in MetaCore (**Supplementary Table 6**). Three (*CCR2, ERBB3,* and *FGFR2)* of the seven "over-connected" shared DEGs coding for receptor proteins (localized at the cell membrane) were selected for further investigations. All three were found to be interactive hubs by interactome and network analysis (**Figure 5**). A literature- and Metabase- search with the term "discoid lupus erythematosus" allowed an investigation into existing as well as emerging therapies in CLE/DLE. A drug analysis on all three receptors revealed CCR2 to be targeted by drugs that are currently in clinical trials for treatment of other related diseases. see **Supplementary Table 7** for a list of existing, emerging, and experimental as well as the newly proposed therapeutic agents, along with relevant literature and source documentation.

Validation Studies

We further evaluated the expression of 8 genes shown to be dysregulated by microarray analysis in CCLE/DLE by RT-qPCR (qPCR) (**Table 1** and **Figure 6**). Included among the 8 was *CCR2,* which we propose as a potential drug target in CCLE therapy. The qPCR experiments demonstrate a relative level of gene expression consistent with our microarray data for all eight DEGs. Genes such as *CCR2, IFI30, OAS1, OAS2,* and *STAT1* and *TNFAIP3* are over-expressed in CCLE/DLE patients as compared to healthy controls. While ERBB3 and FGFR2 exhibited overall low levels of expression, the trend in downward expression (case vs. controls) was also similar to our microarray analysis.

DISCUSSION

Development of a Disease "Roadmap"

Our new *in silico* analyses reveal a more enhanced composite of disease pathomechanisms operative in CCLE. In the proposed disease road-map schema (**Figure 3**), the three phases are not necessarily mutually exclusive, with specific components potentially operative in two, or all three phases across the spectrum. Below, we break down the three broad phases: (1) initiation, (2) amplification, (3) target damage, and dissect the linked disease relevant biological pathway/process (**Figure 2**) to discuss a model for pathobiology in the context of recognized systemic (blood) and local (skin) disturbances.

Initiation

Several well-known trigger factors e.g., UV light, medications, smoking are associated with cutaneous lupus (4, 9, 54–57), all of which could contribute to enhanced autoantigen display to the immune system. Theoretically, this could occur via increased keratinocyte apoptosis, autoantigen translocation to the keratinocyte cell surface, and/or a decreased clearance of apoptotic debris as in SLE (58), causing self-antigens (e.g., nucleosomes) to persist in the extracellular environment, enabling recognition by autoreactive cells (59–65). The skin has been speculated to be the site of autoimmune initiation for both cutaneous and systemic disease in genetically susceptible individuals (56, 57, 66).

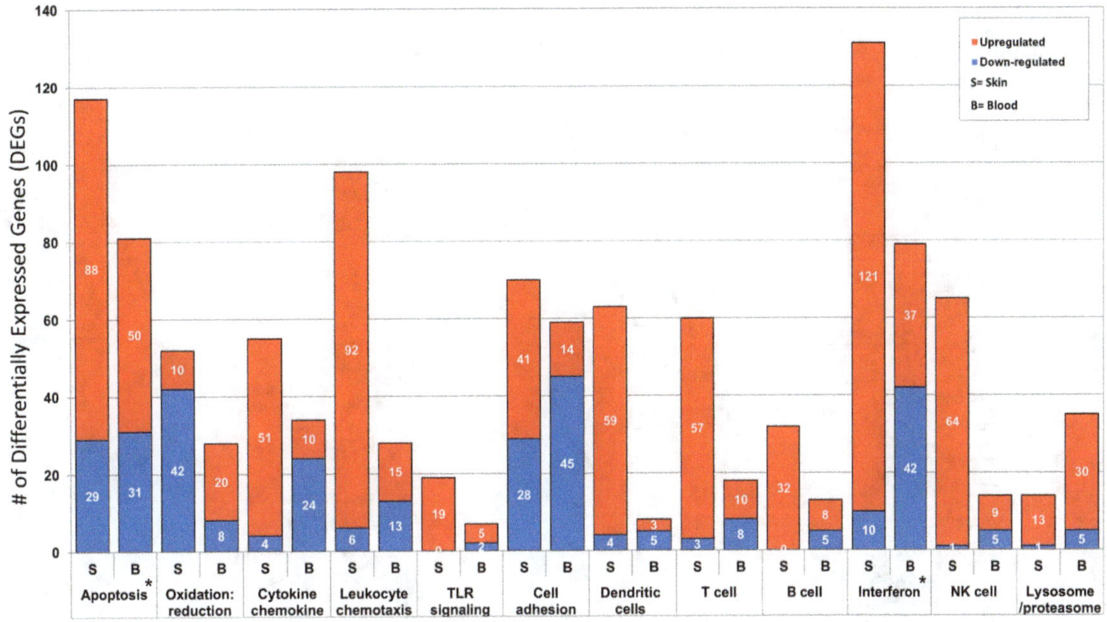

FIGURE 2 | Functional annotation and pathway analysis of the DEGs from CCLE-blood and lesional skin. The two transcriptional profiles reveal several enriched disease-related Gene Ontology (GO) biological processes. We break down the number of DEGs (up- and down-regulated) included in some of the shared disease related processes such as: apoptosis, oxidation: reduction, cytokine chemokine, leukocyte chemotaxis, TLR signaling, cell adhesion, dendritic cells, T cell, B cell, type I interferon, NK cells and lysosome/proteasome. The most prominent signatures for interferon and apoptosis in both profiles are marked with a star (*).

Apoptosis

The potential significance of apoptosis in CLE is underscored by several observations including an increase in the number of UV induced apoptotic keratinocytes found in lesional skin (54, 67). In our analysis, a larger number of dysregulated genes were associated with apoptosis in lesional skin (117 with 75% UP) as compared to peripheral blood (81 with 61% UP), emphasizing enhanced apoptosis (particularly in the skin) as a prominent signature of the disease. Both pro- and anti-apoptotic molecules are dysregulated simultaneously in both environments (21, 22), underscoring the complex and epistatic nature of the apoptotic cascade. It might also indicate redundancies of contributors to apoptosis, perhaps including involvement of diverse cell types (e.g., keratinocytes and lymphocytes) relevant to lupus pathology.

Oxidation: Reduction

Increased upregulation (71% of the 28 DEGs) in oxidative and nitrosative stress related processes in CCLE peripheral blood demonstrated in our dataset is similar to past observations in both SLE and CLE (68–71), underscoring the possibility of post-translational modification of auto-proteins/peptides, rendering them altered and able to provoke the autoimmune reaction.

Cytokines, Chemokine, and Leukocyte Chemotaxis

UV radiation is known to induce the production of numerous pro-inflammatory cytokines in the skin and contributes to the marked photosensitivity observed in CCLE (56, 72). These cytokines can promote translocation of intracellular autoantigens to the surface of epidermal keratinocytes (13, 73). We find higher numbers of upregulated DEGs (93%) associated with cytokine-chemokine related processes in lesional skin as opposed to blood (70% DOWN), perhaps reflecting an influx of cytokine producing cells at the local site of pathology. This may be particularly important as these mediators are short lived and local effects could be tissue specific and different from systemic effects (74).

Pattern Recognition Receptor (PRR) Signaling

We discovered 19 genes (100% UP) related to PRR to be activated in lesional skin, as opposed to 7 (71% UP) in peripheral blood. Upregulation of TLR-4 expression was previously demonstrated in affected tissue of CLE patients (75). PRRs participate in the recognition of both extrinsic and endogenous danger-associated conserved molecular patterns, and thus bridge innate and adaptive immune responses.

Amplification of Immune Response

CCLE is characterized by an increase in local mediators of inflammation in the skin. These effects in turn induce changes which include induction of adhesion molecules that are needed for the migration and sequestration of activated lymphocytes and leukocytes to the skin (76). Accumulating apoptotic debris may also bolster autoantigen presentation by Langerhans cells (LCs) to T cells (77). Binding of autoantibodies to keratinocytes could then further expose self-antigens and promote cytokine release to continue and amplify the autoimmune response. T cell reactivity may in turn promote B cell activation and production

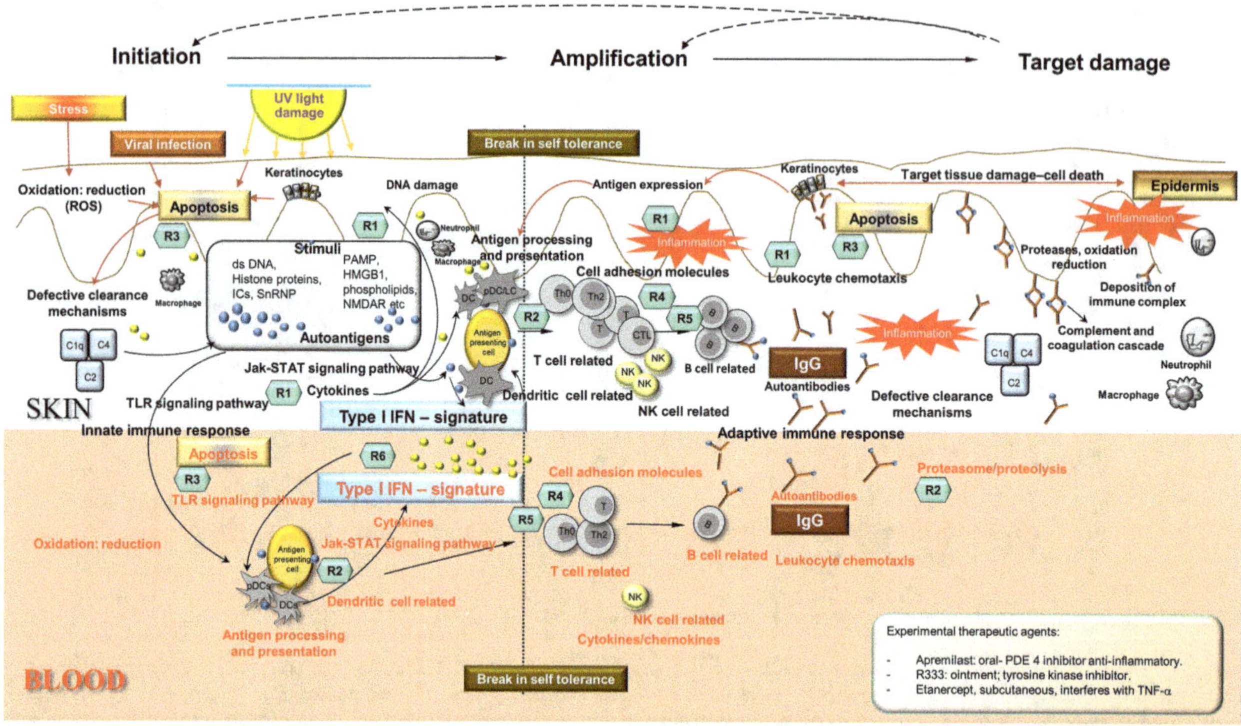

FIGURE 3 | Disease Road Map. Enriched disease-related pathways and processes found in skin and blood profiles underlie three distinct phases in the autoimmune response in CCLE: (i) initiation, (ii) amplification of the immune response, and (iii) target damage in the skin, that are not mutually exclusive. The shared disease-related processes over-represented in skin and blood are as follows: apoptosis, oxidation reduction, cell adhesion, cytokine chemokine activity, leukocyte chemotaxis, NK cell, TLR signaling, dendritic cells, T cell, B cell activation, Interferon signature, lysosome and proteasome, antigen processing and presentation, complement cascade among others (see also **Figure 2**). Potential molecular targets of some of the existing and emerging drugs R (*n*) have been identified in the schematic according to mechanism of action presently used for CLE/DLE treatment. Some experimental drugs have also been included (see inserted box). Drugs used in CLE/DLE treatment R(*n*) (teal hexagons): *Topical agents:* R1 = corticosteroids fluocinonide, R-salbutamol sulfate (anti-inflammatory, acting upon cytokines and leukocytes) *Systemic agents:* R1 = glucocorticoids, R2 = hydroxychloroquine (antimalarial) (acting upon MHC presentation and lysosome pH, anti-inflammatory), R3 = thalidomide, lenalidomide, CC 11050 (TNF-α inhibitors, apoptosis), R4 = methotrexate MTX (acts on T cell proliferation), R5 = pimecrolimus (calcineurin inhibitor, down-regulating T cell activity) TRX-1, AMG 557 (humanized mAbs act as T cell regulators), R6 = humanized mAbs AMG 811 (anti-IFNα) and sirukumab (acts on pro-inflammatory cytokines such as IL-6). Ds, double stranded; UV, ultraviolet; PAMP, pathogen-associated molecular pattern; HMGB1, high mobility group protein B1; ICs, nucleic acid containing immune complexes; NMDAR, N-methyl-D-aspartate receptor; C1q, complement component 1; q subcomponent; C2, complement component 2; C4, complement component 4; DC, dendritic cells; pDC, plasmacytoid DC; LC, Langerhans cells; T, T cells; B, B cells; Th, T helper cells; Th0, T helper cells 0; CTL, cytotoxic T lymphocytes; IgG, immunoglobulin G; NK, natural killer cells; IFN, interferon; TLR, toll-like receptor; PDE4, phosphodiesterase-4; TNF, tumor necrosis factor.

of autoantibodies specific to previously sequestered or altered molecules.

Cell Adhesion

Progression of lupus is facilitated by the local generation of adhesion molecules and expression of their ligands in inflammatory cells (78, 79). In the present study, we demonstrate nearly equal numbers of dysregulated genes linked to cell adhesion in both skin and blood, but observe 59% UP in lesional skin as compared to 76% DOWN in peripheral blood.

Dendritic Cells (DC)

Antigen presentation by *immature* DCs may lead to T cell anergy due to lack of co-stimulation, a mechanism by which certain (self) antigens may evade immune responsiveness (80, 81). We observe much higher numbers of activated genes associated with skin-dendritic cells (94% UP of 63 DEGs), as compared to only 8 DEGs (63% DOWN) in the peripheral blood, underscoring clear patho-mechanistic differences in the two environments.

HLA Region

CLE susceptibility (in patients positive for anti-Ro) is linked to the major histocompatibility complex (MHC) on chromosome 6, including genes for human leukocyte antigens (HLA), complement components, and tumor necrosis factor (TNF) (12, 21, 82–84). We found the top enriched KEGG pathway associated with the 87 DEGs overlapping between CCLE-skin and blood profiles to be antigen processing and presentation (**Supplementary Table 8**) skewed toward activation in both skin (92% UP) and blood (79% UP). Of the twelve DEGs mapping to chromosome 6, *CSNK2B*, and *CDKN1A* are reported as potential CLE-associated susceptibility locus (16) and associated with SLE (85), respectively (**Supplementary Table 3**). The precise influence of the HLA region on CCLE is not clear as of yet, but is

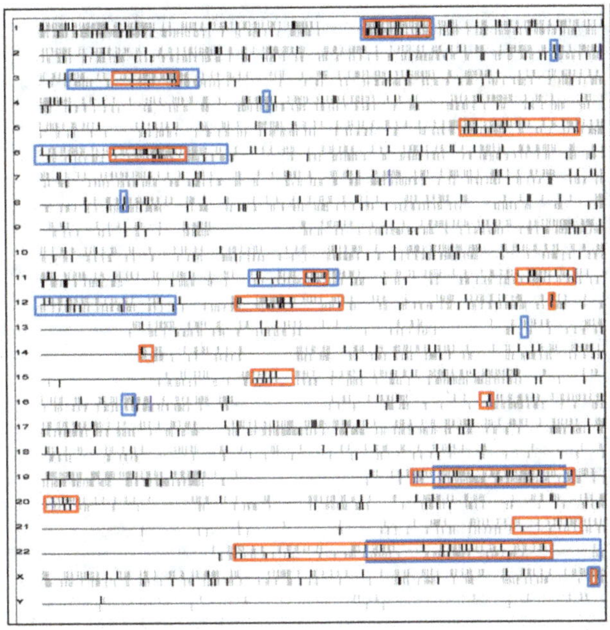

A

Chr	Skin	Blood	Common (skin and blood)	SLE/CLE Loci
1	1q21.2-1q24	1q21-1q25.1	*AIM2, ANP32E, CD48, EFNA1*	*AIM2, FCGR3A, FCGR2A*
2	2q37.1			
3	3p14.3-3p25	3p21.2-p22.3	*CCR2*	
4	4q21-4q21.2			
5		5q31.1-q35		*CD14*
6	6p12.1-6p25	6p21.1-p23	*CAP2, PSMB8*	*MICB, HLA-A. HLA-DOB, TNF, TNXB, CSNK2B, CDKINA,*
7				
8	8p21.3-8p21.2			
9				
10				
11	11p11.2-11q13.4	11q12-q13; 11q23.1-q24.3	*FEN1*	*FEN1*
12	12p11-12p13	12q12-q15; 12q24.31		*C1R, STAT2*
13	13q32-13q33			
14		14q11.2		
15		15q15.1-q21.1		
16	16p13.3	16q22.1-q22.3		
17				
18				
19	19q13-19q13.41	19q13-19q13.4	*ECH1*	
20		20p13		
21		21q22.2-q22.3		
22	22q12-22q13.3	22q11.21-q13.31	*LGALS2, TST, APOBEC3G*	*HMOX1*
X	Xq28	Xq28		
Y				

B

FIGURE 4 | Chromosomal locations of transcriptional "hot spots" found in CCLE-associated blood and lesional skin signatures. **(A)** CCLE blood gene expression data is leveraged to identify transcriptional "hot-spots" in chromosomes where DEGs map with statistically increased frequency. Each horizontal line corresponds to one chromosome. Chromosomal locations of CCLE blood molecular signature are colored in bold black vertical bars vs. the non-differentially expressed genes which are gray. The vertical bars above and below the horizontal lines represent genes either on the forward or reverse strand. Sixteen significant stretches at p-value ≤ 0.001 are considered to be transcriptionally active "hot spots" using the CCLE blood profile (red boxes). Thirteen "hot spots" associated with CCLE lesional skin signature (blue boxes) from our previous study, have been overlaid on the blood chromosomal map revealing seven regions of overlap (bold). **(B)** Twelve genes in the overlapping "hot spots" (including ***CCR2***) were shared between the skin and blood profiles. The seven overlapping "hot spots" also include 14 DEGs from skin (blue), blood (red) and both milieus (purple), which have been previously reported as potential disease loci in SLE. *TNF* is a skin-DEG that is previously described as a putative disease locus for both SLE as well as CLE. *CSNK2B* is a blood-DEG that has been described as a disease locus in CLE.

likely related to its well-defined role in antigen presentation and activation/selection of T cells in the pathogenesis of LE (86–91).

T Cell Response

Our analysis uncovered 60 DEGs (95% UP) in skin and 18 (56% UP) in blood (**Figure 2**) that are involved in T cell related processes such as -activation, -differentiation, -selection, -proliferation, -receptor signaling and -thymic selection, thus implicating a similarly activated T cell mediated autoimmune reaction in CCLE as well.

B Cells

Although B cell hyperactivity and the production of autoantibodies in LE appears to be T cell driven (92, 93), breaking of B cell tolerance without the support of T cells has been reported as well (94). Given that 55–75 % of B cell receptors on human immature B cells are self-reactive, maintenance of B cell tolerance is vital for thwarting the production of autoantibodies with potential disease causing specificities (95). We observed 32 DEGs (100% UP) in lesional skin and 13 (62% UP) in blood associated with B cell antigen receptor engagement.

Interferon

Cytokines play a crucial role in modulating the immune response to foreign and self-antigens, both in the initiation and amplification of the immune response in CCLE. A prominent IFN-α signature in dermal lesions of SLE patients, suggests that the skin acts as a reservoir for IFN producing cells with the ability to promote autoimmunity (96–98). This appears to be a central theme in cutaneous lupus as well (99). In this analysis, we demonstrate a stronger IFN signature in CCLE skin (that is predominantly upregulated) as compared to peripheral blood. This may indicate a potential shift in the engagement of this key cytokine pathway as a pathogenic mediator from the blood to the skin in CCLE patients. **Supplementary Figure 1** demonstrates one such over-represented and activated canonical pathway linked to IFN signaling, with more upregulated genes in the skin than from blood. A more comprehensive picture of the role of various IFN family members in disease pathogenesis will emerge as detailed demographics such as disease onset, age, organs involved, and therapy are taken into consideration.

Target Damage

The pathology in CLE is one of inflammatory lichenoid reaction in which basal keratinocytes that express surface self-antigens are the chief center of damage (100). Global gene expression data revealing dysregulated apoptosis, inflammation, complement system as well as lysosome and proteasome associated breakdown processes in skin and blood from CCLE patients serves to support the model for the creation, accumulation and presentation of

Protein Function	IDs in active data set	Object name	Actual	n	R	N	Expected	Ratio	z-score	* p-value
"Over-connected" Receptors	***CCR2***	**CCR2**	**14**	**1665**	**49**	**38444**	**2.12**	**6.60**	**8.34**	**1.3E-08**
	ERBB3	ErbB3	21	1665	129	38444	5.59	3.76	6.68	1.7E-07
	FGFR2	FGFR2	20	1665	127	38444	5.50	3.64	6.33	5.7E-07

A

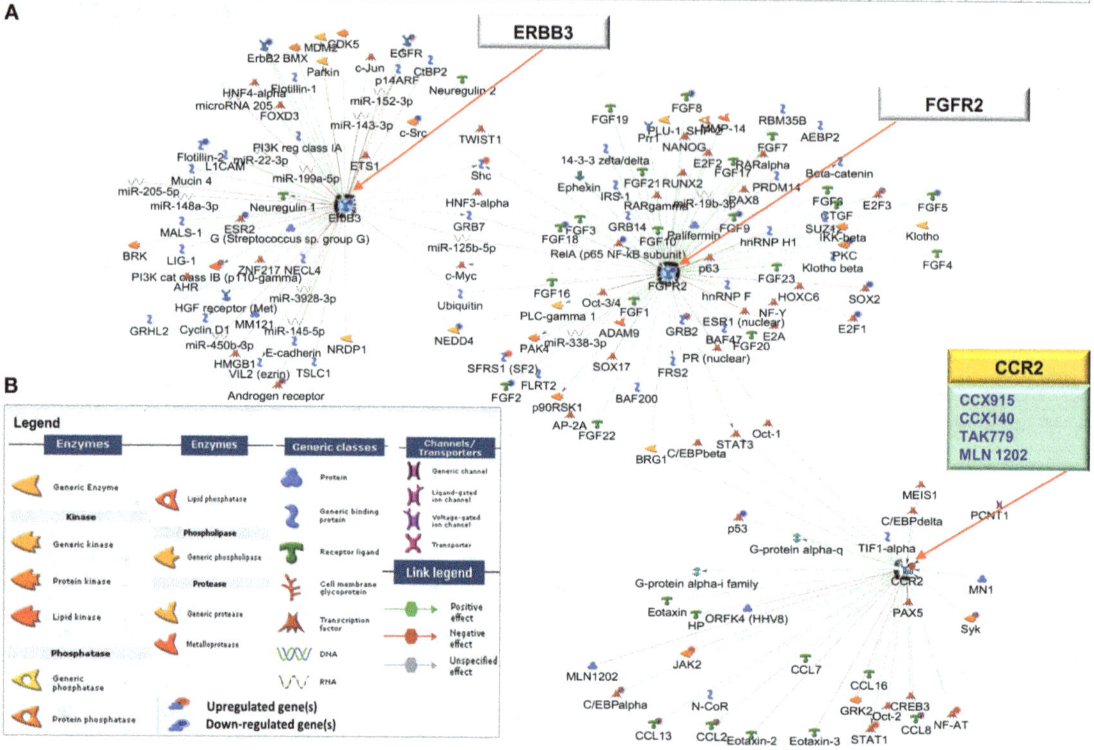

FIGURE 5 | Interactive receptor proteins CCR2, ERBB3 and FGFR2. **(A)** We focused on three receptor proteins (CCR2, ERBB3, and FGFR2) that were considered "over-connected" when the number of observed interactions (actual) was greater than the number of expected interactions accompanied by (significant) low *p*-values (*) and high z-scores **(B)** Algorithms in MetaCore are used to generate networks using the expand by single interaction in both upstream and downstream directions. Interactions within the network reveal all 3 receptors as central hubs connected to each other as well as with a large number of curated interactions with both positive (green) and negative effect (red) to and from (arrow direction) several objects in the CCLE-skin profile as well the larger human proteome database. The individual CCLE-DEGs and proteins in the metabase are representated as nodes of different shapes (see legend) with connections/interactions to one another. Drug target analysis revealed 4 drugs (teal box) that target one of the receptor proteins CCR2, (yellow). All 4 drugs are currently being used in the clinic to treat other closely related diseases (see **Supplementary Table 7**). Explanation of columns: Actual, number of network objects in the activated signatures which interact with the chosen object; *n*, number of network objects in experimental datasets; *R*, number of network objects in the activated background list which interact with the chosen object; *N*, total number of protein-based objects in the activated background list; Expected, mean of hypergeometric distribution; Ratio, connectivity ratio (Actual/Expected); z-score, (Actual-Expected)/(standard deviation); *p*-value: probability to have the value of Actual by chance under null hypothesis of no over-connectivity. Star (*) denotes significant *p*-values.

autoantigens to the immune system to be at the heart of the disease (101–103). Dysregulated apoptosis and clearance processes might be significant for both initiating the autoimmune response as well as for the ultimate damage to the skin, demonstrating how various phases of the disease might be mutually non-exclusive.

Apoptosis/NK Cells and Inflammation

The role of defects in the apoptotic pathway has been discussed previously in the context of disease initiation, but may be relevant for ultimate target damage as well. Multiple apoptotic pathways are involved in both CCLE skin and blood. We observed upregulated markers from both the extrinsic (death receptor related) and intrinsic pathway (stress related) in blood and skin. An understanding of the molecular events that regulate cell death at both the skin and systemic level is essential for clarification of pathogenesis in the disease.

In addition to UV induction of apoptosis, cellular cytotoxic mechanisms involving CTLs, and natural killer (NK) cells have also been implicated in CLE (4, 104–107). Our analysis finds several more NK cell associated genes (65 DEGs, mostly UP) in the CCLE lesional skin than in the blood profile (14 DEGs, mostly UP), with 7 DEGs shared between the two environments. Inflammatory response also included more activated genes in the skin (90% of 144 DEGs UP) than in the blood (78% of 14 DEGs UP).

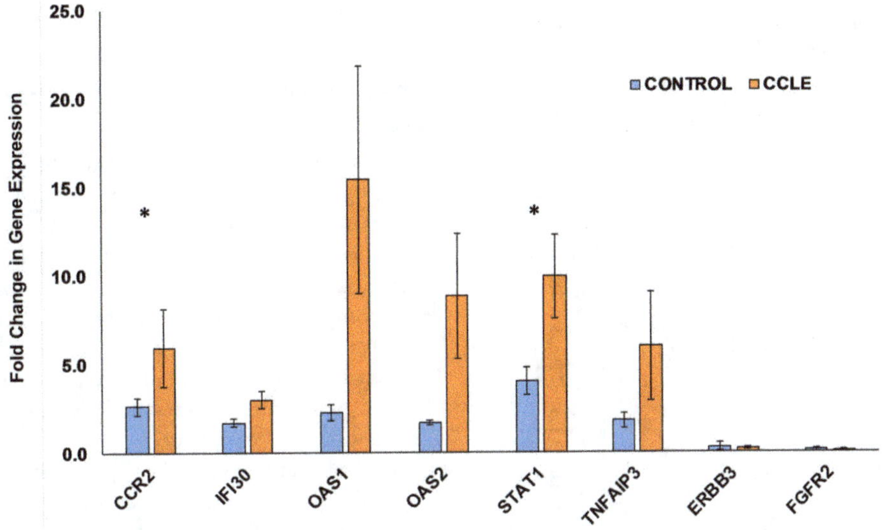

FIGURE 6 | Quantifying gene expression by RT-qPCR. Gene expression for the eight DEGs: *CCR2, IFI30, OAS1, OAS2, STAT1, TNFAIP3, ERBB3,* and *FGFR2,* within both the CCLE skin and blood signatures were quantified using RT-qPCR. Data is normalized to the housekeeping gene β-actin (*ACTB*). Fold change in gene expression in peripheral blood (presented as bar graphs with S.E.M) is calculated using the $2^{-\Delta\Delta Ct}$ method and represent duplicate runs of 5 biological replicates each of CCLE (DLE)-patients and healthy control individuals. Fold change in expression (between case and controls) of *CCR2* and *STAT1* trended toward significant (*p-value = 0.055 and 0.053, respectively). CCLE, chronic cutaneous lupus erythematosus/discoid lupus erythematosus; S.E.M., standard error of the mean.

Complement

The complement cascade is known to be involved in opsonization of apoptotic cells for efficient clearance by phagocytosis, in the absence of which apoptotic cells may remain longer in the system to stimulate autoantibody production (108). This aberration in the clearing mechanism could be associated with both initiation as well as the target damage stage of the autoimmune reaction. In the present study, we observe many more dysregulated genes related to the complement cascade in lesional skin (such as *C2, C1R, C1QB, C3AR1, C4A /// C4B, CD59, CFB, CFD, ERCC6 /// PGBD3,* and *ITGB2* among others; 89% UP) than in blood (*C4BPB, CFHR3, FANCC PLAU, IGHG1.* and *ITGB2;* 83% DOWN). Another effect of complement activation can be apoptosis through cellular events (109), and could be yet another explanation of the increased apoptosis observed in lesional skin over blood (described earlier).

Lysosome/Proteasome

Ubiquitin-mediated proteasomal proteolysis constitutes the intracellular protein-degradation apparatus involved in several cellular functions such as cell cycle, cell differentiation, immune and inflammatory response, stress signaling and apoptosis among others. Upregulated genes (*CTSB, CTSC, CTSH, CTSZ,* and *CTSL*) from the cathepsin related protease family, as well as 15 other members of the proteasome family (all involved in proteolysis), were skewed toward the blood than in skin. The evidence supporting enhanced activation of proteolytic markers in peripheral blood over skin of CCLE patients indicates effective processing of peptides in the systemic milieu to enable MHC I and II mediated autoantigen presentation in the disease, which could lead back to amplification of the immune response and serve as a feedback mechanism in the disease.

Overall, our investigations offer a global comprehensive viewpoint of CCLE-associated transcriptional changes that may be particularly relevant for understanding disease mechanisms and identification of biomarkers relevant to disease progression.

Genetics

We have reported a significant, but not complete overlap between our CCLE expression data and previously reported SLE transcriptional data, indicating that while these two conditions are related, they are also clearly distinct (110). Five of the twelve shared DEGs (described above) in the overlapping CCLE skin and blood "hot spot" regions (*AIM2, CD48, CCR2, FEN1,* and *LGALS2*) also overlap with previously reported SLE associated genes expression or GWAS studies. The remaining seven common DEGs in the two profiles (*ANP32E, EFNA1, CAP2, PSMB8, ECH1, TST,* and *APOBEC3G*) that do not overlap with SLE may thus represent CCLE specific genes. *CSNK2B* (casein kinase 2, beta polypeptide), in the CCLE-blood "hot spot" within the MHC region of chromosome 6, and *APOC1*, mapping to the "hot spot" on chromosome 19 in CCLE-skin have also previously been reported as potential gene markers of CLE (16, 111).

Although the pathogenetic relationship between DLE and SLE is still unclear, our comparative CCLE skin and blood analyses supports the existence of both overlapping as well as distinct genetic susceptibilities and mechanisms relevant to the development of systemic as well as cutaneous LE as discussed previously (4, 21, 22, 110, 112, 113). Furthermore, the DEGs mapping to the "hot spots" which do not overlap with SLE and/or

TABLE 1 | Quantifying gene expression.

#	Gene symbol	Forward primer sequence	Reverse primer sequence	Prod size	Microarray (fold change)				qPCR (fold change) (Blood)			
					Skin	*p*-value	Blood	*p*-value	Control	±S.E.M	CCLE/DLE	±S.E.M
1	*CCR2**	GAGGCATAGGGCAGTGAGAG	GCAATCCTACAGCCAAGAGC	269	1.8	0.031	1.6	0.006	2.64	0.49	5.98	2.19
2	*IFI30*	TGACCATTGTCTGCATGGAA	TCCATGATAGTGTCTGGCGA	100	3.9	0.0006	2	0.027	1.72	0.21	3.02	0.46
3	*OAS1*	CAACTCTGCATCTACTGGACAAAG	AAGTTTCCTGTAGGGTCCGC	125	2.6	0.0001	6	0.001	2.3	0.47	15.42	6.44
4	*OAS2*	TTGACAACCGTCCTGGAAAA	GTAAGCAGCTCCAGGGCATA	121	2.6	0.007	1.9	0.007	1.71	0.17	8.84	3.52
5	*STAT1**	TCAGAAGTGCTGAGTTGGCA	GTCCACGGAATGAGACCATC	125	4.2	0.002	2.2	0.043	4.05	0.78	9.94	2.34
6	*TNFAIP3*	TCAACTGGTGTCGAGAAGTCC	ACGCCCCACATGTACTGAGA	97	2.1	0.003	1.5	0.048	1.81	0.41	6	3.06
7	*ERBB3*	GAACATTCGCCCAACCTTTA	ACGTGGCCGATTAAGTGTTC	279	−2.3	0.003	−1.2	0.041	0.29	0.22	0.22	0.07
8	*FGFR2*	CAGAATGGATAAGCCAGCCA	GCTTGAACGTTGGTCTCTGG	95	−2	0.016	−1.3	0.049	0.12	0.12	0.1	0.03

Differential gene expression in peripheral blood measured by RT-qPCR. Intron-spanning primers were chosen for CCR2, IFI30, OAS1, OAS2, STAT1, TNFAIP3, ERBB3, and FGFR2, which are dysregulated genes within the CCLE skin and blood signatures. Q-PCR data is normalized to the housekeeping gene β-actin (ACTB). Fold changes in expression (with S.E.M) are calculated using the $2^{-\Delta\Delta Ct}$ *method relative to one sample of the control taken as unity and represent duplicate runs of 5 biological replicates each of CCLE (DLE)-patients and healthy controls. Fold change in expression (between case and control blood samples) of CCR2 and STAT1 trended toward significance with p-values = 0.055 and 0.053, respectively (*starred). Gene expression values from the microarray data are included as fold change in gene expression in skin and blood associated with* $p \leq 0.05$. *CCLE, chronic cutaneous lupus erythematosus/Discoid lupus erythematosus; S.E.M., standard error of the mean (see also* ***Figure 6****).*

are previously identified as CLE susceptibility loci potentially represent specific association to the cutaneous disease.

Therapeutic Considerations—Current and Future

Currently, no consensus or evidence based therapeutic regimen exists for CCLE. Moreover, very few well-controlled trials have systematically evaluated commonly used treatments for CLE (114–118). Disease management in CCLE begins with precise diagnosis and a treatment plan that can only be decided upon after comprehensive evaluation and recording of patient clinical and laboratory data. This includes immunological, clinical presentation, race, sex, age of onset, disease flares history, family history, past therapy failures, and histopathology of a skin biopsy among others.

Topical and systemic glucocorticoids, antimalarials, methotrexate and thalidomide are the standard of care in SLE, and are used in cutaneous disease as well. All treatments must be accompanied by intermittent re-evaluation of the patients to screen disease prognosis. The overall choices in therapy are discussed very briefly.

Tacrolimus (calcineurin inhibitor), may be a good substitute for those patients who respond poorly to topical corticosteroids (119). Antimalarial drugs (oral) such as chloroquine and quinacrine are also considered the first line of systemic CLE therapy (120–122). In refractory CLE that does not respond well to antimalarial therapy, the addition of medications that generally suppress the immune system is required. These include: methotrexate (123), mycophenolate mofetil (124), oral retinoids such as acitretin (125, 126), dapsone (127), as well as intravenous immunoglobulin (IVIG) (128, 129), Thalidomide and its structural analogs have also been used to treat recalcitrant CLE, with success in some cases (130). Trials assessing monoclonal antibodies such as sifalimumab and belimumab in CLE are on-going but mostly found to be effective in SLE with mucocutaneous involvement (131, 132).

We have mapped many of the drugs that are currently in clinical use for CCLE to their targets of influence in the "disease road map" based on mechanism of action (please refer to **Figure 3**). GO enrichment analyses of our transcriptional profiles reveal enhanced and activated leukocyte chemotaxis and B cell activation in skin more so than blood. This might explain the observed efficacy of the preventive topical corticosteroids (CS) treatments (114), since they bind to specific cytoplasmic receptors resulting in the inhibition of leukocyte infiltration at the site of inflammation. CS are equally effective in both humoral- and T cell mediated diseases (133). Over-represented disease-related processes such as lysosome/proteasome degradation in blood, as well as NK cells, and antigen processing and presentation in both skin and blood are expected to be the target of antimalarials (hydroxychloroquine or chloroquine), that are known to alter pH in lysosomes (134), modify TLR activation (135) and inhibit antigen presentation. We observe activated T cell related processes in CLE skin and blood analyses which are the predicted targets for several immunosuppressant medications such as methotrexate, a T cell proliferation inhibitor used in the treatment of recalcitrant CLE (123). Thalidomide and analog lenalidomide effectively target TNF-α in UV-induced apoptosis, thus decreasing inflammation. Prominent apoptotic signatures in both skin and blood presumably indicate effective use of these drugs, but they are not the drug of choice in cutaneous lupus due to potential serious side effects. Experimental therapeutic agents include azathropine, (anti-purine metabolite); apremilast, (phosphodiesterase-4 inhibitor); R333 (topical JAK/spleen tyrosine kinase inhibitor acting as an anti-inflammatory molecule), and etanercept (TNF-α inhibitor). Many of these agents are linked to clinical trials (**Supplementary Table 7**).

Clearly, healthcare is moving toward tailoring medicines/therapy targeting specific molecules in individual patients whose expression profiles are known. Our genome-wide transcriptome study is a representation of gene regulation in a highly balanced system of networks and pathways underlying CCLE. Disruption of any of the pathways by primary or secondary drug targeting offers unique treatment opportunities (136). Overall, our new *in silico* analyses identified a novel target, *CCR2* which is a key link to prominent disease related pathways and processes that merits further investigation for potential use in future therapy of CLE.

Chemokine (C-C motif) receptor2 (*CCR2*) encodes two isoforms of a receptor for monocyte chemoattractant protein-1 (MCP-1), which specifically mediates monocyte chemotaxis in inflammatory diseases such as rheumatoid arthritis. *CCR2* maps to the overlapping CCLE skin (FC = 1.8) and blood (FC = 1.6) "hot spot" on chromosome 3. Additionally, previous reports have found a positive correlation with increased gene expression in SLE (137, 138). This makes *CCR2* (implicated in the damaging inflammation underlying autoimmune and inflammatory diseases) a good potential therapeutic target candidate in cutaneous lupus as well. We discovered three xenobiotics: CCX915, CCX140 (clinical trials- phase I and II), and TAK779 (preclinical) that have been used to target the extracellular region of *CCR2*. CCX915 is a highly selective inhibitor of the *CCR2* chemokine receptor in multiple sclerosis and other autoimmune and inflammatory diseases. Preclinical data show that CCX140 selectively inhibits CCR2-mediated migration of monocytes and does not inhibit migration mediated by other chemokine receptors, even when the compound is given at high doses. This high degree of target specificity is an important safety feature that may allow CCX140 to be effective while avoiding unwanted side effects. We also discovered one highly specific humanized monoclonal antibody MLN1202 (clinical trial-Phase II) that interrupts MCP-1 binding to *CCR2*. These drugs (CCX915, CCX140-B, TAK779, and MLN 1202) have been used in the past in treatment of rheumatoid arthritis, diabetes mellitus, multiple sclerosis (139) and cardiovascular diseases with a modicum of success (140, 141) (**Supplementary Table 7**).

SUMMARY

Overall, the present study represents the first comparative analyses of CCLE skin and blood transcriptional profile along with "interactome-" "network-" "drug target-" analyses. The data is integrated and synthesized within the milieu of current literature on SLE/CCLE. We hypothesize a "disease road-map" demonstrating a coordinated orchestration of the autoimmune response in CCLE reflected in three phases: (1) initiation, (2) amplification, and (3) target damage in skin. *In -silico* interactome analyses was conducted to identify potential key functional players associated with the skin disease. Our careful and systematic downstream analyses of the CCLE skin and blood transcriptional data not only allowed us to uncover potential crucial contributors to the metabolic changes linked to the skin disease, but to select the best potential target candidate for future therapy.

Chemokine (C-C motif) receptor2 (*CCR2)* is the only molecule within the scope of our bioinformatics-guided analyses that fits all criteria we used to prioritize it as a potential drug target: (a) included as CCLE-DEG (blood and skin) by *microarray analysis.* The observed upregulation in case vs. control (blood) and lesional vs. non-lesional (skin) were accompanied by low e-values of $\leq$ 0.05, (b) overexpressed in disease vs. control peripheral blood by RT-*qPCR analysis, in a separate set of samples as those used in the microarray analysis,* (c) enriched in lupus-related pathways and processes by *ontology enrichment analyses,* (d) "over-connected" functional molecule by *interactome analysis,* (e) a reaction hub by *network analysis,* (f) mapped to chromosome 3 in an overlapping skin/blood transcriptional "hot spot" by *chromosome mapping analysis,* and (g) targeted by drugs that are currently being used to treat other diseases such as inflammatory and immune diseases by *drug target analysis.*

In summary, the present study, based on genome-wide gene expression aims to integrate clinical, genetic and bioinformatics data to bridge the gap between the laboratory and clinical management of patients. Information and evidence garnered from this report potentially impacts future clinical decision-making through the definition of actionable diagnostic and prognostic markers of the disease and the illumination of disease related pathways relevant to therapeutic response. Finally, we present the exciting possibility of designing potential new clinical trials (with a shorter cycle time due to pre-resolved regulatory issues) in the treatment of CCLE using *repurposed drugs* that target the CCLE related receptor, CCR2.

ETHICS STATEMENT

We have followed ethical conduct of research according to the Weill Cornell Medical College Institutional Review Board: WCM IRB# 0998-398. Signed consent forms were obtained from all patient and healthy control individuals before obtaining punch biopsies or performing blood draws.

AUTHOR CONTRIBUTIONS

RD-R contributed to experimentation, data analyses, research, conceptualizing, and writing of the manuscript and editing. AS contributed to design and procurement of samples for microarray and editing of manuscript.

ACKNOWLEDGMENTS

We thank Birendra Kumar Sinha, Asha Sinha, and Mita Sinha for continuous guidance and support.

REFERENCES

1. Dey-Rao R, Seiffert-Sinha K, Sinha AA. Genome-wide expression analysis suggests unique disease-promoting and disease-preventing signatures in Pemphigus vulgaris. *Genes Immunity.* (2013) 14:487–99. doi: 10.1038/gene.2013.44
2. McCarty DJ, Manzi S, Medsger TA, Jr, Ramsey-Goldman R, LaPorte RE, Kwoh CK. Incidence of systemic lupus erythematosus. Race and gender differences. *Arthritis Rheum.* (1995) 38:1260–70. doi: 10.1002/art.1780380914
3. Young NA, Wu LC, Burd CJ, Friedman AK, Kaffenberger BH, Rajaram MV, et al. Estrogen modulation of endosome-associated toll-like receptor 8: an IFNalpha-independent mechanism of sex-bias in systemic lupus erythematosus. *Clin Immunol.* (2014) 151:66–77. doi: 10.1016/j.clim.2014.01.006
4. Werth VP. Cutaneous lupus: insights into pathogenesis and disease classification. *Bull NYU Hosp Joint Dis.* (2007) 65:200–4.
5. Zahn S, Graef M, Patsinakidis N, Landmann A, Surber C, Wenzel J, et al. Ultraviolet light protection by a sunscreen prevents interferon-driven skin inflammation in cutaneous lupus erythematosus. *Exp Dermatol.* (2014) 23:516–8. doi: 10.1111/exd.12428
6. Gallego H, Crutchfield CE, 3rd, Lewis EJ, Gallego HJ. Report of an association between discoid lupus erythematosus and smoking. *Cutis.* (1999) 63:231–4.
7. Walling HW, Sontheimer RD. Cutaneous lupus erythematosus: issues in diagnosis and treatment. *Am J Clin Dermatol.* (2009) 10:365–81. doi: 10.2165/11310780-000000000-00000
8. Kuhn A, Sontheimer RD. Cutaneous lupus erythematosus: molecular and cellular basis of clinical findings. *Curr Direct Autoimmunity.* (2008) 10:119–40. doi: 10.1159/000131451
9. Szczech J, Samotij D, Werth VP, Reich A. Trigger factors of cutaneous lupus erythematosus: a review of current literature. *Lupus.* (2017) 26:791–807. doi: 10.1177/0961203317691369
10. Suarez A, Lopez P, Mozo L, Gutierrez C. Differential effect of IL10 and TNF{alpha} genotypes on determining susceptibility to discoid and systemic lupus erythematosus. *Ann Rheum Dis.* (2005) 64:1605–10. doi: 10.1136/ard.2004.035048
11. Lopez-Tello A, Rodriguez-Carreon AA, Jurado F, Yamamoto-Furusho JK, Castillo-Vazquez M, Chavez-Munoz C, et al. Association of HLA-DRB1*16 with chronic discoid lupus erythematosus in Mexican mestizo patients. *Clin Exp Dermatol.* (2007) 32:435–8. doi: 10.1111/j.1365-2230.2007.02391.x
12. Millard TP, McGregor JM. Molecular genetics of cutaneous lupus erythematosus. *Clin Exp Dermatol.* (2001) 26:184–91. doi: 10.1046/j.1365-2230.2001.00793.x
13. Lee HJ, Sinha AA. Cutaneous lupus erythematosus: understanding of clinical features, genetic basis, and pathobiology of disease guides therapeutic strategies. *Autoimmunity.* (2006) 39:433–44. doi: 10.1080/08916930600886851
14. Fowler JF, Callen JP, Stelzer GT, Cotter PK. Human histocompatibility antigen associations in patients with chronic cutaneous lupus erythematosus. *J Am Acad Dermatol.* (1985) 12(1 Pt 1):73–7. doi: 10.1016/S0190-9622(85)70012-6
15. Knop J, Bonsmann G, Kind P, Doxiadis I, Vogeler U, Doxiadis G, et al. Antigens of the major histocompatibility complex in patients with chronic discoid lupus erythematosus. *Br J Dermatol.* (1990) 122:723–8. doi: 10.1111/j.1365-2133.1990.tb06258.x
16. Kunz M, Konig IR, Schillert A, Kruppa J, Ziegler A, Grallert H, et al. Genome-wide association study identifies new susceptibility loci for cutaneous lupus erythematosus. *Exp Dermatol.* (2015) 24:510–5. doi: 10.1111/exd.12708
17. Millard TP, Ashton GH, Kondeatis E, Vaughan RW, Hughes GR, Khamashta MA, et al. Human Ro60 (SSA2) genomic organization and sequence alterations, examined in cutaneous lupus erythematosus. *Br J Dermatol.* (2002) 146:210–5. doi: 10.1046/j.1365-2133.2002.04618.x
18. Meyer O, Hauptmann G, Tappeiner G, Ochs HD, Mascart-Lemone F. Genetic deficiency of C4, C2 or C1q and lupus syndromes. Association with anti-Ro (SS-A) antibodies. *Clin Exp Immunol.* (1985) 62:678–84.
19. Osmola A, Namysl J, Jagodzinski PP, Prokop J. Genetic background of cutaneous forms of lupus erythematosus: update on current evidence. *J Appl Genet.* (2004) 45:77–86.
20. Ziemer M, Milkova L, Kunz M. Lupus erythematosus. Part II: clinical picture, diagnosis and treatment. *J Deutschen Dermatologischen Gesellschaft = J German Soc Dermatol.* (2014) 12:285–301; quiz 2. doi: 10.1111/ddg.12254
21. Dey-Rao R, Smith JR, Chow S, Sinha AA. Differential gene expression analysis in CCLE lesions provides new insights regarding the genetics basis of skin vs. systemic disease. *Genomics.* (2014) 104:144–55. doi: 10.1016/j.ygeno.2014.06.003
22. Dey-Rao R, Sinha AA. Genome-wide transcriptional profiling of chronic cutaneous lupus erythematosus (CCLE) peripheral blood identifies systemic alterations relevant to the skin manifestation. *Genomics.* (2015) 105:90–100. doi: 10.1016/j.ygeno.2014.11.004
23. Dey-Rao R, Sinha AA. Genome-wide transcriptional profiling data from skin of chronic cutaneous lupus erythematosus (CCLE) patients. *Data Brief.* (2015) 4:47–9. doi: 10.1016/j.dib.2015.02.024
24. Dey-Rao R, Sinha AA. Genome-wide transcriptional profiling data from chronic cutaneous lupus erythematosus (CCLE) peripheral blood. *Data Brief.* (2015) 2:39–41. doi: 10.1016/j.dib.2014.11.006
25. Coda AB, Icen M, Smith JR, Sinha AA. Global transcriptional analysis of psoriatic skin and blood confirms known disease-associated pathways and highlights novel genomic "hot spots" for differentially expressed genes. *Genomics.* (2012) 100:18–26. doi: 10.1016/j.ygeno.2012.05.004
26. Coda AB, Qafalijaj Hysa V, Seiffert-Sinha K, Sinha AA. Peripheral blood gene expression in alopecia areata reveals molecular pathways distinguishing heritability, disease and severity. *Genes Immun.* (2010) 11:531–41. doi: 10.1038/gene.2010.32
27. Bickel DR. Degrees of differential gene expression: detecting biologically significant expression differences and estimating their magnitudes. *Bioinformatics.* (2004) 20:682–8. doi: 10.1093/bioinformatics/btg468
28. Huang da W, Sherman BT, Lempicki RA. Systematic and integrative analysis of large gene lists using DAVID bioinformatics resources. *Nat Protoc.* (2009) 4:44–57. doi: 10.1038/nprot.2008.211
29. Shmelkov E, Tang Z, Aifantis I, Statnikov A. Assessing quality and completeness of human transcriptional regulatory pathways on a genome-wide scale. *Biol Direct.* (2011) 6:15. doi: 10.1186/1745-6150-6-15
30. Bessarabova M, Ishkin A, JeBailey L, Nikolskaya T, Nikolsky Y. Knowledge-based analysis of proteomics data. *BMC Bioinform.* (2012) 13(Suppl. 16):S13. doi: 10.1186/1471-2105-13-S16-S13
31. Harley JB, Alarcon-Riquelme ME, Criswell LA, Jacob CO, Kimberly RP, Moser KL, et al. Genome-wide association scan in women with systemic lupus erythematosus identifies susceptibility variants in ITGAM, PXK,

KIAA1542 and other loci. *Nat Genet.* (2008) 40:204–10. doi: 10.1038/ng.81

32. Clancy RM, Marion MC, Kaufman KM, Ramos PS, Adler A, Harley JB, et al. Identification of candidate loci at 6p21 and 21q22 in a genome-wide association study of cardiac manifestations of neonatal lupus. *Arthritis Rheumat.* (2010) 62:3415–24. doi: 10.1002/art.27658
33. Hom G, Graham RR, Modrek B, Taylor KE, Ortmann W, Garnier S, et al. Association of systemic lupus erythematosus with C8orf13-BLK and ITGAM-ITGAX. *N Engl J Med.* (2008) 358:900–9. doi: 10.1056/NEJMoa0707865
34. Han JW, Zheng HF, Cui Y, Sun LD, Ye DQ, Hu Z, et al. Genome-wide association study in a Chinese Han population identifies nine new susceptibility loci for systemic lupus erythematosus. *Nature genetics.* (2009) 41:1234–7. doi: 10.1038/ng.472
35. Yang W, Shen N, Ye DQ, Liu Q, Zhang Y, Qian XX, et al. Genome-wide association study in Asian populations identifies variants in ETS1 and WDFY4 associated with systemic lupus erythematosus. *PLoS Genet.* (2010) 6:e1000841. doi: 10.1371/journal.pgen.1000841
36. Okada Y, Shimane K, Kochi Y, Tahira T, Suzuki A, Higasa K, et al. A genome-wide association study identified AFF1 as a susceptibility locus for systemic lupus eyrthematosus in Japanese. *PLoS Genet.* (2012) 8:e1002455. doi: 10.1371/journal.pgen.1002455
37. Li R, Yang W, Zhang J, Hirankarn N, Pan HF, Mok CC, et al. Association of CD247 with systemic lupus erythematosus in Asian populations. *Lupus.* (2012) 21:75–83. doi: 10.1177/0961203311422724
38. Chung SA, Taylor KE, Graham RR, Nititham J, Lee AT, Ortmann WA, et al. Differential genetic associations for systemic lupus erythematosus based on anti-dsDNA autoantibody production. *PLoS Genet.* (2011) 7:e1001323. doi: 10.1371/journal.pgen.1001323
39. Yang J, Yang W, Hirankarn N, Ye DQ, Zhang Y, Pan HF, et al. ELF1 is associated with systemic lupus erythematosus in Asian populations. *Hum Mol Genet.* (2011) 20:601–7. doi: 10.1093/hmg/ddq474
40. Kariuki SN, Franek BS, Kumar AA, Arrington J, Mikolaitis RA, Utset TO, et al. Trait-stratified genome-wide association study identifies novel and diverse genetic associations with serologic and cytokine phenotypes in systemic lupus erythematosus. *Arthritis Res Ther.* (2010) 12:R151. doi: 10.1186/ar3101
41. Graham RR, Cotsapas C, Davies L, Hackett R, Lessard CJ, Leon JM, et al. Genetic variants near TNFAIP3 on 6q23 are associated with systemic lupus erythematosus. *Nat Genet.* (2008) 40:1059–61. doi: 10.1038/ng.200
42. Kozyrev SV, Abelson AK, Wojcik J, Zaghlool A, Linga Reddy MV, Sanchez E, et al. Functional variants in the B-cell gene BANK1 are associated with systemic lupus erythematosus. *Nat Genet.* (2008) 40:211–6. doi: 10.1038/ng.79
43. Cervino AC, Tsinoremas NF, Hoffman RW. A genome-wide study of lupus: preliminary analysis and data release. *Ann N Y Acad Sci.* (2007) 1110:131–9. doi: 10.1196/annals.1423.015
44. Deng Y, Tsao BP. Genetic susceptibility to systemic lupus erythematosus in the genomic era. *Nat Rev Rheumatol.* (2010) 6:683–92. doi: 10.1038/nrrheum.2010.176
45. Wu Z, Siadaty MS, Riddick G, Frierson HF, Jr., Lee JK, Golden W, et al. A novel method for gene expression mapping of metastatic competence in human bladder cancer. *Neoplasia.* (2006) 8:181–9. doi: 10.1593/neo.05727
46. Luo H, Zhao X, Wan X, Huang S, Wu D. Gene microarray analysis of the lncRNA expression profile in human urothelial carcinoma of the bladder. *Int J Clin Exp Med.* (2014) 7:1244–54.
47. Dey-Rao R, Sinha AA. Vitiligo blood transcriptomics provides new insights into disease mechanisms and identifies potential novel therapeutic targets. *BMC Genom.* (2017) 18:109. doi: 10.1186/s12864-017-3510-3
48. Dey-Rao R, Sinha AA. Interactome analysis of gene expression profile reveals potential novel key transcriptional regulators of skin pathology in vitiligo. *Genes Immun.* (2016) 17:30–45. doi: 10.1038/gene.2015.48
49. Dey-Rao R, Sinha AA. A genomic approach to susceptibility and pathogenesis leads to identifying potential novel therapeutic targets in androgenetic alopecia. *Genomics.* (2017) 109:165–76. doi: 10.1016/j.ygeno.2017.02.005
50. Reiner A, Yekutieli D, Benjamini Y. Identifying differentially expressed genes using false discovery rate controlling procedures. *Bioinformatics.* (2003) 19:368–75. doi: 10.1093/bioinformatics/btf877
51. Livak KJ, Schmittgen TD. Analysis of relative gene expression data using real-time quantitative PCR and the 2(-Delta Delta C(T)) Method. *Methods.* (2001) 25:402–8. doi: 10.1006/meth.2001.1262
52. Ito T, Chiba T, Yoshida M. Exploring the protein interactome using comprehensive two-hybrid projects. *Trends Biotechnol.* (2001) 19(10 Suppl.):S23–7. doi: 10.1016/S0167-7799(01)01790-5
53. Ideker T, Ozier O, Schwikowski B, Siegel AF. Discovering regulatory and signalling circuits in molecular interaction networks. *Bioinformatics.* (2002) 18(Suppl. 1):S233–40. doi: 10.1093/bioinformatics/18.suppl_1.S233
54. Norris DA, Whang K, David-Bajar K, Bennion SD. The influence of ultraviolet light on immunological cytotoxicity in the skin. *Photochem Photobiol.* (1997) 65:636–46. doi: 10.1111/j.1751-1097.1997.tb01905.x
55. Petri M. Dermatologic lupus: hopkins lupus cohort. *Semin Cutan Med Surg.* (1998) 17:219–27. doi: 10.1016/S1085-5629(98)80017-5
56. Sontheimer RD. Photoimmunology of lupus erythematosus and dermatomyositis: a speculative review. *Photochem Photobiol.* (1996) 63:583–94. doi: 10.1111/j.1751-1097.1996.tb05660.x
57. Kuhn A, Wenzel J, Weyd H. Photosensitivity, apoptosis, and cytokines in the pathogenesis of lupus erythematosus: a critical review. *Clin Rev Allergy Immunol.* (2014) 47:148–62. doi: 10.1007/s12016-013-8403-x
58. Rekvig OP, Van der Vlag J. The pathogenesis and diagnosis of systemic lupus erythematosus: still not resolved. *Semin Immunopathol.* (2014) 36:301–11. doi: 10.1007/s00281-014-0428-6
59. Yu C, Chang C, Zhang J. Immunologic and genetic considerations of cutaneous lupus erythematosus: a comprehensive review. *J Autoimmun.* (2013) 41:34–45. doi: 10.1016/j.jaut.2013.01.007
60. Lin JH, Dutz JP, Sontheimer RD, Werth VP. Pathophysiology of cutaneous lupus erythematosus. *Clin Rev Allergy Immunol.* (2007) 33:85–106. doi: 10.1007/s12016-007-0031-x
61. Baima B, Sticherling M. Apoptosis in different cutaneous manifestations of lupus erythematosus. *Br J Dermatol.* (2001) 144:958–66. doi: 10.1046/j.1365-2133.2001.04182.x
62. Charles PJ. Defective waste disposal: does it induce autoantibodies in SLE? *Ann Rheum Dis.* (2003) 62:1–3. doi: 10.1136/ard.62.1.1-a
63. Herrmann M, Voll RE, Zoller OM, Hagenhofer M, Ponner BB, Kalden JR. Impaired phagocytosis of apoptotic cell material by monocyte-derived macrophages from patients with systemic lupus erythematosus. *Arthritis Rheumat.* (1998) 41:1241–50. doi: 10.1002/1529-0131(199807)41:7<1241::AID-ART15>3.0.CO;2-H
64. Baumann I, Kolowos W, Voll RE, Manger B, Gaipl U, Neuhuber WL, et al. Impaired uptake of apoptotic cells into tingible body macrophages in germinal centers of patients with systemic lupus erythematosus. *Arthritis Rheumat.* (2002) 46:191–201. doi: 10.1002/1529-0131(200201)46:1<191::AID-ART10027>3.0.CO;2-K
65. Gaipl US, Munoz LE, Grossmayer G, Lauber K, Franz S, Sarter K, et al. Clearance deficiency and systemic lupus erythematosus (SLE). *J Autoimmun.* (2007) 28:114–21. doi: 10.1016/j.jaut.2007.02.005
66. Kuhn A, Beissert S. Photosensitivity in lupus erythematosus. *Autoimmunity.* (2005) 38:519–29. doi: 10.1080/08916930500285626
67. Kuhn A, Herrmann M, Kleber S, Beckmann-Welle M, Fehsel K, Martin-Villalba A, et al. Accumulation of apoptotic cells in the epidermis of patients with cutaneous lupus erythematosus after ultraviolet irradiation. *Arthritis Rheumat.* (2006) 54:939–50. doi: 10.1002/art.21658
68. Wang G, Pierangeli SS, Papalardo E, Ansari GA, Khan MF. Markers of oxidative and nitrosative stress in systemic lupus erythematosus: correlation with disease activity. *Arthritis Rheumat.* (2010) 62:2064–72. doi: 10.1002/art.27442
69. Zahn S, Graef M, Barchet W, Bieber T, Tuting T, Wenzel J. Nitrosative stress: a hallmark of the junctional inflammation in cutaneous lupus erythematosus. *Clin Exp Dermatol.* (2013) 38:96–7. doi: 10.1111/j.1365-2230.2012.04472.x
70. Morgan PE, Sturgess AD, Davies MJ. Increased levels of serum protein oxidation and correlation with disease activity in systemic lupus erythematosus. *Arthritis Rheumat.* (2005) 52:2069–79. doi: 10.1002/art.21130
71. Ryan BJ, Eggleton P. Detection and characterization of autoantibodies against modified self-proteins in SLE sera after exposure to reactive

oxygen and nitrogen species. *Methods Mol Biol.* (2014) 1134:163–71. doi: 10.1007/978-1-4939-0326-9_12

72. Norris DA. Pathomechanisms of photosensitive lupus erythematosus. *J Invest Dermatol.* (1993) 100:58S–68S. doi: 10.1038/jid.1993.25
73. Dorner T, Hucko M, Mayet WJ, Trefzer U, Burmester GR, Hiepe F. Enhanced membrane expression of the 52 kDa Ro(SS-A) and La(SS-B) antigens by human keratinocytes induced by TNF alpha. *Ann Rheum Dis.* (1995) 54:904–9. doi: 10.1136/ard.54.11.904
74. Schroder JM. Cytokine networks in the skin. *J Invest Dermatol.* (1995) 105(1 Suppl.):20S–4S. doi: 10.1038/jid.1995.5
75. Elloumi N, Fakhfakh R, Ayadi L, Sellami K, Abida O, Ben Jmaa M, et al. The increased expression of toll-like receptor 4 in renal and skin lesions in lupus erythematosus. *J Histochem Cytochem.* (2017) 65:389–98. doi: 10.1369/0022155417709234
76. Middleton MH, Norris DA. Cytokine-induced ICAM-1 expression in human keratinocytes is highly variable in keratinocyte strains from different donors. *J Invest Dermatol.* (1995) 104:489–96. doi: 10.1111/1523-1747.ep12605923
77. Albert ML, Sauter B, Bhardwaj N. Dendritic cells acquire antigen from apoptotic cells and induce class I-restricted CTLs. *Nature.* (1998) 392:86–9. doi: 10.1038/32183
78. Nakatani K, Yoshimoto S, Asai O, Sakan H, Terada M, Saito Y, et al. Enhanced expression of the soluble form of E-selectin attenuates progression of lupus nephritis and vasculitis in MRL/lpr mice. *Immunity Inflamm Dis.* (2013) 1:37–46. doi: 10.1002/iid3.6
79. Lasky LA. Selectin-carbohydrate interactions and the initiation of the inflammatory response. *Ann Rev Biochem.* (1995) 64:113–39. doi: 10.1146/annurev.bi.64.070195.000553
80. Steinman RM, Nussenzweig MC. Avoiding horror autotoxicus: the importance of dendritic cells in peripheral T cell tolerance. *Proc Natl Acad Sci USA.* (2002) 99:351–8. doi: 10.1073/pnas.231606698
81. Dhodapkar MV, Steinman RM, Krasovsky J, Munz C, Bhardwaj N. Antigen-specific inhibition of effector T cell function in humans after injection of immature dendritic cells. *J Exp Med.* (2001) 193:233–8. doi: 10.1084/jem.193.2.233
82. McCauliffe DP. Cutaneous lupus erythematosus. *Semin Cutan Med Surg.* (2001) 20:14–26. doi: 10.1053/sder.2001.23091
83. Werth VP, Dutz JP, Sontheimer RD. Pathogenetic mechanisms and treatment of cutaneous lupus erythematosus. *Curr Opin Rheumatol.* (1997) 9:400–9. doi: 10.1097/00002281-199709000-00005
84. Jlajla H, Sellami MK, Sfar I, Laadhar L, Zerzeri Y, Abdelmoula MS, et al. New C1q mutation in a Tunisian family. *Immunobiology.* (2014) 219:241–6. doi: 10.1016/j.imbio.2013.10.010
85. Kim K, Sung YK, Kang CP, Choi CB, Kang C, Bae SC. A regulatory SNP at position–899 in CDKN1A is associated with systemic lupus erythematosus and lupus nephritis. *Genes Immunity.* (2009) 10:482–6. doi: 10.1038/gene.2009.5
86. Mihara M, Fukui H, Koishihara Y, Saito M, Ohsugi Y. Immunologic abnormality in NZB/W F1 mice. Thymus-independent expansion of B cells responding to interleukin-6. *Clin Exp Immunol.* (1990) 82:533–7. doi: 10.1111/j.1365-2249.1990.tb05485.x
87. Shoenfeld Y, Mozes E. Pathogenic anti-DNA idiotype (16/6 Id) in systemic lupus erythematosus. *Rheumatol Int.* (1991) 11:91–3. doi: 10.1007/BF00304494
88. Datta SK. Production of pathogenic antibodies: cognate interactions between autoimmune T and B cells. *Lupus.* (1998) 7:591–6. doi: 10.1191/096120398678920703
89. Lu L, Kaliyaperumal A, Boumpas DT, Datta SK. Major peptide autoepitopes for nucleosome-specific T cells of human lupus. *J Clin Invest.* (1999) 104:345–55. doi: 10.1172/JCI6801
90. Kind P, Lehmann P, Plewig G. Phototesting in lupus erythematosus. *J Invest Dermatol.* (1993) 100:53S–7S. doi: 10.1111/1523-1747.ep12355594
91. Freutel S, Gaffal E, Zahn S, Bieber T, Tuting T, Wenzel J. Enhanced CCR5+/CCR3+ T helper cell ratio in patients with active cutaneous lupus erythematosus. *Lupus.* (2011) 20:1300–4. doi: 10.1177/0961203311409267
92. Bresnihan B, Jasin HE. Suppressor function of peripheral blood mononuclear cells in normal individuals and in patients with systemic lupus erythematosus. *J Clin Invest.* (1977) 59:106–16. doi: 10.1172/JCI108607
93. Fauci AS, Steinberg AD, Haynes BF, Whalen G. Immunoregulatory aberrations in systemic lupus erythematosus. *J Immunol.* (1978) 121:1473–9.
94. Kouskoff V, Lacaud G, Nemazee D. T cell-independent rescue of B lymphocytes from peripheral immune tolerance. *Science.* (2000) 287:2501–3. doi: 10.1126/science.287.5462.2501
95. Wardemann H, Yurasov S, Schaefer A, Young JW, Meffre E, Nussenzweig MC. Predominant autoantibody production by early human B cell precursors. *Science.* (2003) 301:1374–7. doi: 10.1126/science.1086907
96. Blomberg S, Eloranta ML, Cederblad B, Nordlin K, Alm GV, Ronnblom L. Presence of cutaneous interferon-alpha producing cells in patients with systemic lupus erythematosus. *Lupus.* (2001) 10:484–90. doi: 10.1191/096120301678416042
97. Seery JP, Carroll JM, Cattell V, Watt FM. Antinuclear autoantibodies and lupus nephritis in transgenic mice expressing interferon gamma in the epidermis. *J Exp Med.* (1997) 186:1451–9. doi: 10.1084/jem.186.9.1451
98. Jacob CO, van der Meide PH, McDevitt HO. *In vivo* treatment of (NZB X NZW)F1 lupus-like nephritis with monoclonal antibody to gamma interferon. *J Exp Med.* (1987) 166:798–803. doi: 10.1084/jem.166.3.798
99. Crow MK. Interferon pathway activation in systemic lupus erythematosus. *Curr Rheumatol Rep.* (2005) 7:463–8. doi: 10.1007/s11926-005-0053-4
100. Pinkus H. Lichenoid tissue reactions. A speculative review of the clinical spectrum of epidermal basal cell damage with special reference to erythema dyschromicum perstans. *Arch Dermatol.* (1973) 107:840–6. doi: 10.1001/archderm.1973.01620210008002
101. Gaipl US, Kuhn A, Sheriff A, Munoz LE, Franz S, Voll RE, et al. Clearance of apoptotic cells in human SLE. *Curr Direct Autoimmunity.* (2006) 9:173-87. doi: 10.1159/000090781
102. Kuhn A, Krammer PH, Kolb-Bachofen V. Pathophysiology of cutaneous lupus erythematosus–novel aspects. *Rheumatology.* (2006) 45(Suppl. 3):iii14–6. doi: 10.1093/rheumatology/kel284
103. Cohen PL, Caricchio R, Abraham V, Camenisch TD, Jennette JC, Roubey RA, et al. Delayed apoptotic cell clearance and lupus-like autoimmunity in mice lacking the c-mer membrane tyrosine kinase. *J Exp Med.* (2002) 196:135–40. doi: 10.1084/jem.20012094
104. Henkart PA. Lymphocyte-mediated cytotoxicity: two pathways and multiple effector molecules. *Immunity.* (1994) 1:343–6. doi: 10.1016/1074-7613(94)90063-9
105. Grassi M, Capello F, Bertolino L, Seia Z, Pippione M. Identification of granzyme B-expressing CD-8-positive T cells in lymphocytic inflammatory infiltrate in cutaneous lupus erythematosus and in dermatomyositis. *Clin Exp Dermatol.* (2009) 34:910–4. doi: 10.1111/j.1365-2230.2009.03297.x
106. Lieberman J. The ABCs of granule-mediated cytotoxicity: new weapons in the arsenal. *Nat Rev Immunol.* (2003) 3:361–70. doi: 10.1038/nri1083
107. Fogagnolo L, Soares TC, Senna CG, Souza EM, Blotta MH, Cintra ML. Cytotoxic granules in distinct subsets of cutaneous lupus erythematosus. *Clin Exp Dermatol.* (2014) 39:835–9. doi: 10.1111/ced.12428
108. Fishelson Z, Attali G, Mevorach D. Complement and apoptosis. *Mol Immunol.* (2001) 38:207–19. doi: 10.1016/S0161-5890(01)00055-4
109. Uwai M, Terui Y, Mishima Y, Tomizuka H, Ikeda M, Itoh T, et al. A new apoptotic pathway for the complement factor B-derived fragment Bb. *J Cell Physiol.* (2000) 185:280–92. doi: 10.1002/1097-4652(200011)185:2<280::AID-JCP13>3.0.CO;2-L
110. Sinha AA, Dey-Rao R. Genomic Investigation of lupus in the skin. *J Invest Dermatol Sympos Proc.* (2017) 18:S75–S80. doi: 10.1016/j.jisp.2016.09.002
111. Calderon C, Zucht HD, Kuhn A, Wozniacka A, Szepietowski JC, Nyberg F, et al. A multicenter photoprovocation study to identify potential biomarkers by global peptide profiling in cutaneous lupus erythematosus. *Lupus.* (2015) 24:1406–20. doi: 10.1177/0961203315596077
112. Zhang YP, Wu J, Han YF, Shi ZR, Wang L. Pathogenesis of cutaneous lupus erythema associated with and without systemic lupus erythema. *Autoimmunity Rev.* (2017) 16:735–42. doi: 10.1016/j.autrev.2017.05.009
113. Merola JF, Prystowsky SD, Iversen C, Gomez-Puerta JA, Norton T, Tsao P, et al. Association of discoid lupus erythematosus with other clinical manifestations among patients with systemic lupus erythematosus. *J Am Acad Dermatol.* (2013) 69:19–24. doi: 10.1016/j.jaad.2013.02.010
114. Jessop S, Whitelaw DA, Delamere FM. Drugs for discoid lupus erythematosus. *Cochr Database Syst Rev.* (2009) 4:CD002954. doi: 10.1002/14651858.CD002954.pub2

115. Tzung TY, Liu YS, Chang HW. Tacrolimus vs. clobetasol propionate in the treatment of facial cutaneous lupus erythematosus: a randomized, double-blind, bilateral comparison study. *Br J Dermatol.* (2007) 156:191–2. doi: 10.1111/j.1365-2133.2006.07595.x
116. Jemec GB, Ullman S, Goodfield M, Bygum A, Olesen AB, Berth-Jones J, et al. A randomized controlled trial of R-salbutamol for topical treatment of discoid lupus erythematosus. *Br J Dermatol.* (2009) 161:1365–70. doi: 10.1111/j.1365-2133.2009.09330.x
117. Chang AY, Werth VP. Treatment of cutaneous lupus. *Curr Rheumatol Rep.* (2011) 13:300–7. doi: 10.1007/s11926-011-0180-z
118. Callen JP. Management of "refractory" skin disease in patients with lupus erythematosus. *Best Pract Res Clin Rheumatol.* (2005) 19:767–84. doi: 10.1016/j.berh.2005.05.003
119. Kuhn A, Gensch K, Haust M, Schneider SW, Bonsmann G, Gaebelein-Wissing N, et al. Efficacy of tacrolimus 0.1% ointment in cutaneous lupus erythematosus: a multicenter, randomized, double-blind, vehicle-controlled trial. *J Am Acad Dermatol.* (2011) 65:54–64, e1–2. doi: 10.1016/j.jaad.2010.03.037
120. Frances C, Cosnes A, Duhaut P, Zahr N, Soutou B, Ingen-Housz-Oro S, et al. Low blood concentration of hydroxychloroquine in patients with refractory cutaneous lupus erythematosus: a French multicenter prospective study. *Arch Dermatol.* (2012) 148:479–84. doi: 10.1001/archdermatol.2011.2558
121. Cavazzana I, Sala R, Bazzani C, Ceribelli A, Zane C, Cattaneo R, et al. Treatment of lupus skin involvement with quinacrine and hydroxychloroquine. *Lupus.* (2009) 18:735–9. doi: 10.1177/0961203308101714
122. Fruchter R, Kurtzman DJB, Patel M, Merola J, Franks AG, Jr., Vleugels RA, et al. Characteristics and alternative treatment outcomes of antimalarial-refractory cutaneous lupus erythematosus. *JAMA Dermatol.* (2017) 153:937–9. doi: 10.1001/jamadermatol.2017.1160
123. Wenzel J, Brahler S, Bauer R, Bieber T, Tuting T. Efficacy and safety of methotrexate in recalcitrant cutaneous lupus erythematosus: results of a retrospective study in 43 patients. *Br J Dermatol.* (2005) 153:157–62. doi: 10.1111/j.1365-2133.2005.06552.x
124. Gammon B, Hansen C, Costner MI. Efficacy of mycophenolate mofetil in antimalarial-resistant cutaneous lupus erythematosus. *J Am Acad Dermatol.* (2011) 65:717–21. doi: 10.1016/j.jaad.2010.08.011
125. Ruzicka T, Sommerburg C, Goerz G, Kind P, Mensing H. Treatment of cutaneous lupus erythematosus with acitretin and hydroxychloroquine. *Br J Dermatol.* (1992) 127:513–8. doi: 10.1111/j.1365-2133.1992.tb14851.x
126. Kuhn A, Patsinakidis N, Luger T. Alitretinoin for cutaneous lupus erythematosus. *J Am Acad Dermatol.* (2012) 67:e123–6. doi: 10.1016/j.jaad.2011.10.030
127. Klebes M, Wutte N, Aberer E. Dapsone as second-line treatment for cutaneous lupus erythematosus? a retrospective analysis of 34 patients and a review of the literature. *Dermatology.* (2016) 232:91–6. doi: 10.1159/000441054
128. Lampropoulos CE, Hughes GR, DP DC. Intravenous immunoglobulin in the treatment of resistant subacute cutaneous lupus erythematosus: a possible alternative. *Clin Rheumatol.* (2007) 26:981–3. doi: 10.1007/s10067-006-0222-5
129. Ky C, Swasdibutra B, Khademi S, Desai S, Laquer V, Grando SA. Efficacy of intravenous immunoglobulin monotherapy in patients with cutaneous lupus erythematosus: results of proof-of-concept study. *Dermatol Rep.* (2015) 7:5804. doi: 10.4081/dr.2015.5804
130. Cortes-Hernandez J, Torres-Salido M, Castro-Marrero J, Vilardell-Tarres M, Ordi-Ros J. Thalidomide in the treatment of refractory cutaneous lupus erythematosus: prognostic factors of clinical outcome. *Br J Dermatol.* (2012) 166:616–23. doi: 10.1111/j.1365-2133.2011.10693.x
131. Khamashta M, Merrill JT, Werth VP, Furie R, Kalunian K, Illei GG, et al. Sifalimumab, an anti-interferon-alpha monoclonal antibody, in moderate to severe systemic lupus erythematosus: a randomised, double-blind, placebo-controlled study. *Ann Rheum Dis.* (2016) 75:1909–16. doi: 10.1136/annrheumdis-2015-208562
132. Narain S, Furie R. Update on clinical trials in systemic lupus erythematosus. *Curr Opin Rheumatol.* (2016) 28:477–87. doi: 10.1097/BOR.0000000000000311
133. Nickoloff BJ, Nestle FO. Recent insights into the immunopathogenesis of psoriasis provide new therapeutic opportunities. *J Clin Invest.* (2004) 113:1664–75. doi: 10.1172/JCI200422147
134. Kalia S, Dutz JP. New concepts in antimalarial use and mode of action in dermatology. *Dermatol Ther.* (2007) 20:160–74. doi: 10.1111/j.1529-8019.2007.00131.x
135. Lafyatis R, York M, Marshak-Rothstein A. Antimalarial agents: closing the gate on Toll-like receptors? *Arthritis Rheumat.* (2006) 54:3068–70. doi: 10.1002/art.22157
136. Menche J, Sharma A, Kitsak M, Ghiassian SD, Vidal M, Loscalzo J, et al. Disease networks. Uncovering disease-disease relationships through the incomplete interactome. *Science.* (2015) 347:1257601. doi: 10.1126/science.1257601
137. Mandel M, Gurevich M, Pauzner R, Kaminski N, Achiron A. Autoimmunity gene expression portrait: specific signature that intersects or differentiates between multiple sclerosis and systemic lupus erythematosus. *Clin Exp Immunol.* (2004) 138:164–7. doi: 10.1111/j.1365-2249.2004.02587.x
138. Li YM, Chen ZQ, Yao X, Yang AZ, Li AS, Liu DM, et al. mRNA expression of chemokine receptors on peripheral blood mononuclear cells and correlation with clinical features in systemic lupus erythematosus patients. *Chin Med Sci J Chung-kuo i hsueh k'o hsueh tsa chih Chin Acad Med Sci.* (2010) 25:162–8.
139. Hamann I, Zipp F, Infante-Duarte C. Therapeutic targeting of chemokine signaling in Multiple Sclerosis. *J Neurol Sci.* (2008) 274:31–8. doi: 10.1016/j.jns.2008.07.005
140. Vergunst CE, Gerlag DM, Lopatinskaya L, Klareskog L, Smith MD, van den Bosch F, et al. Modulation of CCR2 in rheumatoid arthritis: a double-blind, randomized, placebo-controlled clinical trial. *Arthritis Rheumat.* (2008) 58:1931–9. doi: 10.1002/art.23591
141. Proudfoot AE. Is CCR2 the right chemokine receptor to target in rheumatoid arthritis? *Arthritis Rheumat.* (2008) 58:1889–91. doi: 10.1002/art.23590

18

Nucleic Acid Immunity in the Pathogenesis of Cutaneous Lupus Erythematosus

*Claudia Günther**

Department of Dermatology, University Hospital Carl Gustav Carus, Technical University Dresden, Dresden, Germany

***Correspondence:** Claudia Günther claudia.guenther@uniklinikum-dresden.de*

Cutaneous lupus erythematosus can be a devastating painful and mutilating disease that is associated with an inflammatory response in the skin driven by type I interferon activation. Clearance defects in the extra- and intracellular space lead to an enhanced prevalence of nucleic acids that represent danger signals for the innate immune system. Self nucleic acids can stimulate DNA and RNA sensors that have originally evolved to ensure viral defense. Their activation can induce a type I interferon dominated response in resident skin cells, macrophages and dendritic cells that subsequently progresses to adaptive immune stimulation. The genetic exploration of rare monogenic type I interferon driven diseases helped to identify these pathogenic concepts. Based on a genetic susceptibility lupus patients are more vulnerable to environmental trigger factors such as UV-irradiation that can provoke inflammation with local tissue destruction and eventually systemic disease. Understanding of these pathogenic concepts is a prerequisite for development of targeted therapies.

Keywords: nucleic acid immunity, cutaneous lupus erythematosus, innate immunity, nucleic acid sensors, type I interferon

INTRODUCTION

Lupus erythematosus is a chronic relapsing autoimmune disease with a varying spectrum of clinical manifestations ranging from sole cutaneous involvement to fatal multi-organ disease (1). The wide clinical range of cutaneous symptoms includes a diverse spectrum from acute rash, discoid lupus, cold induced chilblain lesions to succulent subcutaneous infiltrates resembling lupus tumidus (2, 3). Cutaneous lupus can occur with or without systemic involvement. Patients with systemic lupus erythematosus (SLE) frequently develop skin lesions. Disease flares can be induced by external trigger factors among which viral infections, UV-irradiation and smoking are the most important (1). Cutaneous inflammation is characterized by a perivascular and periadnexial lymphohistiocytic infiltration accompanied by an interphase dermatitis and variable epidermal involvement. This lymphocyte activation is a hallmark of adaptive immune stimulation. T cells provide help for activation of autoantigen specific B cells and producing autoantibodies. In patients with lupus erythematosus the target structures of these autoantibodies are proteins associated with nucleic acids (1). Immune complexes containing autoantibodies to nucleic acid binding proteins and nucleic acids are frequently deposited along the basement membrane zone of the skin and the concentration of autoantibodies against double stranded DNA (dsDNA) correlates with systemic involvement and disease activity. This clinical association points to the importance of the immune reaction to nucleic acids during the course of disease.

Cutaneous lupus lesions are characterized by prominent upregulation of type I interferons (IFN) and type I IFN induced proteins and chemokines in the skin (4). Type I IFNs are primarily produced during innate immune recognition of viral nucleic acids for antiviral defense. They lead to a broad immune stimulation know as antiviral state that can overcome immune tolerance mechanism.

This review aims to provide an overview on the role of innate immune processes caused by disturbances in the normal restriction and regulation of the nucleic acid metabolism in the pathogenesis of cutaneous lupus erythematosus.

NUCLEIC ACID SENSING

The defense against viral infections is in great part dependent on recognition of viral nucleic acids by pattern recognition receptors (PRRs) of the innate immune system (5). They developed during millions of years to protect primates and their ancestors from viral attack. The system of PRRs includes membrane, endoplasmic, and cytoplasmatic subtypes specific for either ribonucleic acid (RNA) or deoxyribonucleic acid (DNA) (6) (**Figure 1**). Cell surface and endosomal membranes of most cells are equipped with Toll like receptors (TLRs) that recognize bacterial wall components or nucleic acids. TLR3 is located at the cell surface of some tissue cells such as fibroblasts and in the endosome to recognize dsRNA. The endosomal receptors TLR7 and TLR8 recognize single stranded RNA. TLR9, expressed by plasmacytoid dendritic cells and B cells, is the only TLR recognizing dsDNA in the endosome. In the cytosol the RIG-I-like receptor (RLR) family of RNA sensors (retinoic acid inducible gene I (RIG-I) and melanoma differentiation associated gene 5 (MDA5 or IFIH1) recognize short or long stretches of dsRNA, respectively (6).

The molecules absent in melanoma 2 (AIM2), cyclic GMP–AMP synthetase (cGAS) or IFN inducible protein 16 (IFI16) can sense dsDNA in the cytosol (**Figure 1**). cGAS binds to dsDNA but can also be activated by structured ssDNA (7, 8). cGAS activation catalyzes the synthesis of cyclic GMP-AMP (cGAMP) from ATP and GTP (9). The second messenger cGAMP binds to the endoplasmic-reticulum (ER)-membrane adaptor stimulator of interferon induced genes (STING) and induces trafficking of STING to the ER/Golgi apparatus where it activates the tyrosine binding kinase 1 (TBK1) (9) (**Figure 1**). TBK1 phosphorylates the transcription factor IRF3 that enters the nucleus and induces type I IFN expression (9).

Activation of AIM2 by long dsDNA leads to oligomerization of AIM2 and subsequent formation of an inflammasome in the cytosol. The activation of the AIM2 inflammasome results in caspase 1 activation and the release of the proinflammatory cytokine IL-1beta (10, 11) (**Figure 1**). The dsDNA sensor IFI16 is located in the nucleus under steady state conditions but can be translated to the cytoplasm following UV-irradiation (12). IFI16 mediated recognition of viral DNA can also induce inflammasome formation and IL-1beta activation (12). In addition, during herpes simplex virus type 1 infection IFI16 was described to interact with STING leading to IRF3 dependent type I IFN induction (12). However, other reports describe that IFI16 is dispensable for type I IFN induction following cytomegalovirus infection (13).

Type I IFN is the dominating cytokine induced in the signaling cascade of most nucleic acid sensing PRRs. They directly or indirectly induce transcription factors that upregulate the expression of antiviral effector proteins, chemokines and cytokines mediating the antiviral defense (6). Type I IFNs include multiple subtypes such as IFNbeta and IFNalpha subtypes, depending on species, as well as the lesser-known IFNkappa secreted by keratinocytes (14). Type I IFNs can be produced by all nucleated cells and all cells can respond to type I IFNs through the type I IFN receptor (IFNAR), which binds all subtypes (15) and translates its signal through the Janus kinase 1 and tyrosine kinase (Tyk) 2 (16).

All of these antiviral sensors are not specific for viral nucleic acids but can also be activated by self RNA or DNA (14). This is relevant for an induction of anti-tumor immunity. Self-DNA from dying tumor cells has been shown to induce a STING-dependent immunity that is important for induction of a type I IFN stimulated anti-tumor defense (17, 18).

Under steady state conditions the DNA metabolism needs to be tightly regulated to prevent immune activation by self nucleic acids that would result in autoimmunity (6). Several nucleases and nucleic acid modifying enzymes ensure this task. Normally, DNA is located in the nucleus and mitochondria. DNAse I degrades free DNA that reaches the extracellular space. DNAse II eliminates intracellular DNA from the lysosomal compartment and DNAse III (also designated TREX1) protects the cytoplasm from DNA accumulation. In the nucleus, free ssDNA is bound by RAD51, and replication protein A (RPA) to prevent its translocation to the cytoplasm (19).

Any disturbance in the tightly regulated nucleic acid metabolism and the antiviral defense can lead to chronic type I IFN stimulation that will continuously alert the immune system resulting in an antiviral state. In genetically susceptibly individuals such chronic immune stimulation can lead to the development of autoimmunity.

LESSONS LEARNED FROM MONOGENIC DISEASES

Monogenic diseases are caused by a single mutation in a respective gene. This allows to understand the role of a mutated protein in the disease process and its impact on the clinical phenotype. The first reported monogenic diseases that helped to elucidate the pathogenesis of SLE were complement deficiencies (20). Homozygous deficiency in C1q is associated with childhood onset of classical discoid lupus, Raynaud's phenomenon, non-scarring alopecia, oral ulceration, and cerebral vasculitis (21, 22). A loss of complement supports the formation of large insoluble immune complexes formed by nucleic acids and autoantibodies (20). These immune complexes facilitate the uptake and recognition of nucleic acids by immune cells (23).

In the last years, monogenic diseases associated with type I IFN upregulation were described as interferonopathies

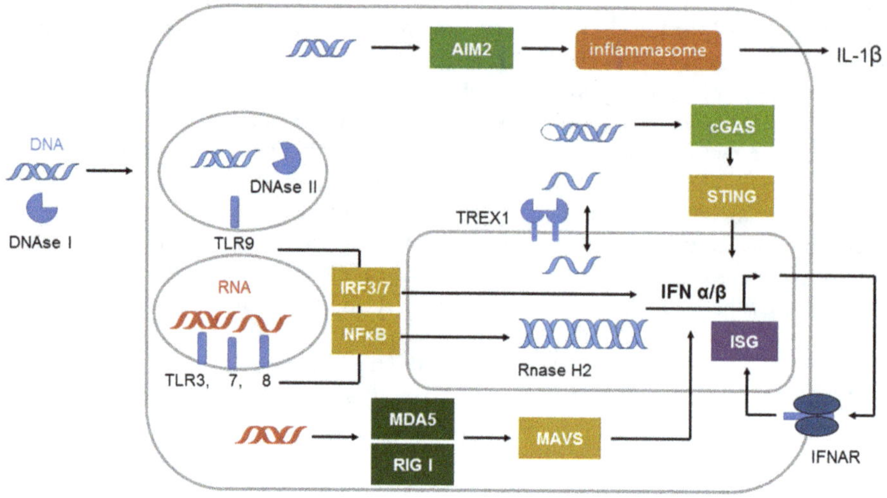

FIGURE 1 | Immune sensing pathways for RNA and DNA in the cell. The compartmentalization of nucleic acids in the cells is strictly regulated. Unrestricted RNA and DNA in the cytosol is a danger signal and can be sensed by specific receptors. The cytosolic immune receptor cyclic GMP–AMP synthetase (cGAS) detects long double-stranded DNA (dsDNA) or highly structured single-stranded DNA (ssDNA) in a special conformation. cGAS signals via STING to induce type I IFN induction. dsDNA can also be recognized by the inflammasome sensor AIM2 leading to IL-1β secretion. Cytosolic DNA is efficiently degraded by 3′ repair exonuclease 1 (TREX1) located in the outer nuclear membrane. DNAse II is restricting DNA in the endolysosome. Endosomal DNA can be detected by Toll-like receptor 9 (TLR9). TLR9 signals via interferon (IFN)-regulatory factor 7 (IRF7) and nuclear factor-κB (NF-κB) to induce type I IFN. dsRNA is detected by TLR3 and TLR7, whereas single-stranded RNA (ssRNA) is sensed by TLR7 and TLR8 in the endosome. These receptors signal via adaptor proteins to induce interferon (IFN)-regulatory factor 3 (IRF3)–IRF7 and type I IFN production and via nuclear factor-κB (NF-κB) to induce proinflammatory cytokines. The cytosolic sensors melanoma differentiation associated gene 5 (MDA5) and retinoic acid inducible gene I (RIG-I) detect dsRNA. Both signal through mitochondrial antiviral signaling protein (MAVS) to induce type I IFN production.

(24). Interferonopathies are caused by mutations that often affect genes involved in nucleic acid metabolism and nucleic acid sensing pathways. Only some mutations have been clinically associated with lupus. The other cause specific disease phenotypes that can share clinical signs and symptoms such as cutaneous ulcerations or livedo with lupus (25). Understanding the pathogenesis of such interferonopathies might help to elucidate the multiple pathogenic pathways that can cause the wide clinical spectrum of lupus erythematosus (26, 27).

Aicardi Goutières Syndrome

One of the main interferonopathy leading to an improved understanding of the induction of autoimmune disorders and especially lupus is Aicardi Goutières syndrome (28, 29). Aicardi Goutières syndrome is a rare encephalopathy of childhood and infancy that may mimic congenital viral infection (29). Affected children suffer from early onset of seizures and fever leading to mental retardation. Many patients show features of systemic autoimmunity especially SLE such as antinuclear and anti-DNA autoantibodies, arthritis as well as cold induced chilblain lupus lesions on acral locations (30).

Aicardi Goutières syndrome is genetically heterogeneous and can be based on mainly biallelic mutations in 7 different genes, that are all involved in nucleic acid metabolism or enhanced type I interferon sensing (31). The first mutations described were detected in the three prime repair exonuclease 1 (Trex1, DNase III) (32). TREX1 is a cytoplasmic exonuclease that degrades ssDNA as single oligonucleotides or overhangs in dsDNA (33, 34). It safeguards the cytosol from accumulation of nucleic acids and thereby prevents the activation of innate nucleic acid sensors by self DNA (33). TREX1 deficiency causes cellular stress and DNA damage response (33). During this process, ssDNA that cannot be retained in the nucleus due to exhaustion of the nucleic binding capacity, escapes into the cytosol and stimulates a cGAS dependent chronic type I IFN response (19, 35). Heterozygous TREX1 mutations enhance the risk for the development of SLE (36).

Other mutations inducing Aicardi Goutières syndrome affect any of the three subunits of the ribonuclease H2 (RNaseH2) (37). The nuclear enzyme is responsible for removing ribonucleotides misincorporated in the DNA and acts on RNA/DNA hybrids (38). Mutations in RNaseH2 lead to cell stress and an increase in DNA damage that is associated with an increased type I interferon production predisposing to autoimmunity and SLE (39).

Further mutations can affect the SAM Domain and HD Domain 1 (SAMHD1) controlling the building blocks of DNA, the nucleotide triphosphate pool in the cell (40). Mutations can also affect the adenosin deaminase, RNA-specific (ADAR), important for RNA editing and gain of function mutations of the cytosolic RNA sensor MDA5 (IFIH1) (31). Mutations in ADAR have been described associated with discoid lupus erythematosus (41) and IFIH1 is a risk gene for SLE (42).

STING-Associated Vasculopathy, Infantile-Onset

STING-associated vasculopathy, infantile-onset (SAVI) is an autoinflammatory disease starting in early childhood with a vasculopathy causing erythematous, pustular, or blistering infiltrates with scaling on acral locations such as the cheeks, ears, nose, and digits that may even lead to necrotizing skin lesions resulting in mutilation and scarring (43). The symptoms worsened in cold weather. Patients may develop low-grade fever flares and inflammatory interstitial lung disease associated with lung fibrosis. They also had low titer antinuclear or antiphospholipid autoantibodies. The disease is caused by a heterozygous *de novo* gain of function mutation in STING-signaling resulting in a constitutive activation of the IFNB promoter and upregulation of type I IFN stimulated genes (ISG) in blood. Interestingly, a single family with SAVI and lupus-like features due to a dominant STING mutation was reported (44).

Familial Chilblain Lupus

Familial chilblain lupus is a rare autosomal dominant monogenic form of lupus erythematosus based on heterozygous mutations in TREX1, SAMHD1, or STING (45–47). The disease is characterized by cold induced livoid infiltrates on acral locations that tend to ulcerate and occur since early childhood (48, 49). Systemic involvement is possible and includes arthritis, antinuclear antibodies, and cytopenias. Type I IFNs are upregulated in skin and blood of the patients (50, 51). Patient fibroblasts with TREX1 mutation respond to cold exposure with cellular stress, senescence, and ISG induction (52).

CANDLE Syndrome

Chronic atypical neutrophilic dermatosis with lipodystrophy and elevated temperature (CANDLE) is an autosomal recessive inherited autoinflammatory disease (53). Starting in infancy, patients suffer from fever accompanied by a widespread, violaceous and often annular, cutaneous eruption. Further symptoms are partial lipodystrophy, hepatomegaly, joint contractions with muscle atrophy and arthralgias. An interferon signature has been found in blood of affected patients. CANDLE is caused by homozygous mutations in PSMB8 encoding proteasome subunit β type 8, which functions as the chymotrypsin-like catalytic subunit of the immunoproteasome and is involved in processing of antigens presented by MHC class-I (54). A recent genome wide imputation approach identified a rare variation in PSMB8 as candidate gene for SLE in a European ancestry population (55).

Childhood-Onset Polyarteritis Nodosa—ADA2 Deficiency

Childhood-onset polyarteritis nodosa is an autosomal recessive disease caused by biallelic mutations of CECR1 (cat eye syndrome chromosome region, candidate 1), encoding extracellular deaminase 2 (ADA2) that deaminates adenosine to inosine (56). A defect in this nucleosid modification induced monocyte-macrophage polarization toward the M1 subset. This inflammatory subset impaired vascular integrity (56). All the patients presented with recurrent fevers and livedo racemosa in early childhood (56, 57). Cutaneous involvement included erythematous nodules and plaques that healed with scars or tissue necrosis leading to mutilation.

DNAse I

Homozygous mutations in DNAse I impair restriction of DNA in the extracellular space. Affected patients suffered from childhood onset SLE with fever, generalized rash, kidney involvement, and prominent autoantibodys directed against dsDNA, and Ro (58). Furthermore, mutations in one of the three human homologs of DNase I, DNase 1L3, caused SLE with onset during childhood, autoantibody formation and nephritis (59).

DNAse II

Patients with biallelic mutations in DNase II and a functional loss of this lysosomal endonuclease develop an autoinflammatory disease state with pancytopenia, deforming arthropathy, glomerulonephritis, mild learning difficulties in school, cutaneous ulcerations, and vasculitis like skin lesions starting in early childhood (60). Deficiency of DNase II in fibroblasts was associated with enhanced expression of ISGs. This ISG upregulation was also detectable in blood indicating the importance of type I IFN in the induction of the clinical symptoms. Variants in DNaseII showed weak associations with the risk of nephritis among korean SLE patients (61).

IMPLICATIONS FOR MULTIFACTORIAL CUTANEOUS LUPUS ERYTHEMATOSUS

Healthy skin has a regular turnover of keratinocytes and is continuously exposed to cell damaging influences such as irradiation. The daily occurring ubiquitous cell debris needs to be safely eliminated by normal immune processes. This process is ensured by several mechanisms that are crucial for the maintenance of self tolerance (1). Phagocytes can recognize and engulf apoptotic cells by altered cell membrane components or self antigens opsonized by autoantibodies or complement components (1). In addition, nucleases degrade circulating nucleic acids. Defective clearance mechanisms result in secondary necrosis and release of self antigens that can be accessed by innate immune cells (62). Lesional lupus skin biopsies characteristically show an interface dermatits with a varying number of dyskeratotic dying keratinocytes. It has been described that such apoptotic cell debris was present for prolonged time in lupus lesions indicating a defect in apoptotic clearance (63). Due to a defect in phagocytes of SLE patients such apoptotic debris can be found in germinal centers attached to follicular dendritic cells that can present autoantigens (64, 65). In addition, mutations in the genes encoding the complement components and impairing regular clearance are among the strongest risk factors for the development of SLE including cutaneous involvement (20). Furthermore, defects in DNAse I, that breaks down extracellular DNA, are associated with lupus erythematosus (66).

If nucleic acids are not removed from the extracellular space, they can serve as autoantigens. Especially if they are complexed with antimicrobial peptides such as LL37, autoantibodies, or the architectural chromosomal protein and proinflammatory mediator high mobility group box protein 1 (HMGB1), nucleic acids are immunogenic, protected from degradation and foster

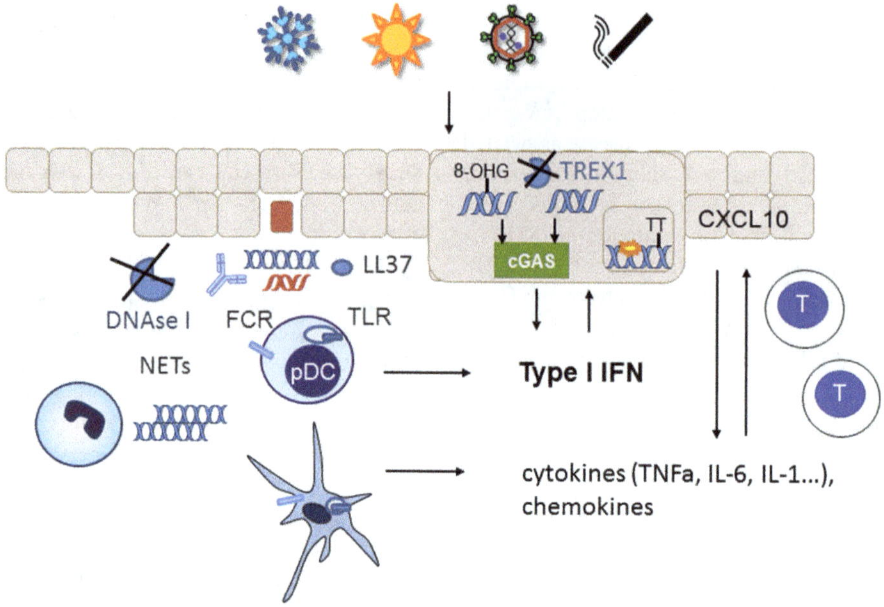

FIGURE 2 | Nucelic acid immunity in the pathogenesis of cutaneous lupus erythematosus. Cutaneous lupus lesions frequently show apoptotic keratinocytes and nucleic acids complexed with autoantibodies along the basement membrane zone (blue DNA, red RNA). In patients with defects in nucleic acids clearance such as complement defects or impaired function of DNase I these nucleic acids can be taken up by immune cells such as plasmacytoid (pDC) or myeloid dendritic cells and sensed by TLRs. Neutrophils can extrude additional DNA into the extracellular space. Phagocytosis of nucleic acids is enhanced by immuncomplexes, complexation with antimicrobial peptides such as LL37 and supported by FC-receptors. The resulting cytokine and chemokine production stimulates an adaptive immune response with infiltration of T cells into the skin. Environmental trigger factors such as UV-irradition or smoking induce DNA damage and reactive oxygen species that can cause oxidation of DNA. The 8-hydroxyguanosine (8-OHG) modification protects DNA against degradation by TREX1. The unrestricted DNA can accumulate in the cytoplasm and induce cGAS stimulation leading to type I IFN induction. In patients with deficiency in TREX1 intracellular DNA can accumulate as danger signal. Other mutations such as RNAseH2 cause ribonucleotide accumulation in DNA that predisposes to cyclobutanpyrimide formation after UV-irradiation and thereby enhance cellular stress.

the uptake by monocytes/macrophages and dendritic cells (67–70) (**Figure 2**). The latter engulf immune complexes in their endosomal compartments where they can access nucleic acid sensing TLRs (**Figure 2**). Monocytes and myeloid dendritic cells can sense RNA by TLR 7 and 8 that results in NFkappa B and TNF alpha upregulation (71). Recognition of HMGB1 nucleosome complexes by TLR2 can further potentiate this cytokine induction that mediates the stimulation of the adaptive immune system (70). TLR3, expressed by tissue resident keratinocytes and fibroblasts senses self RNA that can lead to local type I IFN induction. Plasmacytoid dendritic cells can sense dsDNA by TLR9 and stimulate a robust type I IFN response after the uptake of immune complexes or DNA bound to antimicrobial peptides (23). An accumulation of plasmacytoid dendritic cells was reported in certain types of cutaneous lupus (72) (**Figure 2**).

In addition to unrestricted cellular debris as source of extracellular self-nucleic acids an intense active extrusion of DNA by leukocytes has been described in SLE patients (73). These neutrophil extracellular traps are a known danger signals in SLE and their deposition has also been described in cutaneous lupus lesions (74) (**Figure 2**). In addition, it has been reported that neutrophils from SLE patients contained elevated levels of oxidized mitochondrial DNA compared with healthy controls (75). Those neutrophils could not degrade the DNA by mitophagy or lysosomal degradation but eventually extruded the oxidized mitochondrial DNA upon stimulation with RNP autoantibodies (76). The modified mitochondrial DNA was a potent immune stimulus for plasmacytoid dendritic cells (76) and was suggested to induce a STING dependent systemic type I IFN induction in mice (75).

Furthermore, accumulation of intracellular cytoplasmic DNA has been observed in epithelial cells of cutaneous lupus lesions (77) (**Figure 2**). Normally, this DNA should be eliminated by TREX1. However, UV-induced oxidative DNA-modification has been shown to render DNA resistant to degradation by the cytoplasmic DNAse TREX1 (78). UV-irradiation is one of the most important trigger factors for the discoid and tumidus forms of cutaneous lupus and relevant for induction of acute and subacute cutaneous lupus and SLE. Impaired restriction of modified DNA in the cytoplasm upon UV-irradiation could therefore be a relevant disease trigger factor and pathogenic mechanism for cutaneous lupus. Deficiency of TREX1 due to heterogeneous mutations is an additional risk factor for the development of photosensitive forms of SLE (36). In those patients, DNA accumulates in the cytoplasm due to incomplete restriction by TREX1 and can trigger the cGAS-STING pathway leading to type I IFN activation (**Figure 2**).

UV irradiation is also relevant in the pathogenesis of lupus in patients with SLE and mutations in any of the three subunits of RNase H2 (39). This nuclear enzyme is responsible for eliminating misincorporated ribonucleotides from DNA (79). Mutations that impair this function lead to an enhanced number of ribonucleotides in DNA. Ribonucleotide containing dsDNA has different steric properties that facilitate the formation of cyclobutanpyrimidine dimers in DNA upon UV-irradiation (39). These cyclobutanpyrimidine dimers are among the most frequent UV- induced DNA lesions that need to be eliminated by the DNA repair machinery (80). In RNaseH2 deficient cells from lupus patients UV irradiation causes enhanced DNA damage that consequently led to a prolonged and elevated type I IFN response especially if other trigger factors such as extracellular nucleic acids are present (39) (**Figure 2**).

Activation of the type I IFN pathway is a hallmark of all cutaneous lupus lesions and can be demonstrated by activation of myxovirus resistence protein A (MXA) and the expression of type I IFN induced chemokines such as CXCL10 in the skin. Keratinocytes from SLE patients have been shown to be primed by type I IFNs suggesting continuous type I IFN production in the skin of lupus patients (81, 82). Type I IFNs can also induce expression of inflammasome components such as AIM2 and IFI16. Inflammasome activation in keratinocytes *in vitro* can lead to upregulation IL-18. This cytokine is detectable in lupus lesions and can induce MHC class II expression and CXCL10 upregulation (83). However, inflammasomes also negatively regulate the type I IFN pathway (84). The relevance of these interactions for cutaneous inflammation in lupus is not fully understood.

Chemokines like CXCL10 have the potential to recruit T cells into the skin (4, 85) (**Figure 2**). Their influx is accompanied by histiocytes, dendritic cells and eventually neutrophils, which fuel the immunologic response and lead to tissue destruction, swelling, and erythema.

In conclusion, stimulation of an immune response based on activation of innate nucleic acid sensors in tissue resident or immune cells of the skin seems to be an important pathogenic pathway in the induction of cutaneous lupus and might have implications for disseminating systemic disease. The understanding of pathogenic concepts in lupus might allow a categorization of disease subtypes based on etiology. Phenotype genotype correlations revealed that patients with genetic defects in complement components or DNAse I leading to an enhanced prevalence of extracellular DNA are often affected by severe discoid lupus, exanthemas, and prominent kidney involvement (20). Patients with mutations in TREX1 accumulate intracellular DNA and frequently suffer from chilblain lupus but less frequent organ involvement (50, 86). Future detailed genetic analysis in random lupus patients might substantiate this subtyping and help to develop individual therapies. The currently used drugs include corticosteroids, hydroxychloroquine, and methotrexate (3, 87). They have broad anti-inflammatory effects but were not approved for cutaneous lupus. Hydroxychloroquine impairs nucleic acid sensing by building complexes with DNA or RNA (88). It had effectivity in a population of patients with cutaneous lupus and type I IFN signature whereas hydroxychloroquine refractory patients harbored increased numbers of TNF alpha secreting myeloid dendritic cells and required additional quinacrine treatment (89). This further indicates the clinical variability of the immunologic response in cutaneous lupus patients and underlines the need for detailed pathogenic exploration and personalized medicine. Inhibitors of type I IFN and type I IFN receptor have shown clinical efficacy for cutaneous lupus in phase II clinical trials (90, 91). Furthermore, the janus kinase inhibitors that interfere with signal transduction of the type I IFN receptor have shown effectivity in single patients with cutaneous chilblain lupus (47, 52, 92). These therapeutic efforts may pave the way for new treatment options in future. A detailed understanding of disease pathogenesis is a prerequisite for this development.

AUTHOR CONTRIBUTIONS

CG wrote the text and designed the figures.

ACKNOWLEDGMENTS

The discussions with the cooperating researchers in the TRR237 nucleic acid immunity are gratefully acknowledged.

REFERENCES

1. Liu Z, Davidson A. Taming lupus-a new understanding of pathogenesis is leading to clinical advances. *Nat Med.* (2012) 18:871–882. doi: 10.1038/nm.2752
2. Kuhn A, Landmann A. The classificration and diagnosis of cutaneous lupus erythematosus. *J Autoimmun.* (2014) 48–49:14–9. doi: 10.1016/j.jaut.2014.01.021
3. Hejazi EZ, Werth VP. Cutaneous lupus erythematosus: an update on pathogenesis, diagnosis and treatment. *Am J Clin Dermatol.* (2016) 17:135–46. doi: 10.1007/s40257-016-0173-9
4. Wenzel J, Zahn S, Mikus S, Wiechert A, Bieber T, Tuting T. The expression pattern of interferon-inducible proteins reflects the characteristic histological distribution of infiltrating immune cells in different cutaneous lupus erythematosus subsets. *Br J Dermatol.* (2007) 157:752–7. doi: 10.1111/j.1365-2133.2007.08137.x
5. Medzhitov R, Janeway CA Jr. Innate immunity: the virtues of a nonclonal system of recognition. *Cell.* (1997) 91:295–8. doi: 10.1016/S0092-8674(00)80412-2
6. Schlee M, Hartmann G. Discriminating self from non-self in nucleic acid sensing. *Nat Rev Immunol.* (2016) 16:566–80. doi: 10.1038/nri.2016.78
7. Andreeva L, Hiller B, Kostrewa D, Lassig C, de Oliveira Mann CC, Jan Drexler D, et al. cGAS senses long and HMGB/TFAM-bound U-turn DNA by forming protein-DNA ladders. *Nature.* (2017) 549, 394–8. doi: 10.1038/nature23890
8. Herzner AM, Hagmann CA, Goldeck M, Wolter S, Kubler K, Wittmann S, et al. Sequence-specific activation of the DNA sensor cGAS by Y-form DNA structures as found in primary HIV-1 cDNA. *Nat Immunol.* (2015) 16:1025–33. doi: 10.1038/ni.3267

9. Chen Q, Sun L, Chen ZJ. Regulation and function of the cGAS-STING pathway of cytosolic DNA sensing. *Nat Immunol.* (2016) 17:1142–9. doi: 10.1038/ni.3558
10. Fernandes-Alnemri T, Yu JW, Datta P, Wu J, Alnemri ES. AIM2 activates the inflammasome and cell death in response to cytoplasmic DNA. *Nature.* (2009) 458:509–513. doi: 10.1038/nature07710
11. Hornung V, Ablasser A, Charrel-Dennis M, Bauernfeind F, Horvath G, Caffrey DR, et al. AIM2 recognizes cytosolic dsDNA and forms a caspase-1-activating inflammasome with ASC. *Nature.* (2009) 458:514–8. doi: 10.1038/nature07725
12. Caneparo V, Landolfo S, Gariglio M, De Andrea M. The absent in melanoma 2-like receptor IFN-inducible protein 16 as an inflammasome regulator in systemic lupus erythematosus: the dark side of sensing microbes. *Front Immunol.* (2018) 9:1180. doi: 10.3389/fimmu.2018.01180
13. Gray EE, Winship D, Snyder JM, Child SJ, Geballe AP, Stetson DB. The AIM2-like receptors are dispensable for the interferon response to intracellular DNA. *Immunity.* (2016) 45:255–66. doi: 10.1016/j.immuni.2016.06.015
14. Pichlmair A, Reis e Sousa C. Innate recognition of viruses. *Immunity.* (2007) 27:370–83. doi: 10.1016/j.immuni.2007.08.012
15. Stark GR, Kerr IM, Williams BR, Silverman RH, Schreiber RD. How cells respond to interferons. *Annu Rev Biochem.* (1998) 67:227–64. doi: 10.1146/annurev.biochem.67.1.227
16. Schwartz DM, Kanno Y, Villarino A, Ward M, Gadina M, O'Shea JJ. JAK inhibition as a therapeutic strategy for immune and inflammatory diseases. *Nat Rev Drug Discov.* (2017) 16:843–62. doi: 10.1038/nrd.2017.201
17. Woo SR, Corrales L, Gajewski TF. Innate immune recognition of cancer. *Annu Rev Immunol.* (2015) 33:445–74. doi: 10.1146/annurev-immunol-032414-112043
18. Woo SR, Fuertes MB, Corrales L, Spranger S, Furdyna MJ, Leung MY, et al. STING-dependent cytosolic DNA sensing mediates innate immune recognition of immunogenic tumors. *Immunity.* (2014) 41:830–42. doi: 10.1016/j.immuni.2014.10.017
19. Wolf C, Rapp A, Berndt N, Staroske W, Schuster M, Dobrick-Mattheuer M, et al. RPA and Rad51 constitute a cell intrinsic mechanism to protect the cytosol from self DNA. *Nat Commun.* (2016) 7:11752. doi: 10.1038/ncomms11752
20. Manderson AP, Botto M, Walport MJ. The role of complement in the development of systemic lupus erythematosus. *Annu Rev Immunol.* (2004) 22:431–56. doi: 10.1146/annurev.immunol.22.012703.104549
21. Walport MJ, Davies KA, Botto M. C1q and systemic lupus erythematosus. *Immunobiology.* (1998) 199:265–85. doi: 10.1016/S0171-2985(98)80032-6
22. Stone NM, Williams A, Wilkinson JD, Bird G. Systemic lupus erythematosus with C1q deficiency. *Br J Dermatol.* (2000) 142:521–4. doi: 10.1046/j.1365-2133.2000.03369.x
23. Means TK, Latz E, Hayashi F, Murali MR, Golenbock DT, Luster AD. Human lupus autoantibody-DNA complexes activate DCs through cooperation of CD32 and TLR9. *J Clin Invest.* (2005) 115:407–17. doi: 10.1172/JCI200523025
24. Crow YJ. Type I interferonopathies: a novel set of inborn errors of immunity. *Ann NY Acad Sci.* (2011) 1238:91–8. doi: 10.1111/j.1749-6632.2011.06220.x
25. Lee-Kirsch MA. The Type I interferonopathies. *Annu Rev Med.* (2017) 68:297–315. doi: 10.1146/annurev-med-050715-104506
26. Baechler EC, Batliwalla FM, Karypis G, Gaffney PM, Ortmann WA, Espe KJ, et al. Interferon-inducible gene expression signature in peripheral blood cells of patients with severe lupus. *Proc Natl Acad Sci USA.* (2003) 100:2610–15. doi: 10.1073/pnas.0337679100
27. Alperin JM, Ortiz-Fernandez L, Sawalha AH. Monogenic lupus: a developing paradigm of disease. *Front Immunol.* (2018) 9:2496. doi: 10.3389/fimmu.2018.02496
28. Crow YJ, Rehwinkel J. Aicardi-Goutieres syndrome and related phenotypes: linking nucleic acid metabolism with autoimmunity. *Hum Mol Genet.* (2009) 18:R130–6. doi: 10.1093/hmg/ddp293
29. Aicardi J, Goutieres F. A progressive familial encephalopathy in infancy with calcifications of the basal ganglia and chronic cerebrospinal fluid lymphocytosis. *Ann Neurol.* (1984) 15:49–54. doi: 10.1002/ana.410150109
30. Ramantani G, Kohlhase J, Hertzberg C, Innes AM, Engel K, Hunger S, et al. Expanding the phenotypic spectrum of lupus erythematosus in Aicardi-Goutieres syndrome. *Arthritis Rheum.* (2010) 62:1469–77. doi: 10.1002/art.27367
31. Crow YJ, Manel N. Aicardi-Goutieres syndrome and the type I interferonopathies. *Nat Rev Immunol.* (2015) 15:429–40. doi: 10.1038/nri3850
32. Crow YJ, Hayward BE, Parmar R, Robins P, Leitch A, Ali M, et al. Mutations in the gene encoding the 3'-5' DNA exonuclease TREX1 cause Aicardi-Goutieres syndrome at the AGS1 locus. *Nat Genet.* (2006) 38:917–20. doi: 10.1038/ng1845
33. Yang YG, Lindahl T, Barnes DE. Trex1 exonuclease degrades ssDNA to prevent chronic checkpoint activation and autoimmune disease. *Cell.* (2007) 131:873–86. doi: 10.1016/j.cell.2007.10.017
34. Mazur DJ, Perrino FW. Identification and expression of the TREX1 and TREX2 cDNA sequences encoding mammalian 3'->5' exonucleases. *J Biol Chem.* (1999) 274:19655–60. doi: 10.1074/jbc.274.28.19655
35. Gao D, Li T, Li XD, Chen X, Li QZ, Wight-Carter M, Chen ZJ. Activation of cyclic GMP-AMP synthase by self-DNA causes autoimmune diseases. *Proc Natl Acad Sci USA.* (2015) 112:E5699–705. doi: 10.1073/pnas.1516465112
36. Lee-Kirsch MA, Gong M, Chowdhury D, Senenko L, Engel K, Lee YA, et al. Mutations in the gene encoding the 3'-5' DNA exonuclease TREX1 are associated with systemic lupus erythematosus. *Nat Genet.* (2007) 39:1065–7. doi: 10.1038/ng2091
37. Crow YJ, Leitch A, Hayward BE, Garner A, Parmar R, Griffith E, et al. Mutations in genes encoding ribonuclease H2 subunits cause Aicardi-Goutieres syndrome and mimic congenital viral brain infection. *Nat Genet.* (2006) 38:910–6. doi: 10.1038/ng1842
38. Reijns MA, Rabe B, Rigby RE, Mill P, Astell KR, Lettice LA, et al. Enzymatic removal of ribonucleotides from DNA is essential for mammalian genome integrity and development. *Cell.* (2012) 149:1008–22. doi: 10.1016/j.cell.2012.04.011
39. Gunther C, Kind B, Reijns MA, Berndt N, Martinez-Bueno M, Wolf C, et al. Defective removal of ribonucleotides from DNA promotes systemic autoimmunity. *J Clin Invest.* (2015) 125:413–24. doi: 10.1172/JCI78001
40. Rice GI, Bond J, Asipu A, Brunette RL, Manfield IW, Carr IM, et al. Mutations involved in Aicardi-Goutieres syndrome implicate SAMHD1 as regulator of the innate immune response. *Nat Genet.* (2009) 41:829–32. doi: 10.1038/ng.373
41. Al-Saif F, Alhumidi A, Alhallaf RA. Dyschromatosis symmetrica hereditaria with cutaneous lupus erythematosus and hyperthyroidism. *Int Med Case Rep J.* (2017) 10:149–52. doi: 10.2147/IMCRJ.S132489
42. Wang C, Ahlford A, Laxman N, Nordmark G, Eloranta ML, Gunnarsson I, et al. Contribution of IKBKE and IFIH1 gene variants to SLE susceptibility. *Genes Immun.* (2013) 14:217–22. doi: 10.1038/gene.2013.9
43. Liu Y, Jesus AA, Marrero B, Yang D, Ramsey SE, Montealegre Sanchez GA, Tenbrock K, et al. Activated STING in a vascular and pulmonary syndrome. *N Engl Med J.* (2014) 371:507–18. doi: 10.1056/NEJMoa1312625
44. Jeremiah N, Neven B, Gentili M, Callebaut I, Maschalidi S, Stolzenberg MC, et al. Inherited STING-activating mutation underlies a familial inflammatory syndrome with lupus-like manifestations. *J Clin Invest.* (2014) 124:5516–20. doi: 10.1172/JCI79100
45. Lee-Kirsch MA, Chowdhury D, Harvey S, Gong M, Senenko L, Engel K, et al. A mutation in TREX1 that impairs susceptibility to granzyme A-mediated cell death underlies familial chilblain lupus. *J Mol Med.* (2007) 85:531–7. doi: 10.1007/s00109-007-0199-9
46. Ravenscroft JC, Suri M, Rice GI, Szynkiewicz M, Crow YJ. Autosomal dominant inheritance of a heterozygous mutation in SAMHD1 causing familial chilblain lupus A. *Am J Med Genet A.* (2011) 155A:235–7. doi: 10.1002/ajmg.a.33778
47. Konig N, Fiehn C, Wolf C, Schuster M, Cura Costa E, Tungler V, et al. Familial chilblain lupus due to a gain-of-function mutation in STING. *Ann Rheum Dis.* (2017) 76:468–72. doi: 10.1136/annrheumdis-2016-209841
48. Gunther C, Meurer M, Stein A, Viehweg A, Lee-Kirsch MA. Familial chilblain lupus–a monogenic form of cutaneous lupus erythematosus due to a heterozygous mutation in TREX1. *Dermatology.* (2009) 219:162–6. doi: 10.1159/000222430
49. Lee-Kirsch MA, Gong M, Schulz H, Ruschendorf F, Stein A, Pfeiffer C, et al. Familial chilblain lupus, a monogenic form of cutaneous lupus erythematosus, maps to chromosome 3p. *Am J Hum Genet.* (2006) 79:731–7. doi: 10.1086/507848

50. Gunther C, Berndt N, Wolf C, Lee-Kirsch MA. Familial chilblain lupus due to a novel mutation in the exonuclease III domain of 3' repair exonuclease 1 (TREX1). *JAMA Dermatol.* (2015) 151:426–31. doi: 10.1001/jamadermatol.2014.3438
51. Peschke K, Friebe F, Zimmermann N, Wahlicht T, Schumann T, Achleitner M, et al. Deregulated Type I IFN response in TREX1-associated familial chilblain lupus. *Invest Dermatol J.* (2014) 134:1456–9. doi: 10.1038/jid.2013.496
52. Zimmermann N, Wolf C, Schwenke R, Luth A, Schmidt F, Engel K, et al. Assessment of clinical response to janus kinase inhibition in patients with familial chilblain lupus and TREX1 mutation. *JAMA Dermatol.* (2019) 155:342–6. doi: 10.1001/jamadermatol.2018.5077
53. Torrelo A, Patel S, Colmenero I, Gurbindo D, Lendinez F, Hernandez A, Lopez-Robledillo JC, et al. Chronic atypical neutrophilic dermatosis with lipodystrophy and elevated temperature (CANDLE) syndrome. *J Am Acad Dermatol.* (2010) 62:489–95. doi: 10.1016/j.jaad.2009.04.046
54. Agarwal AK, Xing C, DeMartino GN, Mizrachi D, Hernandez MD, Sousa AB, et al. PSMB8 encoding the beta5i proteasome subunit is mutated in joint contractures, muscle atrophy, microcytic anemia, and panniculitis-induced lipodystrophy syndrome. *Am J Hum Genet.* (2010) 87:866–72. doi: 10.1016/j.ajhg.2010.10.031
55. Martínez-Bueno M, Alarcón-Riquelme ME. Exploring impact of rare variation in systemic lupus erythematosus by a genome wide imputation approach. *Front Immunol.* (2019) 10:258. doi: 10.3389/fimmu.2019.00258
56. Zhou Q, Yang D, Ombrello AK, Zavialov AV, Toro C, Zavialov AV, et al. Early-onset stroke and vasculopathy associated with mutations in ADA2. *N Engl J Med.* (2014) 370:911–20. doi: 10.1056/NEJMoa1307361
57. Skrabl-Baumgartner A, Plecko B, Schmidt WM, Konig N, Hershfield M, Gruber-Sedlmayr U, et al. Autoimmune phenotype with type I interferon signature in two brothers with ADA2 deficiency carrying a novel CECR1 mutation. *Pediatr Rheumatol Online J.* (2017) 15:67. doi: 10.1186/s12969-017-0193-x
58. Dainichi T, Koga H, Tsuji T, Ishii N, Ohyama B, Ueda A, et al. From anti-p200 pemphigoid to anti-laminin gamma1 pemphigoid. *Dermatol J.* (2010) 37:231–8. doi: 10.1111/j.1346-8138.2009.00793.x
59. Al-Mayouf SM, Sunker A, Abdwani R, Abrawi SA, Almurshedi F, Alhashmi N, et al. Loss-of-function variant in DNASE1L3 causes a familial form of systemic lupus erythematosus. *Nat Genet.* (2011) 43:1186–8. doi: 10.1038/ng.975
60. Rodero MP, Tesser A, Bartok E, Rice GI, Della Mina E, Depp M, et al. Type I interferon-mediated autoinflammation due to DNase II deficiency. *Nat Commun.* (2017) 8:2176. doi: 10.1038/s41467-017-01932-3
61. Shin HD, Park BL, Cheong HS, Lee HS, Jun JB, Bae SC. DNase II polymorphisms associated with risk of renal disorder among systemic lupus erythematosus patients. *J Hum Genet.* (2005) 50:107. doi: 10.1007/s10038-004-0227-3
62. Rosen A, Casciola-Rosen L. Autoantigens as substrates for apoptotic proteases: implications for the pathogenesis of systemic autoimmune disease. *Cell Death Diff.* (1999) 6:6–12. doi: 10.1038/sj.cdd.4400460
63. Kuhn A, Herrmann M, Kleber S, Beckmann-Welle M, Fehsel K, Martin-Villalba A, et al. Accumulation of apoptotic cells in the epidermis of patients with cutaneous lupus erythematosus after ultraviolet irradiation. *Arthritis Rheum.* (2006) 54:939–50. doi: 10.1002/art.21658
64. Kuenkele S, Beyer TD, Voll RE, Kalden JR, Herrmann M. Impaired clearance of apoptotic cells in systemic lupus erythematosus: challenge of T and B cell tolerance. *Curr Rheumatol Rep.* (2003) 5:175–7. doi: 10.1007/s11926-003-0061-1
65. Herrmann M, Voll RE, Zoller OM, Hagenhofer M, Ponner BB, Kalden JR. Impaired phagocytosis of apoptotic cell material by monocyte-derived macrophages from patients with systemic lupus erythematosus. *Arthritis Rheum.* (1998) 41:1241–50. doi: 10.1002/1529-0131(199807)41:7<1241::AID-ART15>3.0.CO;2-H
66. Martinez-Valle F, Balada E, Ordi-Ros J, Bujan-Rivas S, Sellas-Fernandez A, Vilardell-Tarres M. DNase 1 activity in patients with systemic lupus erythematosus: relationship with epidemiological, clinical, immunological and therapeutical features. *Lupus.* (2009) 18:418–23. doi: 10.1177/0961203308098189
67. Lande R, Gregorio J, Facchinetti V, Chatterjee B, Wang YH, Homey B, et al. Plasmacytoid dendritic cells sense self-DNA coupled with antimicrobial peptide. *Nature.* (2007) 449:564–9. doi: 10.1038/nature06116
68. Munoz LE, Janko C, Chaurio RA, Schett G, Gaipl US, Herrmann M. IgG opsonized nuclear remnants from dead cells cause systemic inflammation in SLE. *Autoimmunity.* (2010) 43:232–5. doi: 10.3109/08916930903510930
69. Tian J, Avalos AM, Mao SY, Chen B, Senthil K, Wu H, et al. Toll-like receptor 9-dependent activation by DNA-containing immune complexes is mediated by HMGB1 and RAG*Nat Immunol E.* (2007) 8:487–96. doi: 10.1038/ni1457
70. Urbonaviciute V, Furnrohr BG, Meister S, Munoz L, Heyder P, De Marchis F, et al. Induction of inflammatory and immune responses by HMGB1-nucleosome complexes: implications for the pathogenesis of SLE. *J Exp Med.* (2008) 205:3007–18. doi: 10.1084/jem.20081165
71. Hansel A, Gunther C, Baran W, Bidier M, Lorenz HM, Schmitz M, et al. Human 6-sulfo LacNAc (slan) dendritic cells have molecular and functional features of an important pro-inflammatory cell type in lupus erythematosus. *Autoimmun J.* (2013) 40:1–8. doi: 10.1016/j.jaut.2012.07.005
72. Farkas L, Beiske K, Lund-Johansen F, Brandtzaeg P, Jahnsen FL. Plasmacytoid dendritic cells (natural interferon- alpha/beta-producing cells) accumulate in cutaneous lupus erythematosus lesions. *Am Pathol J.* (2001) 159:237–43. doi: 10.1016/S0002-9440(10)61689-6
73. Leffler J, Martin M, Gullstrand B, Tyden H, Lood C, Truedsson L, et al. Neutrophil extracellular traps that are not degraded in systemic lupus erythematosus activate complement exacerbating the disease. *J Immunol.* (2012) 188:3522–31. doi: 10.4049/jimmunol.1102404
74. Villanueva E, Yalavarthi S, Berthier CC, Hodgin JB, Khandpur R, Lin AM, et al. Netting neutrophils induce endothelial damage, infiltrate tissues, and expose immunostimulatory molecules in systemic lupus erythematosus. *J Immunol.* (2011) 187:538–52. doi: 10.4049/jimmunol.1100450
75. Lood C, Blanco LP, Purmalek MM, Carmona-Rivera C, De Ravin SS, Smith CK, et al. Neutrophil extracellular traps enriched in oxidized mitochondrial DNA are interferogenic and contribute to lupus-like disease. *Nat Med.* (2016) 22:146–53. doi: 10.1038/nm.4027
76. Caielli S, Athale S, Domic B, Murat E, Chandra M, Banchereau R, et al. Oxidized mitochondrial nucleoids released by neutrophils drive type I interferon production in human lupus. *J Exp Med.* (2016) 213:697–713. doi: 10.1084/jem.20151876
77. Scholtissek B, Zahn S, Maier J, Klaeschen S, Braegelmann C, Hoelzel M, et al. Immunostimulatory endogenous nucleic acids drive the lesional inflammation in cutaneous lupus erythematosus. *J Invest Dermatol.* (2017) 137:1484–92. doi: 10.1016/j.jid.2017.03.018
78. Gehrke N, Mertens C, Zillinger T, Wenzel J, Bald T, Zahn S, et al. Oxidative damage of DNA confers resistance to cytosolic nuclease TREX1 degradation and potentiates STING-dependent immune sensing. *Immunity.* (2013) 39:482–95. doi: 10.1016/j.immuni.2013.08.004
79. Nick McElhinny SA, Kumar D, Clark AB, Watt DL, Watts BE, Lundstrom EB, et al. Genome instability due to ribonucleotide incorporation into DNA. *Nat Chem Biol.* (2010) 6:774–81. doi: 10.1038/nchembio.424
80. Rastogi RP, Richa, Kumar A, Tyagi MB, Sinha RP. Molecular mechanisms of ultraviolet radiation-induced DNA damage and repair. *Nucleic Acids J.* (2010) 2010:592980. doi: 10.4061/2010/592980
81. Tsoi LC, Hile GA, Berthier CC, Sarkar MK, Reed TJ, Liu J, et al. Hypersensitive IFN responses in lupus keratinocytes reveal key mechanistic determinants in cutaneous lupus. *J Immunol.* (2019) 202:2121–30. doi: 10.4049/jimmunol.1800650
82. Sarkar MK, Hile GA, Tsoi LC, Xing X, Liu J, Liang Y, et al. Photosensitivity and type I IFN responses in cutaneous lupus are driven by epidermal-derived interferon kappa. *Ann Rheum Dis.* (2018) 77:1653–64. doi: 10.1136/annrheumdis-2018-213197
83. Wittmann M, Macdonald A, Renne J. IL-18 and skin inflammation. *Autoimmun Rev.* (2009) 9:45–8. doi: 10.1016/j.autrev.2009.03.003
84. Choubey D, Panchanathan R. Absent in Melanoma 2 proteins in SLE. *Clin Immunol.* (2017) 176:42–8. doi: 10.1016/j.clim.2016.12.011
85. Wenzel J, Worenkamper E, Freutel S, Henze S, Haller O, Bieber T, et al. Enhanced type I interferon signalling promotes Th1-biased inflammation in cutaneous lupus erythematosus. *Pathol J.* (2005) 205:435–42. doi: 10.1002/path.1721
86. Gunther C, Hillebrand M, Brunk J, Lee-Kirsch MA. Systemic involvement in TREX1-associated familial chilblain lupus. *J Am Acad Dermatol.* (2013) 69:e179–81. doi: 10.1016/j.jaad.2013.04.020

87. Kuhn A, Aberer E, Bata-Csorgo Z, Caproni M, Dreher A, Frances C, et al. S2k guideline for treatment of cutaneous lupus erythematosus - guided by the European Dermatology Forum (EDF) in cooperation with the European Academy of Dermatology and Venereology (EADV). *J Eur Acad Dermatol Venereol.* (2017) 31:389–404. doi: 10.1111/jdv.14053
88. Kuznik A, Bencina M, Svajger U, Jeras M, Rozman B, Jerala R. Mechanism of endosomal TLR inhibition by antimalarial drugs and imidazoquinolines. *Immunol J.* (2011) 186:4794–804. doi: 10.4049/jimmunol.1000702
89. Zeidi M, Kim HJ, Werth VP. Increased myeloid dendritic cells and TNF-alpha expression predicts poor response to hydroxychloroquine in cutaneous lupus erythematosus. *J Invest Dermatol.* (2019) 139:324–32. doi: 10.1016/j.jid.2018.07.041
90. Khamashta M, Merrill JT, Werth VP, Furie R, Kalunian K, Illei GG, et al. C.D.s. investigators, Sifalimumab, an anti-interferon-alpha monoclonal antibody, in moderate to severe systemic lupus erythematosus: a randomised, double-blind, placebo-controlled study. *Ann Rheum Dis.* (2016) 75:1909–16. doi: 10.1136/annrheumdis-2015-208562
91. Furie R, Khamashta M, Merrill JT, Werth VP, Kalunian K, Brohawn P, et al. Anifrolumab, an anti-interferon-alpha receptor monoclonal antibody, in moderate-to-severe systemic lupus erythematosus. *Arthritis Rheumatol.* (2017) 69:376–86. doi: 10.1002/art.39962
92. Wenzel J, van Holt N, Maier J, Vonnahme M, Bieber T, Wolf D. JAK1/2 inhibitor ruxolitinib controls a case of chilblain lupus erythematosus. *J Invest Dermatol.* (2016) 136:1281–3. doi: 10.1016/j.jid.2016.02.015

19

A Retrospective Study of Patient-Reported Data of Bullous Pemphigoid and Mucous Membrane Pemphigoid From a US-Based Registry

Janet Lee[1†], *Kristina Seiffert-Sinha*[1†], *Kristopher Attwood*[2] *and Animesh A. Sinha*[1*]

[1] *Department of Dermatology, Jacobs School of Medicine and Biomedical Sciences, University at Buffalo, Buffalo, NY, United States,* [2] *Department of Biostatistics and Bioinformatics, Roswell Park Cancer Institute, Buffalo, NY, United States*

Correspondence:
Animesh A. Sinha
aasinha@buffalo.edu

† These authors have contributed equally to this work

Bullous pemphigoid (BP) and mucous membrane pemphigoid (MMP) are rare chronic autoimmune disorders characterized by subepidermal blistering. For the United States, there is a limited amount of studies in BP and MMP that address disease demographics and clinical data. In order to more comprehensively examine disease demographics and clinical factors, we performed a retrospective analysis of patient-reported data of 138 BP and 165 MMP patients enrolled in the International Pemphigus & Pemphigoid Foundation (IPPF) disease registry from 2010–2016. Patient-reported data was compared to Physician/Investigator reported data generated in our own local patient population (Western New York; 19 BP and 43 MMP patients). We confirm a female predominance in BP (M:F ratio 1:2.1) and MMP (M:F ratio 1:4.3), and a late onset within the 6th decade of life (average age at diagnosis, 59.1 ± 17.5 years for BP and 54.8 ± 11.2 years for MMP). MMP patients were significantly more likely to have a delay in diagnosis >12 months than BP patients (38 vs. 21%, respectively). Similar to other autoimmune conditions, a large number of BP (34%) and MMP (35%) patients present with other co-existing autoimmune disorders, with the most common being thyroid disease for both groups. Increased illness activity was paralleled by an increase in severe limitations of daily activities. The vast majority of of both BP and MMP patients received high intensity immunosuppression (49%). However, the majority of BP patients reported therapy with prednisone combined with other immunosuppressants (40%), while the majority of MMP patients received immunosuppressants other than prednisone (55%). With the exception of age at diagnosis, the clinical and demographic findings from both the national and local datasets were largely consistent with each other, and support those reported in other countries.

Keywords: bullous pemphigoid, mucous membrane pemphigoid, cicatricial pemphigoid, ocular cicatricial pemphigoid, clinical characteristics, autoimmune comorbidity

INTRODUCTION

Among autoimmune blistering diseases bullous Pemphigoid (BP) is the most common, with an estimated incidence of 10 cases per million population (pmp) per year in the United States (US) and between 4.5 and 14 cases/pmp per year in central Europe (1, 2). BP is characterized by the presence of IgG autoantibodies against two hemidesmosomal proteins (BP180 and BP230) located in the epithelial basement membrane zone, leading to the characteristic clinical picture of tense cutaneous blisters. It is primarily a disease of the elderly with a higher prevalence in females than males (2, 3). BP has been associated with several neuropsychiatric disorders such as Parkinson's disease, dementia, stroke, and multiple sclerosis (4, 5) and with autoimmune diseases such as diabetes mellitus and psoriasis (6–9).

Mucous membrane pemphigoid (MMP), also known as cicatricial pemphigoid (CP), is an uncommon autoimmune blistering disease that primarily affects the mucous membranes such as the oral cavity and ocular mucosa. Ocular cicatricial pemphigoid (OCP) is a delineation of MMP that includes ocular manifestations but can also affect extraocular mucous membranes and non-mucosal skin. While blisters can heal without scarring, they often do heal with scars that can lead to permanent disfigurement and complications such as dysphagia and blindness. MMP and its variants are characterized by the presence of autoantibodies to the basement membrane zone at the epidermal-subepidermal junction of mucous membranes and occasionally skin. Autoantibodies are directed against several target antigens including BP180, BP230, laminin 332, laminin 311, a6b4 integrin, and type VII collagen (10). MMP is more common in women, and usually occurs in the fifth and sixth decades of life (10). The annual incidence was estimated to be between 0.9 and 1.3 new cases/pmp in Germany and France 2 decades ago, but has seen a rise by 2 cases/pmp in the following decade (11).

The rare nature of both diseases makes the collection of epidemiologic data with a substantial number of patients a laborious and challenging process. Presently, there is a lack of larger nationwide studies in the US assessing disease characteristics of BP and MMP. While several studies have examined mortality rates of BP in the US population (3, 12–14), studies on autoimmune comorbidities have mainly come from Europe (15) and Asia (1, 6, 8, 9). The exception is a recent large-scale cross-sectional study by Ren et al. that examined comorbitidies (not specifically autoimmune) based on discharge diagnosis codes in hospitalized patients with either a primary or secondary diagnosis of BP across the US (16). However, there was potential for misclassification of diagnosis codes for comorbidities, and clinical characteristics such as the disease severity for patients with either a primary or secondary diagnosis of BP were not assessed. To our knowledge, there have not been any reported national cohort studies performed to assess the clinical characteristics of MMP in the US.

This study presents the first nationwide analysis in the US to evaluate the clinical characteristics of BP and MMP and it's variants through a patient-reported registry established by the International Pemphigus & Pemphigoid Foundation (IPPF). We also compared the data obtained from the IPPF patient registry with data collected in conjunction with sample procurement for our local autoimmune bullous disease biorepository in which the data entry was curated by trained medical professionals. With the exception of age of onset, which was significantly lower than expected in the population participating the IPPF registry, our findings largely confirm those of previous epidemiologic studies in BP and MMP conducted in other countries including lesion location and medications. Additionally, our study reveals previously unknown information regarding delay in diagnosis, autoimmune comorbidity, and correlation between disease activity and limitations in daily activities.

MATERIALS AND METHODS

Study Population and Data Collection

Patients diagnosed with BP or MMP that enrolled in a patient registry hosted by the IPPF between 4/14/2010 and 6/8/2016 were included in this study. The disease registry consisted of a 38-item self-reported survey of demographic information and disease characteristics that was available either online through the IPPF website at http://www.pemphigus.org/research/registry/ or via a mailed form if they did not have internet access (English and Spanish versions were available) (17). The survey was compliant with HIPAA (US Health Insurance Portability and Accountability Act of 1996). Data was exported from SurveyGizmo or from written input to Excel format and analyzed in a retrospective fashion.

Out of all patients responding to the IPPF registry, we included a total of 138 individuals with a diagnosis of BP and 165 individuals with a diagnosis of MMP including its variant OCP. Data from these individuals was used for constant variable analysis. In addition, both the BP and MMP groups included patients who had submitted >1 survey response to the disease registry months to years after the previous entry ($n = 13$ for BP and 11 for MMP/OCP). We included original and repeat entries for the analysis of variable disease parameters including co-existing autoimmune disorders, lesion location, disease activity, and medical care.

Since the registry contains patient-reported data and there is a potential of misclassification/re-call bias, a retrospective analysis of physician/investigator-reported data from a local biorepository-associated database of biopsy-confirmed cases of BP and MMP hosted in the corresponding author's laboratory was also carried out to corroborate the findings from the IPPF disease registry. The study was reviewed and approved by the University at Buffalo Institutional Review Board (IRB# 456887). Patients enrolled in the local biorepository were diagnosed based on standard clinical, biopsy (H&E and direct immunoflourescence) and serological parameters, including anti-BP180 and -BP230 levels and indirect immunoflourescence on salt-split skin. For comparability with the IPPF registry, data collected and analyzed in this study from the local biorepository was limited to patients enrolled between the years of 2008 and 2016. We included a total of 19 individuals with a diagnosis of BP and 43 individuals with a diagnosis of MMP. Again, there were a few patients who had provided data and samples more than once months to years after their first intake ($n = 2$ for BP and 11 for MMP/OCP). As before, repeat entry inclusion was only utilized for analyzing variable disease parameters and was excluded from analyzing constant variables such as demographic information and age at diagnosis.

Statistical Analysis

For descriptive analyses, continuous variables are reported as means and standard deviations (SD), whereas all categorical variables are reported with percentages. All comparisons for categorical outcome variables utilized the Fisher's exact test, and the Mann-Whitney U-test was used for all continuous outcome variables. For all analyses, results were considered statistically significant at the $p \leq 0.05$ level.

RESULTS

Patients and Demographics

IPPF Patient Registry

BP patients had a significantly higher mean age at diagnosis than MMP patients (59.1 vs. 54.8 years, $p = 0.001$). There was no significant difference between males and females in terms of age of diagnosis in either the BP or the MMP groups ($p = 0.21$ and $p = 0.40$, respectively). A female predominance was observed in both groups, however, this was much more pronounced in the MMP group (ratio 4.3:1) than the BP group (ratio 2.1:1). The majority of both BP and MMP patients were Caucasian (85 and 90%) and from the US (81 and 88%) (**Table 1**).

For BP patients, the delay in diagnosis from the first occurrence of lesions was <3 months for 52 patients (38%), 3–6 months in 33 patients (24%), 6–12 months in 24 patients (17%), and >12 months in 29 patients (21%). For MMP patients, 27 (16%) had a delay in diagnosis of <3 months, 41 (25%) 3–6 months, 35 (21%) 6–12 months, and 62 (38%) >12 months. BP patients had a significantly higher chance to be diagnosed early (<3 months) than MMP/OCP patients (38 vs. 16%, $p < 0.0001$), while MMP patients had a significantly higher delay in diagnosis >12 months than BP patients (38 vs. 21%, respectively, $p = 0.002$).

Local Biorepository

The mean age of onset was considerably higher in BP than MMP patients (74.2 vs. 58.8 years, $p < 0.001$). There was no significant difference between age at the time of diagnosis and sex for either BP or MMP groups ($p = 0.15$, $p = 0.93$, respectively). The female:male ratio for MMP patients was higher than for BP patients (2.3:1 vs. 1.4:1, respectively). The majority of patients were Caucasian from both BP (74%) and MMP (79%) groups. All patients for both groups were from the US (**Table 1**). The mean delay in diagnosis for the 19 BP patients was 1.1 ± 2.3 years; for the 43 MMP patients it was 2.0 ± 4.6 years (delay in diagnosis information was not available for 2 BP patients and 3 MMP patients).

TABLE 1 | Baseline characteristics for BP and MMP for IPPF registry and local biorepository patients.

	IPPF registry patients		Local biorepository patients		Comparison: IPPF vs. local	
	BP ($n = 138$)	MMP ($n = 165$)	BP ($n = 19$)	MMP ($n = 43$)	BP (p-value)	MMP (p-value)
Age, mean (±SD), years	61.9 (16.6)[a]	58.0 (10.5)[b]	76.2 (13.2)	62.2 (9.4)[d]	<0.039	0.36
Age at diagnosis, mean (±SD), years	59.1 (17.5)[a]	54.8 (11.2)[b]	74.2 (14.0)	58.8 (9.9)	<0.001	0.02
Male	61.1 (18.3)	57.0 (12.7)	68.9 (11.6)	57.8 (11.2)		
Female	58.2 (17.1)	54.2 (10.8)	78.0 (14.8)	59.2 (9.4)		
Female, *n* (%)	93 (67)	134 (81)	11 (58)	30 (70)	0.444	0.141
Ethnicity, *n* (%)					0.319	0.062
Caucasian (non-Ashkenazi Jewish)	117 (85)	149 (90)	14 (74)	34 (79)		
Ashkenazi	6 (4)	2 (1)	3 (16)	4 (9)		
South Asian	2 (1)	2 (1)	1 (5)	1 (2)		
Hispanic	2 (1)	5 (3)	1 (5)	0		
African American	2 (1)	0 (0)	0	1 (2)		
Asian	5 (4)	3 (2)	0	1 (2)		
Other	4 (3)	4 (2)	0	1 (2)		
Unknown			0	1 (2)		
Country, *n* (%)						
United States	112 (81)	145 (88)				
Other[c]	26 (19)	20 (12)				

[a] *7 patients had no recorded birthdate and date of diagnosis.*

[b] *2 patients had no recorded birthdate and date of diagnosis.*

[c] *Other country (n) for BP patients: Australia (2), Brazil (1), Canada (8), Congo (1), India (2), New Zealand (1), Sweden (1), UK (9), unable to be determined (1). Other country (n) for MMP/OCP patients: Argentina (1), Canada (6), Denmark (1), Greece (1), Italy (1), Norway (1), UK (9).*

[d] *If a patient had multiple intakes, the average of the patient's age over all intakes was used.*

The mean age as well as the mean age of diagnosis was significantly lower in the IPPF registry population when compared with the local biorepository patients, with roughly 15 years difference for the BP patients and 4 years difference for the MMP patients. There were no significant differences in terms of sex and age in the two databases (**Table 1**).

Disease Characteristics

Co-existing Autoimmune Disorders

In the IPPF survey, 52 (34%) of BP patients and 62 (35%) of MMP patients reported co-existing autoimmune disorder(s). Since an individual patient could have >1 co-existing autoimmune disorder, a total of 72 co-existing autoimmune disorders were recorded among BP patients, and a total of 89 co-existing autoimmune disorders were recorded among MMP patients. In the local biorepository, 5 (24%) BP patients reported 7 co-existing autoimmune disorders and 27 (50%) MMP patients reported 35 co-existing autoimmune disorder(s). The percentage of patients afflicted by at least one of the respective co-existing autoimmune diseases are presented in **Figure 1**. The most common co-existing autoimmune disorder reported for both BP (**Figure 1A**) and MMP (**Figure 1B**) patients was thyroid disease.

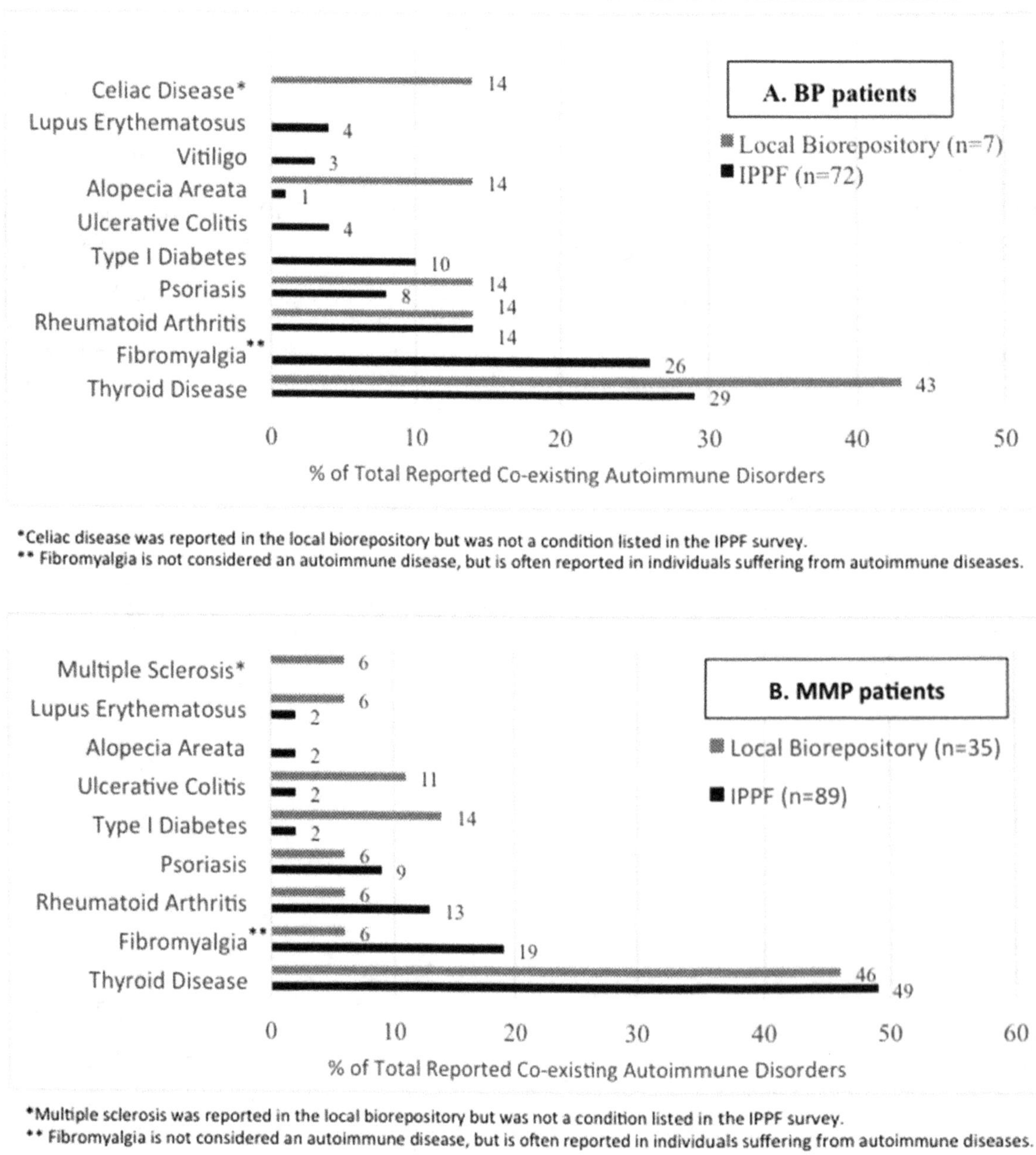

FIGURE 1 | Autoimmune disease comorbidies. The percentages of specific co-existing autoimmune disorders out of all patient-reported autoimmune comorbidities are listed for the IPPF disease registry as well as the local biorepository population among **(A)** BP and **(B)** MMP patients.

Lesion Location

The location of current lesions was analyzed for both BP and MMP patients with active disease only. The majority of BP patients in both the IPPF registry and local biorepository listed their current lesion location as cutaneous only. However, the local biorepository had no patients showing mucosal only lesions with a diagnosis of BP, while 13% the IPPF registry patients reported mucosal only lesions (**Figures 2A,B**). The vast majority of MMP patients reported (**Figure 2A**) or objectively presented with (**Figure 2B**) mucosal only lesions. Only a small number of patients reported cutaneous only lesions. For the local dataset, we were able to confirm that the two patients that presented with cutaneous only lesions had a history of previous mucosal involvement. In order to assess what type of lesions patients can present with over the course of their disease, history of lesion location was determined for IPPF patients by combining data from both current lesions and past lesions. The self-reported results for history of lesion location in the IPPF registry were almost identical to the self-reported results for current lesions (for BP: 59% cutaneous only, 27% mucocutaneous, and 14% mucosal only; for MMP: 1% cutaneous only, 31% mucocutaneous, and 68% mucosal only).

Disease Activity

Patients in the IPPF survey were asked to determine their "global illness activity" defined by the following six choices: (i) no lesions and taking medication, (ii) no lesions and not taking medication, (iii) ongoing transient lesions (lasting <1 week) and taking medication, (iv) ongoing transient lesions and not taking medication, (v) repetitive lesion flares, and (vi) poor or no response to treatment. Using the guidelines established by Murrell et al. (18, 19), we defined the absence of lesions (= no lesions) as complete remission with or without therapy, ongoing transient lesions as partial remission with or without therapy, and repetitive lesion flares and poor or no response to treatment as no remission (active).

The breakdown for disease activity is presented in **Figure 3** (IPPF registry BP: 21% complete remission, 30% partial remission, and 48% active disease; IPPF registry MMP: 17% complete remission, 31% partial remission, and 52% active disease).

Disease activity was also analyzed in terms of limitations in daily activities, defined by the following four choices: (i) none, (ii) mild, (iii) moderate, and (iv) severe. For BP patients, the majority of patients with complete remission reported no

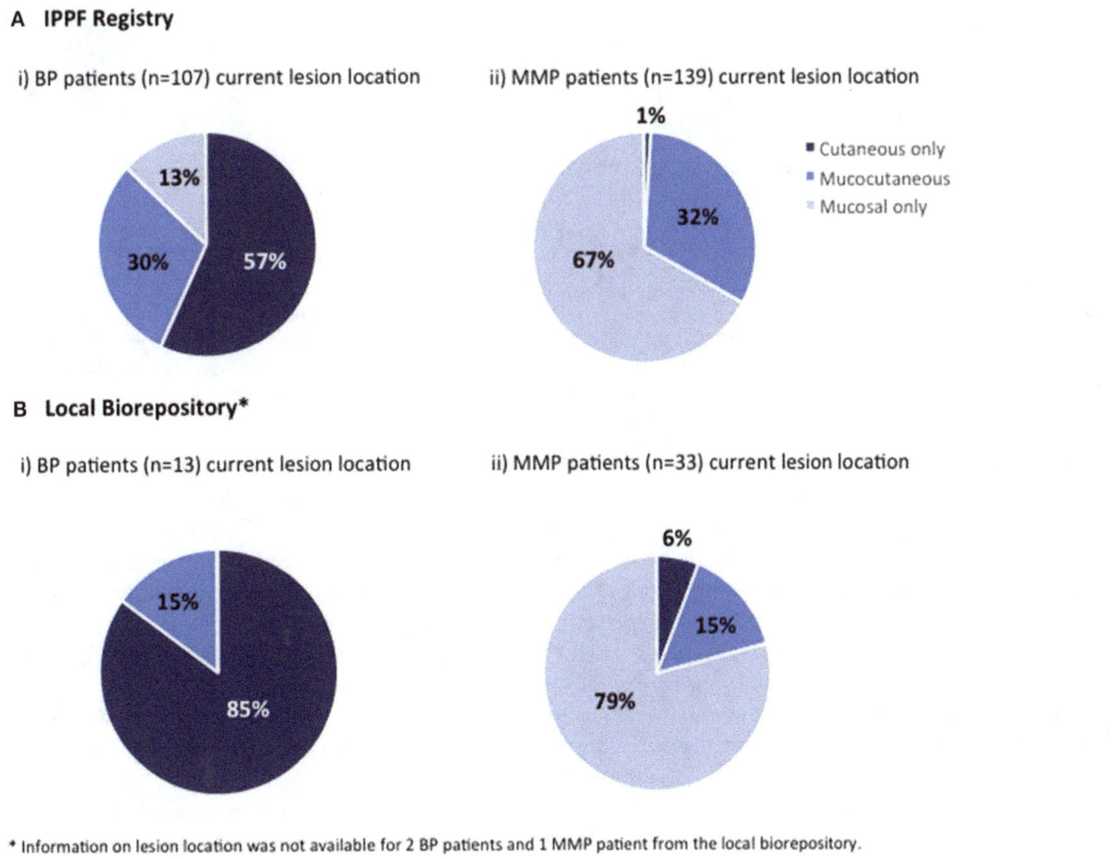

FIGURE 2 | Lesion location. Patients were divided by lesion location into those who at the time of enrollment experienced mucosal lesions only, cutaneous lesions only or both mucosal and cutaneous lesions (mucocutaneous); (**A**-i) BP patients in the IPPF registry, (**A**-ii) MMP in the IPPF registry, (**B**-i) BP patients in the local biorepository, (**B**-ii) MMP patients in the local biorepository.

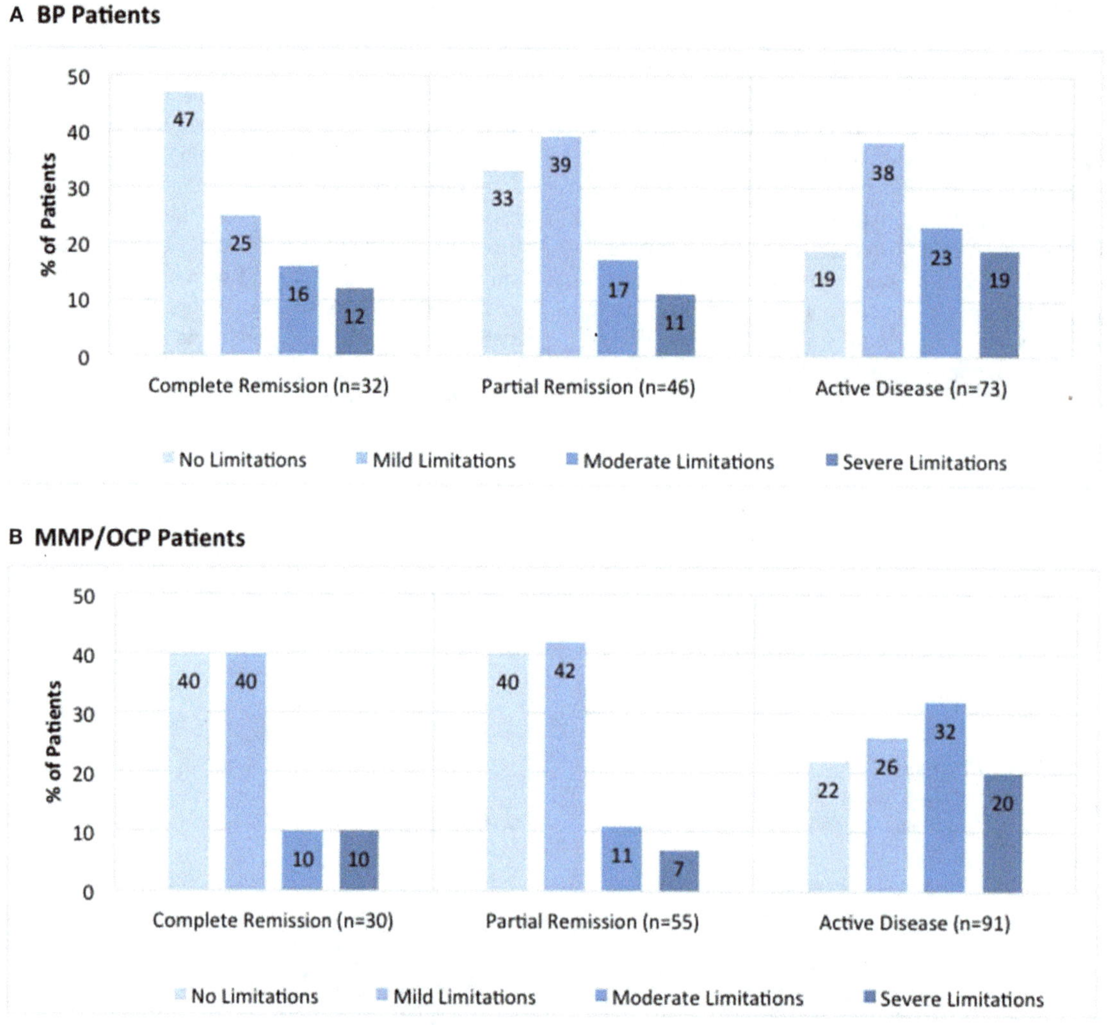

FIGURE 3 | Distribution of limitations in daily activities due to lesions by global illness activity. BP patients **(A)** and MMP patients **(B)** from the IPPF registry were categorized into different groups of global illness activity consisting of either complete remission, partial remission, or active disease. For each group of global illness activity, limitations in daily activity due to lesions classified as either no limitations, mild limitations, moderate limitations, or severe limitations were analyzed. Limitation in daily activities are listed as percent limitation among all patients in a given illness activity group.

limitations in daily activities whereas the majority of those with active disease reported mild limitations in daily activities (**Figure 3A**). There was a significant difference in the number of patients that reported "no limitations in daily activities" between the complete remission and active disease groups (47 vs. 19%, $p = 0.005$). In MMP patients, the majority of patients with complete remission was split between no limitations and mild limitations in daily activities, whereas the majority of those with active disease reported moderate limitations in daily activities (**Figure 3B**). There was a significant difference in the number of patients that reported "moderate limitations in daily activities" between the complete remission and active disease groups for MMP patients (10 vs. 32%, $p = 0.02$).

Medical Care

Among BP patients in the IPPF registry, the vast majority were managed by a dermatologist only, or a by a dermatologist and dentist. Only 10% of patient saw a dentist or other specialty physicians without the involvement of a dermatologist (**Figure 4A**). Among MMP patients, however, less than two-thirds were managed by a dermatologist only, or by a dermatologist and dentist. Forty percent of patients were managed by dentists and/or other specialty physicians without the involvement of a dermatologist (**Figure 4B**).

To compare differing levels of treatment in patient groups distinguished by levels of disease activity, therapy status was defined according to previously published consensus definitions as defined by Murrell et al. (18, 19): (i) no therapy, (ii) minimal therapy, or (iii) more than minimal therapy (anything greater than minimal therapy). Since patients did not report their weight in the IPPF survey, mean weights with respect to age, sex, and ethnicity according to the CDC were used in order to determine the level of treatment (minimal vs. greater than minimal) (20). Regardless of disease activity, the

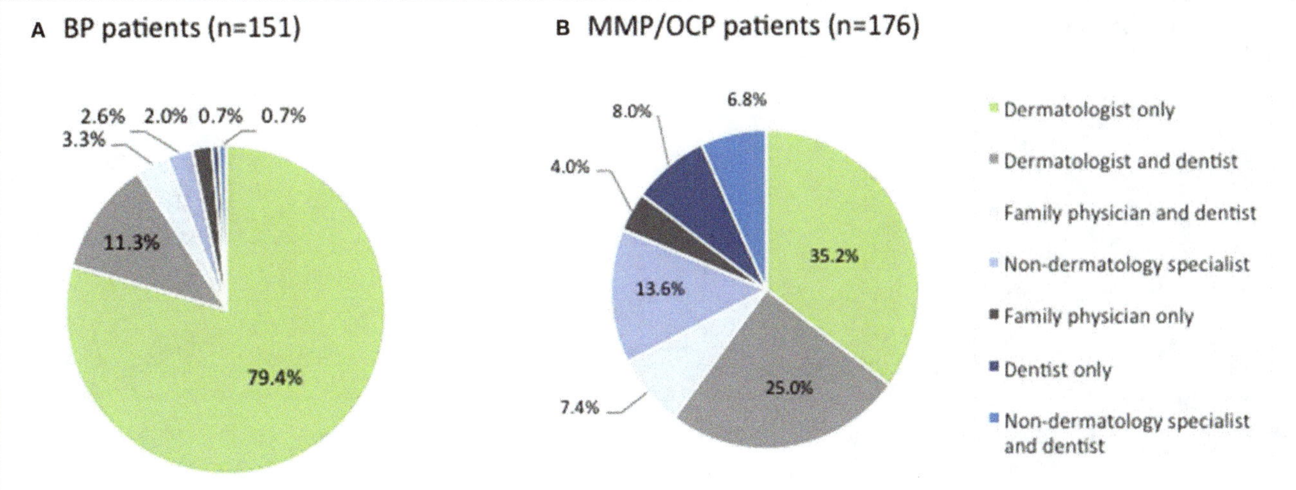

FIGURE 4 | Distribution of medical provider care. BP **(A)** and MMP **(B)** patients from the IPPF registry were analyzed in terms of medical provider care. Percentages list the type of provider or combination of providers consulted for the respective skin condition out of all patients reporting medical care.

TABLE 2 | Level of treatment for IPPF registry and local biorepository patients.

	IPPF registry patients		Local biorepository patients	
	BP (n = 151)	MMP (n = 176)	BP (n = 21)	MMP (n = 54)
No treatment, n (%)	30 (20)	38 (22)	6 (29)	11 (20)
Minimal treatment, n (%)	43 (28)	37 (21)	4 (19)	12 (22)
More than minimal treatment, n (%)	74 (49)	87 (49)	10 (48)	27 (50)
Unable to be determined[a,b], n (%)	4 (3)	14 (8)	1 (5)	4 (7)

[a]*Medication descriptions were not available for 3 BP patients and 13 MMP patients in the IPPF registry, and for 1 BP patient and 1 MMP patient in the local biorepository.*
[b]*Classification of treatment was unable to be determined for 1 BP patient and 1 MMP patient in the IPPF registry, and for 3 MMP patients in the local biorepository.*

TABLE 3 | Medication use for IPPF registry and local biorepository patients.

	IPPF registry patients		Local biorepository patients	
	BP (n = 121)[a]	MMP (n = 138)[b]	BP (n = 15)[a]	MMP (n = 43)[b]
Prednisone only, n (%)	27 (22)	11 (8)	2 (13)	5 (12)
Prednisone + immunosuppressive agent(s) or other adjunct therapies[c], n (%)	48 (40)	38 (28)	8 (53)	10 (23)
Immunosuppressive agent(s) or other adjunct therapies[d], n (%)	43 (36)	76 (55)	4 (27)	27 (63)

[a]*Medications not available for 3 BP patients in the IPPF registry and 1 BP patient in the local biorepository.*
[b]*Medications not available for 13 MMP patients in the IPPF registry and 1 BP patient in the local biorepository.*
[c]*Immunosuppressive agent(s) or other adjunct therapies including: topical steroids, azathioprine, mycophenolate mofetil, cyclophosphamide, cyclosporine, dapsone, tetracyclines, nicotinamide, methotrexate, rituximab, etanercept, IVIg, intralesional injections.*
[d]*All therapies that did not include the use of prednisone, including: topical steroids, azathioprine, mycophenolate mofetil, cyclophosphamide, cyclosporine, dapsone, tetracyclines, nicotinamide, methotrexate, rituximab, etanercept, adalimumab, IVIg.*

majority of patients enrolled in the IPPF repository reported being on more than minimal therapy, followed by minimal and no treatment. Similar results were obtained for patients in the local biorepository (**Table 2**). Amongst BP patients receiving therapy, immunosuppressive and other adjunct therapy was prescribed in the vast majority (76%) of cases, almost equally divided into a group with and without prednisone. In the MMP group, on the other hand, therapy with immunosuppressive and other adjunct agents but without prednisone was most common (55%) (**Table 3**). Again, the distribution of therapeutic regimens was similar in the local biorepository, with the exception of higher degrees of prednisone use in conjunction with other immunosuppressive or adjunct therapies for the BP population (**Table 3**). As expected, a higher percentage of patients in remission were off therapy in both the BP as well as the MMP group (41 and 38%, respectively), while only 8 or 14% of BP or MMP patients with active disease reported being off therapy (**Figure 5**).

DISCUSSION

There have been limited large-scale studies performed to date that have analyzed BP in the US. Although mortality rates of BP have been investigated in the US (3, 12, 14, 21), few studies have assessed comorbidities or other clinical characteristics of this disease. This study sought to improve our understanding of the clinical patterns of these chronic diseases, by using both the IPPF patient registry with large numbers of patients providing self-reported data and a local clinician-annotated biorepository and associated database for comparison.

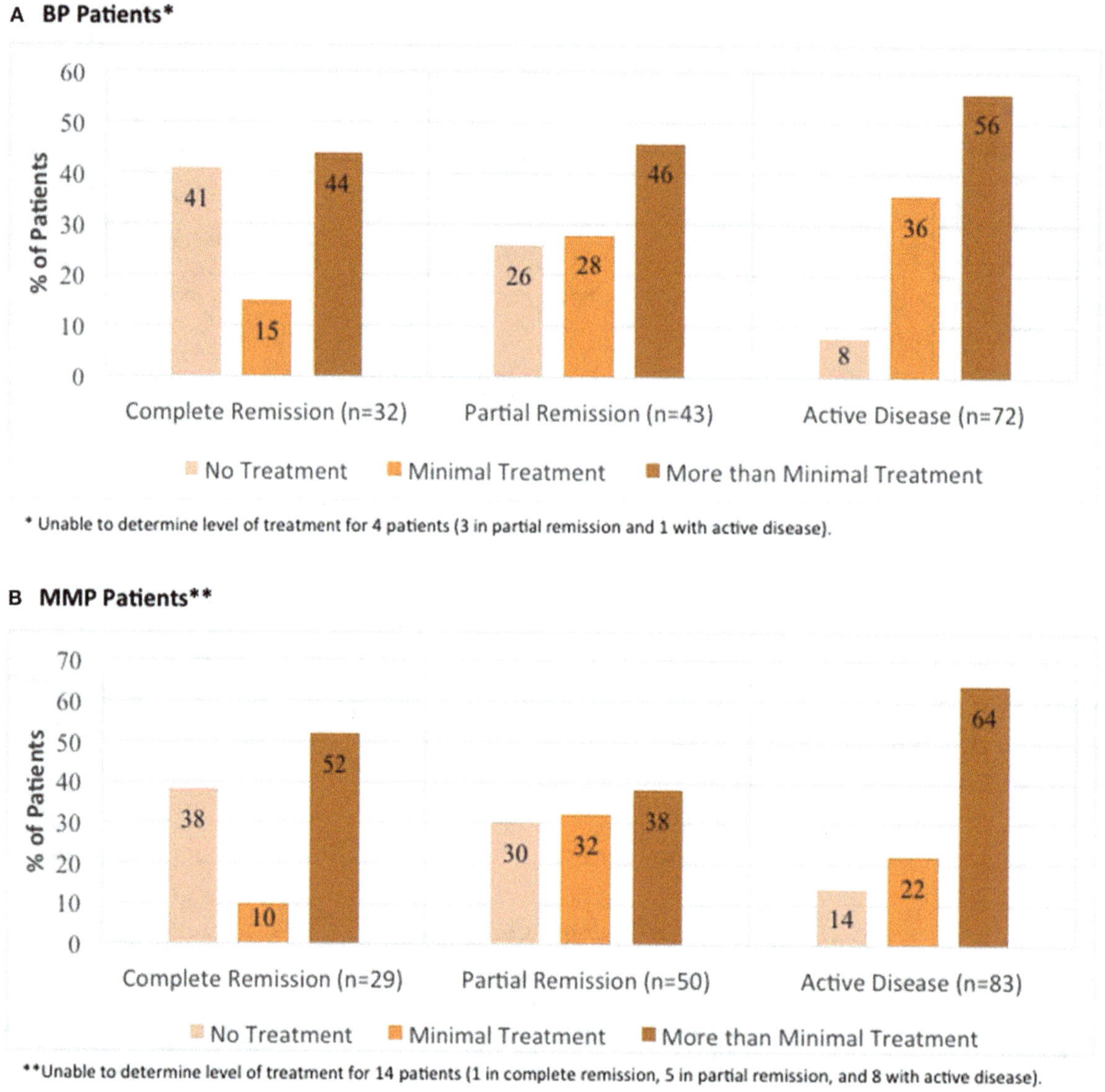

FIGURE 5 | Distribution of level of treatment by global illness activity. BP patients **(A)** and MMP patients **(B)** from the IPPF registry were categorized into different groups of global illness activity consisting of either complete remission, partial remission, or active disease. For each group of global illness activity, level of treatment classified as either no treatment, minimal treatment, or more than minimal treatment was analyzed.

The mean age at diagnosis for BP has been reported to range from 64 to 82.6 years in Europe, Asia, and Africa (22), whereas previous studies in the US have reported a range from 74.5 to 77 years (3, 12, 14). The data in the literature is consistent with the mean age of diagnosis of 74.2 ± 14.0 years from the local biorepository. Interestingly, the IPPF survey showed a significantly lower age of diagnosis (59.1 ± 17.5 years). Since the IPPF study was mainly collected online, the lower age at enrollment and lower age of diagnosis may be due to participation by a slighter younger, more "computer-savvy" demographic. However, both the IPPF registry and local biorepository data on sex distribution was consistent with previous studies that report a higher incidence of BP in females, with female to male ratios typically ranging from 1.04–5.1:1 (22). In MMP, the mean age of diagnosis has been described to occur mainly in the fifth or sixth decade of life (23), i.e., at a slightly younger age than in BP. Our data supports this notion, with a mean age of diagnosis for MMP patients in the 6th decade of life in both datasets. Consistent with the literature that states a female to male ratio of nearly 2:1 (10), MMP patients in both databases studied here displayed a marked female predominance, at levels almost twice of those in observed in BP.

Although patients will routinely report a delay in diagnosis before definitive diagnosis, little is known about the actual time from developing first symptoms to diagnosis for BP and MMP. Data from both the IPPF registry as well as the local biorepository indicate that, generally, BP patients have a shorter delay in diagnosis than MMP patients. Limited data in the literature support these findings with diagnosis delays in BP being on average less than a year (12), while they average more than a year for cicatricial pemphigoid (24). Not surprisingly, the period from the onset of lesions to the first hospitalization was found to be inversely correlated with body surface area (25). A possible explanation for the greater delay in diagnosis may be that patients with cutaneous lesions are more likely to seek the attention of a dermatologist, while patients with mucosal lesions only may not see a dermatologist at all or not until after diagnosis. This assumption is supported by the data on medical care summarized in this study with only 9.3% of BP patients, but 39.8% of MMP patients not being in dermatological care. Our data highlights the continuing need for educational outreach to other medical specialties.

Overall, autoimmune disease has been reported to affect 7.6–9.4% of the population (26, 27), with these individuals at an increased risk of developing a second autoimmune disease (27). In our analysis, a high prevalence of comorbidities, particularly autoimmune thyroid disease, was observed in both the IPPF survey and local biorepository for both BP and MMP patient groups. To our knowledge, few other studies in the US have assessed autoimmune comorbidities in relation to BP, and found associations with diabetes mellitus type 1 (7), SLE, celiac disease, multiple sclerosis, rheumatoid arthritis (RA) and hypothyroidism (16).

Studies from Asian countries such as Taiwan, China, Thailand, and Japan have shown some association between BP and psoriasis (6, 9), and between BP and diabetes mellitus (1, 7, 8, 28). However, European studies from the United Kingdom and Portugal found no statistical differences in autoimmune disorders in general or diabetes mellitus in particular between the BP and control groups (15, 29).

Autoimmune associations for MMP subforms are a matter of debate, showing either no additional risk of autoimmune disorders in patients with OCP (30), or demonstrating associations between OCP and RA (31), and CP with pernicious anemia (32). Our findings are in line with data on autoimmune comorbidities in Pemphigus vulgaris (33) that also showed a predominance of thyroid autoimmunity in the patient population and suggested that common genetic elements across clinically distinct autoimmune diseases may underlie autoimmune susceptibility.

In terms of lesion location, the majority of BP patients reported cutaneous only, followed by mucocutaneous, and mucosal only lesions in the IPPF patient registry, while patients in the local biorepository showed no mucosal only lesions. Prior studies from other countries have shown mucosal lesions for BP patients to either be rare with studies reporting 1.6% (28) or 5.3% (34), while others have stated higher values such as 14.3% (29), 15% (8), and 26.92% (25). For MMP patients, the majority of lesions were located on mucosal surfaces with the IPPF patient registry reporting 67% for mucosal only and the local biorepository showing 79% mucosal only.

A prior quality of life study in autoimmune bullous diseases reported that patients with mucosal involvement had a poorer quality of life than those without (35). Similarly, our findings show that a higher percentage of MMP patients with active disease reported moderate to severe limitations in daily activities compared to those with active BP. Not surprisingly, we found that increased illness activity was paralleled by an increase in moderate-to-severe limitations of daily activities. There have been a number of tools developed to assess the quality of life in patients with BP and MMP such as the Short Form Health Survey, Dermatology Life Quality Index (DLQI), and the Autoimmune Bullous Disease Quality of Life (ABQOL) questionnaire (36). However, data available regarding the usage of these tools and their outcomes is sparse. A small-scale study using the DLQI score indicated "severe impairment" of life quality, with a greater impact related to symptoms and feelings, and daily and leisure activities in BP (37). Our findings suggest that quality of life tools may be useful in clinical settings to assess disease impact.

In terms of treatment, the vast majority of patients received high intensity immunosuppression. While the majority of BP patients reported therapy with oral prednisone combined with other immunosuppressants, the majority of MMP patients received immunosuppressants other than oral prednisone. This is largely consistent with previous studies that have shown systemic corticosteroids, or a combination of systemic corticosteroids with another immunosuppressant to be the most commonly used medications in patients with BP (3, 6, 8, 29, 34, 38).

The strengths of this study include a considerable sample size that is representative of a national patient population (80% of registrants in the IPPF survey and 100% of the patients in the local biorepository were US citizens) and the collaboration between researchers, patients and a not for profit patient support organization (the IPPF). A potential limitation is the self-reporting (including the potential absence of diagnosis confirmation by a physician) and potential recall bias of patient data, particularly in regards to lesion location in the IPPF registry. Prospective studies where biopsies, salt split skin, and antibody levels are analyzed for all patients and correlated with lesion location will be useful to confirm the validity of lesional subtypes reported here. However, we compared the patient self-reported data of the IPPF patient registry to our laboratory biorepository in which data entry was curated by medical professionals in order to corroborate self-reported data and find that, with the exception of age at diagnosis, the findings from both the IPPF and our laboratory biorepository correlate well. We acknowledge that there is a risk for selection bias toward younger populations (particularly with the online format utilized for the IPPF registry), so that older patients with and without neurodegenerative diseases may not be reached. Unfortunately, comorbidities including neurologic diseases or malignancies were not assessed. In the light of newer studies showing support for an association between BP and neurologic diseases (4, 5) these conditions should be included in future questionnaires. Although the present study shows a potential association for patients with either BP or MMP with autoimmune thyroid disease, further studies need to be done to assess the validity and disease relevance of this relationship.

ETHICS STATEMENT

This study was carried out in accordance with the recommendations of the Institutional Review Board of the University at Buffalo for patients enrolled in the local biorepository and the Western Institutional Review board for patients enrolled in the IPPF registry with written informed consent from all subjects. All subjects gave written informed consent in accordance with the Declaration of Helsinki. The protocol was approved by the Institutional Review Board of the University at Buffalo and the Western Institutional Review board.

AUTHOR CONTRIBUTIONS

KS-S and AS designed the study and enrolled the local patients included in this study. JL performed data analysis. JL, KS-S and AS wrote the manuscript. KA performed statistical analyses.

ACKNOWLEDGMENTS

The authors would like to thank the International Pemphigus & Pemphigoid Foundation for providing de-identified data from the IPPF registry. We also thank both our local patient population as well as the patients participating in the IPPF study for providing their time and data.

REFERENCES

1. Kuo CC, Yang FC, Yang MH, Lee DD. Predicting the onset of bullous pemphigoid with co-morbidities: a survey based on a nationwide medical database. In: *Paper Presented at the Bioinformatics and Biomedicine (BIBM), 2013 IEEE International Conference* (2013). Shanghai.
2. Oh D, Zhao C, Murrell D. A review of case–control studies on the risk factors for the development of autoimmune blistering diseases. *J Eur Acad Dermatol Venereol.* (2016) 30:595–603. doi: 10.1111/jdv.13386
3. Colbert RL, Allen DM, Eastwood D, Fairley JA. Mortality rate of bullous pemphigoid in a US medical center. *J Investig Dermatol.* (2004) 122:1091–5. doi: 10.1111/j.0022-202X.2004.22504.x
4. Bastuji-Garin S, Joly P, Lemordant P, Sparsa A, Bedane C, Delaporte E, et al. Risk factors for bullous pemphigoid in the elderly: a prospective case–control study. *J Investig Dermatol.* (2011) 131:637–43. doi: 10.1038/jid.2010.301
5. Langan SM, Groves RW, West J. The relationship between neurological disease and bullous pemphigoid: a population-based case–control study. *J Investig Dermatol.* (2011) 131:631–6. doi: 10.1038/jid.2010.357
6. Chen Y, Wu C, Lin M, Chen T, Liao K, Chen Y, et al. Comorbidity profiles among patients with bullous pemphigoid: a nationwide population-based study. *Br J Dermatol.* (2011) 165:593–9. doi: 10.1111/j.1365-2133.2011.10386.x
7. Chuang T-Y, Korkij W, Soltani K, Clayman J, Cook J. Increased frequency of diabetes mellitus in patients with bullous pemphigoid: a case-control study. *J Am Acad Dermatol.* (1984) 11:1099–102. doi: 10.1016/S0190-9622(84)70266-0
8. Kulthanan K, Chularojanamontri L, Tuchinda P, Sirikudta W, Pinkaew S. Prevalence and clinical features of Thai patients with bullous pemphigoid. *Asian Pac J Allergy Immunol.* (2011) 29:66–72.
9. Ohata C, Ishii N, Koga H, Fukuda S, Tateishi C, Tsuruta D, et al. Coexistence of autoimmune bullous diseases (AIBDs) and psoriasis: a series of 145 cases. *J Am Acad Dermatol.* (2015) 73:50–5. doi: 10.1016/j.jaad.2015.03.016
10. Taylor J, McMillan R, Shephard M, Setterfield J, Ahmed R, Carrozzo M, et al. World workshop on oral medicine VI: a systematic review of the treatment of mucous membrane pemphigoid. *Oral Surg Oral Med Oral Pathol Oral Radiol.* (2015) 120:161–71.e120. doi: 10.1016/j.oooo.2015.01.024
11. Kridin, K. Subepidermal autoimmune bullous diseases: overview, epidemiology, and associations. *Immunol Res.* (2018). 66:6–17 doi: 10.1007/s12026-017-8975-2
12. Brick KE, Weaver CH, Lohse CM, Pittelkow MR, Lehman JS, Camilleri MJ, et al. Incidence of bullous pemphigoid and mortality of patients with bullous pemphigoid in Olmsted County, Minnesota, 1960 through 2009. *J Am Acad Dermatol.* (2014) 71:92–9. doi: 10.1016/j.jaad.2014.02.030
13. Risser J, Lewis K, Weinstock MA. Mortality of bullous skin disorders from 1979 through 2002 in the United States. *Arch Dermatol.* (2009) 145:1005–8. doi: 10.1001/archdermatol.2009.205
14. Parker SR, Dyson S, Brisman S, Pennie M, Swerlick RA, Khan, R, et al. Mortality of bullous pemphigoid: an evaluation of 223 patients and comparison with the mortality in the general population in the United States. *J American Acad Dermatol.* (2008) 59:582–8. doi: 10.1016/j.jaad.2008.07.022
15. Taylor G, Venning V, Wojnarowska F, Welch K. Bullous pemphigoid and autoimmunity. *J Am Acad Dermatol.* (1993) 29:181–4. doi: 10.1016/0190-9622(93)70164-O
16. Ren Z, Hsu D, Brieva J, Silverberg N, Langan S, Silverberg J. Hospitalization, inpatient burden and comorbidities associated with bullous pemphigoid in the USA. *Br J Dermatol.* (2017) 176:87–99. doi: 10.1111/bjd.14821
17. Shah AA, Seiffert-Sinha K, Sirois D, Werth VP, Rengarajan B, Zrnchik W, et al. Development of a disease registry for autoimmune bullous diseases: initial analysis of the pemphigus vulgaris subset. *Acta Derm Venereol.* (2015) 95:86–90. doi: 10.2340/00015555-1854
18. Murrell DF, Daniel BS, Joly P, Borradori L, Amagai M, Hashimoto T, et al. Definitions and outcome measures for bullous pemphigoid: recommendations by an international panel of experts. *J Am Acad Dermatol.* (2012) 66:479–85. doi: 10.1016/j.jaad.2011.06.032
19. Murrell DF, Marinovic B, Caux F, Prost C, Ahmed R, Wozniak K, et al. Definitions and outcome measures for mucous membrane pemphigoid: recommendations of an international panel of experts. *J Am Acad Dermatol.* (2015) 72:168–74. doi: 10.1016/j.jaad.2014.08.024
20. Fryar CD, Gu Q, Ogden CL. Anthropometric reference data for children and adults: United States, 2007–2010. National Center for Health Statistics. *Vital Health Stat.* (2012) 11:1–48. Available online at: https://www.cdc.gov/nchs/data/series/sr_11/sr11_252.pdf
21. Bystryn JC, Rudolph JL. Why is the mortality of bullous pemphigoid greater in Europe than in the US. *J Invest Dermatol.* (2005) 124:xx–xxi. doi: 10.1111/j.0022-202X.2005.23677.x
22. Alpsoy E, Akman-Karakas A, Uzun S. Geographic variations in epidemiology of two autoimmune bullous diseases: pemphigus and bullous pemphigoid. *Arch Dermatol Res.* (2015) 307:291–8. doi: 10.1007/s00403-014-1531-1
23. Ata-Ali Mahmud F, Ata-Ali Mahmud FJ. Pemphigus vulgaris and mucous membrane pemphigoid: update on etiopathogenesis, oral manifestations and managementy *J Clin Exp Dent.* (2011) 3:e246–50. doi: 10.4317/jced.3.e246
24. Laskaris G, Sklavounou A, Stratigos J. Bullous pemphigoid, cicatricial pemphigoid, and pemphigus vulgaris: a comparative clinical survey of 278 cases. *Oral Surg Oral Med Oral Pathol.* (1982) 54:656–62. doi: 10.1016/0030-4220(82)90080-9
25. Serwin AB, Musialkowska E, Piascik M. Incidence and mortality of bullous pemphigoid in north-east Poland (Podlaskie Province), 1999–2012: a retrospective bicentric cohort study. *Int J Dermatol.* (2014) 53:e432–7. doi: 10.1111/ijd.12492
26. Cooper GS, Bynum ML, Somers EC. Recent insights in the epidemiology of autoimmune diseases: improved prevalence estimates and

understanding of clustering of diseases. *J Autoimmun.* (2009) 33:197–207. doi: 10.1016/j.jaut.2009.09.008

27. Somers EC, Thomas SL, Smeeth L, Hall AJ. Are individuals with an autoimmune disease at higher risk of a second autoimmune disorder? *Am J Epidemiol.* (2009) 169:749–55. doi: 10.1093/aje/kwn408
28. Chan K, Ho H. Bullous pemphigoid: a 7-year survey on 75 Chinese patients in Hong Kong. *Hong Kong J Dermatol Venereol.* (2006) 45:71–4.
29. Teixeira VB, Cabral R, Brites MM, Vieira R, Figueiredo A. Bullous pemphigoid and comorbidities: a case-control study in Portuguese patients. *An Bras Dermatol.* (2014) 89:274–8. doi: 10.1590/abd1806-4841.20142516
30. Anzaar F, Cabrita F, Ahmed M, Foster CS. The frequency of other autoimmune disorders in patients with ocular cicatricial pemphigoid. *Acta Ophthalmol.* (2012) 90:e253–4. doi: 10.1111/j.1755-3768.2011.02174.x
31. Olsen KE, Holland EJ. The association between ocular cicatricial pemphigoid and rheumatoid arthritis. *Cornea.* (1998) 17:504–7. doi: 10.1097/00003226-199809000-00007
32. Nayar M, Wojnarowska F, Venning V, Taylor C. Association of autoimmunity and cicatricial pemphigoid: is there an immunogenetic basis? *J Am Acad Dermatol.* (1991) 25:1011–5. doi: 10.1016/0190-9622(91)70299-H
33. Parameswaran A, Attwood K, Sato R, Seiffert-Sinha K, Sinha A. (2015). Identification of a new disease cluster of pemphigus vulgaris with autoimmune thyroid disease, rheumatoid arthritis and type I diabetes. *Br. J. Dermatol.* 172, 729–38. doi: 10.1111/bjd.13433
34. Cai S, Allen J, Lim Y, Chua S, Tan S, Tang M. Mortality of bullous pemphigoid in S ingapore: risk factors and causes of death in 359 patients seen at the National Skin Centre. *Br J Dermatol.* (2014) 170:1319–26. doi: 10.1111/bjd.12806
35. Cianchini G, Paradisi A, Murrell DF. Quality of life in autoimmune blistering diseases. In: DF Murrell, editor. *Blistering Diseases.* Berlin; Heidelberg: Springer (2015). p. 623–31.
36. Sebaratnam DF, Okawa J, Payne A, Murrell DF, Werth VP. Reliability of the autoimmune bullous disease quality of life (ABQOL) questionnaire in the USA. *Qual Life Res.* (2015) 24:2257–60. doi: 10.1007/s11136-015-0965-z
37. Penha MÁ, Farat JG, Miot HA, Barraviera SRCS. Quality of life index in autoimmune bullous dermatosis patients. *An Bras Dermatol.* (2015) 90:190–4. doi: 10.1590/abd1806-4841.20153372
38. Adam B. Bullous diseases: a 7-year survey of experience with 77 patients. *Ann Acad Med Singapore.* (1983) 12:19–25.

Emerging Topical and Systemic JAK Inhibitors in Dermatology

*Farzan Solimani, Katharina Meier and Kamran Ghoreschi**

Department of Dermatology, Venereology and Allergology, Charité—Universitätsmedizin Berlin, Berlin, Germany

***Correspondence:**
Kamran Ghoreschi
kamran.ghoreschi@charite.de

Accumulating data on cellular and molecular pathways help to develop novel therapeutic strategies in skin inflammation and autoimmunity. Examples are psoriasis and atopic dermatitis, two clinically and immunologically well-defined disorders. Here, the elucidation of key pathogenic factors such as IL-17A/IL-23 on the one hand and IL-4/IL-13 on the other hand profoundly changed our therapeutic practice. The knowledge on intracellular pathways and governing factors is shifting our attention to new druggable molecules. Multiple cytokine receptors signal through Janus kinases (JAKs) and associated signal transducer and activators of transcription (STATs). Inhibition of JAKs can simultaneously block the function of multiple cytokines. Therefore, JAK inhibitors (JAKi) are emerging as a new class of drugs, which in dermatology can either be used systemically as oral drugs or locally in topical formulations. Inhibition of JAKs has been shown to be effective in various skin disorders. The first oral JAKi have been recently approved for the treatment of rheumatoid arthritis and psoriatic arthritis. Currently, multiple inhibitors of the JAK/STAT pathway are being investigated for skin diseases like alopecia areata, atopic dermatitis, dermatomyositis, graft-versus-host-disease, hidradenitis suppurativa, lichen planus, lupus erythematosus, psoriasis, and vitiligo. Here, we aim to discuss the immunological basis and current stage of development of JAKi in dermatology.

Keywords: inflammatory skin diseases, JAK (Janus kinase), JAK inhibition, pathophysiology, immunopathogenesis, autoimmune skin diseases, JAK/STAT pathway

INTRODUCTION

The classification of skin diseases and their treatment options are becoming more and more complex. While for a long period of time the morphology of diseased skin was prominent for disease classification and therapeutic procedures, we now have the methodologies for a deep analysis of molecular processes and immunological pattern analysis responsible for the pathophysiological alterations. These advances enlarged our therapeutic repertoire in dermatology remarkably. Deep analysis of skin biopsies allows us to define pathophysiological factors like cytokines, receptors or signaling molecules that are ultimately present at different levels in distinct skin diseases (1–3). This ultimately leads to the identification of new targets and, if these targets are druggable, to new treatments. One striking example of the aforementioned process is the development of a therapeutic variety with monoclonal antibodies (mabs) and small molecules in the treatment of psoriasis (PSO). Traditionally, PSO was treated with topical corticosteroids or dithranol, with phototherapy or immunosuppressive drugs such as cyclosporine. Nowadays, patients with this chronic inflammatory disease are frequently treated with biologicals, either of the first generation (anti-TNF) or the second generation (anti-IL-17/anti-IL-23) (4–7). In recent years, our better understanding of further inflammatory skin diseases such as lupus erythematosus

(LE), lichen planus (LP) or atopic dermatitis (AD) also resulted in the development of novel treatment strategies (8–11). At the same time, we have gained more insight into the role of proteins propagating the intracellular effects of activated cytokine receptors (12). Again, when we pay attention to PSO, small molecules like dimethylfumarate or apremilast are good examples of intracellularly acting compounds that interfere directly or indirectly with signaling pathways (13). Most recently, first inhibitors of signaling proteins directly linked to cytokine receptors have been introduced into the clinics for treating patients with psoriatic arthritis (tofacitinib) and rheumatoid arthritis (tofacitinib and baricitinib). These inhibitors target so-called Janus kinases (JAKs), a family of four proteins: JAK1, JAK2, JAK3, and TYK2 (12). These proteins modulate the inflammatory process by activation of intracytoplasmic transcription factors called signal transducer and activator of transcription (STAT). Once activated, these proteins form dimers, translocate into the nucleus and either positively or negatively modulate the expression of thousands of different genes (12, 14) (**Figure 1**). Since JAK inhibition is not only restricted to systemic drugs administrated orally but has also been developed as a topical treatment option, it is not surprising that inhibitors of JAKs are receiving growing attention from dermatologists and are tested as systemic and/or topical treatment options in various skin diseases (15).

THE JAK FAMILY AND THEIR FUNCTION

The importance of protein kinases and their crucial enzymatic activity was initially determined in 1966 by the work of Krebs and Fischer who showed the essential role of phosphorylation as a mechanism of cell physiology (16). The primary function of protein kinases is to transfer phosphate groups from adenosine triphosphate (ATP) or guanosine triphosphate (GTP) to the hydroxyl groups of amino acids of their protein targets (12). This mechanism is also important for cytokine receptors, which lack intrinsic enzymatic activity (**Figure 2**). In principle, the binding of cytokines to their receptors typically initiates an inflammatory signal (**Figure 1**). A large group of cytokines composed of central interleukins (IL) such as IL-2, IL-6, IL-12, IL-21, IL-22, IL-23, or interferons such as IFN-γ interacts with so-called type I and II cytokine receptors (**Figure 2**). Both of these receptor types lack intrinsic enzyme activity and strongly rely on JAKs for signal transduction (17). After binding, recruited JAKs initiate a

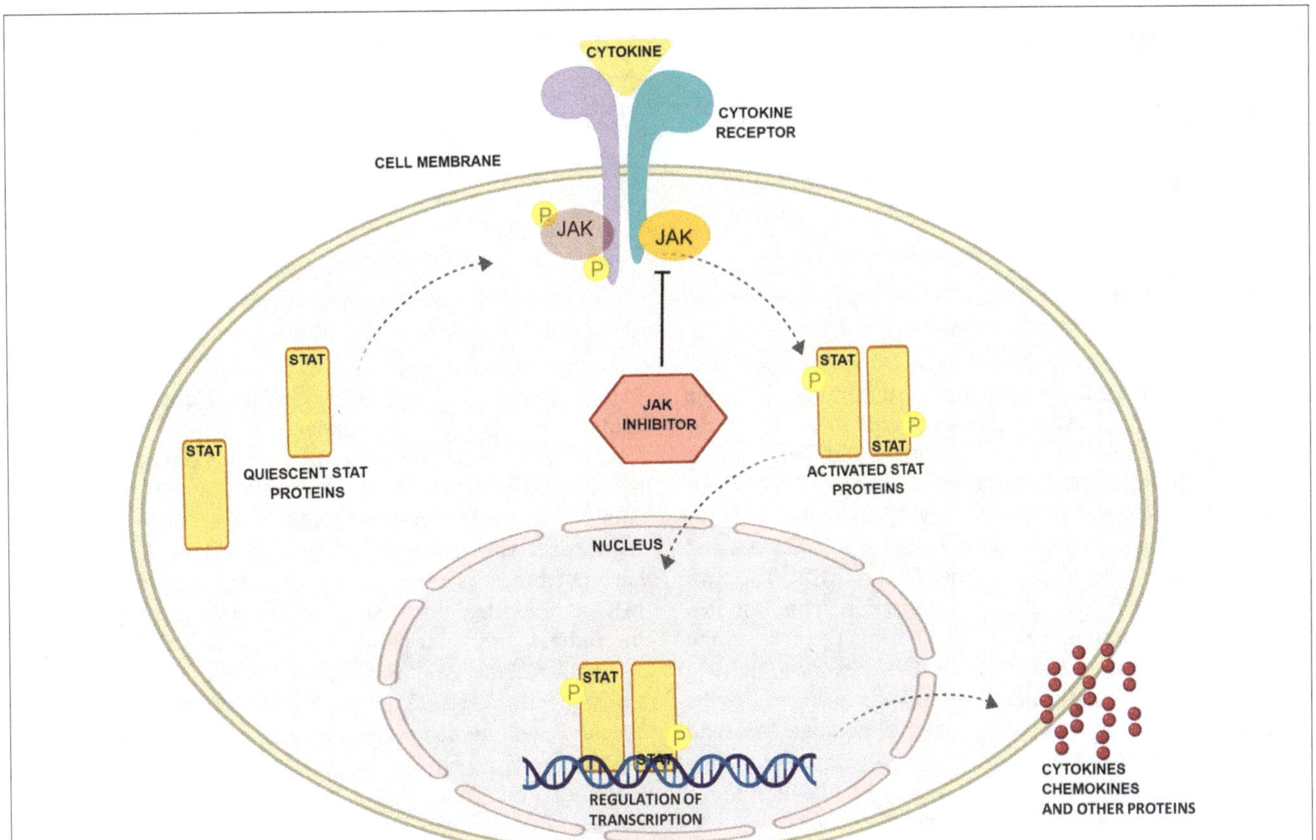

FIGURE 1 | Schematic presentation of the JAK/STAT pathway and the role of JAK inhibitory drugs. Binding of cytokines to receptors, which rely on the JAK/STAT pathway for signal transduction, leads to phosphorylation of JAK and STAT proteins. The latter dimerize, translocate into the nucleus and regulate the expression of inflammatory factors. JAK inhibitors (JAKi) prevent JAK phsophorylation and STAT activation. Figure was created with the help of Biorender.com.

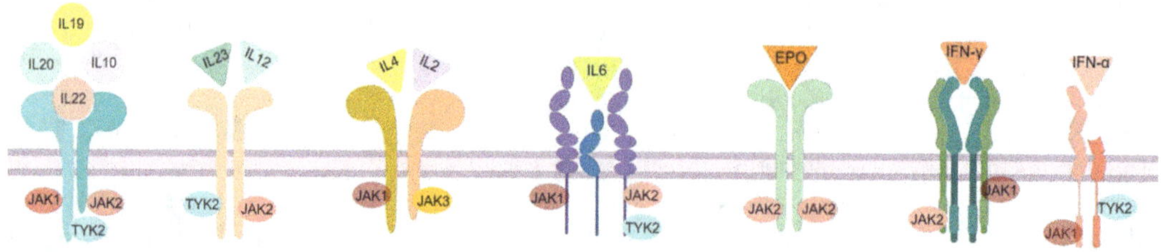

	IL-10 family receptor	Cytokine sharing the IL-12Rβ1	Cytokine receptor sharing the γ-chain	Cytokine receptor sharing the gp130	Homodimeric cytokine receptor	IFN-γ receptor	IFN-α receptor
PAN-JAK INHIBITORS delgocitinib, peficitinib	+	+	+	+	+	+	+
JAK1 JAK3 INHIBITORS tofacitinib, ATI-501, ATI-502	+	-	+	+	-	+	+
JAK1 JAK2 INHIBITORS baricitinib, upadacitinib, CTP-543, ruxolitinib	+	+	+	+	+	+	+
JAK1 TYK2 INHIBITORS PF06700841	+	+	+	+	-	+	+
JAK1 INHIBITORS itacitinib, solcitinib, filgotinib, PF-04965842, INCB054707	+	-	+	+	-	+	+
JAK2 INHIBITORS pecritinib, GSK2586184	+	+	-	+	+	+	-
JAK3 INHIBITORS PF-06651600	-	-	+	-	-	-	-
TYK2 INHIBITORS PF-06835375, PF-06826647, BMS986165	+	+	-	+	-	-	+

FIGURE 2 | Selectivity of JAKi toward type I and type II cytokine receptors. JAKi display different capacities to block cytokine receptor signaling. Pan-JAK inhibitors for example have a broad inhibitory effect, while drugs, which target selectively JAK3 or TYK2 have a more limited mode of action (+, inhibition; -, no inhibition). Figure was created with the help of Biorender.com.

signaling pathway from cellular membrane that ultimately should end in the nucleus: cytokine receptors of type I and II undergo oligomerization, leading to the recruitment of JAKs, which (auto-)phosphorylate tyrosine residues including such within the receptor chains (**Figure 1**). Successively, STAT proteins will be recruited, which then bind to the phosphorylated residues and become activated due to phosphorylation by JAKs. The now activated STAT proteins undergo dimerization. This last step enables the translocation of STAT proteins into the nucleus and the modulation of gene expression (14). Interestingly, most of cytokine receptors use a combination of JAKs for their activity; this could therefore hamper the idea of targeting single JAKs and instead favor a rationale for the use of pan-JAKi under certain settings. However, one should consider that toxicities may limit a strong and ubiquitous JAK blockade (**Table 1**).

JAK DEFICIENCY IN HUMANS AND MICE

The crucial role of JAKs and the relevance of their function can be observed in patients with mutations in genes encoding JAKs or in mice carrying JAK mutations. Here, we will briefly summarize some loss of function (LOF) mutations of JAKs found in humans or by genetic manipulation of mice. Functional deletion of JAK1 or JAK2 in mice results in perinatal or embryonic lethality, respectively. Likewise, reports regarding individuals with deficiency of either JAK1 or JAK2 proteins have not been described, indicating that functional JAK1 and JAK2 are required for embryonic development and survival. In contrast, JAK3 knockout (KO) mice and TYK2 KO mice are both viable. JAK3 is widely expressed in immune cells. Consequently, JAK3 KO mice present a strong reduction of T and B cell numbers and residual immune cells show an impaired activity, exposing mice to multiple infections (18). In agreement with these findings, mutations within the JAK3 gene can present in humans as severe combined immunodeficiency syndrome (SCID) (19, 20). Patients with SCID lack T, NK and diverse B cell populations in the peripheral blood. As a result of this mutation, these patients are constantly exposed to a risk of bacterial, fungal or viral infections (21). The devastating effect on lymphocytes explains the crucial role of JAK3 in

TABLE 1 | Selected adverse effects observed under treatment with JAK inhibitors.

Frequent adverse events observed under treatment with JAK inhibitors
Infections
- Nasopharyngitis
- Upper respiratory tract infections
- Urinary tract infections
Herpes virus reactivation
- Herpes Zoster
- Lip/oral herpes simplex infections
Gastrointestinal disorders
- Nausea
- Diarrhea
Blood/serum changes
- Elevation of liver enzymes [aspartate aminotransferase (AST). alanine aminotransferase (ALT)]
- Hyperlipidemia (increase in cholesterol, triglycerides)
- Increase in bilirubine
- Increase in creatine phosphokinase
Blood cell count alteration
- Decrease in hemoglobin level
- Decrease in white blood cell count
- Neutropenia
Rare adverse events reported under treatment with JAK inhibitors
- Thromboembolic events
- Non-melanoma skin cancers
- Solid cancers

lymphocyte biology. JAK3 is the only JAK protein capable of phosphorylating receptors carrying the γc receptor and this receptor chain is exclusively used by receptors for IL-2, IL-4, IL-7, IL-9, IL-15, and IL-21 (20). LOF mutations within the TYK2 gene are even rarer than JAK3 mutations (22). The few patients reported carrying the mutation show an increased susceptibility for infections, like severe infections of the skin. TYK2 LOF mutations essentially block the signal transduction of the receptors for IL-12, IL-23, and type I IFN (IFN-α/β), resulting in impaired IFN-γ^+ Th1 responses and possibly IL-17^+ Th17 responses (23). Similarly, TYK2 KO mice present a defective response to aforementioned stimuli and have an impaired macrophage activity with increased risk for viral and bacterial infections (24). Based on the selective expression and function of JAK3 in the hematopoietic system, early research focused on the generation of selective JAK3 inhibitors. However, the first inhibitors brought to clinical practice were less selective than expected. The JAK3 inhibitor tofacitinib showed additional activities against JAK1 and to some extent toward JAK2. In contrast, baricitinib is a JAK1/JAK2 inhibitor. However, even these less selective JAKi seem to have acceptable toxicities. Yet, recent efforts in the field of pharmacological chemistry demonstrated that it is possible to generate JAKi with improved selectivity. For instance, second generation JAK3 inhibitors with high selectivity have been synthesized in the last years (25–28). Accumulating data from published studies and ongoing clinical trials will show which type of JAK blockade—low or highly selective compounds—will improve skin diseases without inducing major side effects.

RATIONAL FOR THE USE OF JAKi IN DERMATOLOGY

The perpetuation of inflammation in diseased skin strongly relies on the interaction between cytokines, immune, and tissue cells propagating distinct inflammatory cascades. Some of these immunological processes in the skin, as in PSO or AD, have been deeply elucidated in recent years. The findings led to a radical change of therapeutic approaches. Based on our better understanding of the immunological mechanisms in PSO and AD, a variety of mabs targeting cytokines and small molecules interfering with intracellular signaling pathways have been developed. In this context, it is not surprising that JAKi are gaining increasing attention for the treatment of inflammatory skin diseases (15, 29, 30). Differently than biologics, which target cytokines by intravenous or subcutaneous injection, JAKi target cytokine signaling by either oral or topical administration. The latter way of application may minimize the risk of side effects as observed by systemic JAK inhibition (**Table 1**). Moreover, topical JAKi do not bear the risk of skin atrophy or telangiectasia as observed under long-term use of topical corticosteroids. In the following paragraphs, we aim to present the current position of JAKi in dermatology focusing on inflammatory skin diseases for which JAKi are at least in phase II investigation according to announced trials at clinicaltrials.gov.

ALOPECIA AREATA

Alopecia areata (AA) is the most common immunological cause of hair loss (31). AA can affect both, adults and children. Although certain ethnic groups are more frequently affected than others, the disease does not prefer certain hairs types or color (31). Sudden hair loss is a hallmark of AA. In most of the cases, it appears in a circular well-circumscribed region of the scalp or the beard. AA can eventually lead to the loss of all the hairs of the scalp (alopecia totalis) or, in its most severe form, to the loss of hair of the whole body (alopecia universalis) (31). Frequently, the disease is accompanied by atopic dermatitis or by other autoimmune disorders such as autoimmune thyroiditis (32, 33). AA is determined by the loss of the immune privileged status of the hair follicles, which are then attacked by autoreactive CD8$^+$ T cells and by NK T cells. Remarkably, hair follicles have developed different mechanisms to maintain their privileged immune status. For example, they express molecules such as transforming growth factor (TGF-)β1 and TGF-β2, α melanocyte stimulating hormone (α-MSH) and macrophage migration inhibitory factor (MIF), which hinder activation of T cell and NK T cell functions (31). Additionally, genetic background plays a prominent role in AA. Studies revealed that patients with positive family history for AA have a poorer prognosis and show a recalcitrant disease course often not responding to any treatments (34). Genome-wide-association studies (GWAS) showed the presence of diverse susceptibility loci possibly involved in the pathogenesis of AA like genes encoding for *HLA*, *ULB1*, *IL12RA*, and *PTPN22* (35). *ULB1* encodes for ligands involved in the activation of NKG2D cells, which in C3H/HeJ mice have been shown to

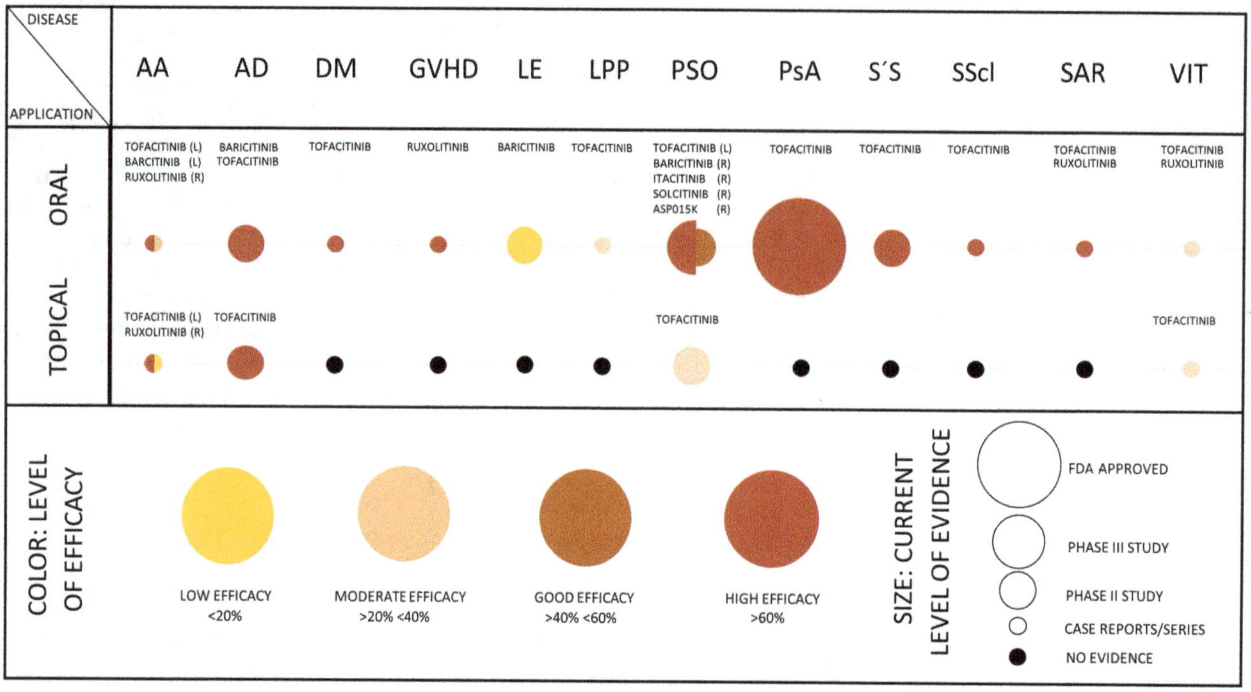

FIGURE 3 | Efficacy of JAKi in dermatology. The scheme summarizes the level of efficacy (as represented by colors) and the level of evidence (as represented by size of circles) in the indicated skin diseases. In diseases, where results from phase II/III studies are available as published, evaluation of JAKi in case series or single case reports was omitted. The scheme was adapted from Eyerich et al. (1). AA, alopecia areata; AD, atopic dermatitis; DM, dermatomyositis; GVHD, graft versus host disease; LE, lupus erythematosus (efficacy on skin lesions); LPP, lichen planopilaris; PSO, psoriasis; PsA, psoriasis arthritis; S'S, Sjögren's syndrome; SScl, systemic sclerosis; SAR, sarcoidosis; VIT, vitiligo; (L), left; and (R), right half of the circle.

be responsible for the destruction of hair follicles (36). Recent findings increased the evidence that JAKs play a crucial role in the pathogenesis of AA. Recipient mice of skin grafted C3H/HeJ mice were treated with mabs targeting IFN-γ, IL-2, and IL-15 each preventing the development of severe AA (36). Furthermore, Xing et al. showed that AA patients and experimental AA mouse models present increased levels of phosphorylated STAT proteins, specifically STAT1, STAT3, and STAT5. These STAT proteins are activated downstream the signals from IFN-γ, IL-2, and IL-15. When using the experimental model of C3H/HeJ mice, systemic treatment with the JAK1/JAK3i tofacitinib or with the JAK1/JAK2i baricitinib protected from hair loss and topical application of tofacitinib stimulated hair regrowth in C3H/HeJ mice (36, 37). In addition, three AA patients were treated orally with the JAK1/JAK2 inhibitor ruxolitinib. This therapeutic approach led to a decrease of $CD8^{+}NKG2D^{+}$ cells and a rapid amelioration of AA (36). Further, microRNAs that influence the expression of the *IL2RA* gene seem to be implicated in AA pathogenesis (38). Although the rationale for treating AA with JAKi is given, the clinical introduction of JAKi for the treatment of AA is still at an early stage (**Figure 3**) (39). Data from phase 2 and 3 studies are needed to clarify the clinical impact of JAKi in patients with AA (**Table 2**; **Figure 3**). Some first clinical experiences with JAKi for the treatment of AA have been published and seem to be promising (40–42). Treatment with oral ruxolitinib showed hair regrowth in 9 out of 12 treated patients without causing severe adverse events. JAK1/JAK2 inhibition by ruxolitinib reduced the expression of cytotoxic markers and IFN-γ expression in lesional skin (43). Similarly, Kennedy-Crispin et al. reported hair regrowth in a subset of patients with AA, AA totalis, or AA universalis treated with tofacitinib 5 mg twice daily. During this study, only low-grade infections were documented (**Table 1**). However, the positive effect on hair regrowth was lost after treatment discontinuation (NCT02197455 and NCT02312882) (44). A recently published case series also reports from the phenomenon of hair loss rebound in AA patients following discontinuation of tofacitinib (45). These first experiences were confirmed by subsequent studies in adults and children using oral or topical JAKi, respectively (46–49). Currently, various double-blind placebo-controlled phase II and III trials testing the efficacy and safety of oral and topical JAKi in AA are ongoing, underlining the growing interest toward these compounds (**Table 2**). One caveat of this promising approach in AA is the preliminary experience that the effect of oral JAKi seems to be timely restricted and hair loss has been reported to reappear upon cessation of pharmacological JAK inhibition in a substantial number of patients (50).

ATOPIC DERMATITIS

Atopic dermatitis (AD) is a common chronic disease of the skin, which severely impairs patient's quality of life. The prevalence

TABLE 2 | Clinical trial program of JAKi in alopecia areata and subtypes according to clinicaltrials.gov.

Disease subtype	Inhibitor	Target	Administration	Phase	Study number
AA AU AT	Tofacitinib	JAK1 JAK3	Topical	Phase II	NCT02812342
	ATI-501	JAK1 JAK3	Oral	Phase II	NCT0359427
	ATI-502	JAK1 JAK3	Topical	Phase II	NCT03759340
AA AT	Ruxolitinib	JAK1 JAK2	Topical	Phase II	NCT02553330
	Baricitinib	JAK1 JAK2	Oral	Phase II/III	NCT03570749
	Tofacitinib	JAK1 JAK3	Oral	Phase IV	NCT03800979
	Tofacitinib	JAK1 JAK3	Oral	Phase II	NCT02299297
	Delgocitinib	PanJAK	Topical	Phase II	NCT02561585
	PF06651600	JAK3	Oral	Phase II	NCT02974868
	PF06700841	JAK1 TYK2			
	PF-06651600	JAK3	Oral	Phase II	NCT03732807
	CTP-543	JAK1 JAK2	Oral	Phase II	NCT03811912
	CTP-543	JAK1 JAK2	Oral	Phase II	NCT03137381
eAA	Delgocitinib	PanJAK	Topical	Phase II	NCT03325296
	ATI-502	JAK1 JAK3	Topical	Phase II	NCT03551821

AA, alopecia areata; AU, alopecia universalis; AT, alopecia totalis; eAA, eyebrows alopecia areata.

TABLE 3 | JAKi tested for atopic dermatitis.

Disease subtype	Inhibitor	Target	Administration	Phase	Study number
AD	Baricitinib	JAK1 JAK2	Oral	Phase III	NCT03334396
	Baricitinib	JAK1 JAK2	Oral	Phase III	NCT03334422
	Upadacitinib	JAK1	Oral	Phase II	NCT02925117
	Upadacitinib	JAK1	Oral	Phase III	NCT03738397
	Upadacitinib	JAK1	Oral	Phase III	NCT03607422
	Ruxolitinib	JAK1 JAK2	Oral	Phase II	NCT03011892
	Ruxolitinib	JAK1 JAK2	Oral	Phase III	NCT03745651
	Delgocitinib	PanJAK	Topical	Phase I	NCT03826901
	Delgocitinib	PanJAK	Topical	Phase II	NCT03725722
	PF-04965842	JAK1 JAK2	Oral	Phase III	NCT03796676
	PF-04965842	JAK1	Oral	Phase III	NCT03422822
	PF-04965842	JAK1	Oral	Phase III	NCT03720470
	PF-04965842	JAK1	Oral	Phase III	NCT03627767
	PF-04965842	JAK1	Oral	Phase II	NCT02780167
	PF-04965842	JAK1	Oral	Phase III	NCT0334960
	PF-04965842	JAK1	Oral	Phase III	NCT03575871
pAD	Upadacitinib	JAK1	Oral	Phase I	NCT03646604

AD, atopic dermatitis; pAD, pediatric atopic dermatitis. Clinical trial program according to clinicaltrials.gov.

of AD is higher in children and adolescents, but the disease can manifest at any age. Clinically, AD is characterized by the presence of pruriginous eczematous lesions, typically on flexural sites (8). In almost 80% of AD patients, skin integrity is altered due to LOF mutations within the gene encoding filaggrin (*FGN*). Impaired *FGN* expression promotes the loss of transepidermal water resulting in xerosis and eczema. The skin barrier dysregulation together with the "atopic" cytokine milieu increases the risk for skin superinfections with bacteria or viruses (51). Historically, AD is thought to be a Th2 dominated disease. Nonetheless, there is growing evidence that the immunological environment of AD is not solely defined by Th2 cells and related cytokines (IL-4, IL-5, IL-10, IL-13, and IL-31) but also by cytokines linked to other Th cell responses such as IFN-γ (Th1), IL17, or IL-22 (Th17) and IL-33 (an alarmin) (8, 52–56). Dupilumab, a mab against IL-4Rα has shown efficacy in a large number of patients and is the first approved biological for AD (57). Nonetheless, the cytokine microenvironment in AD seems to be complex and patients seem to present with different cytokine signatures at different stages. Several mabs are in phase 2/3 development, including mabs neutralizing IL-13 (tralokinumab and lebrikizumab), IL-31 (nemolizumab) (58–60), and IL-33 (etokimab) (61). The neutralization of other cytokines is being tested in patients with AD including secukinumab and ustekinumab, mabs against IL-17A and p40 subunit of IL-23/IL-12, respectively. Given the diversity of cytokines implicated in the inflammatory processes of AD, there is growing interest toward JAKi, which could interfere with the signaling of multiple cytokines simultaneously (62). Tofacitinib and baricitinib are so far the best-studied JAKi in AD (63). The JAK1/JAK3i tofacitinib abrogates IL-4 signaling and the differentiation of Th2 cells (64). Oral tofacitinib has been shown to be effective in patients with moderate to severe AD (65, 66) and topical tofacitinib is effective in mild forms of AD (67). The latter formulation is of special interest in topical AD treatment, which is mostly based on topical corticosteroids or calcineurin inhibitors (67). The JAK1/JAK2i baricitinib is also being tested in AD patients. Guttman-Yassky et al. showed that oral baricitinib at a dose of 2 or 4 mg strongly ameliorates AD, helping patients to spare long-lasting application of topical corticosteroids (68). Other compounds, like the JAK1i oclacitinib or the pan-JAKi JTE-052 showed efficacy when orally administrated in small-sized cohorts (69, 70). Currently, two different phase III studies are investigating the efficacy and safety of oral baricitinib as a monotherapy for AD. Other systemically applied JAKi under clinical investigation for AD include the JAK1 inhibitors upadacitinib (71) and PF-04965842. Topically applied JAKi tested for adult and pediatric AD include the pan-JAKi delgocitinib (LEO124249) (**Table 3**). Positive results, in absence of severe side effects when using topical JAKi, could enormously help young patients in which the application of

TABLE 4 | JAKi trial in patients with dermatomyositis.

Disease type	Inhibitor	Target	Administration	Phase	Study number
DM	Tofacitinib	JAK1 JAK3	Oral	Phase I	NCT03002649

Clinical trial program according to clinicaltrials.gov. DM, dermatomyositis.

topical corticosteroids and systemic immunosuppressive drugs are often precarious.

DERMATOMYOSITIS

Dermatomyositis (DM) is an ab-mediated autoimmune disease, which affects skin and muscles with variating extent (72, 73). A complex auto-ab profile (74) is helpful for diagnosing DM and for estimating the risk for developing distant organ involvement like lung, larynx, gastrointestinal tract, or heart during the disease course. Adult DM is frequently associated with malignancies (75). The pathophysiology is not completely understood, nonetheless multiple studies showed a pivotal role played by IFN-γ producing Th1 cells in DM (72, 76, 77). The standard treatment regimen in DM includes high-dose corticosteroids, non-steroidal immunosuppressants like azathioprine and often requires additional intravenous immunoglobulins (IVIG) (73, 78). In addition, diagnosis and treatment of disease-associated cancer is important. More recently, different case reports and small case studies showed a positive outcome of recalcitrant chronic DM after treatment with either ruxolitinib or tofacitinib (79–82) (**Figure 3**). Remarkably, JAKi seem to have a positive effect on lung involvement in DM (79, 82–84), which often represents a high-risk-mortality complication. The efficacy of tofacitinib is currently under investigation in a small cohort of 10 patients with recalcitrant DM (NCT03002649) (**Table 4**). If JAKi can improve non-cancer associated DM with limited toxicities, this treatment option would be of help and spare long-term use of high dose corticosteroids.

GRAFT-VERSUS-HOST DISEASE

Graf-versus-Host Disease (GVHD) is a serious though common systemic reaction following hematopoietic stem cell transplantation or donor lymphocyte infusion (85). It is caused by donor T lymphocytes activated by host antigens. Different organs may be affected during GVHD and the skin is one of the most commonly targeted organs. Cutaneous GVHD presents in an acute and/or a chronic form. Acute (aGVHD) is clinically characterized by maculopapulous rash, disseminated erythematous skin areas, which can eventually converge in a generalized erythroderma (86). The chronic GVHD (cGVHD) shows a heterogeneous clinical presentation and can develop from the acute form. Lesions often present as LP-like or scleroderma-like lesions, nonetheless the disease can present differently and resemble PSO or keratosis pilaris (86). Immunologically, the aGVHD of the skin shows a T cell infiltration made up mostly by Th2 type cells. In contrast, in cGVHD the skin contains an infiltrate rich in type 1 and type 17 cells. In peripheral blood, cGVHD patients present lower numbers of Treg cells and the expression of their transcription factor FOXP3 is strongly reduced (87, 88). Glucocorticosteroids, both as topical and in oral form together with other immunosuppressants and phototherapy or extracorporeal photopheresis are the mainstay treatment for cGVHD (89). Given the important role of T cells and their associated cytokines, the application of JAKi may theoretically be of benefit for patients with GVHD. Experimental studies showed that pro-inflammatory mediators such as IL-6 and IFN-γ play a major role in the pathogenesis of GVHD (90). Furthermore, polymorphisms on genes encoding for IL-6 and IFN-γ have been associated with disease severity (91, 92). Accordingly, Choi et al. showed that IFN-γ receptor (IFN-γR)-deficient allogeneic Tconv reduced the risk for GVHD in mice (93). They tested the efficacy of ruxolitinib in wild type T cells in two murine MHC mismatched models, showing that inhibition of JAK proteins induce an effect similar to the genetic loss of IFN-γR *in vitro* and *in vivo* (93). Other experimental studies confirmed that JAKi like ruxolitinib (94) or tofacitinib improve or even prevent severe GVHD (95). The benefit of ruxolitinib in preclinical models was translated to humans and, also here, showed improvement of GVHD in six patients (96). After preliminary encouraging results regarding the effect of ruxolitinib in cGVHD in humans (97) (**Figure 3**), different studies are now investigating the possibly beneficial role of JAK inhibition in aGVHD and cGVHD. A multicenter, randomized phase 2 trial has been initiated, to test the efficacy of oral ruxolitinib in steroid-refractory aGVHD (98). The GRAVITAS-301 study (NCT03139604) is investigating the efficacy of itacitinib (a JAK1 inhibitor) in acute GVHD in a randomized, double-blind placebo-controlled phase 3 study. This compound as well as ruxolitinib and baricitinib are currently under investigation in cGVHD (**Table 5**). Most recently, itacitinib even entered two phase I studies for prophylactic use to prevent GVHD after cell stem transplantation (**Table 5**).

HIDRADENITIS SUPPURATIVA

Hidradenitis suppurativa (HS) (also designated as acne inversa) is a chronic debilitating inflammatory skin disease frequently occurring in skin areas with substantial presence of follicles (99). The disorder is characterized by occlusion of follicular ducts with consequent increase in local bacteria. This process evolves in cyst rupture and generalized local tissue inflammation (99). Of note, it is probable that a sublatent skin inflammatory process precedes bacterial accumulation; this could be triggered e.g., by behavioral factors like smoking and obesity, which typically worsen the course of HS (99). Moreover, HS patients often carry mutations in the γ-secretase encoding gene *PSEN* (100). Due to the important role played by bacteria in HS, first line treatments are based on antibiotic therapy with anti-inflammatory properties (101, 102). Nonetheless, recent studies elucidated the role of cytokines present in the inflammatory milieu of HS skin showing an overexpression of IL-17A, IL-26,

TABLE 5 | Clinical trials using JAKi in Graft-versus-Host-Disease according to clinicaltrials.gov.

Disease subtype	Inhibitor	Target	Administration	Phase	Study number
Prophylaxis of GVHD	Itacitinib	JAK1	Oral	Phase I	NCT03320642
	Itacitinib	JAK1	Oral	Phase I	NCT03755414
aGVHD	Ruxolitinib	JAK1 JAK2	Oral	Phase II	NCT02396628
	Ruxolitinib	JAK1 JAK2	Oral	Phase III	NCT02913261
	Ruxolitinib	JAK1 JAK2	Oral	Phase II	NCT03702698
	Ruxolitinib	JAK1 JAK2	Oral	Phase II	NCT03491215
	Ruxolitinib	JAK1 JAK2	Oral	Phase II	NCT02953678
	Itacitinib	JAK1	Oral	Phase I	NCT03497273
	Itacitinib	JAK1	Oral	Phase I/II	NCT03721965
	Itacitinib	JAK1	Oral	Phase III	NCT03139604
	Itacitinib	JAK1	Oral	Phase II	NCT03846479
	Pacritinib	JAK2	Oral	Phase I	NCT02891603
aGVHD cGVHD	Ruxolitinb	JAK1 JAK2	Oral	Phase II	NCT02997280
cGVHD	Baricitinib	JAK1 JAK2	Oral	Phase I/II	NCT02759731
	Itacitinib	JAK1	Oral	Phase III	NCT03584516
	Ruxolitinib	JAK1 JAK2	Oral	Phase II	NCT03616184
	Ruxolitinib	JAK1 JAK2	Oral	n/a	NCT03147742
	Ruxolitinib	JAK1 JAK2	Oral	Phase III	NCT03112603
	Ruxolitinib	JAK1 JAK2	Topical	Phase II	NCT03395340

aGVHD, acute Graft-versus-Host-Disease; cGVHD, chronic graft-versus-host-diseases.

IFN-γ, IL-27, and IL-β, and, a concomitant downregulation of IL-22 (103, 104). This moved the focus of researchers from the role of bacteria to the function of cytokines in HS. Adalimumab, a mab against TNF, is the first biological approved for the treatment of HS (105). Targeting cytokines like IL-1 or IL-17/IL-23 have been reported to have mixed results (37, 106) or are presently under intensive clinical investigation. Given that cytokines are crucial in HS pathogenesis, inhibition of the JAK/STAT pathway could help to regulate the expression of inflammatory factors like IL-6 or IL-23 simultaneously. Clinical studies like NCT03607787 and NCT03569371 are evaluating the safety of INCB054707, a JAK1 inhibitor in HS (**Table 6**).

TABLE 6 | Trials on JAKI in hidradenitis suppurativa according to clinicaltrials.gov.

Disease type	Inhibitor	Target	Administration	Phase	Study number
HS	INCB054707	JAK1	Oral	Phase II	NCT03607487
	INCB054707	JAK1	Oral	Phase II	NCT03569371

HS, hidradenitis suppurativa.

TABLE 7 | Trial on JAKi in lichen planus.

Disease type	Inhibitor	Target	Administration	Phase	Study number
cLP	Ruxolitinib	JAK1 JAK2	Topical	Phase II	NCT03697460

Clinical trial program according to clinicaltrials.gov. cLP, cutaneous lichen planus.

LICHEN PLANUS

LP is a common inflammatory disease of the skin and mucous membranes, clinically characterized by polygonal papules presenting a characteristic white, reticulate on their surface (Wickham striae). Frequently, the oral cavity is affected by LP (OLP) (107). Rarely, LP can affect the scalp, LP planopilaris (LPP), or the nails (nail LP) (107). A classic feature of this inflammatory disorder is the histological presence of a dense T cellular infiltrate disposed in a band like pattern (lichenoid infiltrate) (10). The need of new therapeutic options is given, since LP often presents a challenging chronic recalcitrant course (especially OLP) and the traditional therapeutic options are of limited efficacy. Treatment of LP is mainly based on oral or topical glucocorticosteroids, phototherapy, retinoids or immunosuppressive drugs such as cyclosporine or methotrexate (107). There is growing evidence that LP is a Th1 driven disease (10, 108, 109), although Th17-associated cytokines have also been reported in LP (110–112). A recent study showed that the T cell infiltrate presents high numbers of Th1/Tbet$^+$ cells and the presence of IL-17A$^+$ cells, disposed beneath the basal cells of the epidermis (10). Peripheral Th1/Th17 cell reactive against skin autoantigens further underlines the proposed autoreactive pathophysiology of LP (10). Finally, therapeutic blockade of IL-17 or of IL-23 seems to be a promising approach for the treatment of LP (11). The dominance of IFN-γ in LP skin suggests that JAK inhibition could be a therapeutic option. A small retrospective study consisting of 10 patients with LPP treated with oral tofacitinib as monotherapy or as adjunctive therapy showed mixed clinical efficacy in 8/10 patients (113). According to clinicaltrials.gov, the study NCT03697460 is testing the efficacy of ruxolitinib cream in LP (**Table 7**). It is likely, that JAKi will be a therapeutic option for patients with steroid-refractory LP variants. Given the beneficial effect of tofacitinib on nail PSO (114), a possibly similar effect on nail LP is conceivable. This should be addressed in the future, since nail LP is very painful and cicatrial.

LUPUS ERYTHEMATOSUS

Lupus erythematosus (LE) is a severe, chronic autoimmune ab-mediated disorder with variable clinical presentation and difficult-to-treat clinical course. The disease is widely known for the presence of a butterfly-like rash on the face of affected patients with systemic LE (SLE) (115). Based on the diverse subtypes, LE can be restricted to the organ skin or present a systemic course with manifestation at multiple organs (115). Both environmental and behavioral factors (such as smoking or sun exposure) and genetic factors are meant to play a role in the pathogenesis of LE (115–117). Possibly, gut pathobionts and in general, bacterial and viral stimuli could trigger the onset of the disease (118). In LE there is evidence that multiple cytokines such as IL-16, IL-17, IL-18, and TNF are implicated in the inflammatory process. In any event, type I IFNs are thought to play a major role in LE pathogenesis (119). The latter family of cytokines strongly relies on the JAK/STAT pathway for signal transmission (**Figure 2**). In addition, the role of STAT proteins has been widely investigated (120). The pivotal role of STAT1 in LE has been analyzed in mice and in humans. In the MRL/lpr mouse model, STAT1 is overexpressed in both B and T cells. STAT1 gene silencing ($STAT1^{-/-}$) in this mouse model is accompanied by a decrease of $CD4^{+}$ producing IFN-γ T cells, a milder course of nephritis and a remarkable decrease of auto-ab levels (121–123). In humans diagnosed with LE as in mice, STAT1 is overexpressed in T and B cells. STAT1 levels correlate with clinical disease activity and with the level of expression of IFN-γ-induced genes (124–126). In addition, STAT3 and STAT4 seem to be relevant in the pathogenesis of LE. The lack of STAT3 seems to be protective in a LE murine model (127, 128). In MRL/lpr LE prone mice treatment with tofacitinib led to a decrease of auto-ab production and amelioration of nephritis and skin inflammation. Similarly, two different LE mouse models showed a decrease of several cytokines (IL-12, IL-17A, IFN-γ, and TNF), and a decrease of antinuclear auto-ab levels upon treatment with CEP-33779, a JAK2 inhibitor (129). However, in humans, the JAK1 inhibitor GSK2586184 showed to be ineffective in a small size study of patients with SLE (130). Conversely, baricitinib has been tried in patients with SLE in a double blind, randomized, placebo-controlled phase 2 trial (NCT02708095) (**Figure 3**) (131). Baricitinib was administered at 2 or 4 mg daily. Results showed that the 4 mg dose leads to a consistent clinical improvement in SLE, especially on arthritis. Of note, adverse events were almost comparable to the placebo group (132). At the time of this writing, different compounds targeting different JAKs are under clinical investigation for the treatment of SLE or discoid LE (**Table 8**).

TABLE 8 | Clinical trials of JAKi in systemic and/or discoid lupus erythematosus according to clinicaltrials.gov.

Disease subtype	Inhibitor	Target	Administration	Phase	Study number
SLE	Tofacitinib	JAK1 JAK3	Oral	Phase I	NCT02535689
	Baricitinib	JAK1 JAK2	Oral	Phase III	NCT03843125
	Baricitinib	JAK1 JAK2	Oral	Phase III	NCT03616912
	GSK2586184	JAK1	Oral	Phase II	NCT01777256
	PF06835375	TYK2	Oral	Phase I	NCT03334851
	PF06700841	JAK1 TYK1	Oral	Phase II	NCT03845517
	BMS986165	TYK2	Oral	Phase II	NCT03252587
SLE/DLE	Tofacitinib	JAK1 JAK3	Oral	Phase 1	NCT03159936

SLE, systemic lupus erythematosus; DLE, discoid lupus erythematosus.

PSORIASIS VULGARIS

PSO is a common inflammatory skin disease with well-defined pathogenesis. Based on the research of recent years numerous targeted treatments have been developed for PSO (4). In its classic appearance, this chronic inflammatory disorder presents with erythematous scaly plaques, which are preferentially disposed at extensor sites and in areas of mechanic stress. In addition, scalp, nails and inverse regions are frequently affected. In around 20–30% of cases, patients with PSO also suffer from joint involvement (psoriatic arthritis, PSA) (4). There is a wide range of treatment possibilities for PSO. Topical treatments include glucocorticosteroids, vitamin D derivatives, and dithranol. While phototherapy is becoming less important, oral drugs like methotrexate, acitretin, dimethylfumarate, or apremilast are widely used (4). Cyclosporine should be avoided due to its toxicities compared to the numerous less-toxic alternatives. Besides oral drugs, various biologics have been established for PSO (6). The first generation of antipsoriatic biologics targets TNF. Since PSO is widely accepted as the prototypic Th17 driven disease, multiple second-generation biologics have been approved in the meanwhile. These either neutralize IL-17A, bind its receptor or target IL-23. Although the neutralization of IL-17A is effective in most patients, some patients do not respond. The implication of multiple cytokines like IL-6, IL-22, IL-23, or IFN-γ in psoriasis pathogenesis suggests that the inhibition of JAKs could be a powerful and more profound treatment than a treatment with a single mab. Of note, STAT3 is a key factor in IL-23/Th17 signaling. Active JAKs and active STAT3 are typically found in psoriatic skin (133, 134). The role of IL-23 and Th17 cells has also been studied in the imiquimod (IMQ) PSO mouse model. In this model, silencing of TYK2 by gene targeting abrogated skin inflammation (135). Likewise, the use of JAKi successively ameliorated skin inflammation with a concomitant decrease of cytokine levels in the IMQ PSO mouse model (136). In humans, Krueger et al. showed in a small cohort ($n = 12$) that treatment with tofacitinib (10 mg twice daily) ameliorated PSO and this was accompanied at a molecular level by the decrease of phosphorylated STAT1 and STAT3. Similarly, tofacitinib decreased epidermal thickness, reduced the number of T cells infiltrating the skin and suppressed the IL-23/Th17 pathway (137). These preliminary findings paved the way for JAKi application in humans with PSO. A phase III randomized double-blind placebo-controlled study (NCT01815424) demonstrated the efficacy of tofacitinib at doses of 5 or 10 mg twice daily in patients with moderate to severe PSO (138). The oral PSO trial (OPT) pivotal I and II studies confirmed these positive results by oral tofacitinib in chronic plaque PSO (**Figure 3**). Importantly, only 6% of treated patients experienced adverse events (139). Notably, treatment discontinuation was associated with a risk of relapse; however, re-initiation of the treatment rapidly resolved psoriatic inflammation (140). Another phase III randomized multicenter study showed that the efficacy of tofacitinib 10 mg twice daily is similar to the efficacy of etanercept 50 mg twice weekly in PSO (141). Tofacitinib (5 or 10 mg daily) is also beneficial in nail PSO (114). The OPAL study showed that the JAK1/JAK3i is highly effective in the control of PSA in patients not responding to anti TNF-α treatment. In 2018, tofacitinib 5 mg twice daily was approved by the FDA for the treatment of PSA (142). Under this therapeutic regimen tofacitinib seems to have an acceptable safety profile without severe adverse events even during long-term application (143, 144). Based on the experience with tofacitinib, numerous JAKi are tested as oral drugs or as topical formulation for PSO (**Table 9**) (145–147). So far, the efficacy of topical JAKi for psoriasis is not convincing (148–150). In a double-blind study, topical application of the JAK1/JAK2i ruxolitinib (1 or 1.5%) showed comparable reduction of skin inflammation as calcipotriene 0.005% cream or betamethasone dipropionate 0.05% cream (151). Oral JAKi are more promising. In a randomized, double blind, placebo controlled phase IIb study the JAK1/JAK2i baricitinib at 2, 4, 8, or 10 mg daily dose showed encouraging results in the treatment of moderate to severe PSO (152). Lastly, selective inhibition of TYK2 with the oral compound BMS-986165 seems to be another very promising therapeutic option for the treatment of PSO. In a phase II trial BMS-986165 given at 3, 6, 9, or 12 mg daily over a period of 12 weeks resulted in an impressive clearing of PSO compared to placebo (153). According to clinicaltrials.gov, the number of registered studies on JAKi for PSO is rapidly growing (**Table 9**). Both oral and topical compounds are currently under clinical investigation for PSO. These include the oral compounds solcitinib, filgotinib, upadacitinib, and delgocitinib (LEO124249), a topical pan-JAKi (154). The selective TYK2 inhibitors PF-06826647 and BMS-986165 are under investigation for PSO or PSO/PSA, respectively (**Table 9**). The expected results from these clinical trials will be a major step toward extending the therapeutic spectrum of PSO and PSA by oral compounds.

VITILIGO

Vitiligo is a skin disease with severe psychological impact on patients. The disease is characterized by the presence of white depigmented skin spots due to melanocytic destruction by self-reactive $CD8^+$ T cells (155). There is an enormous need for effective treatment options since presently the limited treatment modalities are only effective in some patients. Currently, patients with vitiligo are either treated with topical glucocorticosteroids, topical calcineurin inhibitors (off-label), or with phototherapy (narrowband UVB). In addition, systemic administration of glucocorticosteroids or other immunosuppressive drugs are used. Mechanistically, type I immune responses seem to be responsible for the development of vitiligo (156–159). In lesional skin, overexpression of IFN-γ, which translates its intracellular signal through STAT1, and associated chemokines like CXCL10 and its receptor CXCR3 are found (158). The biological relevance of these clinical findings was confirmed in mouse models of vitiligo. For instance, transfusion of $CXCR3^{-/-}$ PMEL T cells in vitiligo prone mice did not evolve to phenotypic alterations. Similarly, interfering with the CXCL10-CXCR3 interaction through targeting of CXCL10 with mabs results in vitiligo reversal in mice with established disease (160). These and other findings helped to elucidate the copious immunological players dominating vitiligo and underlined the crucial role of the JAK/STAT pathway and their related factors in the pathogenesis of this disorder. First small-size case series report from the efficacy of JAKi in vitiligo (161). Rothstein et al. used ruxolitinib 1.5% cream over a period of 20 weeks in a small group of 12

TABLE 9 | JAKi trials in psoriasis vulgaris, psoriatic arthritis and psoriasis inversa according to clinicaltrials.gov.

Disease subtype	Inhibitor	Target	Administration	Phase	Study number
PSO	Ruxolitinib	JAK1 JAK2	Topical	Phase II	NCT00617994
	Peficitinib	PanJAK	Oral	Phase II	NCT01096862
	PF-06826647	TYK2	Oral	Phase II	NCT03895372
	PF-06826647	TYK2	Oral	Phase I	NCT03210961
	PF-06700841	JAK1 TYK2	Topical	Phase II	NCT03850483
	PF-06763809	n/a	Topical	Phase I	NCT03469336
	BMS-986165	TYK2	Oral	Phase III	NCT03624127
	BMS-986165	TYK2	Oral	Phase III	NCT03611751
PSA	Itacitinib	JAK1	Oral	Phase II	NCT01634087
	Upadacitinib	JAK1	Oral	Phase III	NCT03104374
	Upadacitinib	JAK1	Oral	Phase III	NCT03104400
	Tofacitinib	JAK1 JAK3	Oral	Phase III	NCT03736161
	Tofacitinib	JAK1 JAK3	Oral	Phase III	NCT03486457
	Tofacitinib	JAK1 JAK3	Oral	Phase III	NCT01976364
	Filgotinib	JAK1	Oral	Phase II	NCT03320876
	BMS-986165	TYK2	Oral	Phase II	NCT03881059
iPSO	Delgocitinib	PanJAK	Oral	Phase II	NCT02695940

PSO, psoriasis vulgaris; PSA, psoriasis arthritis; iPSO, psoriasis inversa.

TABLE 10 | Clinical trials on JAKi for treating patients with vitiligo according to clinicaltrials.gov.

Disease type	Inhibitor	Target	Administration	Phase	Study number
Vitiligo	Ruxolitinib	JAK1 JAK2	Topical	Phase II	NCT03099304
	Ruxolitinib	JAK1 JAK2	Topical	Phase II	NCT02809976
	ATI-502	JAK1 JAK3	Topical	Phase II	NCT03468855
	PF-06651600 PF-06700841	JAK3 JAK1 TYK2	Oral	Phase II	NCT03715829

patients with vitiligo. They reported successful repigmentation of facial spots, while repigmentation of other anatomical sites showed mixed results (162). Similar results with better responses of facial spots than non-facial spots were reported by a recently published cohort study with 16 patients receiving 2% tofacitinib cream (163). A retrospective case study of 10 patients treated with oral tofacitinib 5 or 10 mg once daily suggests that a combination of phototherapy with JAKi is therapeutically more effective than JAKi monotherapy (164) (**Figure 3**). These reports indicate that JAKi in combination with UV exposure are required for stimulating repigmentation. Currently, different JAKi are under investigation in phase II trials for topical application in patients with vitiligo (**Table 10**).

POSSIBLE FUTURE APPLICATIONS

The introduction of JAKi is enlarging the therapeutic repertoire of dermatologists and is proving efficacy in numerous inflammatory diseases. Disorders like vitiligo or AA are in high need for efficient treatments. Increasing evidence confirming the beneficial role of systemic or topical JAKi in the treatment of these disorders is accumulating. Since the JAK/STAT signaling pathway plays a crucial role for many cytokines (**Figure 2**), a variety of inflammatory dermatological disorders may benefit from this new class of immunomodulators. For instance, lichen sclerosus et atrophicans (LSA) is an inflammatory disorder of skin and genital mucosa associated with severe pruritus and scaring. Many patients do not respond adequately to topical steroids (165). Due to its frequent recalcitrant course, there is an urgent need of new therapeutics for LSA. Inflammatory factors like IFN-γ, CXCL10, and CCR5 are highly expressed in lesional skin, suggesting that LSA is a Th1-dominated disorder (166). Oral or topical application of JAKi could stop the inflammatory circuit in LSA. Case reports on positive effects of JAKi exist for LSA and for patients with other sclerosing skin diseases like morphea, eosinophilic fasciitis, or systemic sclerosis (167, 168). These results are in agreement with experimental findings demonstrating a pivotal role of STAT3 in the activation of profibrotic pathways *in vivo* and *in vitro* (169). JAK inhibitors also improve inflammatory bowel diseases (IBD) like ulcerative colitis. Based on this data, it can be argued that IBD-associated skin diseases such as cheilitis granulomatosa (CG), pyoderma gangrenosum (PG) or erythema nodosum (EN) could also benefit from JAKi. CG shows a similar immunological profile as Crohn's disease with overexpression of IFN-γ (170–172). Patients with CG benefit from drugs such as thalidomide or lenalidomide (173, 174), which suppress Th1 cell responses (175). In contrast, analysis of PG and EN lesional skin revealed overexpression of TNF and STAT3, the latter one suggesting a rationale for the application of JAKi in these diseases (176). Other inflammatory diseases, where the use of JAKi seems to be desirable include sarcoidosis (177–180), and Sjögren's syndrome (SS), autoimmune diseases with strong molecular association to the JAK/STAT signaling pathway (181–184). Patients with blistering skin diseases like bullous pemphigoid, dermatitis herpetiformis Duhring and pemphigus vulgaris may also benefit from JAKi (185–187). JAKi have been shown to inhibit auto-ab production in preclinical models (188). Moreover, different studies highlighted the crucial role of STAT1 and STAT3 in transporting the signals derived from IL-6 and IL-21, two crucial cytokines for germinal centers formation. Lack of IL-6 and IL-21 leads to a strong reduction of T follicular helper (T_{FH}) cell levels and consequently to impaired germinal center formation and suppression of IgG levels, since T_{FH} cells provide unavoidable help for B cells' ab production (189, 190). Due to this preliminary data, JAKi could dramatically improve patients' quality of life in auto-ab-mediated bullous skin disorders, where high doses of oral glucocorticosteroids are currently the therapeutic gold standard and where the need of new therapeutic approaches is high, even though the B cell depleting mAb rituximab has been approved recently (191, 192). Another group of skin disorders that could benefit from JAKi are eczema. Delgocitinib, a pan-JAKi is currently under investigation in patients with chronic hand eczema (**Table 11**) and shows some first promising results (193). In nickel-induced allergic contact dermatitis there is evidence of an important involvement of the JAK/STAT pathway (194). Accordingly, mouse models for contact dermatitis show positive response to treatment with topical tofacitinib (JAK1/JAK3i) (195, 196), thus suggesting a possible application of topical JAKi also in humans. In Behcet's disease, an autoimmune disorder with unsolved pathogenesis experimental studies showed overexpression of Th17 related genes, overexpression of type I IFN-inducible genes and activation of the JAK/STAT pathway (197–199). These first experimental results pave the way for a future tentative application of JAKi in this disorder. Lastly, JAKi could improve autoinflammatory disorders. A patient with synovitis, acne, pustulosis, hyperostosis, and osteitis (SAPHO), has been successfully treated by a combination of methotrexate and oral tofacitinib (200). Similarly, the clinical trials NCT01724580 and NCT02974595 proved efficacy of baricitinib in a small group of patients affected by CANDLE (chronic atypical neutrophilic dermatosis with lipodystrophy and elevated temperatures) and SAVI (stimulator of IFN-genes associated vasculopaty with onset in infancy) (201, 202).

TABLE 11 | Clinical trials of JAKi in chronic hand eczema. cHE, chronic hand eczema according to clinicaltrials.gov.

Disease type	Inhibitor	Target	Administration	Phase	Study number
cHE	Delgocitinib	PanJAK	Topical	Phase II	NCT03683719
	Delgocitinib	PanJAK	Topical	Phase II	NCT02664805

CONCLUDING REMARKS

The introduction of JAKi in dermatology will revolutionize the therapeutic outcome of various inflammatory skin diseases. There is growing evidence that the JAK/STAT signaling pathway is a key pathway in numerous skin disorders. However, we are facing several hurdles. First, the development of selective JAKi was harder than initially thought. First generation JAKi, like tofacitinib and baricitinib, which were thought to be highly selective, target more than one single JAK. This is not necessarily a disadvantage regarding efficacy, but of course may bear a higher risk for toxicities (17). For instance, significant inhibition toward JAK2 leads to anemia. Some unexpected adverse events were also observed when using first generation JAKi (203–205). One example is the increase in cholesterol levels by tofacitinib (144, 206–208), which could be a paradox effect induced by the reduction of inflammation (209). The more recently developed JAKi seem to have improved selectivity (25, 27, 210). The other caveat for treating skin disorders via topical route is to generate formulations that allow small molecules like JAKi to penetrate the skin. Here, improvements like nanocarriers may be helpful (211–213). We still have a high therapeutic need for several skin diseases like vitiligo, AA, AD, LPP, LSA, and others. JAKi as topical formulation or systemic drug could be an outstanding improvement without side effects typically observed when using topical or systemic glucocorticosteroids. Yet, in the majority of the aforementioned skin diseases, we urgently need more evidence and larger double-blind placebo-controlled studies to confirm efficacy and safety of JAKi. The safety profile of JAKi reported so far seems to be acceptable, at least when used as monotherapy. One important question, which could favor the introduction of JAKi in dermatological daily routine, is the comparison of these with the well-established application of mabs. Even though studies directly comparing JAKi with biologicals are widely missing for dermatological indications, the anti-inflammatory properties of JAKi are conceivably profound. Nonetheless, the safety profile of these new compounds compared to the safety profile of mabs seem not to be very different (214–216). Experience from the here discussed studies show that severe adverse events are rare. Common adverse events like infections of the upper respiratory tract or common disturbances such as headache or diarrhea can be frequent, but easy to manage (217–219) (**Table 1; Supplementary Tables 1–3**). The reactivation of herpes zoster infection seems to be more frequent in patients treated with JAKi compared to those receiving biologicals and therefore vaccination prior to treatment initiation should be discussed (220–223). Blood count alterations seem to be reversible and normalize after withdrawal (224, 225) (**Table 1**). Published studies with different JAKi indicate an increased risk for bacterial and viral infections (226–230). From an economic point of view the lower production costs of JAKi compared to mabs may favor their application in dermatology (231). However, the simultaneous inhibition of multiple cytokines by systemic JAKi bears the risk for fatal outcomes during severe infections and possibly also the risk for cancer development on the long run 232). Moreover, the dose and half-life of JAKi is an important issue. It will be crucial to lower the threshold of JAK/STAT activation but not to permanently block this pathway. Notably, another major issue which must be addressed in the future and which is presently unknown is the impact of these drugs on long-term treatments setting. First data from non-dermatological studies will be available soon, but data from longer observational periods after approval for dermatological indications are needed 233–236). This will be important for calculating the risk for both, infectious and tumor diseases (237). In conclusion, JAK inhibitory drugs are emerging as a new and effective treatment for various diseases. So far, the results arouse enthusiasm among dermatologist; nonetheless, further studies will decide about the real-world efficacy and safety profiles of this new class of immunomodulators.

AUTHOR CONTRIBUTIONS

FS and KG designed the manuscript and designed figures and tables. FS, KM, and KG drafted the manuscript and approved the final version of the manuscript. KG revised critically the final version of the manuscript.

REFERENCES

1. Eyerich K, Eyerich S. Immune response patterns in non-communicable inflammatory skin diseases. *J Eur Acad Dermatol Venereol.* (2018) 32:692–703. doi: 10.1111/jdv.14673
2. Yazdi AS, Rocken M, Ghoreschi K. Cutaneous immunology: basics and new concepts. *Semin Immunopathol.* (2016) 38:3–10. doi: 10.1007/s00281-015-0545-x
3. Sabat RWK, Loyal L, Döcke WD, Ghoreschi K. T cell pathology in skin inflammation. *Semin Immunopathol.* (2019) 41:359–77. doi: 10.1007/s00281-019-00742-7
4. Boehncke WH, Schon MP. Psoriasis. *Lancet.* (2015) 386:983–94. doi: 10.1016/S0140-6736(14)61909-7
5. Kopp T, Riedl E, Bangert C, Bowman EP, Greisenegger E, Horowitz A, et al. Clinical improvement in psoriasis with specific targeting of interleukin-23. *Nature.* (2015) 521:222–6. doi: 10.1038/nature 14175
6. Lowes MA, Suarez-Farinas M, Krueger JG. Immunology of psoriasis. *Annu Rev Immunol.* (2014) 32:227–55. doi: 10.1146/annurev-immunol-032713-120225
7. Eberle FC, Bruck J, Holstein J, Hirahara K, Ghoreschi K. Recent advances in understanding psoriasis. *F1000Res.* (2016) 5:770. doi: 10.12688/f1000research.7927.1
8. Weidinger S, Novak N. Atopic dermatitis. *Lancet.* (2016) 387:1109–22. doi: 10.1016/S0140-6736(15)00149-X
9. Tsokos GC, Lo MS, Costa Reis P, Sullivan KE. New insights into the immunopathogenesis of systemic lupus erythematosus. *Nat Rev Rheumatol.* (2016) 12:716–30. doi: 10.1038/nrrheum.2016.186
10. Schmidt T, Solimani F, Pollmann R, Stein R, Schmidt A, Stulberg I, et al. TH1/TH17 cell recognition of desmoglein 3 and bullous pemphigoid antigen 180 in patients with lichen planus. *J Allergy Clin Immunol.* (2018) 142:669–72.e7. doi: 10.1016/j.jaci.2018.02.044
11. Solimani F, Pollmann R, Schmidt T, Schmidt A, Zheng X, Savai R, et al. Therapeutic targeting of Th17/Tc17 cells leads to clinical improvement of lichen planus. *Front Immunol.* (2019) 10:1808. doi: 10.3389/fimmu.2019.01808
12. Ghoreschi K, Laurence A, O'Shea JJ. Janus kinases in immune cell signaling. *Immunol Rev.* (2009) 228:273–87. doi: 10.1111/j.1600-065X.2008.00754.x

13. Bruck J, Dringen R, Amasuno A, Pau-Charles I, Ghoreschi K. A review of the mechanisms of action of dimethylfumarate in the treatment of psoriasis. *Exp Dermatol.* (2018) 27:611–24. doi: 10.1111/exd.13548
14. O'Shea JJ, Schwartz DM, Villarino AV, Gadina M, McInnes IB, Laurence A. The JAK-STAT pathway: impact on human disease and therapeutic intervention. *Annu Rev Med.* (2015) 66:311–28. doi: 10.1146/annurev-med-051113-024537
15. Welsch K, Holstein J, Laurence A, Ghoreschi K. Targeting JAK/STAT signalling in inflammatory skin diseases with small molecule inhibitors. *Eur J Immunol.* (2017) 47:1096–107. doi: 10.1002/eji.201646680
16. Fischer EH, Krebs EG. Relationship of structure to function of muscle phosphorylase. *Fed Proc.* (1966) 25:1511–20.
17. Ghoreschi K, Laurence A, O'Shea JJ. Selectivity and therapeutic inhibition of kinases: to be or not to be? *Nat Immunol.* (2009) 10:356–60. doi: 10.1038/ni.1701
18. Nosaka T, Vandeursen JMA, Tripp RA, Thierfelder WE, Witthuhn BA, Mcmickle AP, et al. Defective lymphoid development in mice lacking Jak3. *Science.* (1995) 270:800–2. doi: 10.1126/science.270.5237.800
19. Pesu M, Candotti F, Husa M, Hofmann SR, Notarangelo LD, O'Shea JJ. Jak3, severe combined immunodeficiency, and a new class of immunosuppressive drugs. *Immunol Rev.* (2005) 203:127–42. doi: 10.1111/j.0105-2896.2005.00220.x
20. Russell SM, Tayebi N, Nakajima H, Riedy MC, Roberts JL, Aman MJ, et al. Mutation of Jak3 in a patient with SCID: essential role of Jak3 in lymphoid development. *Science.* (1995) 270:797–800. doi: 10.1126/science.270.5237.797
21. Macchi P, Villa A, Giliani S, Sacco MG, Frattini A, Porta F, et al. Mutations of Jak-3 gene in patients with autosomal severe combined immune deficiency (SCID). *Nature.* (1995) 377:65–8. doi: 10.1038/377065a0
22. Minegishi Y, Saito M, Morio T, Watanabe K, Agematsu K, Tsuchiya S, et al. Human tyrosine kinase 2 deficiency reveals its requisite roles in multiple cytokine signals involved in innate and acquired immunity. *Immunity.* (2006) 25:745–55. doi: 10.1016/j.immuni.2006.09.009
23. Kreins AY, Ciancanelli MJ, Okada S, Kong XF, Ramirez-Alejo N, Kilic SS, et al. Human TYK2 deficiency: mycobacterial and viral infections without hyper-IgE syndrome. *J Exp Med.* (2015) 212:1641–62. doi: 10.1084/jem.20140280
24. Karaghiosoff M, Neubauer H, Lassnig C, Kovarik P, Schindler H, Pircher H, et al. Partial impairment of cytokine responses in Tyk2-deficient mice. *Immunity.* (2000) 13:549–60. doi: 10.1016/S1074-7613(00)00054-6
25. Forster M, Chaikuad A, Dimitrov T, Doring E, Holstein J, Berger BT, et al. Development, optimization, and structure-activity relationships of covalent-reversible JAK3 inhibitors based on a tricyclic imidazo[5,4-d]pyrrolo[2,3- b]pyridine scaffold. *J Med Chem.* (2018) 61:5350–66. doi: 10.1021/acs.jmedchem.8b00571
26. Forster M, Chaikuad A, Bauer SM, Holstein J, Robers MB, Corona CR, et al. Selective JAK3 inhibitors with a covalent reversible binding mode targeting a new induced fit binding pocket. *Cell Chem Biol.* (2016) 23:1335–40. doi: 10.1016/j.chembiol.2016.10.008
27. Dai J, Yang LX, Addison G. Current status in the discovery of covalent Janus kinase 3 (JAK3) inhibitors. *Mini Rev Med Chem.* (2019) 19:1531. doi: 10.2174/1389557519666190617152011
28. Xu H, Jesson MI, Seneviratne UI, Lin TH, Sharif MN, Xue L, et al. PF-06651600, a dual JAK3/TEC family kinase inhibitor. *ACS Chem Biol.* (2019) 14:1235–42. doi: 10.1021/acschembio.9b00188
29. Szilveszter KP, Nemeth T, Mocsai A. Tyrosine kinases in autoimmune and inflammatory skin diseases. *Front Immunol.* (2019) 10:1862. doi: 10.3389/fimmu.2019.01862
30. Hosking AM, Juhasz M, Mesinkovska NA. Topical Janus kinase inhibitors: a review of applications in dermatology. *J Am Acad Dermatol.* (2018) 79:535–44. doi: 10.1016/j.jaad.2018.04.018
31. Gilhar A, Etzioni A, Paus R. Alopecia areata. *N Engl J Med.* (2012) 366:1515–25. doi: 10.1056/NEJMra1103442
32. Barahmani N, Schabath MB, Duvic M, National Alopecia Areata R. History of atopy or autoimmunity increases risk of alopecia areata. *J Am Acad Dermatol.* (2009) 61:581–91. doi: 10.1016/j.jaad.2009.04.031
33. Chu SY, Chen YJ, Tseng WC, Lin MW, Chen TJ, Hwang CY, et al. Comorbidity profiles among patients with alopecia areata: the importance of onset age, a nationwide population-based study. *J Am Acad Dermatol.* (2011) 65:949–56. doi: 10.1016/j.jaad.2010.08.032
34. Goh C, Finkel M, Christos PJ, Sinha AA. Profile of 513 patients with alopecia areata: associations of disease subtypes with atopy, autoimmune disease and positive family history. *J Eur Acad Dermatol Venereol.* (2006) 20:1055–60. doi: 10.1111/j.1468-3083.2006.01676.x
35. Petukhova L, Duvic M, Hordinsky M, Norris D, Price V, Shimomura Y, et al. Genome-wide association study in alopecia areata implicates both innate and adaptive immunity. *Nature.* (2010) 466:113–7. doi: 10.1038/nature09114
36. Xing L, Dai Z, Jabbari A, Cerise JE, Higgins CA, Gong W, et al. Alopecia areata is driven by cytotoxic T lymphocytes and is reversed by JAK inhibition. *Nat Med.* (2014) 20:1043–9. doi: 10.1038/nm.3645
37. Aaronson DS, Horvath CM. A road map for those who don't know JAK-STAT. *Science.* (2002) 296:1653–5. doi: 10.1126/science.1071545
38. Tafazzoli A, Forstner AJ, Broadley D, Hofmann A, Redler S, Petukhova L, et al. Genome-wide microRNA analysis implicates miR-30b/d in the etiology of alopecia areata. *J Invest Dermatol.* (2018) 138:549–56. doi: 10.1016/j.jid.2017.09.046
39. Phan K, Sebaratnam DF. JAK inhibitors for alopecia areata: a systematic review and meta-analysis. *J Eur Acad Dermatol Venereol.* (2019) 33:850–6. doi: 10.1111/jdv.15489
40. Liu LY, Craiglow BG, Dai F, King BA. Tofacitinib for the treatment of severe alopecia areata and variants: a study of 90 patients. *J Am Acad Dermatol.* (2017) 76:22–8. doi: 10.1016/j.jaad.2016.09.007
41. Craiglow BG, Liu LY, King BA. Tofacitinib for the treatment of alopecia areata and variants in adolescents. *J Am Acad Dermatol.* (2017) 76:29–32. doi: 10.1016/j.jaad.2016.09.006
42. Almutairi N, Nour TM, Hussain NH. Janus kinase inhibitors for the treatment of severe alopecia areata: an open-label comparative study. *Dermatology.* (2019) 235:130–6. doi: 10.1159/000494613
43. Mackay-Wiggan J, Jabbari A, Nguyen N, Cerise JE, Clark C, Ulerio G, et al. Oral ruxolitinib induces hair regrowth in patients with moderate-to-severe alopecia areata. *JCI Insight.* (2016) 1:e89790. doi: 10.1172/jci.insight.89790
44. Kennedy Crispin M, Ko JM, Craiglow BG, Li S, Shankar G, Urban JR, et al. Safety and efficacy of the JAK inhibitor tofacitinib citrate in patients with alopecia areata. *JCI Insight.* (2016) 1:e89776. doi: 10.1172/jci.insight.89776
45. Gordon SC, Abudu M, Zancanaro P, Ko JM, Rosmarin D. Rebound effect associated with JAK inhibitor use in the treatment of alopecia areata. *J Eur Acad Dermatol Venereol.* (2019) 33:e156–e7. doi: 10.1111/jdv.15383
46. Jabbari A, Sansaricq F, Cerise J, Chen JC, Bitterman A, Ulerio G, et al. An open-label pilot study to evaluate the efficacy of tofacitinib in moderate to severe patch-type alopecia areata, totalis, and universalis. *J Invest Dermatol.* (2018) 138:1539–45. doi: 10.1016/j.jid.2018.01.032
47. Bayart CB, DeNiro KL, Brichta L, Craiglow BG, Sidbury R. Topical Janus kinase inhibitors for the treatment of pediatric alopecia areata. *J Am Acad Dermatol.* (2017) 77:167–70. doi: 10.1016/j.jaad.2017.03.024
48. Rachubinski AL, Estrada BE, Norris D, Dunnick CA, Boldrick JC, Espinosa JM. Janus kinase inhibition in Down syndrome: 2 cases of therapeutic benefit for alopecia areata. *JAAD Case Rep.* (2019) 5:365–7. doi: 10.1016/j.jdcr.2019.02.007
49. Craiglow BG. Topical tofacitinib solution for the treatment of alopecia areata affecting eyelashes. *JAAD Case Rep.* (2018) 4:988–9. doi: 10.1016/j.jdcr.2018.07.018
50. Gilhar A, Keren A, Paus R. JAK inhibitors and alopecia areata. *Lancet.* (2019) 393:318–9. doi: 10.1016/S0140-6736(18)32987-8
51. Gao L, Bin L, Rafaels NM, Huang L, Potee J, Ruczinski I, et al. Targeted deep sequencing identifies rare loss-of-function variants in IFNGR1 for risk of atopic dermatitis complicated by eczema herpeticum. *J Allergy Clin Immunol.* (2015) 136:1591–600. doi: 10.1016/j.jaci.2015.06.047
52. Czarnowicki T, Krueger JG, Guttman-Yassky E. Novel concepts of prevention and treatment of atopic dermatitis through barrier and immune manipulations with implications for the atopic march. *J Allergy Clin Immun.* (2017) 139:1723–34. doi: 10.1016/j.jaci.2017.04.004
53. Werfel T, Allam JP, Biedermann T, Eyerich K, Gilles S, Guttman-Yassky E, et al. Cellular and molecular immunologic mechanisms in patients with atopic dermatitis. *J Allergy Clin Immun.* (2016) 138:336–49. doi: 10.1016/j.jaci.2016.06.010
54. Iikura M, Suto H, Kajiwara N, Oboki K, Ohno T, Okayama Y, et al. IL-33 can promote survival, adhesion and cytokine production in human mast cells.

Lab Invest. (2007) 87:971–8. doi: 10.1038/labinvest.3700663

55. Saluja R, Ketelaar ME, Hawro T, Church MK, Maurer M, Nawijn MC. The role of the IL-33/IL-1RL1 axis in mast cell and basophil activation in allergic disorders. *Mol Immunol.* (2015) 63:80–5. doi: 10.1016/j.molimm.2014.06.018
56. Kamijo H, Miyagaki T, Hayashi Y, Akatsuka T, Watanabe-Otobe S, Oka T, et al. Increased interleukin-26 expression promotes Th17 and Th2-associated cytokine production by keratinocytes in atopic dermatitis. *J Invest Dermatol* (2019) doi: 10.1016/j.jid.2019.07.713. [Epub ahead of print].
57. Simpson EL, Akinlade B, Ardeleanu M. Two phase 3 trials of dupilumab versus placebo in atopic dermatitis. *N Engl J Med.* (2017) 376:1090–1. doi: 10.1056/NEJMc1700366
58. Wollenberg A, Howell MD, Guttman-Yassky E, Silverberg JI, Kell C, Ranade K, et al. Treatment of atopic dermatitis with tralokinumab, an anti-IL-13 mAb. *J Allergy Clin Immunol.* (2019) 143:135–41. doi: 10.1016/j.jaci.2018.05.029
59. Kabashima K, Furue M, Hanifin JM, Pulka G, Wollenberg A, Galus R, et al. Nemolizumab in patients with moderate-to-severe atopic dermatitis: Randomized, phase II, long-term extension study. *J Allergy Clin Immunol.* (2018) 142:1121–30.e7. doi: 10.1016/j.jaci.2018.03.018
60. Simpson EL, Flohr C, Eichenfield LF, Bieber T, Sofen H, Taieb A, et al. Efficacy and safety of lebrikizumab (an anti-IL-13 monoclonal antibody) in adults with moderate-to-severe atopic dermatitis inadequately controlled by topical corticosteroids: a randomized, placebo-controlled phase II trial (TREBLE). *J Am Acad Dermatol.* (2018) 78:863–71.e11. doi: 10.1016/j.jaad.2018.01.017
61. Smith D, Helgason H, Sulem P, Bjornsdottir US, Lim AC, Sveinbjornsson G, et al. A rare IL33 loss-of-function mutation reduces blood eosinophil counts and protects from asthma. *PLoS Genet.* (2017) 13:1006659. doi: 10.1371/journal.pgen.1006659
62. Amano W, Nakajima S, Kunugi H, Numata Y, Kitoh A, Egawa G, et al. The Janus kinase inhibitor JTE-052 improves skin barrier function through suppressing signal transducer and activator of transcription 3 signaling. *J Allergy Clin Immunol.* (2015) 136:667–77.e7. doi: 10.1016/j.jaci.2015.03.051
63. He H, Guttman-Yassky E. JAK inhibitors for atopic dermatitis: an update. *Am J Clin Dermatol.* (2019) 20:181–92. doi: 10.1007/s40257-018-0413-2
64. Ghoreschi K, Jesson MI, Li X, Lee JL, Ghosh S, Alsup JW, et al. Modulation of innate and adaptive immune responses by tofacitinib (CP-690,550). *J Immunol.* (2011) 186:4234–43. doi: 10.4049/jimmunol.1003668
65. Levy LL, Urban J, King BA. Treatment of recalcitrant atopic dermatitis with the oral Janus kinase inhibitor tofacitinib citrate. *J Am Acad Dermatol.* (2015) 73:395–9. doi: 10.1016/j.jaad.2015.06.045
66. Morris GM, Nahmias ZP, Kim BS. Simultaneous improvement of alopecia universalis and atopic dermatitis in a patient treated with a JAK inhibitor. *JAAD Case Rep.* (2018) 4:515–7. doi: 10.1016/j.jdcr.2017.12.016
67. Bissonnette R, Papp KA, Poulin Y, Gooderham M, Raman M, Mallbris L, et al. Topical tofacitinib for atopic dermatitis: a phase IIa randomized trial. *Br J Dermatol.* (2016) 175:902–11. doi: 10.1111/bjd.14871
68. Guttman-Yassky E, Silverberg JI, Nemoto O, Forman SB, Wilke A, Prescilla R, et al. Baricitinib in adult patients with moderate-to-severe atopic dermatitis: a phase 2 parallel, double-blinded, randomized placebo-controlled multiple-dose study. *J Am Acad Dermatol.* (2019) 80:913–21.e9. doi: 10.1016/j.jaad.2018.01.018
69. Haugh IM, Watson IT, Alan Menter M. Successful treatment of atopic dermatitis with the JAK1 inhibitor oclacitinib. *Proc (Bayl Univ Med Cent)* (2018) 31:524–5. doi: 10.1080/08998280.2018.1480246
70. Nakagawa H, Nemoto O, Yamada H, Nagata T, Ninomiya N. Phase 1 studies to assess the safety, tolerability and pharmacokinetics of JTE-052 (a novel Janus kinase inhibitor) ointment in Japanese healthy volunteers and patients with atopic dermatitis. *J Dermatol.* (2018) 45:701–9. doi: 10.1111/1346-8138.14322
71. Vazquez ML, Kaila N, Strohbach JW, Trzupek JD, Brown MF, Flanagan ME, et al. Identification of N-{cis-3-[Methyl(7H-pyrrolo[2,3-d]pyrimidin-4-yl)amino]cyclobutyl}propane-1-sulfo namide (PF-04965842): a selective JAK1 clinical candidate for the treatment of autoimmune diseases. *J Med Chem.* (2018) 61:1130–52. doi: 10.1021/acs.jmedchem.7b01598
72. Thompson C, Piguet V, Choy E. The pathogenesis of dermatomyositis. *Br J Dermatol.* (2018) 179:1256–62. doi: 10.1111/bjd.15607
73. Selva-O'Callaghan A, Pinal-Fernandez I, Trallero-Araguas E, Milisenda JC, Grau-Junyent JM, Mammen AL. Classification and management of adult inflammatory myopathies. *Lancet Neurol.* (2018) 17:816–28. doi: 10.1016/S1474-4422(18)30254-0
74. Fujimoto M, Watanabe R, Ishitsuka Y, Okiyama N. Recent advances in dermatomyositis-specific autoantibodies. *Curr Opin Rheumatol.* (2016) 28:636–44. doi: 10.1097/BOR.0000000000000329
75. Zhang W, Jiang SP, Huang L. Dermatomyositis and malignancy: a retrospective study of 115 cases. *Eur Rev Med Pharmacol Sci.* (2009) 13:77–80.
76. Greenberg SA, Pinkus JL, Pinkus GS, Burleson T, Sanoudou D, Tawil R, et al. Interferon-alpha/beta-mediated innate immune mechanisms in dermatomyositis. *Ann Neurol.* (2005) 57:664–78. doi: 10.1002/ana.20464
77. Greenberg SA, Sanoudou D, Haslett JN, Kohane IS, Kunkel LM, Beggs AH, et al. Molecular profiles of inflammatory myopathies. *Neurology.* (2002) 59:1170–82. doi: 10.1212/WNL.59.8.1170
78. Dalakas MC, Illa I, Dambrosia JM, Soueidan SA, Stein DP, Otero C, et al. A controlled trial of high-dose intravenous immune globulin infusions as treatment for dermatomyositis. *N Engl J Med.* (1993) 329:1993–2000. doi: 10.1056/NEJM199312303292704
79. Hornig J, Weinhage T, Schmidt LH, Buerke B, Schneider U, Pavenstadt H, et al. Response of dermatomyositis with lung involvement to Janus kinase inhibitor treatment. *Z Rheumatol.* (2018) 77:952–7. doi: 10.1007/s00393-018-0565-8
80. Hornung T, Janzen V, Heidgen FJ, Wolf D, Bieber T, Wenzel J. Remission of recalcitrant dermatomyositis treated with ruxolitinib. *N Engl J Med.* (2014) 371:2537–8. doi: 10.1056/NEJMc1412997
81. Kurtzman DJ, Wright NA, Lin J, Femia AN, Merola JF, Patel M, et al. Tofacitinib citrate for refractory cutaneous dermatomyositis: an alternative treatment. *JAMA Dermatol.* (2016) 152:944–5. doi: 10.1001/jamadermatol.2016.0866
82. Wendel S, Venhoff N, Frye BC, May AM, Agarwal P, Rizzi M, et al. Successful treatment of extensive calcifications and acute pulmonary involvement in dermatomyositis with the Janus-Kinase inhibitor tofacitinib - a report of two cases. *J Autoimmun.* (2019) 100:131–6. doi: 10.1016/j.jaut.2019.03.003
83. Chen Z, Wang X, Ye S. Tofacitinib in amyopathic dermatomyositis-associated interstitial lung disease. *N Engl J Med.* (2019) 381:291–3. doi: 10.1056/NEJMc1900045
84. Kurasawa K, Arai S, Namiki Y, Tanaka A, Takamura Y, Owada T, et al. Tofacitinib for refractory interstitial lung diseases in anti-melanoma differentiation-associated 5 gene antibody-positive dermatomyositis. *Rheumatology.* (2018) 57:2114–9. doi: 10.1093/rheumatology/key188
85. Aractingi S, Chosidow O. Cutaneous graft-versus-host disease. *Arch Dermatol.* (1998) 134:602–12. doi: 10.1001/archderm.134.5.602
86. Hymes SR, Alousi AM, Cowen EW. Graft-versus-host disease: part I. Pathogenesis and clinical manifestations of graft-versus-host disease. *J Am Acad Dermatol.* (2012) 66:515.e1–18. doi: 10.1016/j.jaad.2011.11.960
87. Bruggen MC, Klein I, Greinix H, Bauer W, Kuzmina Z, Rabitsch W, et al. Diverse T-cell responses characterize the different manifestations of cutaneous graft-versus-host disease. *Blood.* (2014) 123:290–9. doi: 10.1182/blood-2013-07-514372
88. Zorn E, Kim HT, Lee SJ, Floyd BH, Litsa D, Arumugarajah S, et al. Reduced frequency of FOXP3+ CD4+CD25+ regulatory T cells in patients with chronic graft-versus-host disease. *Blood.* (2005) 106:2903–11. doi: 10.1182/blood-2005-03-1257
89. Ghoreschi K, Thomas P, Penovici M, Ullmann J, Sander CA, Ledderose G, et al. PUVA-bath photochemotherapy and isotretinoin in sclerodermatous graft-versus-host disease. *Eur J Dermatol.* (2008) 18:667–70. doi: 10.1684/ejd.2008.0517
90. Imamura M, Hashino S, Kobayashi H, Kubayashi S, Hirano S, Minagawa T, et al. Serum cytokine levels in bone marrow transplantation: synergistic interaction of interleukin-6, interferon-gamma, and tumor necrosis factor-alpha in graft-versus-host disease. *Bone Marrow Transplant.* (1994) 13:745–51.
91. Lin MT, Storer B, Martin PJ, Tseng LH, Gooley T, Chen PJ, et al. Relation of an interleukin-10 promoter polymorphism to graft-versus-host disease and survival after hematopoietic-cell transplantation. *N Engl J Med.* (2003) 349:2201–10. doi: 10.1056/NEJMoa022060

92. Cavet J, Dickinson AM, Norden J, Taylor PR, Jackson GH, Middleton PG. Interferon-gamma and interleukin-6 gene polymorphisms associate with graft-versus-host disease in HLA-matched sibling bone marrow transplantation. *Blood.* (2001) 98:1594–600. doi: 10.1182/blood.V98.5.1594
93. Choi J, Ziga ED, Ritchey J, Collins L, Prior JL, Cooper ML, et al. IFNgammaR signaling mediates alloreactive T-cell trafficking and GVHD. *Blood.* (2012) 120:4093–103. doi: 10.1182/blood-2012-01-403196
94. Carniti C, Gimondi S, Vendramin A, Recordati C, Confalonieri D, Bermema A, et al. Pharmacologic inhibition of JAK1/JAK2 signaling reduces experimental murine acute GVHD while preserving GVT effects. *Clin Cancer Res.* (2015) 21:3740–9. doi: 10.1158/1078-0432.CCR-14-2758
95. Okiyama N, Furumoto Y, Villarroel VA, Linton JT, Tsai WL, Gutermuth J, et al. Reversal of CD8 T-cell-mediated mucocutaneous graft-versus-host-like disease by the JAK inhibitor tofacitinib. *J Invest Dermatol.* (2014) 134:992–1000. doi: 10.1038/jid.2013.476
96. Spoerl S, Mathew NR, Bscheider M, Schmitt-Graeff A, Chen S, Mueller T, et al. Activity of therapeutic JAK 1/2 blockade in graft-versus-host disease. *Blood.* (2014) 123:3832–42. doi: 10.1182/blood-2013-12-543736
97. Zeiser R, Burchert A, Lengerke C, Verbeek M, Maas-Bauer K, Metzelder SK, et al. Ruxolitinib in corticosteroid-refractory graft-versus-host disease after allogeneic stem cell transplantation: a multicenter survey. *Leukemia.* (2015) 29:2062–8. doi: 10.1038/leu.2015.212
98. von Bubnoff N, Ihorst G, Grishina O, Rothling N, Bertz H, Duyster J, et al. Ruxolitinib in GvHD (RIG) study: a multicenter, randomized phase 2 trial to determine the response rate of Ruxolitinib and best available treatment (BAT) versus BAT in steroid-refractory acute graft-versus-host disease (aGvHD) (NCT02396628). *BMC Cancer.* (2018) 18:1132. doi: 10.1186/s12885-018-5045-7
99. Saunte DML, Jemec GBE. Hidradenitis suppurativa: advances in diagnosis and treatment. *JAMA.* (2017) 318:2019–32. doi: 10.1001/jama.2017.16691
100. Wang B, Yang W, Wen W, Sun J, Su B, Liu B, et al. Gamma-secretase gene mutations in familial acne inversa. *Science.* (2010) 330:1065. doi: 10.1126/science.1196284
101. Mendonca CO, Griffiths CE. Clindamycin and rifampicin combination therapy for hidradenitis suppurativa. *Br J Dermatol.* (2006) 154:977–8. doi: 10.1111/j.1365-2133.2006.07155.x
102. Bettoli V, Join-Lambert O, Nassif A. Antibiotic treatment of hidradenitis suppurativa. *Dermatol Clin.* (2016) 34:81–9. doi: 10.1016/j.det.2015.08.013
103. Hotz C, Boniotto M, Guguin A, Surenaud M, Jean-Louis F, Tisserand P, et al. Intrinsic defect in keratinocyte function leads to inflammation in hidradenitis suppurativa. *J Invest Dermatol.* (2016) 136:1768–80. doi: 10.1016/j.jid.2016.04.036
104. Wolk K, Warszawska K, Hoeflich C, Witte E, Schneider-Burrus S, Witte K, et al. Deficiency of IL-22 contributes to a chronic inflammatory disease: pathogenetic mechanisms in acne inversa. *J Immunol.* (2011) 186:1228–39. doi: 10.4049/jimmunol.0903907
105. Kimball AB, Tzellos T, Calimlim BM, Teixeira HD, Geng Z, Okun MM. Achieving hidradenitis suppurativa response score is associated with significant improvement in clinical and patient-reported outcomes: *post hoc* analysis of pooled data from PIONEER I and II. *Acta Derm Venereol.* (2018) 98:932–7. doi: 10.2340/00015555-3012
106. Blok JL, Li K, Brodmerkel C, Horvatovich P, Jonkman MF, Horvath B. Ustekinumab in hidradenitis suppurativa: clinical results and a search for potential biomarkers in serum. *Br J Dermatol.* (2016) 174:839–46. doi: 10.1111/bjd.14338
107. Le Cleach L, Chosidow O. Clinical practice. Lichen planus. *N Engl J Med·* (2012) 366:723–32. doi: 10.1056/NEJMcp1103641
108. Wenzel J, Scheler M, Proelss J, Bieber T, Tuting T. Type I interferon-associated cytotoxic inflammation in lichen planus. *J Cutan Pathol.* (2006) 33:672–8. doi: 10.1111/j.1600-0560.2006.00527.x
109. Shao S, Tsoi LC, Sarkar MK, Xing X, Xue K, Uppala R, et al. IFN-γ enhances cell-mediated cytotoxicity against keratinocytes via JAK2/STAT1 in lichen planus. *Sci Transl Med.* (2019) 11:eaav7561. doi: 10.1126/scitranslmed.aav7561
110. Chen J, Feng J, Chen X, Xu H, Zhou Z, Shen X, et al. Immunoexpression of interleukin-22 and interleukin-23 in oral and cutaneous lichen planus lesions: a preliminary study. *Mediators Inflamm.* (2013) 2013:801974. doi: 10.1155/2013/801974
111. Piccinni MP, Lombardelli L, Logiodice F, Tesi D, Kullolli O, Biagiotti R, et al. Potential pathogenetic role of Th17, Th0, and Th2 cells in erosive and reticular oral lichen planus. *Oral Dis.* (2014) 20:212–8. doi: 10.1111/odi.12094
112. Shaker O, Hassan AS. Possible role of interleukin-17 in the pathogenesis of lichen planus. *Br J Dermatol.* (2012) 166:1367–8. doi: 10.1111/j.1365-2133.2011.10793.x
113. Yang CC, Khanna T, Sallee B, Christiano AM, Bordone LA. Tofacitinib for the treatment of lichen planopilaris: a case series. *Dermatol Ther.* (2018) 31:e12656. doi: 10.1111/dth.12656
114. Merola JF, Elewski B, Tatulych S, Lan S, Tallman A, Kaur M. Efficacy of tofacitinib for the treatment of nail psoriasis: Two 52-week, randomized, controlled phase 3 studies in patients with moderate-to-severe plaque psoriasis. *J Am Acad Dermatol.* (2017) 77:79–87.e1. doi: 10.1016/j.jaad.2017.01.053
115. Lisnevskaia L, Murphy G, Isenberg D. Systemic lupus erythematosus. *Lancet.* (2014) 384:1878–88. doi: 10.1016/S0140-6736(14)60128-8
116. Dorgham K, Amoura Z, Parizot C, Arnaud L, Frances C, Pionneau C, et al. Ultraviolet light converts propranolol, a nonselective beta-blocker and potential lupus-inducing drug, into a proinflammatory AhR ligand. *Eur J Immunol.* (2015) 45:3174–87. doi: 10.1002/eji.2014 45144
117. Deng Y, Tsao BP. Genetic susceptibility to systemic lupus erythematosus in the genomic era. *Nat Rev Rheumatol.* (2010) 6:683–92. doi: 10.1038/nrrheum.2010.176
118. Manfredo Vieira S, Hiltensperger M, Kumar V, Zegarra-Ruiz D, Dehner C, Khan N, et al. Translocation of a gut pathobiont drives autoimmunity in mice and humans. *Science.* (2018) 359:1156–61. doi: 10.1126/science.aar7201
119. Kuhn A, Wenzel J, Bijl M. Lupus erythematosus revisited. *Semin Immunopathol.* (2016) 38:97–112. doi: 10.1007/s00281-015-0550-0
120. Alunno A, Padjen I, Fanouriakis A, Boumpas DT. Pathogenic and therapeutic relevance of JAK/STAT signaling in systemic lupus erythematosus: integration of distinct inflammatory pathways and the prospect of their inhibition with an oral agent. *Cells.* (2019) 8:E898. doi: 10.3390/cells8080898
121. Dong J, Wang QX, Zhou CY, Ma XF, Zhang YC. Activation of the STAT1 signalling pathway in lupus nephritis in MRL/lpr mice. *Lupus.* (2007) 16:101–9. doi: 10.1177/0961203306075383
122. Hadj-Slimane R, Chelbi-Alix MK, Tovey MG, Bobe P. An essential role for IFN-alpha in the overexpression of Fas ligand on MRL/lpr lymphocytes and on their spontaneous Fas-mediated cytotoxic potential. *J Interferon Cytokine Res.* (2004) 24:717–28. doi: 10.1089/jir.2004. 24.717
123. Yiu G, Rasmussen TK, Ajami B, Haddon DJ, Chu AD, Tangsombatvisit S, et al. Development of Th17-associated interstitial kidney inflammation in lupus-prone mice lacking the gene encoding STAT-1. *Arthritis Rheumatol.* (2016) 68:1233–44. doi: 10.1002/art. 39535
124. Karonitsch T, Feierl E, Steiner CW, Dalwigk K, Korb A, Binder N, et al. Activation of the interferon-gamma signaling pathway in systemic lupus erythematosus peripheral blood mononuclear cells. *Arthritis Rheum.* (2009) 60:1463–71. doi: 10.1002/art.24449
125. Lu MC, Lai NS, Chen HC, Yu HC, Huang KY, Tung CH, et al. Decreased microRNA(miR)-145 and increased miR-224 expression in T cells from patients with systemic lupus erythematosus involved in lupus immunopathogenesis. *Clin Exp Immunol.* (2013) 171:91–9. doi: 10.1111/j.1365-2249.2012.04676.x
126. Menon M, Blair PA, Isenberg DA, Mauri C. A regulatory feedback between plasmacytoid dendritic cells and regulatory B cells is aberrant in systemic lupus erythematosus. *Immunity.* (2016) 44:683–97. doi: 10.1016/j.immuni.2016.02.012
127. Ding C, Chen X, Dascani P, Hu X, Bolli R, Zhang HG, et al. STAT3 signaling in B cells is critical for germinal center maintenance and contributes to the pathogenesis of murine models of lupus. *J Immunol.* (2016) 196:4477–86. doi: 10.4049/jimmunol.1502043
128. Xu Z, Duan B, Croker BP, Morel L. STAT4 deficiency reduces autoantibody production and glomerulonephritis in a mouse model of lupus. *Clin Immunol.* (2006) 120:189–98. doi: 10.1016/j.clim.2006.03.009

129. Lu LD, Stump KL, Wallace NH, Dobrzanski P, Serdikoff C, Gingrich DE, et al. Depletion of autoreactive plasma cells and treatment of lupus nephritis in mice using CEP-33779, a novel, orally active, selective inhibitor of JAK2. *J Immunol.* (2011) 187:3840–53. doi: 10.4049/jimmunol.1101228
130. Kahl L, Patel J, Layton M, Binks M, Hicks K, Leon G, et al. Safety, tolerability, efficacy and pharmacodynamics of the selective JAK1 inhibitor GSK2586184 in patients with systemic lupus erythematosus. *Lupus.* (2016) 25:1420–30. doi: 10.1177/0961203316640910
131. Kubo S, Nakayamada S, Tanaka Y. Baricitinib for the treatment of rheumatoid arthritis and systemic lupus erythematosus: a 2019 update. *Expert Rev Clin Immunol.* (2019) 15:693–700. doi: 10.1080/1744666X.2019.1608821
132. Wallace DJ, Furie RA, Tanaka Y, Kalunian KC, Mosca M, Petri MA, et al. Baricitinib for systemic lupus erythematosus: a double-blind, randomised, placebo-controlled, phase 2 trial. *Lancet.* (2018) 392:222–31. doi: 10.1016/S0140-6736(18)31363-1
133. Sano S, Chan KS, Carbajal S, Clifford J, Peavey M, Kiguchi K, et al. Stat3 links activated keratinocytes and immunocytes required for development of psoriasis in a novel transgenic mouse model. *Nat Med.* (2005) 11:43–9. doi: 10.1038/nm1162
134. Alves de Medeiros AK, Speeckaert R, Desmet E, Van Gele M, De Schepper S, Lambert J. JAK3 as an emerging target for topical treatment of inflammatory skin diseases. *PLoS ONE.* (2016) 11:e0164080. doi: 10.1371/journal.pone.0164080
135. Ishizaki M, Akimoto T, Muromoto R, Yokoyama M, Ohshiro Y, Sekine Y, et al. Involvement of tyrosine kinase-2 in both the IL-12/Th1 and IL-23/Th17 axes *in vivo*. *J Immunol.* (2011) 187:181–9. doi: 10.4049/jimmunol.1003244
136. Works MG, Yin F, Yin CC, Yiu Y, Shew K, Tran TT, et al. Inhibition of TYK2 and JAK1 ameliorates imiquimod-induced psoriasis-like dermatitis by inhibiting IL-22 and the IL-23/IL-17 axis. *J Immunol.* (2014) 193:3278–87. doi: 10.4049/jimmunol.1400205
137. Krueger J, Clark JD, Suarez-Farinas M, Fuentes-Duculan J, Cueto I, Wang CQ, et al. Tofacitinib attenuates pathologic immune pathways in patients with psoriasis: a randomized phase 2 study. *J Allergy Clin Immunol.* (2016) 137:1079–90. doi: 10.1016/j.jaci.2015.12.1318
138. Zhang J, Tsai TF, Lee MG, Zheng M, Wang G, Jin H, et al. The efficacy and safety of tofacitinib in Asian patients with moderate to severe chronic plaque psoriasis: a phase 3, randomized, double-blind, placebo-controlled study. *J Dermatol Sci.* (2017) 88:36–45. doi: 10.1016/j.jdermsci.2017.05.004
139. Papp KA, Menter MA, Abe M, Elewski B, Feldman SR, Gottlieb AB, et al. Tofacitinib, an oral Janus kinase inhibitor, for the treatment of chronic plaque psoriasis: results from two randomized, placebo-controlled, phase III trials. *Br J Dermatol.* (2015) 173:949–61. doi: 10.1111/bjd.14018
140. Bissonnette R, Iversen L, Sofen H, Griffiths CE, Foley P, Romiti R, et al. Tofacitinib withdrawal and retreatment in moderate-to-severe chronic plaque psoriasis: a randomized controlled trial. *Br J Dermatol.* (2015) 172:1395–406. doi: 10.1111/bjd.13551
141. Bachelez H, van de Kerkhof PC, Strohal R, Kubanov A, Valenzuela F, Lee JH, et al. Tofacitinib versus etanercept or placebo in moderate-to-severe chronic plaque psoriasis: a phase 3 randomised non-inferiority trial. *Lancet.* (2015) 386:552–61. doi: 10.1016/S0140-6736(14)62113-9
142. Gladman D, Rigby W, Azevedo VF, Behrens F, Blanco R, Kaszuba A, et al. Tofacitinib for psoriatic arthritis in patients with an inadequate response to TNF inhibitors. *N Engl J Med.* (2017) 377:1525–36. doi: 10.1056/NEJMoa1615977
143. Valenzuela F, Korman NJ, Bissonnette R, Bakos N, Tsai TF, Harper MK, et al. Tofacitinib in patients with moderate-to-severe chronic plaque psoriasis: long-term safety and efficacy in an open-label extension study. *Br J Dermatol.* (2018) 179:853–62. doi: 10.1111/bjd.16798
144. Wolk R, Armstrong EJ, Hansen PR, Thiers B, Lan S, Tallman AM, et al. Effect of tofacitinib on lipid levels and lipid-related parameters in patients with moderate to severe psoriasis. *J Clin Lipidol.* (2017) 11:1243–56. doi: 10.1016/j.jacl.2017.06.012
145. Bissonnette R, Luchi M, Fidelus-Gort R, Jackson S, Zhang H, Flores R, et al. A randomized, double-blind, placebo-controlled, dose-escalation study of the safety and efficacy of INCB039110, an oral janus kinase 1 inhibitor, in patients with stable, chronic plaque psoriasis. *J Dermatolog Treat.* (2016) 27:332–8. doi: 10.3109/09546634.2015.1115819
146. Papp K, Pariser D, Catlin M, Wierz G, Ball G, Akinlade B, et al. A phase 2a randomized, double-blind, placebo-controlled, sequential dose-escalation study to evaluate the efficacy and safety of ASP015K, a novel Janus kinase inhibitor, in patients with moderate-to-severe psoriasis. *Br J Dermatol.* (2015) 173:767–76. doi: 10.1111/bjd.13745
147. Ludbrook VJ, Hicks KJ, Hanrott KE, Patel JS, Binks MH, Wyres MR, et al. Investigation of selective JAK1 inhibitor GSK2586184 for the treatment of psoriasis in a randomized placebo-controlled phase IIa study. *Br J Dermatol.* (2016) 174:985–95. doi: 10.1111/bjd.14399
148. Papp KA, Bissonnette R, Gooderham M, Feldman SR, Iversen L, Soung J, et al. Treatment of plaque psoriasis with an ointment formulation of the Janus kinase inhibitor, tofacitinib: a Phase 2b randomized clinical trial. *BMC Dermatol.* (2016) 16:15. doi: 10.1186/s12895-016-0051-4
149. Ports WC, Khan S, Lan S, Lamba M, Bolduc C, Bissonnette R, et al. A randomized phase 2a efficacy and safety trial of the topical Janus kinase inhibitor tofacitinib in the treatment of chronic plaque psoriasis. *Br J Dermatol.* (2013) 169:137–45. doi: 10.1111/bjd.12266
150. Bagherani N, Smoller BR. Efficacy of topical tofacitinib, a Janus kinase inhibitor, in the treatment of plaque psoriasis. *Dermatol Ther.* (2017) 30:e12467 . doi: 10.1111/dth.12467
151. Punwani N, Scherle P, Flores R, Shi J, Liang J, Yeleswaram S, et al. Preliminary clinical activity of a topical JAK1/2 inhibitor in the treatment of psoriasis. *J Am Acad Dermatol.* (2012) 67:658–64. doi: 10.1016/j.jaad.2011.12.018
152. Papp KA, Menter MA, Raman M, Disch D, Schlichting DE, Gaich C, et al. A randomized phase 2b trial of baricitinib, an oral Janus kinase (JAK) 1/JAK2 inhibitor, in patients with moderate-to-severe psoriasis. *Br J Dermatol.* (2016) 174:1266–76. doi: 10.1111/bjd.14403
153. Papp K, Gordon K, Thaci D, Morita A, Gooderham M, Foley P, et al. Phase 2 trial of selective tyrosine kinase 2 inhibition in psoriasis. *N Engl J Med.* (2018) 379:1313–21. doi: 10.1056/NEJMoa1806382
154. Tanimoto A, Ogawa Y, Oki C, Kimoto Y, Nozawa K, Amano W, et al. Pharmacological properties of JTE-052: a novel potent JAK inhibitor that suppresses various inflammatory responses *in vitro* and *in vivo*. *Inflamm Res.* (2015) 64:41–51. doi: 10.1007/s00011-014-0782-9
155. Taieb A, Picardo M. Clinical practice. Vitiligo. *N Engl J Med.* (2009) 360:160–9. doi: 10.1056/NEJMcp0804388
156. Grimes PE, Morris R, Avaniss-Aghajani E, Soriano T, Meraz M, Metzger A. Topical tacrolimus therapy for vitiligo: therapeutic responses and skin messenger RNA expression of proinflammatory cytokines. *J Am Acad Dermatol.* (2004) 51:52–61. doi: 10.1016/j.jaad.2003.12.031
157. Harris JE, Harris TH, Weninger W, Wherry EJ, Hunter CA, Turka LA. A mouse model of vitiligo with focused epidermal depigmentation requires IFN-γ for autoreactive CD8(+) T-cell accumulation in the skin. *J Invest Dermatol.* (2012) 132:1869–76. doi: 10.1038/jid.2011.463
158. Rashighi M, Agarwal P, Richmond JM, Harris TH, Dresser K, Su MW, et al. CXCL10 is critical for the progression and maintenance of depigmentation in a mouse model of vitiligo. *Sci Transl Med.* (2014) 6:223ra23. doi: 10.1126/scitranslmed.3007811
159. Wankowicz-Kalinska A, van den Wijngaard RM, Tigges BJ, Westerhof W, Ogg GS, Cerundolo V, et al. Immunopolarization of CD4+ and CD8+ T cells to Type-1-like is associated with melanocyte loss in human vitiligo. *Lab Invest.* (2003) 83:683–95. doi: 10.1097/01.LAB.0000069521.42488.1B
160. Agarwal P, Rashighi M, Essien KI, Richmond JM, Randall L, Pazoki-Toroudi H, et al. Simvastatin prevents and reverses depigmentation in a mouse model of vitiligo. *J Invest Dermatol.* (2015) 135:1080–8. doi: 10.1038/jid.2014.529
161. Relke N, Gooderham M. The use of Janus kinase inhibitors in vitiligo: a review of the literature. *J Cutan Med Surg.* (2019) 23:298–306. doi: 10.1177/1203475419833609
162. Rothstein B, Joshipura D, Saraiya A, Abdat R, Ashkar H, Turkowski Y, et al. Treatment of vitiligo with the topical Janus kinase inhibitor ruxolitinib. *J Am Acad Dermatol.* (2017) 76:1054–60.e1. doi: 10.1016/j.jaad.2017.02.049
163. Mobasher P, Guerra R, Jiayang Li S, Frangos J, Ganesan AK, Huang V. Open label pilot study of 2% tofacitinib for the treatment of refractory vitiligo. *Br J Dermatol.* (2019). doi: 10.1111/bjd.18606
164. Liu LY, Strassner JP, Refat MA, Harris JE, King BA. Repigmentation in vitiligo using the Janus kinase inhibitor tofacitinib may require concomitant light exposure. *J Am Acad Dermatol.* (2017) 77:675–682.e1. doi: 10.1016/j.jaad.2017.05.043

165. Fistarol SK, Itin PH. Diagnosis and treatment of lichen sclerosus an update. *Am J Clin Dermatol.* (2013) 14:27–47. doi: 10.1007/s40257-012-0006-4
166. Terlou A, Santegoets LA, van der Meijden WI, Heijmans-Antonissen C, Swagemakers SM, van der Spek PJ, et al. An autoimmune phenotype in vulvar lichen sclerosus and lichen planus: a Th1 response and high levels of microRNA-155. *J Invest Dermatol.* (2012) 132(3 Pt 1):658–66. doi: 10.1038/jid.2011.369
167. Deverapalli SC, Rosmarin D. The use of JAK inhibitors in the treatment of progressive systemic sclerosis. *J Eur Acad Dermatol Venereol.* (2018) 32:e328. doi: 10.1111/jdv.14876
168. Kim SR, Charos A, Damsky W, Heald P, Girardi M, King BA. Treatment of generalized deep morphea and eosinophilic fasciitis with the Janus kinase inhibitor tofacitinib. *JAAD Case Rep.* (2018) 4:443–5. doi: 10.1016/j.jdcr.2017.12.003
169. Chakraborty D, Sumova B, Mallano T, Chen CW, Distler A, Bergmann C, et al. Activation of STAT3 integrates common profibrotic pathways to promote fibroblast activation and tissue fibrosis. *Nat Commun.* (2017) 8:1130. doi: 10.1038/s41467-017-01236-6
170. DeFilippis EM, Feldman SR, Huang WW. The genetics of pyoderma gangrenosum and implications for treatment: a systematic review. *Br J Dermatol.* (2015) 172:1487–97. doi: 10.1111/bjd.13493
171. Nasifoglu S, Heinrich B, Welzel J. Successful therapy for pyoderma gangrenosum with a Janus kinase 2 inhibitor. *Br J Dermatol.* (2018) 179:504–5. doi: 10.1111/bjd.16468
172. Freysdottir J, Zhang S, Tilakaratne WM, Fortune F. Oral biopsies from patients with orofacial granulomatosis with histology resembling Crohn's disease have a prominent Th1 environment. *Inflamm Bowel Dis.* (2007) 13:439–45. doi: 10.1002/ibd.20023
173. Thomas P, Walchner M, Ghoreschi K, Rocken M. Successful treatment of granulomatous cheilitis with thalidomide. *Arch Dermatol.* (2003) 139:136–8. doi: 10.1001/archderm.139.2.136
174. Solimani F, Eming R, Juratli HA, Scarsella L, Gschnell M, Pfutzner W. Successful treatment of cheilitis granulomatosa with lenalidomide. *J Eur Acad Dermatol Venereol.* (2019) 33:e357–e9. doi: 10.1111/jdv.15654
175. McHugh SM, Rifkin IR, Deighton J, Wilson AB, Lachmann PJ, Lockwood CM, et al. The immunosuppressive drug thalidomide induces T helper cell type 2 (Th2) and concomitantly inhibits Th1 cytokine production in mitogen- and antigen-stimulated human peripheral blood mononuclear cell cultures. *Clin Exp Immunol.* (1995) 99:160–7. doi: 10.1111/j.1365-2249.1995.tb05527.x
176. Vavricka SR, Galvan JA, Dawson H, Soltermann A, Biedermann L, Scharl M, et al. Expression patterns of TNFα, MAdCAM1, and STAT3 in intestinal and skin manifestations of inflammatory bowel disease. *J Crohns Colitis.* (2018) 12:347–54. doi: 10.1093/ecco-jcc/jjx158
177. Zhou T, Casanova N, Pouladi N, Wang T, Lussier Y, Knox KS, et al. Identification of Jak-STAT signaling involvement in sarcoidosis severity via a novel microRNA-regulated peripheral blood mononuclear cell gene signature. *Sci Rep.* (2017) 7:4237. doi: 10.1038/s41598-017-0 4109-6
178. Damsky W, Thakral D, Emeagwali N, Galan A, King B. Tofacitinib treatment and molecular analysis of cutaneous sarcoidosis. *N Engl J Med.* (2018) 379:2540–6. doi: 10.1056/NEJMoa1805958
179. Damsky W, Thakral D, McGeary MK, Leventhal J, Galan A, King B. Janus kinase inhibition induces disease remission in cutaneous sarcoidosis and granuloma annulare. *J Am Acad Dermatol.* (2019) doi: 10.1016/j.jaad.2019.05.098. [Epub ahead of print].
180. Wei JJ, Kallenbach LR, Kreider M, Leung TH, Rosenbach M. Resolution of cutaneous sarcoidosis after Janus kinase inhibitor therapy for concomitant polycythemia vera. *JAAD Case Rep.* (2019) 5:360–1. doi: 10.1016/j.jdcr.2019.02.006
181. Davies R, Sarkar I, Hammenfors D, Bergum B, Vogelsang P, Solberg SM, et al. Single cell based phosphorylation profiling identifies alterations in toll-like receptor 7 and 9 signaling in patients with primary sjogren's syndrome. *Front Immunol.* (2019) 10:281. doi: 10.3389/fimmu.2019.00281
182. Fox RI. Sjogren's syndrome. *Lancet.* (2005) 366:321–31. doi: 10.1007/3-211-27377-8_13
183. Davies R, Hammenfors D, Bergum B, Vogelsang P, Gavasso S, Brun JG, et al. Aberrant cell signalling in PBMCs upon IFN-α stimulation in primary Sjogren's syndrome patients associates with type I interferon signature. *Eur J Immunol.* (2018) 48:1217–27. doi: 10.1002/eji.201747213
184. Liew SH, Nichols KK, Klamerus KJ, Li JZ, Zhang M, Foulks GN. Tofacitinib (CP-690,550), a Janus kinase inhibitor for dry eye disease: results from a phase 1/2 trial. *Ophthalmology.* (2012) 119:1328–35. doi: 10.1016/j.ophtha.2012.01.028
185. Juczynska K, Wozniacka A, Waszczykowska E, Danilewicz M, Wagrowska-Danilewicz M, Wieczfinska J, et al. Expression of the JAK/STAT signaling pathway in bullous pemphigoid and dermatitis herpetiformis. *Mediators Inflamm.* (2017) 2017:6716419. doi: 10.1155/2017/6716419
186. Tavakolpour S. Tofacitinib as the potent treatment for refractory pemphigus: a possible alternative treatment for pemphigus. *Dermatol Ther.* (2018) 31:e12696. doi: 10.1111/dth.12696
187. Sarny S, Hucke M, El-Shabrawi Y. Treatment of mucous membrane pemphigoid with janus kinase inhibitor baricitinib. *JAMA Ophthalmol.* (2018) 136:1420–2. doi: 10.1001/jamaophthalmol.2018.3789
188. Onda M, Ghoreschi K, Steward-Tharp S, Thomas C, O'Shea JJ, Pastan IH, et al. Tofacitinib suppresses antibody responses to protein therapeutics in murine hosts. *J Immunol.* (2014) 193:48–55. doi: 10.4049/jimmunol.1400063
189. Choi YS, Eto D, Yang JA, Lao C, Crotty S. Cutting edge: STAT1 is required for IL-6-mediated Bcl6 induction for early follicular helper cell differentiation. *J Immunol.* (2013) 190:3049–53. doi: 10.4049/jimmunol.1203032
190. Ma CS, Avery DT, Chan A, Batten M, Bustamante J, Boisson-Dupuis S, et al. Functional STAT3 deficiency compromises the generation of human T follicular helper cells. *Blood.* (2012) 119:3997–4008. doi: 10.1182/blood-2011-11-392985
191. Amber KT, Maglie R, Solimani F, Eming R, Hertl M. Targeted therapies for autoimmune bullous diseases: current status. *Drugs.* (2018) 78:1527–48. doi: 10.1007/s40265-018-0976-5
192. Didona D, Maglie R, Eming R, Hertl M. Pemphigus: current and future therapeutic strategies. *Front Immunol.* (2019) 10:1418. doi: 10.3389/fimmu.2019.01418
193. Worm M, Bauer A, Elsner P, Mahler V, Molin S, Nielsen TSS. Efficacy and safety of topical delgocitinib in patients with chronic hand eczema: data from a randomised, double-blind, vehicle-controlled Phase 2a study. *Br J Dermatol.* (2019). doi: 10.1111/bjd.18469
194. Bechara R, Antonios D, Azouri H, Pallardy M. Nickel sulfate promotes IL-17A producing CD4+ T cells by an IL-23-dependent mechanism regulated by TLR4 and Jak-STAT pathways. *J Invest Dermatol.* (2017) 137:2140–8. doi: 10.1016/j.jid.2017.05.025
195. Fujii Y, Sengoku T. Effects of the Janus kinase inhibitor CP-690550 (tofacitinib) in a rat model of oxazolone-induced chronic dermatitis. *Pharmacology.* (2013) 91:207–13. doi: 10.1159/000347184
196. Fukuyama T, Ehling S, Cook E, Baumer W. Topically administered Janus-kinase inhibitors tofacitinib and oclacitinib display impressive antipruritic and anti-inflammatory responses in a model of allergic dermatitis. *J Pharmacol Exp Ther.* (2015) 354:394–405. doi: 10.1124/jpet.115.223784
197. Puccetti A, Fiore PF, Pelosi A, Tinazzi E, Patuzzo G, Argentino G, et al. Gene expression profiling in behcet's disease indicates an autoimmune component in the pathogenesis of the disease and opens new avenues for targeted therapy. *J Immunol Res.* (2018) 2018:4246965. doi: 10.1155/2018/4246965
198. Takeuchi M, Kastner DL, Remmers EF. The immunogenetics of Behcet's disease: a comprehensive review. *J Autoimmun.* (2015) 64:137–48. doi: 10.1016/j.jaut.2015.08.013
199. Tulunay A, Dozmorov MG, Ture-Ozdemir F, Yilmaz V, Eksioglu-Demiralp E, Alibaz-Oner F, et al. Activation of the JAK/STAT pathway in Behcet's disease. *Genes Immun.* (2015) 16:170–5. doi: 10.1038/gene. 2014.64
200. Yang Q, Zhao Y, Li C, Luo Y, Hao W, Zhang W. Case report: successful treatment of refractory SAPHO syndrome with the JAK inhibitor tofacitinib. *Medicine.* (2018) 97:e11149. doi: 10.1097/MD.00000000000 11149
201. Sanchez GAM, Reinhardt A, Ramsey S, Wittkowski H, Hashkes PJ, Berkun Y, et al. JAK1/2 inhibition with baricitinib in the treatment of autoinflammatory interferonopathies. *J Clin Invest.* (2018) 128:3041–52. doi: 10.1172/JCI98814
202. Kim H, Brooks KM, Tang CC, Wakim P, Blake M, Brooks SR, et al. Pharmacokinetics, pharmacodynamics, and proposed dosing of the Oral JAK1 and JAK2 inhibitor baricitinib in pediatric and young adult CANDLE and SAVI patients. *Clin Pharmacol Ther.* (2018) 104:364–73.

doi: 10.1002/cpt.936
203. Verden A, Dimbil M, Kyle R, Overstreet B, Hoffman KB. Analysis of spontaneous postmarket case reports submitted to the FDA regarding thromboembolic adverse events and JAK inhibitors. *Drug Saf.* (2018) 41:357–61. doi: 10.1007/s40264-017-0622-2
204. Tarp S, Eric Furst D, Boers M, Luta G, Bliddal H, Tarp U, et al. Risk of serious adverse effects of biological and targeted drugs in patients with rheumatoid arthritis: a systematic review meta-analysis. *Rheumatology.* (2017) 56:417–25. doi: 10.1093/rheumatology/kew442
205. Scott IC, Hider SL, Scott DL. Thromboembolism with Janus kinase (JAK) Inhibitors for rheumatoid arthritis: how real is the risk? *Drug Saf.* (2018) 41:645–53. doi: 10.1007/s40264-018-0651-5
206. Sands BE, Taub PR, Armuzzi A, Friedman GS, Moscariello M, Lawendy N, et al. Tofacitinib treatment is associated with modest and reversible increases in serum lipids in patients with ulcerative colitis. *Clin Gastroenterol Hepatol.* (2019) doi: 10.1016/j.cgh.2019.04.059. [Epub ahead of print].
207. Novikova DS, Udachkina HV, Markelova EI, Kirillova IG, Misiyuk AS, Demidova NV, et al. Dynamics of body mass index and visceral adiposity index in patients with rheumatoid arthritis treated with tofacitinib. *Rheumatol Int.* (2019) 39:1181–9. doi: 10.1007/s00296-019-04303-x
208. Saeed I, McLornan D, Harrison CN. Managing side effects of JAK inhibitors for myelofibrosis in clinical practice. *Expert Rev Hematol.* (2017) 10:617–25. doi: 10.1080/17474086.2017.1337507
209. Perez-Baos S, Barrasa JI, Gratal P, Larranaga-Vera A, Prieto-Potin I, Herrero-Beaumont G, et al. Tofacitinib restores the inhibition of reverse cholesterol transport induced by inflammation: understanding the lipid paradox associated with rheumatoid arthritis. *Br J Pharmacol.* (2017) 174:3018–31. doi: 10.1111/bph.13932
210. Hammaren HM, Virtanen AT, Abraham BG, Peussa H, Hubbard SR, Silvennoinen O. Janus kinase 2 activation mechanisms revealed by analysis of suppressing mutations. *J Allergy Clin Immunol.* (2019) 143:1549–59.e6. doi: 10.1016/j.jaci.2018.07.022
211. Lademann J, Richter H, Meinke MC, Lange-Asschenfeldt B, Antoniou C, Mak WC, et al. Drug delivery with topically applied nanoparticles: science fiction or reality. *Skin Pharmacol Physiol.* (2013) 26:227–33. doi: 10.1159/000351940
212. Lademann J, Richter H, Schanzer S, Meinke MC, Darvin ME, Schleusener J, et al. Follicular penetration of nanocarriers is an important penetration pathway for topically applied drugs. *Hautarzt.* (2019) 70:185–92. doi: 10.1007/s00105-018-4343-y
213. Lademann J, Schaefer H, Otberg N, Teichmann A, Blume-Peytavi U, Sterry W. Penetration of microparticles into human skin. *Hautarzt.* (2004) 55:1117–9. doi: 10.1007/s00105-004-0841-1
214. Fleischmann R, Mysler E, Hall S, Kivitz AJ, Moots RJ, Luo Z, et al. Efficacy and safety of tofacitinib monotherapy, tofacitinib with methotrexate, and adalimumab with methotrexate in patients with rheumatoid arthritis (ORAL Strategy): a phase 3b/4, double-blind, head-to-head, randomised controlled trial. *Lancet.* (2017) 390:457–68. doi: 10.1016/S0140-6736(17)31618-5
215. Taylor PC, Keystone EC, van der Heijde D, Weinblatt ME, Del Carmen Morales L, Reyes Gonzaga J, et al. Baricitinib versus placebo or adalimumab in rheumatoid arthritis. *N Engl J Med.* (2017) 376:652–62. doi: 10.1056/NEJMoa1608345
216. van Vollenhoven RF, Fleischmann R, Cohen S, Lee EB, Garcia Meijide JA, Wagner S, et al. Tofacitinib or adalimumab versus placebo in rheumatoid arthritis. *N Engl J Med.* (2012) 367:508–19. doi: 10.1056/NEJMoa1112072
217. Mueller RB, Hasler C, Popp F, Mattow F, Durmisi M, Souza A, et al. Effectiveness, tolerability, and safety of tofacitinib in rheumatoid arthritis: a retrospective analysis of real-world data from the St. Gallen and Aarau cohorts. *J Clin Med.* (2019) 8:E1548. doi: 10.3390/jcm8101548
218. Ma C, Lee JK, Mitra AR, Teriaky A, Choudhary D, Nguyen TM, et al. Systematic review with meta-analysis: efficacy and safety of oral Janus kinase inhibitors for inflammatory bowel disease. *Aliment Pharmacol Ther.* (2019) 50:5–23. doi: 10.1111/apt.15297
219. Winthrop KL, Park SH, Gul A, Cardiel MH, Gomez-Reino JJ, Tanaka Y, et al. Tuberculosis and other opportunistic infections in tofacitinib-treated patients with rheumatoid arthritis. *Ann Rheum Dis.* (2016) 75:1133–8. doi: 10.1136/annrheumdis-2015-207319
220. Curtis JR, Xie F, Yun H, Bernatsky S, Winthrop KL. Real-world comparative risks of herpes virus infections in tofacitinib and biologic-treated patients with rheumatoid arthritis. *Ann Rheum Dis.* (2016) 75:1843–7. doi: 10.1136/annrheumdis-2016-209131
221. Winthrop KL, Wouters AG, Choy EH, Soma K, Hodge JA, Nduaka CI, et al. The safety and immunogenicity of live zoster vaccination in patients with rheumatoid arthritis before starting tofacitinib: a randomized phase II trial. *Arthritis Rheumatol.* (2017) 69:1969–77. doi: 10.1002/art.40187
222. Almanzar G, Kienle F, Schmalzing M, Maas A, Tony HP, Prelog M. Tofacitinib modulates the VZV-specific CD4+ T cell immune response *in vitro* in lymphocytes of patients with rheumatoid arthritis. *Rheumatology.* (2019) 58:2051–60. doi: 10.1093/rheumatology/kez175
223. Winthrop KL, Yamanaka H, Valdez H, Mortensen E, Chew R, Krishnaswami S, et al. Herpes zoster and tofacitinib therapy in patients with rheumatoid arthritis. *Arthritis Rheumatol.* (2014) 66:2675–84. doi: 10.1002/art.38745
224. Weinhold KJ, Bukowski JF, Brennan TV, Noveck RJ, Staats JS, Lin L, et al. Reversibility of peripheral blood leukocyte phenotypic and functional changes after exposure to and withdrawal from tofacitinib, a Janus kinase inhibitor, in healthy volunteers. *Clin Immunol.* (2018) 191:10–20. doi: 10.1016/j.clim.2018.03.002
225. Shi JG, Chen X, Lee F, Emm T, Scherle PA, Lo Y, et al. The pharmacokinetics, pharmacodynamics, and safety of baricitinib, an oral JAK 1/2 inhibitor, in healthy volunteers. *J Clin Pharmacol.* (2014) 54:1354–61. doi: 10.1002/jcph.354
226. Chen Y, Gong FY, Li ZJ, Gong Z, Zhou Z, Ma SY, et al. A study on the risk of fungal infection with tofacitinib (CP-690550), a novel oral agent for rheumatoid arthritis. *Sci Rep.* (2017) 7:6779. doi: 10.1038/s41598-017-07261-1
227. Lussana F, Cattaneo M, Rambaldi A, Squizzato A. Ruxolitinib-associated infections: a systematic review and meta-analysis. *Am J Hematol.* (2018) 93:339–47. doi: 10.1002/ajh.24976
228. Strand V, Ahadieh S, French J, Geier J, Krishnaswami S, Menon S, et al. Systematic review and meta-analysis of serious infections with tofacitinib and biologic disease-modifying antirheumatic drug treatment in rheumatoid arthritis clinical trials. *Arthritis Res Ther.* (2015) 17:362. doi: 10.1186/s13075-015-0880-2
229. Curtis JR, Xie F, Yang S, Bernatsky S, Chen L, Yun H, et al. Risk for herpes zoster in tofacitinib-treated rheumatoid arthritis patients with and without concomitant methotrexate and glucocorticoids. *Arthritis Care Res.* (2019) 71:1249–54. doi: 10.1002/acr.23769
230. Colombel JF. Herpes zoster in patients receiving JAK inhibitors for ulcerative colitis: mechanism, epidemiology, management, and prevention. *Inflamm Bowel Dis.* (2018) 24:2173–82. doi: 10.1093/ibd/izy150
231. Kotyla PJ. Are Janus kinase inhibitors superior over classic biologic agents in RA patients? *Biomed Res Int.* (2018) 2018:7492904. doi: 10.1155/2018/7492904
232. Curtis JR, Lee EB, Kaplan IV, Kwok K, Geier J, Benda B, et al. Tofacitinib, an oral Janus kinase inhibitor: analysis of malignancies across the rheumatoid arthritis clinical development programme. *Ann Rheum Dis.* (2016) 75:831–41. doi: 10.1136/annrheumdis-2014-205847
233. Harigai M, Takeuchi T, Smolen JS, Winthrop KL, Nishikawa A, Rooney TP, et al. Safety profile of baricitinib in Japanese patients with active rheumatoid arthritis with over 1.6 years median time in treatment: an integrated analysis of Phases 2 and 3 trials. *Mod Rheumatol.* (2019) 20:1–8. doi: 10.1080/14397595.2019.1583711
234. Sandborn WJ, Panes J, D'Haens GR, Sands BE, Su C, Moscariello M, et al. Safety of tofacitinib for treatment of ulcerative colitis, based on 4.4 years of data from global clinical trials. *Clin Gastroenterol Hepatol.* (2019) 17:1541–50. doi: 10.1016/j.cgh.2018.11.035
235. Wollenhaupt J, Lee EB, Curtis JR, Silverfield J, Terry K, Soma K, et al. Safety and efficacy of tofacitinib for up to 9.5 years in the treatment of rheumatoid arthritis: final results of a global, open-label, long-term extension study. *Arthritis Res Ther.* (2019) 21:89. doi: 10.1186/s13075-019-1866-2

236. Cohen SB, Tanaka Y, Mariette X, Curtis JR, Lee EB, Nash P, et al. Long-term safety of tofacitinib for the treatment of rheumatoid arthritis up to 8.5 years: integrated analysis of data from the global clinical trials. *Ann Rheum Dis.* (2017) 76:1253–62. doi: 10.1136/annrheumdis-2016-210457
237. Winthrop KL. The emerging safety profile of JAK inhibitors in rheumatic disease. *Nat Rev Rheumatol.* (2017) 13:234–43. doi: 10.1038/nrrheum.2017.23

21

Non-Invasive Approaches for the Diagnosis of Autoimmune/Autoinflammatory Skin Diseases—A Focus on Psoriasis and *Lupus erythematosus*

Anna Berekméri[1,2], Ana Tiganescu[3], Adewonuola A. Alase[1], Edward Vital[1,2], Martin Stacey[4†] and Miriam Wittmann[1,2†]*

[1] Faculty of Medicine and Health, Leeds Institute of Rheumatic and Musculoskeletal Medicine, University of Leeds, Leeds, United Kingdom, [2] Leeds Biomedical Research Centre, National Institute for Health Research, Leeds Teaching Hospitals, Leeds, United Kingdom, [3] Faculty of Medicine and Health, Leeds Institute of Cardiovascular and Metabolic Medicine, University of Leeds, Leeds, United Kingdom, [4] Faculty of Biological Sciences, School of Molecular and Cellular Biology, University of Leeds, Leeds, United Kingdom

***Correspondence:**
Miriam Wittmann
m.wittmann@leeds.ac.uk

† Joint senior authors

The traditional diagnostic gold standard for inflammatory skin lesions of unclear etiology is dermato-histopathology. As this approach requires an invasive skin biopsy, biopsy processing and analysis by specialized histologists, it is a resource intensive approach requiring trained healthcare professionals. In many health care settings access to this diagnostic approach can be difficult and outside emergency cases will usually take several weeks. This scenario leads to delayed or inappropriate treatment given to patients. With dramatically increased sensitivity of a range of analysis systems including mass spectrometry, high sensitivity, multiplex ELISA based systems and PCR approaches we are now able to "measure" samples with unprecedented sensitivity and accuracy. Other important developments include the long-term monitoring of parameters using microneedle approaches and the improvement in imaging systems such as optical coherence tomography. In this review we will focus on recent achievements regarding measurements from non-invasive sampling, in particular from plucked hair and skin tape-strips which seem well suited for the diagnosis of lupus erythematosus and psoriatic inflammation, respectively. While these approaches will not replace clinical observation—they can contribute to improved subgroup diagnosis, stratified therapeutic approaches and have great potential for providing molecular and mechanistic insight in to inflammatory skin diseases.

Keywords: lupus, psoriasis, skin inflammation, tape stripping, hair follicle

INTRODUCTION

Traditionally, the diagnosis of autoimmune and inflammatory skin diseases relies on the visual assessment by experienced dermatologists as well as dermato-histopathology. Descriptive diagnosis of skin biopsies is normally based on conventional histological staining but may also include direct immunofluorescence for the detection of antibody and complement deposits. Depending on the underlying disease, blood results in particular regarding circulating auto-antibodies directed against structural epidermal components (pemphigus, pemphigoid) or anti-nuclear antibodies can give certainty regarding the underlying disease. However, as blood focused diagnostics can often be negative for cutaneous disease manifesting, key information must often be derived from analysis of skin tissue itself.

So why are changes or additions to the established diagnostic approach for inflammatory skin disease required? There are a number of reasons. Firstly, due to the non-systemic nature of many skin diseases, reliable serum biomarkers may simply be non-existent or unreliable. Secondly, the use of skin biopsies as a diagnostic tool is an invasive procedure and not always readily available in many health systems or local situations. Skin biopsies require specialized, trained health care professionals, laboratory and histology staff (dermatohistopathologists) and the time to perform biopsies in addition to the wait for result reporting, can in clinical reality often be weeks. Furthermore, as many primary health care settings lack access to specialist dermatology care, approaches suitable for general practitioners (GP) would be very welcome to support diagnostic pathways.

Apart from costs, time and staff availability, an important issue comes from the recognized need and ambition to move forward in the field of stratified medicine (also referred to as personalized medicine, precision medicine). This approach aims to recognize sub-types of diseases outside the traditional morphology based categories, allowing optimized treatment choices and thus preventing the current "trial and error" approach to identify which treatment actually works best for which patient. For this to become a reality for a wide range of patients, researchers, and clinicians need to start thinking of alternatives to conventional approaches and embrace new molecular analysis tools, parameters not traditionally included in dermatology diagnosis, and easy, non-invasive approaches. Ideally, these approaches would not require highly-trained specialists to perform and analyse results, results would be available within the first presentation of the patient ("point-of-care" diagnostic) and would allow repeated diagnostic assessment over time.

While confirming the diagnosis of cutaneous lupus erythematosus (LE) can be challenging due to the wide variety of possible lesion morphologies, the diagnosis of psoriasis is usually directed by pathognomonic clinical presentation. So why is there a need to additional approaches regarding psoriatic inflammation? Diagnostic challenges occur for lesions which do not fall into the typical plaque type psoriasis or display minimal pathology; however, they are important to diagnose due to the existence of co-morbidities such as psoriatic arthritis and cardiovascular disease. Lesions in certain anatomical locations such as palmoplantar, retro-auricular, outer ear canal and scalp can also be challenging for both GP and trained dermatologists, and in particular skin fold lesions can often be misdiagnosed as fungal infection and treated without success with anti-fungals.

In this review we endeavor to give an overview of existing non-invasive techniques and highlight major recent advances demonstrating their potential as next generation diagnostics and as powerful tools to provide cellular and molecular insights in to inflammatory skin diseases.

IMAGING

Recent developments in imaging and imagining analysis techniques have added to our ability to assess real time changes in the skin. The most widely used imaging technique in standard care dermatology for suspicious and/or pigmented lesions is dermatoscopy. Dermatoscopy standards are developed by the international dermatoscopy society (dermoscopy-ids.org) and the approach has also been successfully used to support diagnosis of inflammatory skin conditions [for review: (1–3)]. Dermatoscopy needs training, although machine learning based analysis tools are successfully being developed in particular for cancerous lesions, and is usually performed in dermatology settings.

While this review does not specifically focus on imaging techniques, the following innovative approaches have to be mentioned, although they do require significant financial investments. A recent development, not yet introduced into clinical settings is Raster Scanning Optoacoustic Mesoscopy (RSOM) (4). This technique also termend photoacoustic mesoscopy is based on ultra-broadband (10–180 MHz) detection, achieves tissue resolution of 4 μm axially and 20 μm laterally and importantly can visualize vascular patterns in dermal skin compartments. A number of studies have collected images from human skin including eczema, psoriasis and nail fold changes in scleroderma capillaries (4, 5). This imaging approach can distinguish between intra- and subepidermal morphology features typical for eczema or psoriasis lesions (5).

By contrast, optical coherence tomography (OCT), which can deliver similar morphology information [detailed comparison of OCT vs. RSOM is given in (4)], has been used in a wide range of skin lesions, in particular in neoplastic ones to assess invasiveness and depth of the tumor. OCT uses light to capture sub-micrometer resolution and creates three-dimensional images from upper skin layers. The method is based on low-coherence interferometry employing near-infrared light. The use of relatively long wavelength light allows it to penetrate 1–2 mm into the tissue. This method generates detailed 3D data on skin surface roughness, tissue density, and vascular network in addition to non-invasive measurement of architectural features such as epidermal thickness. This technology is already being utilized as a biomarker for scleroderma and systemic sclerosis (6–8), preclinical diagnosis of palmar hyperkeratosis (9) and to evaluate wound re-epithelialization (10).

In psoriasis, OCT can detect all common psoriasis nail changes including leukonychia/white spots, pitting/localized surface irregularities, diffuse surface waving, onycholysis, and subungual hyperkeratosis (11). Studies evaluating psoriatic plaque vascular morphology are also beginning to surface, although are currently limited by low cohort numbers (12, 13).

In cutaneous LE, OCT has been shown to correlate with histological features of disease including hyperkeratosis, epidermal atrophy, and edema (14). More recently available higher resolution OCT has also been found to be of value for the diagnosis of autoimmune blistering skin diseases. However, to date—this technique is considered auxiliary to skin biopsies in this disease group (15, 16) and larger trials are not available yet.

Unfortunately, at present, costly hardware, expertise and time required to analyzed skin lesions is likely to limit the use of OCT to the research setting and specialist clinics.

Microcirculatory abnormalities are found in many inflammatory skin diseases. High Resolution Laser Doppler imaging (LDI) is a single-probe, non-invasive imaging method that can quantify total local microcirculatory blood perfusion, including capillaries, arterioles, venules, and shunting vessels. Similarly to ultrasound, it is based on the Doppler effect. Briefly, when low-level light is directed onto the skin, a fraction of this light penetrates the skin and interacts with both the static tissue and the moving red blood cells (RBCs). The light that is reflected from this static tissue remains unchanged in wavelength. The light that is scattered from the moving RBCs undergoes a change in wavelength. This backscattered light is then collected by the photodetector of LDI system to provide a signal or reading that is proportional to the speed and density of the moving RBCs (17). Alteration in peripheral blood flow (as measured by LDI) has been shown to correlate with inflammation in skin psoriasis (18). More recently, our group showed that in cutaneous LE, LDI showed better correlation with histology than clinical assessment using the local Cutaneous LE Disease Area and Severity Index (CLASI) or a physician's visual analog scale (19).

FUNCTIONAL SKIN TESTING

Trans-Epidermal Water Loss

Trans-epidermal water loss (TEWL) is a validated measure of skin epidermal permeability barrier function, measured with a non-invasive Tewameter® probe (20, 21). Evaporation of water from the skin occurs as part of normal skin metabolism. As barrier function is disrupted, water loss increases. TEWL measures the density gradient of the water evaporation from the skin, expressed as evaporation rate ($g/h/m^2$). In addition to resting TEWL, epidermal function can be assessed by measuring TEWL recovery over time following barrier disruption by repeated tape stripping (20).

Although atopic eczema is best recognized for its barrier defects clinical and molecular evidence suggest that barrier defects play a role in psoriatic disease pathogenesis (22–25). Further, experimental skin barrier disruption leads to several psoriasis-like features including epidermal hyperproliferation, production of pro-inflammatory cytokines, increased inflammatory infiltrate, elevated vascular endothelial growth factor and consequently, increased vascularization (26–29). Conversely, glucocorticoid/corticosteroid therapy reverses many of these features to restore normal barrier function (23, 30). Glucocorticoids also help to maintain the barrier function by directly promoting keratinocyte differentiation pathways (31, 32) which result in a paradoxical improvement in barrier function (33). Interestingly, a recent transcriptomic study found a >90% deficit in expression of the glucocorticoid-activating enzyme 11β-hydroxysteroid dehydrogenase type 1 in psoriatic plaques (34) which has also recently been shown to modulate epidermal barrier integrity (35).

Several small clinical studies have employed TEWL as a measure of treatment efficacy in psoriasis (36–40). However, the use of TEWL as a diagnostic tool has not been studied in detail due to a lack of specificity, as other skin conditions such as eczema also present with impaired epidermal barrier function (41, 42). A recent study by Ye et al. used TEWL to demonstrate differences in barrier recovery between stable and progressive forms of psoriasis in uninvolved skin sites (43). Further studies in larger cohorts are required to fully assess the auxiliary value of TEWL as a non-invasive diagnostic or disease activity measure in psoriasis.

TEWL is mainly examined in diseases with epidermal involvement. Thus, LE which shows inflammatory activity around the basement membrane area may not show significant changes in TEWL but this is currently unexplored.

Skin Elasticity

Skin elasticity is typically measured by a non-invasive Cutometer® probe (or similar method) which utilizes negative pressure to aspirate a small section of skin. The distance the skin travels is affected by its elastic properties and this is recorded as a series of parameters (44). This has been utilized to measure elasticity in skin disorders characterized by stiffness such as scleroderma and systemic sclerosis (45–47).

A limited number of studies have assessed changes in skin elasticity in psoriasis. Differences in total elastic and plastic deformation were found between psoriasis, dermatitis, and lichen planus patients and within patient groups compared to uninvolved sites, with psoriasis exhibiting the greatest superficial stiffness (48). This could be partly due to psoriasis exhibiting a relatively greater epidermal hyperproliferation and lower hydration than dermatitis and lichen planus (48, 49).

As with TEWL, changes in elasticity were also detected between uninvolved sites in patients with psoriasis and skin from healthy volunteers (50).

Skin elasticity in LE has not been studied in detail but reports indicate differential elastic fiber staining compared to lichen planopilaris which is challenging to distinguish clinically in the later stages (51), suggesting this non-invasive method merits further investigation in LE.

However, the lack of molecular information obtained through this method and variability caused by factors such as age, sun-exposure, anatomical location, and ethnicity are likely to prevent this method being widely used for personalized diagnostics.

EPIDERMAL SAMPLING

Non-invasive Sampling of Skin Epithelium via Tape Stripping

Non-invasive sampling of skin epithelium via tape stripping uses adhesive tapes to "strip" the superficial layers of the skin, peeling of layers tape by tape. This method has been widely used over the last decade in research settings; however with increased sensitivity of detection methods and the given ease of sampling—this approach becomes more interesting for clinical diagnostic pathways.

Different types of tapes are available, the most widely used being the acrylic-based (D-Squame discs—1.4 cm diameter, CuDerm, Dallas, TX, USA or 2.2 cm diameter, Monaderm,

Monaco), and synthetic rubber-based tapes (Adhesive Research, Glen Rock, PA) but other tapes, such as Barrier (Mölnlycke, Allerod, Denmark) and cellophane tapes (Nichiban Co, Tokyo, Japan) are also utilized. Tapes are placed on the skin with gentle pressure for 2–10 s, and then removed with a quick movement. D-squame pressure applicator (Monaderm) can be used to standardize pressure (225 g/cm^2). It has been shown that due to the stronger adhesion of corneocytes toward the stratum granulosum, the protein content of tapes decreases in parallel with the increase of tape number/depth of penetration (52, 53). Studies examining the depth of skin removed by tape stripping techniques indicate that in case of healthy skin, depending on anatomical location, at least 30 consecutive tapes are needed to remove the stratum corneum (SC) via D-Squame tapes (54, 55). We have confirmed these results by applying 50 sequential half cut D-Squame discs to a healthy skin area. Simultaneous visualization of the taped and non-taped area was performed with OCT imaging, examining the skin surface roughness and epidermal thickness (**Figure 1**).

Sample collection can be followed by mRNA or protein isolation from pooled tapes. The composition of buffers for protein extraction differ, however most contain Triton-X100 and protease inhibitor cocktails. Sonication steps can be applied in order to improve the yield of extracted protein.

Skin-taping requires no special preparation of the skin and no anesthetic. In the authors view the largest advantage of tape stripping is that it allows for direct sampling of the pathologically involved skin (lesional skin). In contrast to biopsies, which are not a preferred option in pediatric settings and at certain anatomical sites due to their invasiveness and potential for scar formation, tape stripping can be repeatedly performed at any anatomical site, independent of age and location (56–58).

A potential disadvantage of tape stripping lies in the difficulty of sampling standardization. Quantity and quality of sampled skin may differ not only between individuals, but also intra-individually due to differences in epidermal thickness, skin hydration and intercellular adherence (52, 59–62). A study on RNA yield when sampling healthy skin at different locations demonstrated considerable inter- as well as intra-individual variations (mean RNA mass = 11 ng ± 3.6 from the forearm, and = 91 ng ± 31 from the back, when using 12 consecutive tapes). The authors indicated that rather than corneocytes, other associated cells (specialized keratinocytes, components of adnexal structures) are the main source of RNA recovered by tapes. In addition, a variable distribution in the normal baseline mRNA expression of pro-inflammatory IL-8 and TNFα was demonstrated, which could contribute to differences in disease specific anatomical predilection sites. The study highlights that despite the distinct epidermal characteristics at different sites, mRNA expression can be internally normalized to combined housekeeping gene expression levels, as they are relatively uniformly distributed (63).

Healthy skin sampling is limited to the stratum corneum (SC), however this is often not the case in pathologically involved skin, where inflammation influences not only the morphology [hyperproliferative epidermis with thickened SC in psoriasis vs. reduced SC thickness with increased corneocyte cohesion in acute eczema compared to healthy and non-lesional skin (64)], but also the cellular composition within the epidermis, barrier defects at the level of tight junctions and the basement membrane, thus allowing "leakiness" of serum components into the epidermal compartment. Therefore, the authors believe, that the term "stratum corneum sampling/harvesting" should be avoided when referring to tape stripping in diseased skin, as one cannot be certain which layers of the epidermis are collected. Moreover, additional variations can result from different sampling techniques (e.g., applied pressure, duration, the dynamic of tape removal, precise reapplication at the same site) (61, 65, 66).

Studies focusing on transcriptomic profiling of lesional and non-lesional skin material obtained by non-invasive tape stripping are limited in number. In an early study Morhenn et al. used 20 subsequent acrylic based tapes describing distinct RNA cytokine profiles in allergic and irritant contact dermatitis using ribonuclease protection assay (67). Follow up work by Wong et al. demonstrated that the application of four rubber based tapes is sufficient to obtain adequate amount of RNA, suitable for RT-PCR and amplification for microarray analysis. However, the yield of RNA from healthy skin is low compared to inflamed skin (68). To date, only one study focusing on the "taped" mRNA profile in psoriasis showed an upregulation of TNFα, IFNγ, KRT-16, CD2, IL-23A, IL-12B, and VEGF in psoriatic lesions (69). Interestingly, this study found stronger expression of five of these mRNA levels in tape stripping material compared to punch biopsy material from adjacent sites. This highlights that although tape-striping does not sample the deeper layers of the skin, it may have an advantage in detecting epithelial diagnostic biomarkers in diseases with epidermal involvement.

However, overall there are noteworthy limitations for the use of skin tape-strip sampling for transcriptomic analysis as the quantity and quality of RNA obtained is suboptimal. This is due to the skin surface being particularly rich in RNAases and due to the fact that RNA degradation is a natural process of skin differentiation as cells mature into corneocytes. This makes the method prone to false negative results. A recent study by Dyjack et al. (70) reported an ~40% failure rate in RNA isolation from non-lesional atopic dermatitis (AD) tape samples, compared to the 86% isolation success rate from lesional AD skin. Of interest, transcriptome (RNAseq)—proteome (LC-MS/MS) correlation based on full thickness skin biopsy material from lesional and non-lesional psoriatic skin demonstrated an only modest correlation (71). A clear advantage of focusing on protein detection in diagnostic approaches is their stability and the ease to measure their concentration in a timely manner.

Recent evidence suggests that protein sampling of the epidermis via tape stripping is a surprisingly efficient method to detect and study a range of mediators, from structural proteins to antimicrobial peptides, chemokines, and cytokines contributing to disease pathomechanisms, using traditional ELISA, western blot and Multiplex bead-based technologies where available. Furthermore, studies analyzing protein extracts from tape stripping with highly sensitive mass spectrometry (MS) techniques are emerging as an unbiased approach to examine disease entities not only from the perspective of

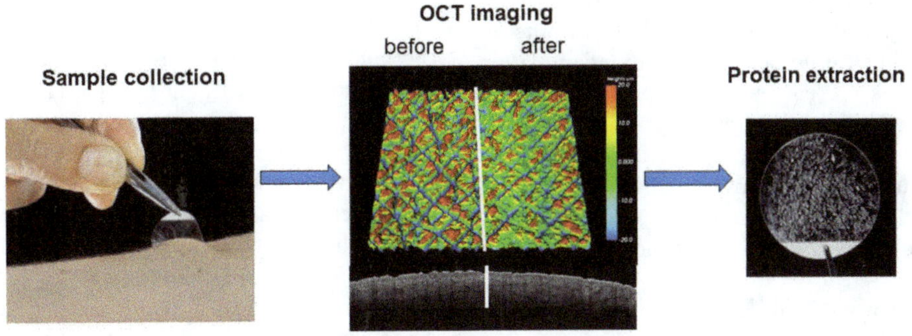

FIGURE 1 | Imaging of a 4 mm volar skin surface area of a healthy forearm with optical coherence tomography (OCT) after application of 50 tape stripes on the right side of the area reveals smoothening of the skin roughness. OCT imaging confirms that sampling of healthy skin remains at the level of the cornified layer and doesn't penetrate deeper than the uppermost layer of the epidermis.

disease subtype diagnosis, but importantly the detection of differentially expressed proteins can also provide potential mechanistic insight into the initiation and maintenance of these inflammatory diseases.

One of the most comprehensive tape stripping studies focusing on healthy vs. psoriatic skin identified 140 proteins expressed in lesional psoriatic skin by combining tape sampling and MS analysis (72). Compared to healthy, significant upregulation of 20 proteins were found, amongst them proteins playing role in keratinocyte differentiation, antimicrobial activity, cell-cell and cell-matrix interactions, protease inhibition and in signaling pathways (FABP5, fatty acid-binding protein; CALML5, calmodulin-like protein 5; NGAL, neutrophil gelatinase-associated lipocalin, elafin, S100A7 "psoriasin," α-enolase, galectin-7 (members of the serpin family, 14-3-3-protein sigma). Zn-α-2-glycoprotein was the only protein found to be downregulated in lesional vs. healthy samples. Although promising, many of the mediators found upregulated in psoriatic lesional tape samples compared to healthy have also been described to be also upregulated in tape harvested lesional AD skin, such as galectin-7, Serpin and S100 family members, FABP5 and α-enolase (73–76). Galectin-7 expressed in the SC has been previously studied as an indicator of skin barrier disruption in eczema (77), and serpin B3 has been highlighted as a potential biomarker for atopic inflammation (73, 78), although serpin family members seem to play a pathophysiological role in psoriatic inflammation as well (79, 80).

Additionally, Mehul et al. (72) were able to quantify known pathophysiological chemokines in psoriatic tape samples, including CXCR3 ligands (CXCL10, CXCL11) which are involved in the chemotaxis of IFNγ expressing lymphocytes) and CCL20 which acts on CCR6^{+} IL-17 producing leukocytes (72, 81, 82). Tape sampling of psoriatic skin also detects strong expression of the neutrophil chemoattractants CXCL1 (GROα) and CXCL8 (IL-8) (72, 83). This is in line with the neutrophilic infiltrate known to characterize psoriatic skin lesions (84, 85). Unlike in protein extracts from full thickness biopsies, CXCL1 was also detectable in non-lesional tape samples (72). The same study found low expression but detectable levels of IL-17 pathway cytokines including IL12p40 subunit which is part of both IL-12 and IL-23, IL17A, and IL17F in psoriatic lesional tape samples. According to the authors' experience, in contrast to epidermal chemokines, detection of lymphokines in tape stripped samples from lesional skin is not very reliable probably due to disease activity dependent differences in lymphocyte infiltration into the upper skin layers.

There are a number of studies focusing on atopic inflammation vs. healthy skin which identified elevated CCL17 (TARC) and TSLP in tape harvested material with correlations to disease severity (86, 87). However, none of the mentioned investigations directly compared lesional skin from different diseases which leaves interpretation on whether detected molecules are disease specific or just general inflammation markers open to discussion.

We have recently (88) compared tape harvested proteins expressed in psoriatic and atopic eczema inflammation with comparable lesion scores (e.g., local inflammatory intensity), non-lesional and healthy skin. The study identified increase expression of IL-36γ, a pro-inflammatory IL-1 family member, as a surprisingly robust biomarker for psoriatic inflammation. These results are in line with previous research which showed significantly enhanced IL-36γ mRNA expression in psoriasis biopsy material compared to healthy skin and recognized IL-36γ as an important cytokine in the pathogenesis of psoriatic inflammation (89–91). Other previously described markers including CCL20, CXCL1, and CXCL8, were also strongly increased in lesional psoriatic samples compared to eczema but were not as reliable as IL-36γ in discriminating the two entities.

Lesional psoriatic skin is well described to overexpress antimicrobial peptides (AMPs) in the outermost layers of the skin. Thus, non-invasive surface sampling is ideally suited study their expression in different conditions. AMPs measured via tape stripping (92, 93) but also "washing fluid" (94, 95) obtained from the skin surface confirmed significantly higher expression levels of hBD2 in both lesional psoriatic and eczematous skin compared to healthy controls. To date, there is no published tape stripping data regarding hBD3 expression in psoriasis, although increased secretion of hBD3 and RNase7 have been shown in non-lesional AD compared to healthy skin (96). Markedly elevated S100 family members (S100A7, S100A8, S100A9) expression which contribute to antimicrobial defense but are also an indicator of inflammation at epithelial surfaces, have been reported in psoriatic lesional SC (72). Identification of fecal calprotectin (formed by a heteromeric complex of two subunits, S100A8 and S100A9) is currently used as a routine non-invasive diagnostic tool to distinguish inflammatory bowel disease (IBD) from irritable bowel syndrome, to follow up disease activity and predict disease relapse (97).

All skin diseases showing epidermal inflammation present with some degree of pruritus, which is well recognized to be a complex phenomenon. Neuropeptides which can impact on release of histamine, vasoactive mediators and pro-inflammatory cytokines and play a role in itch. Keratinocytes are the main source of the neurotrophic nerve growth factor (NGF), a regulator of sensory nerves innervating the skin and which can induce lymphocyte activation and keratinocyte proliferation (98, 99). NGF has been recognized to be upregulated in both atopic and psoriatic lesional skin, and correlates positively with the severity of itch (100, 101). A study focusing on AD has shown that NGF is measurable in tape collected samples, and that its levels correlate with disease and itch severity and are found reduced following treatment (102). IL-31 also called the "pruritic cytokine"—which is currently targeted by biologics approach in clinical studies—can be successfully measured in psoriatic lesional SC (72).

Metabolomics is an exciting newly emerging field. Recent data using skin and serum samples suggest that perturbations in the glycolysis and amino acid metabolic pathways may play an important role in the pathogenesis of psoriasis (103, 104). So far there is a lack of studies combining tape stripping with examining metabolomics data, although this could represent a valuable future approach.

Other Approaches for Epidermal Sampling

Other approaches for epidermal sampling include—as mentioned above—washing buffer approaches which seems to be particularly suitable to monitor the *in vivo* secretion of AMP (94, 95).

Epidermal material can also be obtained by scraping of the skin surface with a surgical blade. For psoriasis lesions, this approach allows detection of chemokines, growth factors including VEGF and IL-1 family members (104). However, this sampling methods seems difficult to standardize.

Suction blister (105) has been successfully used in research settings to allow protein measurement of interstitial fluid from lesional skin—however this approach seems less suitable for clinical practice as it is time intense and requires special setups and training. A promising approach suitable for point of care diagnostic is the analysis of interstitial fluid by means of microneedle patches (106). This approach is being used for continuous glucose monitoring and drug bioavailability. This method has not yet been applied to inflammatory skin conditions.

HAIR FOLLICLE ANALYSIS

Hair follicles are generally referred to as an "appendage" located in the skin (107, 108). Hair biologists however consider the hair follicle an "end organ," with its own complex microenvironment (109). The hair producing segment of the hair follicle is constantly being renewed from a stem cell pool (110–112). The hair follicle is mainly composed of keratinocytes that make up the hair shaft as well as the inner and outer root sheaths. The hair follicle also has a specialized mesenchymal population referred to as dermal papilla (DP) (112) which play a role in regulating the activities of keratinocytes in forming a follicle and hair shaft. The hair follicle stages include anagen (active growth), catagen (degeneration of the lower follicle), telogen (quiescence), and then regeneration (108, 112).

The bulge region of the hair follicle is located in an area of the outer root sheath just beneath the sebaceous gland and is believed to be the reservoir for epidermal stem cells in the hair follicle (113). This region shows features of an immunologically privileged (IP) site (114). Some of the critical features indicating collapse of immune privilege, which goes along with inflammatory alopecia conditions, is the expression of MCH I and other related molecules, downregulation of CK15, E-cadherin and increased expression of genes associated with epithelial-mesenchymal transition, such as vimentin, fibronectin, and SLUG (115).

Cutaneous Lupus

Cutaneous lupus can present as an organ specific disease localized only to the skin or can occur as a manifestation of a systemic disease (116). The subtype of CLE that results in permanent scarring is the chronic discoid LE (CDLE) (117). CDLE lesions appear frequently on the scalp, with resultant permanent scar and irreversible hair loss (118, 119). The pathogenesis of CDLE involves accumulation of apoptotic materials, resulting in secondary necrosis and the activation of the interferon (IFN) pathway by nucleic materials, leading to inflammation and the recruitment of cytotoxic, IFNγ-producing $CD8^+$ T cells. The recruitment of the cells to the bulge region of the hair follicles coupled with collapse of immune privilege ultimately leads to permanent hair loss and atrophic scarring (120). A key feature in LE is high expression of IFN and IFN stimulated genes (ISGs), such as myxovirus protein A (Mx1), IFN inducible protein 6 (IFI6), guanylate binding protein 1 (GBP-1), CXCL9, and CXCL10 (121–123). In addition to high IFN expression, IFN-induced expression of MHC I and MHC I pathway-related molecule, such as beta 2 microglobulin (β2M) has been reported in *ex vivo* human scalp skin culture (124, 125). IFNs have anti-proliferative properties on skin cells (126) and this may explain the reduced proliferation and neovascularization reported in CDLE cells and tissues, and may be major contributors to the scarring outcome (127).

The current gold standard for diagnosis of connective tissue disease manifesting at the skin organ which includes LE is dermato-immunohistopatholog and key features for LE include interface dermatitis i.e., deposition of inflammatory cells at the dermo-epidermal junction, basal cell vacuolization, keratinocytes

TABLE 1 | Characteristics of non-invasive diagnostic approaches.

Method	Current applications	Studying	Advantages	Disadvantages
Tape stripping	Non-invasive sampling of the upper epidermal layers (mainly stratum corneum)	Physiology of the stratum corneum	Non-invasive, no scarring, painless, repeatable, applicable at any anatomical location (e.g., face) and suitable for any age group (including children)	Depth of sampling varies between different skin conditions and different body sites
		Diagnostic markers	Provides valuable molecular information	Need storage access (freezer) and sample transport facility if not processed at site
		Treatment targets	Easy and quick to perform, no special training or professional knowledge is required	
		Disease pathomechanism	Cost effective	
		Disease monitoring	Potential as a non-invasive tool for diagnostic, disease activity and therapeutic response	
		Epidermal wound healing		
		Excretion of endogenous substances		
		Percutaneous absorption of topical treatments—kinetics of drug delivery		
		Treatment efficacy and toxicity (e.g., glucocorticoid therapy)		
	Disruption of the skin barrier	Skin barrier function (TEWL)		
	"Deep" tape stripping = Koebnerisation	Pathophysiology of psoriasis		
Hair plucking	Research	Etiology and pathogenesis of diseases involving the hair follicle (LE, LPP, scarring vs. non-scarring alopecias)	Relatively non-invasive, repeatable, and suitable for any age group (including children)	Variability in the quality of hair follicle obtained
		Wound healing	Provides valuable molecular information	Restricted to patients with presence of "pluckable" hairs; so far only investigated for the scalp
		Therapeutic response	Easy and quick to perform, however, the examiner needs to be able to differentiate anagen from telogen hair	Need for further scientific data
			Potential as a non-invasive tool for diagnostic, disease activity and therapeutic response	Results may depend on hair cycle stage. The same hair cycle stage should be analyzed (e.g., anagen) depending on research question
				Need storage access (freezer) and sample transport facility if not processed at site
Trans-Epidermal Water Loss (TEWL)	Skin epidermal permeability/barrier function	Barrier defects in various pathologies (eczema, psoriasis)	Non-invasive, painless, repeatable, applicable at any anatomical location (e.g., face) and suitable for any age group (including children)	Lack of molecular information—lack of specificity as a diagnostic tool
		Treatment efficacy and toxicity (e.g., glucocorticoid therapy)	Validated measure, quick, and accurate	Need access to the instrument (Tewameter®) and specific software
				Application limited to epidermal pathologies
Skin elasticity	Skin elasticity measurements	Skin disorders characterized by stiffness (scleroderma, systemic sclerosis) and, other pathologies	Non-invasive, painless, repeatable, applicable at any anatomical location (e.g., face) and suitable for any age group (including children)	Lack of molecular information—lack of specificity as a diagnostic tool
		Skin aging		Variability (age, sun-exposure, anatomical location, ethnicity)
		Treatment efficacy and toxicity (e.g., glucocorticoid therapy)		Need access to the instrument (Cutometer®) and specific software

apoptosis, lymphohistiocytic infiltration around appendages and vessels, mucin deposition, basement membrane thickening, and follicular plugging (128, 129). An important differential diagnosis for LE of the scalp is Lichen planopilaris (LPP) which also presents as interface dermatitis in dermatohistopathology and can be difficult to distinguish in some cases. As with LE, current knowledge suggests that scarring in LPP is due to $CD8^+$ T-cell driven attack on the epidermal stem cells of the hair follicles due to collapse of immune privilege (114).

Scalp dermatoscopy can be a useful addition to the diagnostic portfolio in dermatology settings (130). The hair follicle epithelium has been recognized as a valuable tissue for diagnostic purposes. The group of Blume-Peytavi has demonstrated the diagnostic potential of hair follicles obtained by hair plucking or cyanoacrylate surface stripping in androgenic alopecia and seborrheic dermatitis conditions (131–133).

Since the hair follicle is the main target in CDLE, we used 3 5 plucked anagen hair follicles as a non-invasive diagnostic approach (134). We found increased expression of ISGs that are known to play important role in the pathogenesis of the disease (121). Interestingly, we also found increased expression of β2M. Both of these findings have also been made for LPP by Harries et al. (114) who used laser capture microdissection of scalp biopsy to gain hair follicle specific information (114). Of interest, regarding diagnostic difficulties for CDLE vs. LPP lesion, significant contribution of complement activation identifies LE lesions. In our analysis of plucked hair follicle derived epithelium, we found increased expression of C3 in lesional LE in comparison to non-lesional, psoriatic, and healthy hair follicles.

Of interest, despite the hair follicles not being specifically involved in type 2 diabetes, the use of hair follicles as an alternative means of diagnosing the disease has been suggested (135). This hypothesis is hinged on the prolonged shortage of oxygen supply to the hair follicles in hyperglycaemic patients thus leading to hair follicles damage, sparseness of hair, or decreased hair growth speed (136).

Based on our experience, patients are highly acceptant of hair follicle plucking (in our setup 5–10 hairs) for diagnostic or research purposes and are also happy for repeated sampling e.g., to ascertain therapeutic responses. In addition, hair follicle collection does not require specialist training.

CONCLUSION

The need to include analysis of tissue specific responses in precision medicine approaches has been recognized. **Table 1** gives an overview including advantages and limitations of the main approaches discussed in this review. Dermatoscopy and functional skin testing are useful to support diagnostic processes but their use seem to be limited to specialized dermatology department and training is needed for correct use and interpretation.

As highlighted in this review, novel imaging techniques have great potential to allow non-invasive diagnostic by visualizing changes in the epidermal down to the vessel compartment. Access to imaging devices such as OCT and RSOM are however limited to specialized centers due to high costs.

By contrast, epidermal sampling by tape stripping and for the scalp by hair follicle plucking do not need specific training, are easy and fast to perform, suitable for point of care approaches and can give molecular information beyond morphology changes. This could significantly help with disease subgroup identification and importantly provide a molecular understanding of the inflammatory processes behind these diseases and highlight novel targets for future therapeutics. Thus, protein biomarkers detectable with non-invasive epidermal/hair follicle sampling has the potential to direct treatment pathways, follow up disease progression and therapeutic response.

It remains to be demonstrated in well planned prospective studies which compare standard of care diagnostic with the here discussed non-invasive diagnostic approaches if suitable protein biomarker algorithm can be developed with high enough sensitivity and specificity for a range of inflammatory skin conditions to replace current biopsy approaches. Another previously discussed (137) outcome of such studies could be that approaches such as tape stripping cannot fully replace dermatohistopathology but could prove to be of significant support for treatment decision pathways either in primary care setting (e.g., inverse psoriasis vs. fungal infection; palmoplantar eczema vs. psoriasis), in secondary care dermatology (e.g., predicting response to therapy) or in other disciplines such as rheumatology (e.g., supporting the diagnosis of psoriatic arthritis). The potential of epidermal sampling to be developed into a point-of-care test for specific diagnostic problems is given by the ease of sampling. Larger trials and development of robust biomarker algorithms are needed to fully appreciate the value epidermal sampling could have in routine care settings.

AUTHOR CONTRIBUTIONS

All authors contributed to writing the manuscript. AB performed the optical coherence tomography imaging shown in **Figure 1**.

REFERENCES

1. Lacarrubba F, Ardigo M, Di Stefani A, Verzi AE, Micali G. Dermatoscopy and reflectance confocal microscopy correlations in nonmelanocytic disorders. *Dermatol Clin.* (2018) 36:487–501. doi: 10.1016/j.det.2018.05.015
2. Deinlein T, Richtig G, Schwab C, Scarfi F, Arzberger E, Wolf I, et al. The use of dermatoscopy in diagnosis and therapy of nonmelanocytic skin cancer. *J German Soc Dermatol.* (2016) 14:144–51. doi: 10.1111/ddg.12903
3. Lacarrubba F, Verzi AE, Dinotta F, Scavo S, Micali G. Dermatoscopy in inflammatory and infectious skin disorders. *Giorn Italiano Dermatol Venereol.* (2015) 150:521–31.

4. Hindelang B, Aguirre J, Schwarz M, Berezhnoi A, Eyerich K, Ntziachristos V, et al. Non-invasive imaging in dermatology and the unique potential of raster-scan optoacoustic mesoscopy. *J Eur Acad Dermatol Venereol.* (2019) 33:1051–61. doi: 10.1111/jdv.15342
5. Aguirre J, Schwarz M, Garzorz N, Omar M, Buehler A, Eyerich K, et al. Precision assessment of label-free psoriasis biomarkers with ultra-broadband optoacoustic mesoscopy. *Nat Biomed Eng.* (2017) 1:0068. doi: 10.1038/s41551-017-0068
6. Abignano G, Aydin SZ, Castillo-Gallego C, Liakouli V, Woods D, Meekings A, et al. Virtual skin biopsy by optical coherence tomography: the first quantitative imaging biomarker for scleroderma. *Ann Rheum Dis.* (2013) 72:1845–51. doi: 10.1136/annrheumdis-2012-202682
7. Abignano G, Del Galdo F. Quantitating skin fibrosis: innovative strategies and their clinical implications. *Curr Rheumatol Rep.* (2014) 16:404. doi: 10.1007/s11926-013-0404-5
8. Kang T, Abignano G, Lettieri G, Wakefield RJ, Emery P, Del Galdo F. Skin imaging in systemic sclerosis. *Eur J Rheumatol.* (2014) 1:111–6. doi: 10.5152/eurjrheumatol.2014.036
9. Abignano G, Kapadia A, Lettieri G, Goodfield M, Emery P, McGonagle D, et al. Use of optical coherence tomography for the diagnosis of preclinical lesions of circumscribed palmar hypokeratosis. *Clin Exp Dermatol.* (2017) 42:192–5. doi: 10.1111/ced.13027
10. Greaves NS, Benatar B, Whiteside S, Alonso-Rasgado T, Baguneid M, Bayat A. Optical coherence tomography: a reliable alternative to invasive histological assessment of acute wound healing in human skin? *Brit J Dermatol.* (2014) 170:840–50. doi: 10.1111/bjd.12786
11. Abignano G, Laws P, Del Galdo F, Marzo-Ortega H, McGonagle D. Three-dimensional nail imaging by optical coherence tomography: a novel biomarker of response to therapy for nail disease in psoriasis and psoriatic arthritis. *Ann Rheum Dis.* (2017) 76:734. doi: 10.1136/annrheumdis-2017-eular.4157
12. Deegan AJ, Talebi-Liasi F, Song SZ, Li YD, Xu JJ, Men SJ, et al. Optical coherence tomography angiography of normal skin and inflammatory dermatologic conditions. *Lasers Surg Med.* (2018) 50:183–93. doi: 10.1002/lsm.22788
13. Odorici G, Losi A, Ciardo S, Pellacani G, Conti A. Non-invasive evaluation of Secukinumab efficacy in severe plaque psoriasis with confocal microscopy and optical coherence tomography: a case report. *Skin Res Technol.* (2018) 24:160–2. doi: 10.1111/srt.12409
14. Gambichler T, Hyun J, Moussa G, Tomi NS, Boms S, Altmeyer P, et al. Optical coherence tomography of cutaneous lupus erythematosus correlates with histopathology. *Lupus.* (2007) 16:35–8. doi: 10.1177/0961203306074773
15. Mandel VD, Cinotti E, Benati E, Labeille B, Ciardo S, Vaschieri C, et al. Reflectance confocal microscopy and optical coherence tomography for the diagnosis of bullous pemphigoid and pemphigus and surrounding subclinical lesions. *J Eur Acad Dermatol Venereol.* (2018) 32:1562–9. doi: 10.1111/jdv.14795
16. Capocasale G, Panzarella V, Rodolico V, Di Fede O, Campisi G. *In vivo* optical coherence tomography imaging in a case of mucous membrane pemphigoid and a negative Nikolsky's sign. *J Dermatol.* (2018) 45:603–5. doi: 10.1111/1346-8138.14267
17. Wardell K, Jakobsson A, Nilsson GE. Laser Doppler perfusion imaging by dynamic light scattering. *IEEE Trans Biomed Eng.* (1993) 40:309–16. doi: 10.1109/10.222322
18. Hendriks AG, Steenbergen W, Hondebrink E, van Hespen JC, van de Kerkhof PC, Seyger MM. Whole field laser Doppler imaging of the microcirculation in psoriasis and clinically unaffected skin. *J Dermatol Treat.* (2014) 25:18–21. doi: 10.3109/09546634.2013.777382
19. Md Yusof MY, Britton J, Hensor EM, Goodfield M, Wittmann M, Emery P, Vital EM. Laser Doppler imaging: an objective outcome measure for assessment of cutaneous lupus erythematosus. *Ann Rheum Dis.* (2017) 76(Suppl. 2):1019–20. doi: 10.1136/annrheumdis-2017-eular.6784
20. Grubauer G, Elias PM, Feingold KR. Transepidermal water loss: the signal for recovery of barrier structure and function. *J Lipid Res.* (1989) 30:323–33.
21. Alexander H, Brown S, Danby S, Flohr C. Research techniques made simple: transepidermal water loss measurement as a research tool. *J Investig Dermatol.* (2018) 138:2295–300.e1. doi: 10.1016/j.jid.2018.09.001
22. Gottlieb AB, Staiano-Coico L, Cohen SR, Varghese M, Carter DM. Occlusive hydrocolloid dressings decrease keratinocyte population growth fraction and clinical scale and skin thickness in active psoriatic plaques. *J Dermatol Sci.* (1990) 1:93–6. doi: 10.1016/0923-1811(90)90221-X
23. Volden G, Kragballe K, Van De Kerkhof PC, Aberg K, White RJ. Remission and relapse of chronic plaque psoriasis treated once a week with clobetasol propionate occluded with a hydrocolloid dressing versus twice daily treatment with clobetasol propionate alone. *J Dermatolog Treat.* (2001) 12:141–4. doi: 10.1080/09546630152607862
24. Bergboer JGM, Zeeuwen PLJM, Schalkwijk J. Genetics of psoriasis: evidence for epistatic interaction between skin barrier abnormalities and immune deviation. *J Investig Dermatol.* (2012) 132:2320–31. doi: 10.1038/jid.2012.167
25. Friedman SJ. Management of psoriasis-vulgaris with a hydrocolloid occlusive dressing. *Arch Dermatol.* (1987) 123:1046–52. doi: 10.1001/archderm.123.8.1046
26. Proksch E, Feingold KR, Man MQ, Elias PM. Barrier function regulates epidermal DNA-synthesis. *J Clin Investig.* (1991) 87:1668–73. doi: 10.1172/JCI115183
27. Wood LC, Elias PM, Calhoun C, Tsai JC, Grunfeld C, Feingold KR. Barrier disruption stimulates interleukin-1 alpha expression and release from a pre-formed pool in murine epidermis. *J Investig Dermatol.* (1996) 106:397–403. doi: 10.1111/1523-1747.ep12343392
28. Lin TK, Man MQ, Santiago JL, Park K, Roelandt T, Oda Y, et al. Topical antihistamines display potent anti-inflammatory activity linked in part to enhanced permeability barrier function. *J Investig Dermatol.* (2013) 133:469–78. doi: 10.1038/jid.2012.335
29. Elias PM, Arbiser J, Brown BE, Rossiter H, Man MQ, Cerimele F, et al. Epidermal vascular endothelial growth factor production is required for permeability barrier homeostasis, dermal angiogenesis, and the development of epidermal hyperplasia - Implications for the pathogenesis of psoriasis. *Am J Pathol.* (2008) 173:689–99. doi: 10.2353/ajpath.2008.080088
30. Satake K, Amano T, Okamoto T. Low systemic exposure and calcemic effect of calcipotriol/betamethasone ointment in rats with imiquimod-induced psoriasis-like dermatitis. *Eur J Pharmacol.* (2018) 826:31–8. doi: 10.1016/j.ejphar.2018.02.032
31. Lee B, Vouthounis C, Stojadinovic O, Brem H, Im M, Tomic-Canic M. From an enhanceosome to a repressosome: molecular antagonism between glucocorticoids and EGF leads to inhibition of wound healing. *J Mol Biol.* (2005) 345:1083–97. doi: 10.1016/j.jmb.2004.11.027
32. Laurence EB, Christophers E. Selective action of hydrocortisone on postmitotic epidermal cells *in vivo*. *J Investig Dermatol.* (1976) 66:222–9. doi: 10.1111/1523-1747.ep12482145
33. Lin TK, Man MQ, Santiago JL, Scharschmidt TC, Hupe M, Martin-Ezquerra G, et al. Paradoxical benefits of psychological stress in inflammatory dermatoses models are glucocorticoid mediated. *J Investig Dermatol.* (2014) 134:2890–7. doi: 10.1038/jid.2014.265
34. Li BS, Tsoi LC, Swindell WR, Gudjonsson JE, Tejasvi T, Johnston A, et al. Transcriptome analysis of psoriasis in a large case-control sample: RNA-seq provides insights into disease mechanisms. *J Investig Dermatol.* (2014) 134:1828–38. doi: 10.1038/jid.2014.28
35. Tiganescu A, Hupe M, Uchida Y, Mauro T, Elias PM, Holleran WM. Topical 11 beta-hydroxysteroid dehydrogenase type 1 inhibition corrects cutaneous features of systemic glucocorticoid excess in female mice. *Endocrinology.* (2018) 159:547–56. doi: 10.1210/en.2017-00607
36. Berardesca E, Vignoli GP, Farinelli N, Vignini M, Distante F, Rabbiosi G. Noninvasive evaluation of topical calcipotriol versus clobetasol in the treatment of psoriasis. *Acta Derm Venereol.* (1994) 74:302–4.
37. Hagemann I, Proksch E. Topical treatment by urea reduces epidermal hyperproliferation and induces differentiation in psoriasis. *Acta Derm Venereol.* (1996) 76:353–6.
38. Liu M, Li X, Chen XY, Xue F, Zheng J. Topical application of a linoleic acid-ceramide containing moisturizer exhibit therapeutic and preventive benefits for psoriasis vulgaris: a randomized controlled trial. *Dermatol Ther.* (2015) 28:373–82. doi: 10.1111/dth.12259
39. Rajabi-Estarabadi A, Hasanzadeh H, Taheri A, Feldman SR, Firooz A. The efficacy of short-term clobetasol lotion in the treatment of scalp psoriasis. *J Dermatol Treat.* (2018) 29:111–5. doi: 10.1080/09546634.2017.1341616

40. Darlenski R, Hristakieva E, Aydin U, Gancheva D, Gancheva T, Zheleva A, et al. Epidermal barrier and oxidative stress parameters improve during in 311 nm narrow band UVB phototherapy of plaque type psoriasis. *J Dermatol Sci.* (2018) 91:28–34. doi: 10.1016/j.jdermsci.2018.03.011
41. Man G, Elias PM, Man MQ. Therapeutic benefits of enhancing permeability barrier for atopic eczema. *Dermatol Sin.* (2015) 33:84–9. doi: 10.1016/j.dsi.2015.03.006
42. Elias PM, Wakefield JS. Mechanisms of abnormal lamellar body secretion and the dysfunctional skin barrier in patients with atopic dermatitis. *J Allergy Clin Immun.* (2014) 134:781–91.e1. doi: 10.1016/j.jaci.2014.05.048
43. Ye L, Lv CZ, Man G, Song SP, Elias PM, Man MQ. Abnormal epidermal barrier recovery in uninvolved skin supports the notion of an epidermal pathogenesis of psoriasis. *J Investig Dermatol.* (2014) 134:2843–6. doi: 10.1038/jid.2014.205
44. Neto P, Ferreira M, Bahia F, Costa P. Improvement of the methods for skin mechanical properties evaluation through correlation between different techniques and factor analysis. *Skin Res Technol.* (2013) 19:405–16. doi: 10.1111/srt.12060
45. NikkelsTassoudji N, Henry F, PierardFranchimont C, Pierard GE. Computerized evaluation of skin stiffening in scleroderma. *Eur J Clin Investig.* (1996) 26:457–60. doi: 10.1046/j.1365-2362.1996.154303.x
46. Osmola-Mankowska A, Silny W, Danczak-Pazdrowska A, Polanska A, Olek-Hrab K, Sadowska-Przytocka A, et al. "Assessment of chronic sclerodermoid Graft-versus-Host Disease patients, using 20MHz high-frequency ultrasonography and cutometer methods". *Skin Res Technol.* (2013) 19:E417–22. doi: 10.1111/j.1600-0846.2012.00659.x
47. Dobrev HP. In vivo study of skin mechanical properties in patients with systemic sclerosis. *J Am Acad Dermatol.* (1999) 40:436–42. doi: 10.1016/S0190-9622(99)70494-9
48. Yazdanparast T, Yazdani K, Humbert P, Khatami A, Ahmad Nasrollahi S, Hassanzadeh H, et al. Comparison of biophysical, biomechanical and ultrasonographic properties of skin in chronic dermatitis, psoriasis and lichen planus. *Med J Islam Repub Iran.* (2018) 32:108. doi: 10.14196/mjiri.32.108
49. Bovenschen HJ, Seyger MM, Van de Kerkhof PC. Plaque psoriasis vs. atopic dermatitis and lichen planus: a comparison for lesional T-cell subsets, epidermal proliferation and differentiation. *Br J Dermatol.* (2005) 153:72–8. doi: 10.1111/j.1365-2133.2005.06538.x
50. Dobrev H. In vivo study of skin mechanical properties in psoriasis vulgaris. *Acta Derm Venereol.* (2000) 80:263–6. doi: 10.1080/000155500750012135
51. Farzaneh Asadi Kani Z, Nasiri S, Rafiei R, Younespour S. Evaluation of elastic fibers pattern with orcein staining in differential diagnosis of lichen planopilaris and discoid lupus erythematosus. *Acta Med Iran.* (2014) 52:220–7.
52. King CS, Barton SP, Nicholls S, Marks R. The change in properties of the stratum corneum as a function of depth. *Br J Dermatol.* (1979) 100:165–72. doi: 10.1111/j.1365-2133.1979.tb05556.x
53. Clausen M-L, Slotved HC, Krogfelt KA, Agner T. Tape stripping technique for stratum corneum protein analysis. *Sci Rep.* (2016) 6:19918. doi: 10.1038/srep19918
54. Pinkus H. Examination of the epidermis by the strip method of removing horny layers. I. Observations on thickness of the horny layer, and on mitotic activity after stripping. *J Investig Dermatol.* (1951) 16:383–6. doi: 10.1038/jid.1951.45
55. Solberg J, Ulrich NH, Krustrup D, Ahlstrom MG, Thyssen JP, Menne T, et al. Skin tape stripping: which layers of the epidermis are removed? *Contact Dermatitis.* (2018) 80:319–21. doi: 10.1111/cod.13199
56. McAleer MA, Jakasa I, Hurault G, Sarvari P, McLean WHI, Tanaka RJ, et al. Systemic and stratum corneum biomarkers of severity in infant atopic dermatitis include markers of innate and T helper cell-related immunity and angiogenesis. *Br J Dermatol.* (2019) 180:586–96. doi: 10.1111/bjd.17088
57. Hulshof L, Hack DP, Hasnoe QCJ, Dontje B, Jakasa I, Riethmüller C, et al. A minimally invasive tool to study immune response and skin barrier in children with atopic dermatitis. *Br J Dermatol.* (2019) 180:621–30. doi: 10.1111/bjd.16994
58. Furue M. Useful components in the stratum corneum for assessment of atopic dermatitis. *Br J Dermatol.* (2019) 180:457–8. doi: 10.1111/bjd.17117
59. van der Molen RG, Spies F, van 't Noordende JM, Boelsma E, Mommaas AM, Koerten HK. Tape stripping of human stratum corneum yields cell layers that originate from various depths because of furrows in the skin. *Archiv Dermatol Res.* (1997) 289:514–8. doi: 10.1007/s004030050232
60. Black D, Del Pozo A, Lagarde JM, Gall Y. Seasonal variability in the biophysical properties of stratum corneum from different anatomical sites. *Skin Res Technol.* (2000) 6:70–6. doi: 10.1034/j.1600-0846.2000.006002070.x
61. Löffler H, Dreher F, Maibach HI. Stratum corneum adhesive tape stripping: influence of anatomical site, application pressure, duration and removal. *Br J Dermatol.* (2004) 151:746–52. doi: 10.1111/j.1365-2133.2004.06084.x
62. Raj N, Voegeli R, Rawlings AV, Gibbons S, Munday MR, Summers B, et al. Variation in stratum corneum protein content as a function of anatomical site and ethnic group. *Int J Cosmet Sci.* (2016) 38:224–31. doi: 10.1111/ics.12274
63. Wong R, Tran V, Talwalker S, Benson NR. Analysis of RNA recovery and gene expression in the epidermis using non-invasive tape stripping. *J Dermatol Sci.* (2006) 44:81–92. doi: 10.1016/j.jdermsci.2006.08.007
64. Voegeli R, Rawlings AV, Breternitz M, Doppler S, Schreier T, Fluhr JW. Increased stratum corneum serine protease activity in acute eczematous atopic skin. *Br J Dermatol.* (2009) 161:70–7. doi: 10.1111/j.1365-2133.2009.09142.x
65. Breternitz M, Flach M, Präßler J, Elsner P, Fluhr JW. Acute barrier disruption by adhesive tapes is influenced by pressure, time and anatomical location: integrity and cohesion assessed by sequential tape stripping; a randomized, controlled study. *Br J Dermatol.* (2007) 156:231–40. doi: 10.1111/j.1365-2133.2006.07632.x
66. Lademann J, Jacobi U, Surber C, Weigmann HJ, Fluhr JW. The tape stripping procedure – evaluation of some critical parameters. *Eur J Pharmaceut Biopharmaceut.* (2009) 72:317–23. doi: 10.1016/j.ejpb.2008.08.008
67. Morhenn VB, Chang E-Y, Rheins LA. A noninvasive method for quantifying and distinguishing inflammatory skin reactions. *J Am Acad Dermatol.* (1999) 41:687–92. doi: 10.1016/S0190-9622(99)70002-2
68. Wong R, Tran V, Morhenn V, Hung S-p, Andersen B, Ito E, et al. Use of RT-PCR and DNA microarrays to characterize RNA recovered by non-invasive tape harvesting of normal and inflamed skin. *J Investig Dermatol.* (2004) 123:159–67. doi: 10.1111/j.0022-202X.2004.22729.x
69. Benson NR, Papenfuss J, Wong R, Motaal A, Tran V, Panko J, et al. An analysis of select pathogenic messages in lesional and non-lesional psoriatic skin using non-invasive tape harvesting. *J Investig Dermatol.* (2006) 126:2234–41. doi: 10.1038/sj.jid.5700412
70. Dyjack N, Goleva E, Rios C, Kim BE, Bin L, Taylor P, et al. Minimally invasive skin tape strip RNA sequencing identifies novel characteristics of the type 2–high atopic dermatitis disease endotype. *J Allergy Clin Immunol.* (2018) 141:1298–309. doi: 10.1016/j.jaci.2017.10.046
71. Swindell WR, Remmer HA, Sarkar MK, Xing X, Barnes DH, Wolterink L, et al. Proteogenomic analysis of psoriasis reveals discordant and concordant changes in mRNA and protein abundance. *Genome Med.* (2015) 7:86. doi: 10.1186/s13073-015-0208-5
72. Mehul B, Laffet G, Seraidaris A, Russo L, Fogel P, Carlavan I, et al. Noninvasive proteome analysis of psoriatic stratum corneum reflects pathophysiological pathways and is useful for drug profiling. *Br J Dermatol.* (2017) 177:470–88. doi: 10.1111/bjd.15346
73. Broccardo CJ, Mahaffey SB, Strand M, Reisdorph NA, Leung DY. Peeling off the layers: skin taping and a novel proteomics approach to study atopic dermatitis. *J Allergy Clin Immunol.* (2009) 124:1113–5.e1–11. doi: 10.1016/j.jaci.2009.07.057
74. Sakabe J-I, Kamiya K, Yamaguchi H, Ikeya S, Suzuki T, Aoshima M, et al. Proteome analysis of stratum corneum from atopic dermatitis patients by hybrid quadrupole-orbitrap mass spectrometer. *J Allergy Clin Immunol.* (2014) 134:957–60.e8. doi: 10.1016/j.jaci.2014.07.054
75. Winget JM, Finlay D, Mills Kevin J, Huggins T, Bascom C, Isfort RJ, et al. Quantitative proteomic analysis of stratum corneum dysfunction in adult chronic atopic dermatitis. *J Investig Dermatol.* (2016) 136:1732–5. doi: 10.1016/j.jid.2016.03.037
76. Reisdorph N, Armstrong M, Powell R, Quinn K, Legg K, Leung D, et al. Quantitation of peptides from non-invasive skin tapings using isotope dilution and tandem mass spectrometry. *J Chromatogr B.* (2018) 1084:132–40. doi: 10.1016/j.jchromb.2018.03.031

77. Niiyama S, Yoshino T, Yasuda C, Yu X, Izumi R, Ishiwatari S, et al. Galectin-7 in the stratum corneum: a biomarker of the skin barrier function. *Int J Cosmet sci.* (2016) 38:487–95. doi: 10.1111/ics.12326
78. Mitsuishi K, Nakamura T, Sakata Y, Yuyama N, Arima K, Sugita Y, et al. The squamous cell carcinoma antigens as relevant biomarkers of atopic dermatitis. *Clin Exper Allergy.* (2005) 35:1327–33. doi: 10.1111/j.1365-2222.2005.02353.x
79. Takeda A, Higuchi D, Takahashi T, Ogo M, Baciu P, Goetinck PF, et al. Overexpression of serpin squamous cell carcinoma antigens in psoriatic skin. *J Investig Dermatol.* (2002) 118:147–54. doi: 10.1046/j.0022-202x.2001.01610.x
80. Sun Y, Sheshadri N, Zong W-X. SERPINB3 and B4: from biochemistry to biology. *Sem Cell Develop Biol.* (2017) 62:170–7. doi: 10.1016/j.semcdb.2016.09.005
81. Nestle FO, Kaplan DH, Barker J. Psoriasis. *New Engl J Med.* (2009) 361:496–509. doi: 10.1056/NEJMra0804595
82. Nedoszytko B, Sokołowska-Wojdyło M, Ruckemann-Dziurdzinska K, Roszkiewicz J, Nowicki RJ. Chemokines and cytokines network in the pathogenesis of the inflammatory skin diseases: atopic dermatitis, psoriasis and skin mastocytosis. *Postepy Dermatol Alergol.* (2014) 31:84–91. doi: 10.5114/pdia.2014.40920
83. Berekmeri A, Latzko A, Alase A, Macleod T, Ainscough JS, Laws P, et al. Detection of IL-36gamma through noninvasive tape stripping reliably discriminates psoriasis from atopic eczema. *J Allergy Clin Immunol.* (2018) 142:988–91.e4. doi: 10.1016/j.jaci.2018.04.031
84. Gillitzer R, Ritter U, Spandau U, Goebeler M, Bröcker E-B. Differential expression of GRO-α and IL-8 mRNA psoriasis: a model for neutrophil migration and accumulation *in vivo*. *J Investig Dermatol.* (1996) 107:778–82. doi: 10.1111/1523-1747.ep12371803
85. De Rosa G, Mignogna C. The histopathology of psoriasis. *Reumatismo.* (2007) 59(Suppl. 1):46–8. doi: 10.4081/reumatismo.2007.1s.46
86. Morita E, Takahashi H, Niihara H, Dekio I, Sumikawa Y, Murakami Y, et al. Stratum corneum TARC level is a new indicator of lesional skin inflammation in atopic dermatitis. *Allergy.* (2010) 65:1166–72. doi: 10.1111/j.1398-9995.2010.02361.x
87. Sano Y, Masuda K, Tamagawa-Mineoka R, Matsunaka H, Murakami Y, Yamashita R, et al. Thymic stromal lymphopoietin expression is increased in the horny layer of patients with atopic dermatitis. *Clin Exp Immunol.* (2013) 171:330–7. doi: 10.1111/cei.12021
88. D'Erme AM, Wilsmann-Theis D, Wagenpfeil J, Holzel M, Ferring-Schmitt S, Sternberg S, et al. IL-36gamma (IL-1F9) is a biomarker for psoriasis skin lesions. *J Investig Dermatol.* (2015) 135:1025–32. doi: 10.1038/jid.2014.532
89. Muhr P, Zeitvogel J, Heitland I, Werfel T, Wittmann M. Expression of interleukin (IL)-1 family members upon stimulation with IL-17 differs in keratinocytes derived from patients with psoriasis and healthy donors. *Br J Dermatol.* (2011) 165:189–93. doi: 10.1111/j.1365-2133.2011.10302.x
90. Liang Y, Sarkar MK, Tsoi LC, Gudjonsson JE. Psoriasis: a mixed autoimmune and autoinflammatory disease. *Curr Opin Immunol.* (2017) 49:1–8. doi: 10.1016/j.coi.2017.07.007
91. Buhl A-L, Wenzel J. Interleukin-36 in infectious and inflammatory skin diseases. *Front Immunol.* (2019) 10:1162. doi: 10.3389/fimmu.2019.01162
92. Asano S, Ichikawa Y, Kumagai T, Kawashima M, Imokawa G. Microanalysis of an antimicrobial peptide, β-defensin-2, in the stratum corneum from patients with atopic dermatitis. *Br J Dermatol.* (2008) 159:97–104. doi: 10.1111/j.1365-2133.2008.08613.x
93. Clausen ML, Jungersted JM, Andersen PS, Slotved HC, Krogfelt KA, Agner T. Human beta-defensin-2 as a marker for disease severity and skin barrier properties in atopic dermatitis. *Br J Dermatol.* (2013) 169:587–93. doi: 10.1111/bjd.12419
94. Glaser R, Meyer-Hoffert U, Harder J, Cordes J, Wittersheim M, Kobliakova J, et al. The antimicrobial protein psoriasin (S100A7) is upregulated in atopic dermatitis and after experimental skin barrier disruption. *J Investig Dermatol.* (2009) 129:641–9. doi: 10.1038/jid.2008.268
95. Wittersheim M, Cordes J, Meyer-Hoffert U, Harder J, Hedderich J, Glaser R. Differential expression and in vivo secretion of the antimicrobial peptides psoriasin (S100A7), RNase 7, human beta-defensin-2 and−3 in healthy human skin. *Exp Dermatol.* (2013) 22:364–6. doi: 10.1111/exd.12133
96. Clausen M-L, Slotved HC, Krogfelt KA, Agner T. Measurements of AMPs in stratum corneum of atopic dermatitis and healthy skin–tape stripping technique. *Sci Rep.* (2018) 8:1666. doi: 10.1038/s41598-018-20204-8
97. Laserna-Mendieta Emilio J, Lucendo Alfredo J. Faecal calprotectin in inflammatory bowel diseases: a review focused on meta-analyses and routine usage limitations. *Clin Chem Lab Med.* (2019) 57:1295–1307. doi: 10.1515/cclm-2018-1063
98. Raychaudhuri SP, Jiang WY, Farber EM. Psoriatic keratinocytes express high levels of nerve growth factor. *Acta Dermatovenereol Stockholm.* (1998) 78:84–6. doi: 10.1080/000155598433368
99. Pincelli C. Nerve growth factor and keratinocytes: a role in psoriasis. *Eur J Dermatol.* (2000) 10:85–90.
100. Nakamura M, Toyoda M, Morohashi M. Pruritogenic mediators in psoriasis vulgaris: comparative evaluation of itch-associated cutaneous factors. *Br J Dermatol.* (2003) 149:718–30. doi: 10.1046/j.1365-2133.2003.05586.x
101. Dou Y-C, Hagströmer L, Emtestam L, Johansson O. Increased nerve growth factor and its receptors in atopic dermatitis: an immunohistochemical study. *Archiv Dermatol Res.* (2006) 298:31–7. doi: 10.1007/s00403-006-0657-1
102. Yamaguchi J, Aihara M, Kobayashi Y, Kambara T, Ikezawa Z. Quantitative analysis of nerve growth factor (NGF) in the atopic dermatitis and psoriasis horny layer and effect of treatment on NGF in atopic dermatitis. *J Dermatol Sci.* (2009) 53:48–54. doi: 10.1016/j.jdermsci.2008.08.011
103. Yan D, Afifi L, Jeon C, Trivedi M, Chang HW, Lee K, et al. The metabolomics of psoriatic disease. *Psoriasis.* (2017) 7:1–15. doi: 10.2147/PTT.S118348
104. Kang H, Li X, Zhou Q, Quan C, Xue F, Zheng J, et al. Exploration of candidate biomarkers for human psoriasis based on gas chromatography-mass spectrometry serum metabolomics. *Br J Dermatol.* (2017) 176:713–22. doi: 10.1111/bjd.15008
105. Svoboda M, Hlobilová M, Marešová M, Sochorová M, Kováčik A, Vávrová K, et al. Comparison of suction blistering and tape stripping for analysis of epidermal genes, proteins and lipids. *Archiv Dermatol Res.* (2017) 309:757–65. doi: 10.1007/s00403-017-1776-6
106. Kolluru C, Williams M, Yeh JS, Noel RK, Knaack J, Prausnitz MR. Monitoring drug pharmacokinetics and immunologic biomarkers in dermal interstitial fluid using a microneedle patch. *Biomed Microdevices.* (2019) 21:14. doi: 10.1007/s10544-019-0363-3
107. Hardy MH. The secret life of the hair follicle. *Trends Genet.* (1992) 8:55–61. doi: 10.1016/0168-9525(92)90044-5
108. Legue E, Sequeira I, Nicolas JF. Hair follicle renewal: authentic morphogenesis that depends on a complex progression of stem cell lineages. *Development.* (2010) 137:569–77. doi: 10.1242/dev.044123
109. Rishikaysh P, Dev K, Diaz D, Qureshi WM, Filip S, Mokry J. Signaling involved in hair follicle morphogenesis and development. *Int J Mol Sci.* (2014) 15:1647–70. doi: 10.3390/ijms15011647
110. Cotsarelis G, Sun TT, Lavker RM. Label-retaining cells reside in the bulge area of pilosebaceous unit: implications for follicular stem cells, hair cycle, and skin carcinogenesis. *Cell.* (1990) 61:1329–37. doi: 10.1016/0092-8674(90)90696-C
111. Fuchs E, Horsley V. More than one way to skin. *Genes Dev.* (2008) 22:976–85. doi: 10.1101/gad.1645908
112. Morgan BA. The dermal papilla: an instructive niche for epithelial stem and progenitor cells in development and regeneration of the hair follicle. *CSH Perspect Med.* (2014) 4:a015180. doi: 10.1101/cshperspect.a015180
113. Ohyama M, Terunuma A, Tock CL, Radonovich MF, Pise-Masison CA, Hopping SB, et al. Characterization and isolation of stem cell-enriched human hair follicle bulge cells. *J Clin Invest.* (2006) 116:249–60. doi: 10.1172/JCI26043
114. Harries MJ, Meyer K, Chaudhry I, J EK, Poblet E, Griffiths CE, et al. Lichen planopilaris is characterized by immune privilege collapse of the hair follicle's epithelial stem cell niche. *J Pathol.* (2013) 231:236–47. doi: 10.1002/path.4233
115. Imanishi H, Ansell DM, Cheret J, Harries M, Bertolini M, Sepp N, et al. Epithelial-to-mesenchymal stem cell transition in a human organ: lessons from lichen planopilaris. *J Invest Dermatol.* (2018) 138:511–9. doi: 10.1016/j.jid.2017.09.047
116. Robinson ES, Werth VP. The role of cytokines in the pathogenesis of cutaneous lupus erythematosus. *Cytokine.* (2015) 73:326–34. doi: 10.1016/j.cyto.2015.01.031

117. Gronhagen CM, Fored CM, Granath F, Nyberg F. Cutaneous lupus erythematosus and the association with systemic lupus erythematosus: a population-based cohort of 1088 patients in Sweden. *Br J Dermatol.* (2011) 164:1335–41. doi: 10.1111/j.1365-2133.2011.10272.x
118. Al-Refu K, Goodfield M. Hair follicle stem cells in the pathogenesis of the scarring process in cutaneous lupus erythematosus. *Autoimmun Rev.* (2009) 8:474–7. doi: 10.1016/j.autrev.2008.12.015
119. Chung HJ, Goldberg LJ. Histologic features of chronic cutaneous lupus erythematosus of the scalp using horizontal sectioning: emphasis on follicular findings. *J Am Acad Dermatol.* (2017) 77:349–55. doi: 10.1016/j.jaad.2017.02.039
120. Wenzel J, Tuting T. An IFN-associated cytotoxic cellular immune response against viral, self-, or tumor antigens is a common pathogenetic feature in "interface dermatitis". *J Invest Dermatol.* (2008) 128:2392–402. doi: 10.1038/jid.2008.96
121. Zahn S, Rehkamper C, Kummerer BM, Ferring-Schmidt S, Bieber T, Tuting T, et al. Evidence for a pathophysiological role of keratinocyte-derived type III interferon (IFNlambda) in cutaneous lupus erythematosus. *J Invest Dermatol.* (2011) 131:133–40. doi: 10.1038/jid.2010.244
122. Dang W, Xu L, Yin Y, Chen S, Wang W, Hakim MS, et al. IRF-1, RIG-I and MDA5 display potent antiviral activities against norovirus coordinately induced by different types of interferons. *Antiviral Res.* (2018) 155:48–59. doi: 10.1016/j.antiviral.2018.05.004
123. Tretina K, Park ES, Maminska A, MacMicking JD. Interferon-induced guanylate-binding proteins: guardians of host defense in health and disease. *J Exp Med.* (2019) 216:482–500. doi: 10.1084/jem.20182031
124. Meyer KC, Klatte JE, Dinh HV, Harries MJ, Reithmayer K, Meyer W, et al. Evidence that the bulge region is a site of relative immune privilege in human hair follicles. *Br J Dermatol.* (2008) 159:1077–85. doi: 10.1111/j.1365-2133.2008.08818.x
125. Pi LQ, Jin XH, Hwang ST, Lee WS. Effects of calcitonin gene-related peptide on the immune privilege of human hair follicles. *Neuropeptides.* (2013) 47:51–7. doi: 10.1016/j.npep.2012.07.008
126. Alase AA, El-Sherbiny YM, Vital EM, Tobin DJ, Turner NA, Wittmann M. IFNlambda stimulates MxA production in human dermal fibroblasts via a MAPK-dependent STAT1-independent mechanism. *J Invest Dermatol.* (2015) 135:2935–43. doi: 10.1038/jid.2015.317
127. Nyberg F, Fransson J, Stephansson E. Proliferation and effects of UVA irradiation in cultured fibroblasts from lesions in cutaneous lupus erythematosus. *Exp Dermatol.* (2000) 9:53–7. doi: 10.1034/j.1600-0625.2000.009001053.x
128. Fabbri P, Amato L, Chiarini C, Moretti S, Massi D. Scarring alopecia in discoid lupus erythematosus: a clinical, histopathologic and immunopathologic study. *Lupus.* (2004) 13:455–62. doi: 10.1191/0961203304lu1041oa
129. Elman SA, Joyce C, Nyberg F, Furukawa F, Goodfield M, Hasegawa M, et al. Development of classification criteria for discoid lupus erythematosus: results of a Delphi exercise. *J Am Acad Dermatol.* (2017) 77:261–7. doi: 10.1016/j.jaad.2017.02.030
130. Shim WH, Jwa SW, Song M, Kim HS, Ko HC, Kim BS, et al. Dermoscopic approach to a small round to oval hairless patch on the scalp. *Ann Dermatol.* (2014) 26:214–20. doi: 10.5021/ad.2014.26.2.214
131. Pfannes EK, Hadam S, Doge N, Fimmel S, Blume-Peytavi U, Vogt A. Mini-zone cyanoacrylate skin surface stripping: a new method for non-invasive sampling of scalp material. *Exp Dermatol.* (2016) 25:555–6. doi: 10.1111/exd.13006
132. Vogt A, Pfannes EKB, Fimmel S, Hadam S, Andruck A, Kottner J, et al. Infundibular protein and RNA microarray analyses from affected and clinically non-affected scalp in male androgenetic alopecia patients. *Exp Dermatol.* (2017) 26:518–21. doi: 10.1111/exd.13326
133. Schwartz JR, Shah R, Krigbaum H, Sacha J, Vogt A, Blume-Peytavi U. New insights on dandruff/seborrhoeic dermatitis: the role of the scalp follicular infundibulum in effective treatment strategies. *Br J Dermatol.* (2011) 165(Suppl. 2):18–23. doi: 10.1111/j.1365-2133.2011.10573.x
134. Shalbaf M, Alase AA, Berekmeri A, Md Yusof MY, Pistolic J, Goodfield MJ, et al. Plucked hair follicles from patients with chronic discoid lupus erythematosus show a disease-specific molecular signature. *Lupus Sci Med.* (2019) 6:e000328. doi: 10.1136/lupus-2019-000328
135. Miranda JJ, Taype-Rondan A, Tapia JC, Gastanadui-Gonzalez MG, Roman-Carpio R. Hair follicle characteristics as early marker of type 2 diabetes. *Med Hypotheses.* (2016) 95:39–44. doi: 10.1016/j.mehy.2016.08.009
136. Plikus MV, Van Spyk EN, Pham K, Geyfman M, Kumar V, Takahashi JS, et al. The circadian clock in skin: implications for adult stem cells, tissue regeneration, cancer, aging, and immunity. *J Biol Rhythms.* (2015) 30:163–82. doi: 10.1177/0748730414563537
137. Ghosh D, Bernstein JA, Khurana Hershey GK, Rothenberg ME, Mersha TB. Leveraging multilayered "Omics" data for atopic dermatitis: a road map to precision medicine. *Front Immunol.* (2018) 9:2727. doi: 10.3389/fimmu.2018.02727

Permissions

All chapters in this book were first published Frontiers; hereby published with permission under the Creative Commons Attribution License or equivalent. Every chapter published in this book has been scrutinized by our experts. Their significance has been extensively debated. The topics covered herein carry significant findings which will fuel the growth of the discipline. They may even be implemented as practical applications or may be referred to as a beginning point for another development.

The contributors of this book come from diverse backgrounds, making this book a truly international effort. This book will bring forth new frontiers with its revolutionizing research information and detailed analysis of the nascent developments around the world.

We would like to thank all the contributing authors for lending their expertise to make the book truly unique. They have played a crucial role in the development of this book. Without their invaluable contributions this book wouldn't have been possible. They have made vital efforts to compile up to date information on the varied aspects of this subject to make this book a valuable addition to the collection of many professionals and students.

This book was conceptualized with the vision of imparting up-to-date information and advanced data in this field. To ensure the same, a matchless editorial board was set up. Every individual on the board went through rigorous rounds of assessment to prove their worth. After which they invested a large part of their time researching and compiling the most relevant data for our readers.

The editorial board has been involved in producing this book since its inception. They have spent rigorous hours researching and exploring the diverse topics which have resulted in the successful publishing of this book. They have passed on their knowledge of decades through this book. To expedite this challenging task, the publisher supported the team at every step. A small team of assistant editors was also appointed to further simplify the editing procedure and attain best results for the readers.

Apart from the editorial board, the designing team has also invested a significant amount of their time in understanding the subject and creating the most relevant covers. They scrutinized every image to scout for the most suitable representation of the subject and create an appropriate cover for the book.

The publishing team has been an ardent support to the editorial, designing and production team. Their endless efforts to recruit the best for this project, has resulted in the accomplishment of this book. They are a veteran in the field of academics and their pool of knowledge is as vast as their experience in printing. Their expertise and guidance has proved useful at every step. Their uncompromising quality standards have made this book an exceptional effort. Their encouragement from time to time has been an inspiration for everyone.

The publisher and the editorial board hope that this book will prove to be a valuable piece of knowledge for researchers, students, practitioners and scholars across the globe.

List of Contributors

David R. Pearson
Department of Dermatology, University of Minnesota Medical School, Minneapolis, MN, United States

Victoria P. Werth
Corporal Michael J. Crescenz VA Medical Center, Philadelphia, PA, United States
Department of Dermatology, Perelman School of Medicine, University of Pennsylvania, Philadelphia, PA, United States

Bernhard F. Gibbs, Nikolaos Patsinakidis and Ulrike Raap
Division of Experimental Allergy and Immunodermatology, University of Oldenburg, Oldenburg, Germany

Katharina Marie Bach, Julia Busse and Luise Erpenbeck
Department of Dermatology, Venereology and Allergology, University Medical Center Göttingen, Göttingen, Germany

Elsa Neubert
Department of Dermatology, Venereology and Allergology, University Medical Center Göttingen, Göttingen, Germany
Institute of Physical Chemistry, Göttingen University, Göttingen, Germany

Ivan Bogeski
Institute of Cardiovascular Physiology, University Medical Center Göttingen, Göttingen, Germany

Michael P. Schön
Department of Dermatology, Venereology and Allergology, University Medical Center Göttingen, Göttingen, Germany
Lower Saxony Institute of Occupational Dermatology, University Medical Center Göttingen, Göttingen, Germany

Sebastian Kruss
Institute of Physical Chemistry, Göttingen University, Göttingen, Germany
Center for Nanoscale Microscopy and Molecular Physiology of the Brain (CNMPB), Göttingen, Germany

Gyu Tae Park, Yang Woo Kwon, Tae Wook Lee and Seong Gyu Kwon
Department of Physiology, Pusan National University School of Medicine, Yangsan-si, South Korea

Hyun-Chang Ko and Moon Bum Kim
Department of Dermatology, Pusan National University School of Medicine, Yangsan-si, South Korea

Jae Ho Kim
Department of Physiology, Pusan National University School of Medicine, Yangsan-si, South Korea
Research Institute of Convergence Biomedical Science and Technology, Pusan National University Yangsan Hospital, Yangsan-si, South Korea

Farzan Solimani, Robert Pollmann, Thomas Schmidt, Stefan Mühlenbein, Julia Pickert, Verena Eubel, Christian Möbs, Rüdiger Eming and Michael Hertl
Department of Dermatology and Allergology, Philipps-Universität Marburg, Marburg, Germany

Ansgar Schmidt
Department of Pathology, Philipps-Universität Marburg, Marburg, Germany

Xiang Zheng
Max Planck Institute for Heart and Lung Research, Member of the German Center for Lung Research (DZL), Member of the Cardio-Pulmonary Institute (CPI), Bad Nauheim, Germany

Rajkumar Savai
Max Planck Institute for Heart and Lung Research, Member of the German Center for Lung Research (DZL), Member of the Cardio-Pulmonary Institute (CPI), Bad Nauheim, Germany
Department of Internal Medicine, Member of the DZL, Member of CPI, Justus Liebig University, Giessen, Germany

Hiroaki Iwata
Department of Dermatology, Hokkaido University Graduate School of Medicine, Sapporo, Japan

Mayumi Kamaguchi
Department of Dermatology, Hokkaido University Graduate School of Medicine, Sapporo, Japan
Department of Oral Diagnosis and Medicine, Hokkaido University Graduate School of Dental Medicine, Sapporo, Japan

Christian D. Sadik, Ewan A. Langan, Victoria Grätz, Detlef Zillikens and Patrick Terheyden
Department of Dermatology, Allergy, and Venereology, University of Lübeck, Lübeck, Germany

Elias Walter, Franziska Vielmuth, Marie-Therès Wanuske, Matthias Seifert and Jens Waschke
Institute of Anatomy and Cell Biology, Ludwig-Maximilians-Universität München, Munich, Germany

Giovanni Genovese, Emilio Berti and Angelo Valerio Marzano
Dermatology Unit, Fondazione IRCCS Ca' Granda Ospedale Maggiore Policlinico, Milan, Italy
Department of Physiopathology and Transplantation, Università degli Studi di Milano, Milan, Italy

Giovanni Di Zenzo
Molecular and Cell Biology Laboratory, Istituto Dermopatico dell'Immacolata (IDI) IRCCS, Rome, Italy

Emanuele Cozzani
DISSAL Section of Dermatology, Università degli Studi di Genova, Genoa, Italy

Massimo Cugno
Department of Physiopathology and Transplantation, Università degli Studi di Milano, Milan, Italy
Internal Medicine Unit, Fondazione IRCCS Ca' Granda Ospedale Maggiore Policlinico, Milan, Italy

Feng Xu, Gui-qing Li, Jian Chen, Di Yang and Gui-lian Xu
Department of Immunology, Army Medical University (Third Military Medical University), Chongqing, China

Quan-you Zheng
Department of Immunology, Army Medical University (Third Military Medical University), Chongqing, China
Department of Urology, 958th Hospital of PLA, Army Medical University (Third Military Medical University), Chongqing, China

Yu Zhong and Dao-dong Sun
Department of Urology, 958th Hospital of PLA, Army Medical University (Third Military Medical University), Chongqing, China

Shen-ju Liang
Department of Rheumatism and Immunology, Daping Hospital, Army Medical University (Third Military Medical University), Chongqing, China

Na Luo
Department of Dermatology, Southwest Hospital, Army Medical University (Third Military Medical University), Chongqing, China

Shun Wu, You Li, Ming Tang and Ke-qin Zhang
Department of Nephrology, Southwest Hospital, Army Medical University (Third Military Medical University), Chongqing, China

Michael Olbrich, Axel Künstner, Hauke Busch and Anke Fähnrich
Medical Systems Biology, Institute of Experimental Dermatology, University of Lübeck, Lübeck, Germany
Institute of Cardiogenetics, University of Lübeck, Lübeck, Germany

Mareike Witte
Department of Dermatology, University of Lübeck, Lübeck, Germany

Sho Hiroyasu, Christopher T. Turner, Katlyn C. Richardson and David J. Granville
International Collaboration On Repair Discoveries (ICORD), Vancouver Coastal Health Research Institute (VCHRI), Vancouver, BC, Canada
Department of Pathology and Laboratory Medicine, University of British Columbia (UBC), Vancouver, BC, Canada
BC Professional Firefighters' Burn and Wound Healing Group, Vancouver Coastal Health Research Institute (VCHRI), University of British Columbia (UBC), Vancouver, BC, Canada

Luana Caroline Oliveira, Gabriela Canalli Kretzschmar, Andressa Cristina Moraes dos Santos, Carolina Maciel Camargo, Ticiana Della Justina Farias, Maria Luiza Petzl-Erler and Angelica Beate Winter Boldt
Laboratory of Human Molecular Genetics, Department of Genetics, Federal University of Paraná, Curitiba, Brazil

Renato Mitsunori Nisihara
Laboratory of Molecular Immunopathology, Department of Clinical Pathology, Clinical Hospital, Federal University of Paraná, Curitiba, Brazil

Andre Franke and Michael Wittig
Institute of Clinical Molecular Biology, Christian-Albrechts-University of Kiel, Kiel, Germany

Enno Schmidt
Lübeck Institute of Experimental Dermatology, University of Lübeck, Lübeck, Germany
Department of Dermatology, University of Lübeck, Lübeck, Germany

Reinhart Speeckaert, Jo Lambert and Nanja van Geel
Department of Dermatology, Ghent University Hospital, Ghent, Belgium

Annelies Demeyer, Elien Van Nuffel, Griet Baudelet, Yasmine Driege, Marja Kreike, David Muyllaert, Jens Staal and Rudi Beyaert
VIB Center for Inflammation Research, Ghent, Belgium
Department of Biomedical Molecular Biology, Ghent University, Ghent, Belgium

Rama Dey-Rao, Animesh A. Sinha, Janet Lee and Kristina Seiffert-Sinha
Department of Dermatology, Jacobs School of Medicine and Biomedical Sciences, University at Buffalo, Buffalo, NY, United States

Claudia Günther
Department of Dermatology, University Hospital Carl Gustav Carus, Technical University Dresden, Dresden, Germany

Kristopher Attwood
Department of Biostatistics and Bioinformatics, Roswell Park Cancer Institute, Buffalo, NY, United States

Katharina Meier and Kamran Ghoreschi
Department of Dermatology, Venereology and Allergology, Charité—Universitätsmedizin Berlin, Berlin, Germany

Adewonuola A. Alase
Faculty of Medicine and Health, Leeds Institute of Rheumatic and Musculoskeletal Medicine, University of Leeds, Leeds, United Kingdom

Anna Berekméri, Edward Vital and Miriam Wittmann
Faculty of Medicine and Health, Leeds Institute of Rheumatic and Musculoskeletal Medicine, University of Leeds, Leeds, United Kingdom
Leeds Biomedical Research Centre, National Institute for Health Research, Leeds Teaching Hospitals, Leeds, United Kingdom

Ana Tiganescu
Faculty of Medicine and Health, Leeds Institute of Cardiovascular and Metabolic Medicine, University of Leeds, Leeds, United Kingdom

Martin Stacey
Faculty of Biological Sciences, School of Molecular and Cellular Biology, University of Leeds, Leeds, United Kingdom

Index

www.ingramcontent.com/pod-product-compliance
Lightning Source LLC
LaVergne TN
LVHW080952210926
848485LV00004B/828